PRINCIPLES OF PHYSICAL MEDICINE
AND REHABILITATION
IN THE MUSCULOSKELETAL DISEASES

PRINCIPLES OF PHYSICAL MEDICINE AND REHABILITATION IN THE MUSCULOSKELETAL DISEASES

Edited by

JAMES C. LEEK, M.D.
Associate Clinical Professor of Medicine
Division of Rheumatology
Department of Internal Medicine
University of California, Davis, School of Medicine
Davis, California

M. ERIC GERSHWIN, M.D.
Professor of Medicine
Division of Rheumatology
Department of Internal Medicine
University of California, Davis, School of Medicine
Davis, California

WILLIAM M. FOWLER, JR., M.D.
Professor and Former Chairman
Department of Physical Medicine and Rehabilitation
University of California, Davis, School of Medicine
Davis, California

Grune & Stratton, Inc.
Harcourt Brace Jovanovich, Publishers
Orlando   New York   San Diego   Boston   London
San Francisco   Tokyo   Sydney   Toronto

Library of Congress Cataloging-in-Publication Data
Main entry under title:

Principles of physical medicine and rehabilitation in
the musculoskeletal diseases.

Includes bibliographies and index.
1. Arthritics—Rehabilitation.   2. Rheumatism—
Patients—Rehabilitation.   3. Physical therapy.
I. Leek, James C.   II. Gershwin, M. Eric, 1946–
III. Fowler, William M. (William Mayo), 1926–
[DNLM: 1. Arthritis—rehabilitation.   2. Physical
Medicine.   3. Rheumatism—rehabilitation.   WE 344 P957]
RC933.P695   1986   616.7'2306   85-27331
ISBN 0-8089-1773-0

Grune & Stratton, Inc.
Orlando, FL 32887

Distributed in the United Kingdom by
Grune & Stratton, Ltd.
24/28 Oval Road, London NW 1

Library of Congress Catalog Number 85-27331
International Standard Book Number 0-8089-1773-0
Printed in the United States of America
86 87 88 89   10 9 8 7 6 5 4 3 2 1

DEDICATION

To our wives and families for their support and encouragement, and to our patients who have shown us the need and the great potential for rehabilitation in arthritis.

CONTENTS

PREFACE

In recent years there has been an explosion of knowledge in rheumatology and rapid growth in the numbers of practicing rheumatologists. Despite this growth, the vast majority of patients with musculoskeletal diseases are managed largely by primary care physicians. Moreover, a growth in the expertise in the rehabilitation of rheumatic diseases has been slower and less accessible to both the rheumatologist and to the primary care physician. It is clear, however that the application of principles of rehabilitation is a crucial part of the management program to achieve the best outcome in patients with arthritis.

While textbooks dealing with the medical and surgical modalities of therapy for rheumatic diseases are increasingly common, concise, practical information concerning rehabilitation assessment and treatment has been less available to the practicing physician and has even been rather limited in rheumatology training programs. Physicians in both primary care and specialty areas are frequently confronted with a wide variety of rheumatic disorders ranging from rheumatoid arthritis, the most prevalent of the progressive arthritic diseases, to the very common problems of soft tissue rheumatism and back pain.

This book is intended to provide a clinically useful background in the principles and modalities of rehabilitation in the rheumatic diseases. It is organized in two major sections. The first provides an introduction to the concepts of rehabilitation techniques and to the physical modalities involved. This section concludes with discussions of pain management and the psychosocial and vocational aspects of rehabilitation. The second section discusses the application of these concepts and techniques to specific musculoskeletal problems. These chapters are organized by anatomic region.

This book is intended for practitioners and residents in training who deal with common muscular and arthritic diseases including primary care physicians, internists, rheumatologists, orthopedists, and physiatrists.

The concept of physical medicine and rehabilitation in rheumatology is a subject of great recent interest. For example, over the past two years, a special subsection of the American Rheumatism Association in rehabilitation has been created. In addition, the study of PM&R is being made a requirement for education programs in rheumatology throughout the United States. Similarly, rotation in rheumatology are now required for students and housestaff desiring board certification in Physical Medicine and Rehabilitation.

The editors of the volume have had a major interest in developing this volume; all three approach it from different perspectives. Dr. Leek is primarily a clinical rheumatologist and has been director of the Rheumatic Disease Clinics at the University Medical Center. In addition, he coordinates training of housestaff in Rheumatology both in Internal Medicine as well as in Physical Medicine Residency Programs. Dr. Gershwin is Chief of the Division of Rheumatology as well as Director of Education for both Rheumatology and Clinical Immunology at the University. He has helped develop two working manuals for teaching of education programs for housestaff and is director of the UCD Rheumatology Center. Dr. Fowler was previously Chairman of the Department of Physical Medicine and Rehabilitation. Over the past decade his major interests have been in the rehabilitation of muscle diseases and in rheumatic diseases. UCD is unique in having multidisciplinary combined programs and clinics and thus is in a unique position to develop this volume.

Finally the three editors wish to thank Susan Hammel and Nikki Rojo for their secretarial assistance and patience.

James C. Leek
M. Eric Gershwin
William M. Fowler, Jr.

CONTRIBUTORS

Frances Sommer Anderson, Ph.D.
Senior Psychologist
Rusk Institute of Rehabilitation Medicine
New York University Medical Center
New York, New York

John H. Bland, M.D., FACP
Professor of Medicine
University of Vermont College of Medicine
Burlington, Vermont

Steven F. Brena, M.D.
Professor, Anesthesia and Rehabilitation Medicine
Chief, Psychology Unit
Pain Rehabilitation Center
Emory University, School of Medicine
Atlanta, Georgia

Andrei Calin, M.D., MRCP
Consultant Rheumatologist
Royal National Hospital for Rheumatic Diseases
Bath, England

Stanley L. Chapman, M.D.
Senior Associate in Rehabilitation Medicine
Chief, Psychology Unit
Pain Rehabilitation Center
Emory University, School of Medicine
Atlanta, Georgia

Sam C. Colachis, Jr., M.D.
Director of P.M.&R.
St. Luke's Hospital Medical Center
Phoenix, Arizona
Formerly Assistant Professor and Acting Chairman
Department of Physical Medicine and Rehabilitation
UCLA School of Medicine

F. Richard Convery, M.D.
Professor of Surgery
Division of Orthopaedics and Rehabilitation
Department of Surgery
University of California, San Diego
School of Medicine
San Diego, California

Martha Minteer-Convery, M.D.
Associate Clinical Professor
Division of Orthopaedics and Rehabilitation
Department of Surgery
University of California

Richard D. Coutts, M.D.
Clinical Professor of Orthopaedic Surgery
University of California, San Diego
San Diego, California

Barbara J. deLateur, M.D.
Professor
Department of Rehabilitation Medicine
University of Washington, School of Medicine
Seattle, Washington

Arlene Feinblatt, Ph.D.
Senior Psychologist
Rusk Institute of Rehabilitation Medicine
New York University Medical Center
New York, New York

William M. Fowler, Jr., M.D.
Professor and Former Chairman
Department of Physical Medicine and Rehabilitation
University of California, Davis, School of Medicine
Davis, California

Bernard F. Germain, M.D.
Director, Division of Rheumatology
University of South Florida
College of Medicine
Tampa, Florida

M. Eric Gershwin, M.D.
Professor of Medicine
Division of Rheumatology
Department of Internal Medicine
University of California, Davis, School of Medicine
Davis, California

Wayne Gordon, Ph.D.
Assistant Professor of Clinical Rehabilitation
Rusk Institute of Rehabilitation Medicine
New York University Medical Center
New York, New York

Thomas L. Greene, M.D.
Assistant Professor of Orthopaedic Surgery
University of South Florida
College of Medicine
Tampa, Florida

Myron M. Laban, M.D., FACP
Director, Department of P.M.&R.
William Beaumont Hospital
Clinical Associate Professor
Wayne State University
Clinical Professor
Oakland University
Royal Oak, Michigan

James C. Leek, M.D.
Associate Clinical Professor of Medicine
Division of Rheumatology
Department of Internal Medicine
University of California, Davis, School of Medicine
Sacramento, California

David Leffers, M.D.
Assistant Professor of Orthopaedic Surgery
University of South Florida
College of Medicine
Tampa, Florida

Justus F. Lehmann, M.D.
Professor and Chairman
Department of Rehabilitation Medicine
University of Washington, School of Medicine
Seattle, Washington

James S. Lieberman, M.D., F.A.C.P.
Professor/Chair, Physical Medicine and Rehabilitation
Professor, Neurology
University of California, Davis, School of Medicine
Sacramento, California

William P. Maier, M.D.
Fellow in Medicine
Emory University School of Medicine
Atlanta, Georgia

Stanley M. Naguwa, M.D.
Assistant Clinical Professor
Division of Rheumatology
Department of Internal Medicine
University of California, Davis, School of Medicine
Davis, California

Vernon C. Nickel, M.D.
Professor of Orthopaedic Surgery
University of California, San Diego
San Diego, California

Kenneth S. O'Rourke, M.D.
  Resident Physician
  Department of Medicine
  David Grant Medical Center
  Travis Air Force Base, California

Margaret M. Portwood, M.D.
  Assistant Professor of Medicine
  Department of Physical Medicine and Rehabilitation
  University of California, Davis, School of Medicine
  Sacramento, California

John B. Redford, M.D.
  Professor and Chairman
  Department of Rehabilitation Medicine
  University of Kansas, College of Health Sciences
  Kansas City, Kansas

Linda B. Rosker, B.S., O.T.R.
  Assistant Chief of Occupational Therapy
  David Grant Medical Center
  Travis Air Force Base, California

Richard Santore, M.D.
  Assistant Clinical Professor
  Department of Orthopaedic Surgery
  University of California, San Diego
  School of Medicine
  San Diego, California

Hugh A. Smythe, M.D., FRCP (C)
  Professor and Head
  Wellesley Hospital and Rheumatic Disease Unit
  University of Toronto
  Toronto, Ontario

Richard White, M.D.
  Assistant Professor of Medicine
  Division of Rheumatology
  Department of Internal Medicine
  University of California, Davis, School of Medicine
  Sacramento, California

Colon H. Wilson, Jr., M.D.
  Internal Medicine Group of Atlanta
  Formerly Professor
  Division of Rheumatology
  Emory University, School of Medicine
  Atlanta, Georgia

Part 1

Basic Principles and Therapeutic Modalities

James C. Leek
M. Eric Gershwin
William M. Fowler, Jr.

1

The Challenge of Arthritis Rehabilitation: An Overview of Goals, Modalities, and Patient Evaluation

One of the most difficult problems that patients with arthritis and their families face is the reality that they suffer from a chronic disease with little likelihood of spontaneous remission. In fact, the emphasis by physicians has so heavily involved the use of pharmacotherapy and laboratory tests, that most everyone loses sight of the fact that people with arthritis are living with their disease, not dying of it. Indeed, for most people, patients and physicians alike, physical medicine and rehabilitation is a discipline that is applied primarily to patients suffering from strokes or serious injuries. Only a relative few consider physical medicine and rehabilitation an essential component in the management of chronic arthritis.

The national impact of osteoarthritis and rheumatoid arthritis is enormous. Musculoskeletal diseases account for more than 40 percent of all patients referred for vocational rehabilitation. They are the second most frequent cause of outpatient complaints amongst chronic diseases. Musculoskeletal diseases account for 20 percent of all Medicare hospital costs. The number of days of work loss per year for rheumatoid arthritis and osteoarthritis is staggering. None of these data illustrate, however, the social impact of musculoskeletal disease. We tend to lose sight of the young mother with arthritis and morning stiffness who is unable to dress her kids for school. We lose sight of the worker who loses his job for recurrent absence. We lose sight of the marital breakdowns that are nearly twice as frequent in arthritis patients as in the general population.[8] The financial and social hardships are substantial. Patients with stage 3 rheumatoid arthritis lose an average of 60 percent of their income in the first six years of disease.[5] the average lifetime economic cost of rheumatoid arthritis has been estimated to be greater than $20,000.[13] This figure, calculated in 1977 dollars, includes $4400 for medical care expenses and over $16,000 of lost productivity. Thus, in the past, the medical approach to arthritis has been too narrowly focussed in pharmacotherapy rather than on the total management of patients and the preservation of function. In contrast to rheumatoid arthritis, the effect of ankylosing spondylitis on employment is less severe.[6]

PRINCIPLES OF PHYSICAL MEDICINE AND REHABILITATION IN THE MUSCULOSKELETAL DISEASES

Approximately 50 years ago there were only a handful of causes of arthritis that were identified. We now recognize more than a 100 different causes of arthritis. Moreover, although we may congratulate ourselves on the tremendous advances in both diagnosis and treatment of patients, it is clear that we have only begun to scratch the surface. The answer or answers to the management of arthritis will likely remain elusive in the near future.

We believe it is very important to identify as early as possible those patients who will need more intensive follow-up than others. It is essential to predict which patients are more likely to develop functional disability. Involvement by Social service, peer interaction groups, as well as consultation with other disciplines is essential. A patient should not be allowed to become seriously functionally disabled before suggesting vocational rehabilitation. A number of identifiable work factors are important in maintaining employability. Chief among these is autonomy in controlling the pace and content of work activities.[14] Accessibility of the work place is also an important consideration.

Timely referral to specialists in the rehabilitation team is an aspect that cannot be over emphasized. For example, prompt orthopedic evaluation of the adolescent with hip pain is crucial to the outcome of a slipped capital femoral epiphysis. Similarly, if joint replacement is indicated, it should be done at an early opportune time, when the joint prosthesis will offer a functional immediate advantage over the patient's own joint; not done at a time after such serious disability has taken place that little social and personal impact can be gained from such an operation. These considerations are further discussed in Chapter 16.

The goals of physical medicine and rehabilitation are to maintain patients in the most active role possible, using the maximum resources available to the community. Although other textbooks on rehabilitation and rheumatic disease have been written, and specific goals have been outlined by the American Rheumatism Association (ARA), we hope that our approach in this text is different and useful. We believe that physical medicine and arthritis should be discussed in a regional fashion, rather than by going through an exhaustive list of diseases or an encyclopedia of different appliances. The final common pathway, the end denominator of arthritis, is joint destruction. Destruction of a particular joint will have similar functional consequences be it rheumatoid arthritis, osteoarthritis, or septic arthritis. Additional factors including continued inflammatory disease and use of different medications, must obviously be taken into account. However, the goals of joint rehabilitation are not significantly different.

Many physicians hold the belief that musculoskeletal diseases are divided into two large groups: relatively trivial self-limited conditions for which little need be done and severe relentless arthritic diseases for which little effective treatment is available. In the minds of many, rehabilitation is thought of only in regards to patients with the most severe crippling forms of this latter group. In fact, however, the techniques of arthritis rehabilitation are useful in all levels of musculoskeletal diseases. Although the overall need increases with the level of disability, joint protection techniques, for example, are as applicable to the patient with early mild arthritis as they are to those with advanced disease. All aspects of the comprehensive management of the patient with arthritis are a part of the rehabilitation process, in addition to a wide range of activities specifically designed to limit the impact of disease on the patient's quality of life.

A comprehensive rehabilitation program for the arthritis patient should include the precise diagnosis and medical management to control the underlying disease process and measures to limit the effects of the arthritic process on the patient's independence and functional abilities. Key components of this process are relief of pain, maintenance and restoration of joint mobility and strength, prevention of deformity, and provision of adaptive equipment to maintain independence in daily and vocational activities.

In order to plan an effective rehabilitation program, patient evaluation must include assessment of the patient's functional level as well as the usual clinical parameters such as joint inflammation and range of motion. Impairment of function in daily activities is the dominant factor in the impact of arthritis on a patient's life.[2] Traditional measures of disease activity in rheumatic diseases such as rheumatoid arthritis tend to focus on attempts to evaluate activity of the underlying disease (number of painful and swollen joints, sedimentation rate, etc.), which may not correlate well with the patient's functional status.

In addition to determining what activities are limited, it is important to identify the responsible limiting factors (pain, fatigue, weakness, or biomechanical abnormalities such as decreased range of motion or instability may all be contributing features). The functional assessment must then be correlated with other components of the musculoskeletal examination to make effective treatment decisions regarding functional disabilities. The clinical evaluation should also assess prognosis and reversibility of the underlying joint disease.

In the office setting a minimal functional evaluation should include review of limitations in the many activities of daily living (such as eating, dressing, lifting, and personal hygiene), limitation of job activities, and limitations in walking and related mobility activities (such as arising from a chair). For more comprehensive evaluation there are a wide array of functional evaluation scales available. Among the most commonly used is the American Rheumatism Association functional classification,[12] which subdivides functional impairment into four classes (Table 1-1). The distribution of patients with rheumatoid arthritis among the functional classes from several large series of patients are shown in Table 1-2. It should be kept in mind that these are selected series from referral centers and thus reflect a greater severity of disease and disability than is likely to be present in the community at large. Although the ARA classification provides a convenient broad outline of functional ability, it is of limited value in the serial assessment of patients. A much more comprehensive but time consuming approach to functional assessment is the evaluation of activities of daily living generally performed by the occupational therapist. Recently several relatively brief standardized scales for the comprehensive evaluation of functional status in arthritis have been developed and validated. These are the Arthritis Impact Measurement Scale,[7] developed at the Boston University, and the Stanford Arthritis Center Health Assessment Questionnaire.[3] These can be self-administered and take approximately 20 minutes to complete. The parameters evaluated by these scales are

Table 1-1

Functional Classification of Rheumatoid Arthritis (ARA)

Class 1: Able to perform all normal activities
Class 2: Able to adequate perform normal activities despite discomfort or limitation of 1 or more joints.
Class 3: Able to perform few or none of usual activities of occupation and self-care.
Class 4: Largely or totally incapacitated, confined to bed or wheelchair, little or no self-care.

Data from Steinbrocker D, Traeger CH, Batterman RC: Therapeutic Criteria in Rheumatoid Arthritis. JAMA 140:659–662, 1949.

Table 1-2
ARA Functional Class of Patients with Rheumatoid Arthritis at Long-Term Follow-Up

Series	Functional Class%				Approximate Mean Duration of RA
	I	II	III	IV	
Pincus et al (1984)[10]	16	42	34	8	20 years
Scott et al (1983)[11]	30	37	21	12	15 years
Cosh et al (1982)[1]	24	31	39	6	20 years

shown in Table 1-3. These scales, which can be self administered, provide a brief standardized method for the serial evaluation of functional status in patients with rheumatic diseases.

Following the clinical and functional evaluation, a management plan must be developed that addresses not only specific medical measures to control the arthritic process but also includes the use of appropriate regimens of rest, exercise, and the various available physical modalities to relieve pain and maintain musculoskeletal function. Where appropriate assistive devices are employed to further these goals and allow the patient to remain as independent as possible. Assistive devices should not be used as a substitute for measures to improve joint mobility and function.

A critical feature of all management programs is the education of the patient regarding their disease process, the modalities of treatment, and (especially) the principles of joint protection and energy conservation. A large number of educational pamphlets and books are available from the Arthritis Foundation, which can be useful in providing such information to the patient. Compliance with the therapeutic regimen will be enhanced if the patient understands the process and rationale for their treatment. Information concerning appropriate goals and limitation of activity should be provided according to the patient's functional level. Suitable modifications of living and working environment and tasks can be suggested. Relatively minor physical modifications may make major differences in the patient's independence.[4] All members of the rehabilitation team should participate in the educational process, which should be coordinated by the primary physician. Involvement of the occupational and physical therapist is particularly important in

Table 1-3
Components of Several Useful Self-Administered Functional Assessment Measures

Arthritis Impact Measurement Scales[7]	Standford Health Assessment Questionaire[8]
Mobility	Disability Scale
Physical Activity	Dressing and Grooming
Dexterity	Arising
Household Activities	Eating
Activities of Daily Living	Walking
Anxiety	Hygiene
Depression	Reach
Social Activity	Grip
Pain	Activities
	Assistive Devices
	Activities Which Require Assistance
	Pain Scale

teaching and monitoring methods of joint protection, the use of assistive devices, and exercise programs.

The principles of joint protection and energy conservation are the corner stones of management of the patient with arthritis. Energy conservation requires a pragmatic balance between rest and activity, particularly in the systemic rheumatic diseases such as rheumatoid arthritis in which inflammation and complaints of fatigue are important considerations. Rest is also therapeutically effective for joint inflammation. The principles of joint protection are designed to limit stresses on joints, to prevent pain, and protect the inflamed joint against progressive injury and deformity. Leverage can be used to minimize the force necessary for a given task by changing the method or using assistive devices. Joint protection measures are particularly important for actively inflamed joints. Examples of the use of joint protection techniques are provided in Table 1-4.

The use of orthotic and assistive devices are, in effect, applications of joint protection techniques. Splints and braces are used to immobilize or rest involved joints, to provide stability, and prevent or correct deformities. Assistive devices are pieces of equipment that are designed to reduce stress on joints, provide leverage to reduce the force required to accomplish certain tasks, and to limit energy consumption. These include canes, crutches, and walkers, which substantially reduce the weight bearing forces involved in ambulation as well as a variety of special utensils for every day activities that provide mechanical advantage to compensate for impaired function. Examples include enlarging the handles of hand held utensils as well as extension of handles that can compensate for limited range of motion.

Exercise programs are an important part of the rehabilitation plan and serve several functions depending on the stage and activity of disease. Exercise intensity varies from passive exercise performed by a therapist through active assistive exercise in which the patient actively contracts the muscles but is assisted by the therapist to active independent exercise and resistive exercise in which the patient actively contracts the involved muscles

Table 1-4

Joint Protection Techniques[9]

Principle:	Use largest available joint.
Examples:	Use forearm rather than hand grip for lifting or carrying.
	Use palm rather than MCPs for pushing or turning.
	Carry purse by shoulder strap rather than hand grip.
	Lift heavy objects with both hands.
Principle:	Limit force of gravity
Examples:	Working from a sitting position rather than standing decreases force on joints of lower extremities.
	Use of cane or crutches to decrease force on joints of lower extremities.
	Slide heavy objects rather than lifting.
Principle:	Use of most stable position
Examples:	Use of long-handled equipment to avoid bending
	Proper lifting techniques (lifting with the leg muscles while keeping the back straight)
	In patients with swan neck deformities, avoid positions in which MCPs are flexed and PIPs are extended.

Data from Melvin JL: Joint protection training and energy conservation in Melvin JL (ed.) Rheumatic Disease: Occupational therapy and rehabilitation. Philadelphia, F.A. Davis, 1977, pp. 191–206 with or without resistance. The goals of the exercise program are to maintain or improve joint range of motion and to preserve or increase muscle strength. The relative emphasis placed on each of these goals varies with the stage of disease and the degree of inflammation present. During periods of joint inflammation active exercise may increase pain and inflammation. The primary goal in this setting is to maintain joint mobility that is best done by assisted active range of motion exercises. After the inflammatory process is controlled one can plan a more vigorous program of active exercise; eventually the goal is to restore strength lost due to pain and disuse. Exercise periods should be coordinated with appropriate pain relief measures such as analgesic and antiinflammatory drugs and the application of superficial heat.

The application of superficial heat is useful in the relief of pain, stiffness, and muscle spasm. A widely used example of the application of heat to facilitate exercise is the use of paraffin bath treatments for the rheumatoid hand. Hydrotherapy is another example in which the use of superficial heat is combined with the buoyant properties of water that provide support against the force of gravity. The application of cold is also useful in reduction of pain and muscle spasm.

The rehabilitation goal in the management of individuals with musculoskeletal disorders is to restore them to the fullest physical, emotional, social, vocational, and economic usefulness of which they are capable, and to insure that they lead as near a normal life as possible. The rehabilitation program, therefore, should consider the patient's entire needs, and attention to the psychosocial and vocational aspects is as important as the medical and physical treatment of the disability. Specific physical medicine treatment of the musculoskeletal system is primarily symptomatic and directed toward the symptoms and findings of pain, contractures, deformity, and weakness with a goal of maintaining or restoring function. The emphasis should be placed on the remaining ability rather than on the disability. Major objectives are: (1) early establishment of a rehabilitation plan, (2) self-care, (3) maximum use of the hands, (4) ambulation and elevation, (5) restoration of function where possible, (6) anticipation of complications and the development of a program of prevention, and (7) supportive counselling to the patient and family.

Musculoskeletal management is based on an understanding of the natural evolution of each stage of the disease and its patterns of weakness, contractures, and deformity. A knowledge of pathokinetics is essential to the proper timing of therapy and bracing so that measures can be appropriately staged to ensure full use of available strength and function. It should be acknowledged that for most musculoskeletal diseases there is no specific physical treatment. Hence, treatment is symptomatic, goal-oriented, and directed largely toward findings that appear during the course of the disease; pain and tenderness, tightness and contractures, joint involvement and deformity, and weakness. These complications usually result in decreased or lost motor function so translation of improved and specific motor and sensory function into practical activities such as walking and hand use is the final objective. Symptomatic management is often modified by either prognostic categories or disease stages. For example, objectives for rheumatoid arthritis will vary for the acute, subacute and chronic stages of the disease. The aims of management are to relieve pain and inflammation and to carry the individual through the acute stage so that when remission occurs minimal deformity is left or if deformity is unavoidable, the contractures occur in the most functional position. Therefore, the main principles of physical treatment during the acute stage are rest, heat, and gentle assisted active movement. As synovitis is controlled during the subacute stage in rheumatoid arthritis, treatment is primarily directed at maintaining the maximum range of joint movement to prevent joint adhesions and maintaining or restoring muscle strength. Rest is less important than in the acute stage and is concentrated on the maintenance of the joint in a position of function.

Chronic joint disease is characterized by the presence of significant deformities and contractures that may not be reversible. Therapy is directed to maintaining the maximum degree of mobility or to insure that any ankylosis that may occur will do so with the joint in a position of function. Management includes exercise to restore strength and range of motion, splints for maintaining joints in the optimal functional position, traction and plaster casts for progressive correction of joint contractures. Assistive aids for self-care, transfer, writing, and communication become important.

Although consultation with rheumatologists is available in most communities, many of those rheumatologists have had little training in rehabilitation. Moreover specialists in Physical Medicine and Rehabilitation, or physiatrists, as well recognized as being in under supply, although there is now a trend toward rapid growth in the availability of physiatrists and P.M. & R. training programs. Of necessity, therefore, much of the care provided to patients with arthritis will be given by their primary physicians. This is appropriate but requires that the rehabilitation team approach be applied and that all practitioners become familiar with the principles of rehabilitation outlined in this book.

REFERENCES

1. Cosh JA, Rasker JJ: A twenty year follow-up of 100 patients with rheumatoid arthritis. Ann Rheum Dis 41:317, 1982
2. Fries JF: The Assessment of Disability from First to Future Principles. Brit J Rheum 22 (Suppl): 45-58, 1983
3. Fries JF, Spitz P, Kraines RG, et al: Measurement of patient outcome in arthritis. Arthritis Rheum 23:137-145, 1980
4. Liang MH, Partridge AJ, Larson ME, et al: Evaluation of comprehensive rehabilitation services for elderly homebound patients with arthritis and orthopedic disability. Arth Rheum 27:258-266, 1984
5. McDuffie FC: Morbidity impact of rheumatoid arthritis in society. Am J Med 78(Suppl 1A): 1-5, 1985
6. McGuigan LE, Hart HH, Gow PJ, et al: Employment in ankylosing spondylitis. Ann Rheum Dis 43:604-606, 1984
7. Meenan RF, Gertman PM, Mason JH: Measuring health status in arthritis: The arthritis impact measurement scales. Arthritis Rheum 23:146-152, 1980
8. Meenan RF, Yelin EH, Nevitt M, et al: The impact of chronic disease: A sociomedical profile of rheumatoid arthritis. Arth Rheum 24:544-549, 1981
9. Melvin JL: Joint protection training and energy conservation, in Melvin JL (ed.) Rheumatic Disease: Occupational Therapy and Rehabilitation. Philadelphia, F.A. Davis, 1977, pp. 191-206
10. Pincus T, Callahan LF, Sal WG, et al: Severe functional declines, work disability and increased mortality in 75 rheumatoid arthritis patients studies over 9 years. Arthritis Rheum 27:864-8721, 1984
11. Scott DL, Coulton BL, Chapman JH: The long-term effects of treating rheumatoid arthritis. J R Coll Physicians Lond 17:79-85, 1983
12. Steinbrocker D, Traeger CH, Batterman RC: Therapeutic Criteria in Rheumatoid Arthritis. JAMA 140:659-662, 1949
13. Stone CE: The lifetime economic costs of rheumatoid arthritis. J Rheumatol 11:819-827, 1984
14. Yelin E, Meenan R, Nevitt M, et al: Work disability in rheumatoid arthritis: Effects of disease, social and work factors. Ann Intern Med 93:551-556, 1980

Colon H. Wilson, Jr.
William P. Maier

2

Exercise and Mobilization Techniques

The appropriate use of exercise in the management of the rheumatic disorders requires an understanding of the different modalities of exercise, and the effects of each on inflammatory and noninflammatory arthritis as well as specific regional rheumatic disorders. Exercises may be either resistive or nonresistive. Nonresistive exercises are range of motion (ROM) exercises that are performed without resistence. They may be performed passively by a therapist (without effort on the part of the patient) or actively by the patient, with or without assistance by the therapist. Resistive exercises may be isotonic, isometric, or isokinetic. In isotonic exercises the joint is moved through a range of motion against resistence supplied by the therapists muscle power or a weight. Isometric exercise does not allow the joint to move while the muscles are tightened maximally against an immovable resistence. On an isokinetic exercise machine the force is automatically adjusted, causing the torque to remain constant, so that tension remains uniform as the muscle shortens or lengthens. Aerobic exercises are designed to promote oxygen consumption and to promote fitness. The modalities of exercise therapy to be discussed will usually fall into one of the following types; isometric exercises, range of motion exercises, and aerobic types of exercises. In addition to discussion of the role of these exercises, other supportive and adjunctive interventions will be mentioned when appropriate. These adjunctive interventions will include heat and cold modalities, rest, splinting, and nutrition.

The relation and interaction of skeletal muscles and joints form the fundamental units of mammalian locomotion. Locomotion requires, in addition, a connective tissue framework consisting of bone, ligaments, and tendons. Because these structures cross or are contiguous with the joint, processes that disturb joints often involve these structures as well. While some rheumatic diseases may be associated with a primary myopathy (Rheumatoid arthritis,[22] systemic lupus erythematosus,[25] MCTD,[50] scleroderma,[10] and polymyositis and dermatomyositis[43]) the major causes of muscle weakness, fatigue, atrophy, and dysfunction in arthritis is usually an epiphenomenon of diseased joints, and contigous connective tissue structures. Arthropathy results in muscle weakness through a combination of a variety of mechanisms including disuse (caused by pain or functional loss), effusion, and ligamentous and tendinous dysfunction. Because this weakness is an impor-

PRINCIPLES OF PHYSICAL MEDICINE AND REHABILITATION
IN THE MUSCULOSKELETAL DISEASES

tant cause of functional loss to the individual arthritic patient, exercise therapy is used in conjunction with other interventions (removal of effusions, suppression of inflammation with drug therapy, weight control, rest, and surgical procedures) to restore function and to prevent contracture or further functional loss.

An informed approach to designing exercise programs for patients with rheumatic disorders requires an understanding of the physiology of muscle strengthening, muscle atrophy, and the effects of different types of exercise on the inflamed joint. During muscle training the duration required to attain maximal strength is thought to be approximately 4–6 weeks.[43] Conversely, if a muscle is immobilized, it can atrophy up to 30 percent in one week and lose an additional 3 percent of strength every day thereafter.[32,57]

When approaching an inflamed joint this scheme is complicated by several factors. Active isotonic exercise requiring joint movement can increase inflammation and pain in an inflamed joint. Also, in a joint where an effusion is present, increased intraarticular pressures during movement may cause unphysiologic strains on articular surfaces.[27] These increased pressures may hasten cartilage loss and actually cause formation of subchondral cysts, worsening of pain, or frank joint capsule rupture. Because of these factors, when inflammatory arthritis is present isometric strengthening exercises are less painful to accomplish and are preferable physiologically.

Comparative studies have shown that isometric exercises are equivalent to isotonic exercise in muscle training.[33,34,37,38,49] Muscle strength may be just as well developed by small numbers of brief isometric contractions performed on a daily basis. Bearing these factors in mind, the ideal exercise regimen for an arthritic patient with evidence of inflammation would combine conventional range-of-motion exercises, to preserve joint motion, with a program of brief, maximal isometric contractions of the muscles most important for normal function (i.e. quadriceps muscles and deltoid muscles). Clinical studies have documented that such programs are preferable to isotonic exercises not only in arthritic patients but also in others requiring rehabilitation following surgery or trauma.[14]

The presence of a joint effusion presents specific problems for rehabilitation of disturbed muscle. Evidence suggests that in the presence of a significant effusion there is a reflex inhibition of muscle contraction across the joint.[12] This inhibition may negate any possible benefits from a strengthening program. Adequate treatment of effusion, whether by aspiration, rest, or immobilization, combined with antiinflammatory drug therapy, must precede attempts to strengthen the supporting muscles.

In addition to maintaining strength, adequate function requires maintenance of normal range of motion of all joints, thereby preventing contracture. This is accomplished by either active range of motion exercises, with or without assistance, or passive range of motion exercises. These exercises are an intergral part of the management of all inflammatory arthropathies. Figures 2-1 and 2-2 review the standard range of motion exercise program for specific joints. Since most rheumatic problems are chronic or recurring, the patient must be encouraged to continue his or her home program of exercises indefinitely.

An adequate program of rest has long been known to benefit patients with inflammatory arthritis and must be incorporated into any program of exercise and rehabilitation. The importance of rest has been demonstrated both clinically and experimentally.[5] Experienced clinicians have long recognized that excessive fatigue may contribute to an exacerbation of symptoms, therefore, rest periods should be scheduled at intervals in the patient's day between periods of activity. For example a patient with moderately active rheumatoid arthritis would be more easily controlled on a program that incorporates a one hour rest period at the end of each of two four-hour periods of activity.

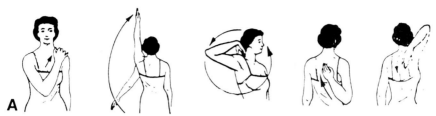

Fig. 2-1.(A)   Illustrated exercise charts are appreciated by patients. In this figure and the following figure are examples of illustrations used in the home exercise instructions given patients at the author's clinic for arthritis. Shoulder: 1, With your fingers pull you arm upward to your shoulder as far as it will go. 2, Try to touch you ear keeping your arm straight. 3, Circle you elbow several times in each direction. 4, Put your hand into the small of your back, then push it as far as you can. 5, Push your hand as far down your back as you can.

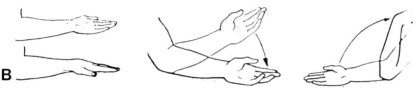

Fig. 2-1.(B)   Elbow: 1, Turn your hand over and try to make your palm touch the table. 2, Straighten your elbow as far as possible. No attempt should be made to force your elbow straight with the other hand or with weights. 3, After pulling you hand back as far as you can, relax a little, then try again.

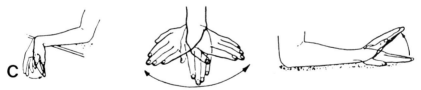

Fig. 2-1.(C)   Wrist: 1, Rest you forearm on a table with your elbow making a right angle. Lift your hand, relax, then lift again. 2, With your forearm and hand flat on a table, move your hand from side to side as far as you can. 3, Pull your hand back as far as you can then relax a little and try again.

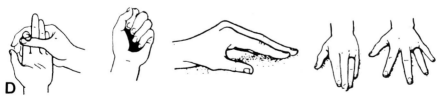

Fig. 2-1.(D)   Fingers: 1, Bend each finger joint individually then all simultaneously. 2, Try gripping a ball of wool tightly. 3, Try to arch your hand while keeping your fingers straight. 4, Put your hand flat on a table, separate your fingers, then squeeze them together again.

13

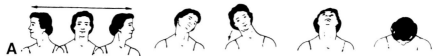

Fig. 2-2.(A)   Exercises for the neck: 1, In the sitting position, twist your head as far as possible in each direction. 2, Sit or stand with your hands on your hips. First circle your head clockwise, then counterclockwise. 3, In the sitting position, try to touch each shoulder with your head. 4, In the sitting position, look behind you as far as possible then look at your toes.

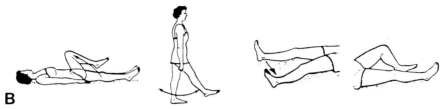

Fig. 2-2.(B)   Hips: 1, Try to bend your knee to your chest; relax a little and try again. 2, Stand on your good leg and swing your other leg backward and forward from your hip. 3, Stretch your affected leg out to one side keeping it straight. 4, Lie on your back. Bend your knee and then move it from side to side across your body.

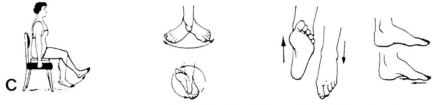

Fig. 2-2.(C)   Knee: 1, Sit with your feet off the floor. Lift your leg and then allow it to return to the bent position SLOWLY. Ankle: 1, Turn your foot inward and then outward as far as possible. 2, Circle your foot several times clockwise, then counterclockwise. Toes: 1, Sit with your legs crossed and your affected leg uppermost. Bend you ankle up and then straighten it, pointing your toe. 2, Stand upright and try to arch your foot while keeping your toes straight and pressed onto the floor.

EXERCISE AND MOBILIZATION TECHNIQUES IN RHEUMATOID ARTHRITIS AND OTHER CHRONIC INFLAMMATORY ARTHRITIDES

Rheumatoid arthritis is a systemic disease characterized by a chronic proliferative, inflammatory reaction in the synovial and subsynovial tissues of the joints, which eventually results in erosion and destruction of joint cartilage, the subchondral bone and the supporting capsular structures. These changes interfere with normal joint function and eventually give rise to typical joint deformities and characteristic radiologic abnormalities. The early clinical presentation is usually that of a symmetrical polyarthritis involving small peripheral joints. With persistence of the disease all synovial joints may become inflamed. Women are affected about three times as frequently as men, with a peak incidence in the third through the fifth decades. The cause of rheumatoid arthritis is unknown, but evidence suggests that it is an immunologic disease.[23]

Rheumatoid arthritis is usually associated with systemic features such as malaise, decreased appetite, morning stiffness, and easy fatigability. The presence of Rheumatoid Factor in approximately 70+ percent of patients, and evidence of a systemic inflammatory process (e.g. an elevated sedimentation rate and a normochromic, normocytic anemia) assist in confirming the diagnosis.[28]

Rheumatoid arthritis may be complicated by a host of extraarticular manifestations that may require special interventions. These include inflammatory eye disease (episcleritis and scleromalacia), Sjogren's syndrome, Felty's syndrome, interstitial pulmonary disease, pleural and pericardial effusions, nerve entrapment syndromes, and vasculitis.[6]

The therapy of rheumatoid arthritis is complex. Treatment of early disease, before erosions are detectable radiologically, is based on the use of antiinflammatory and analgesic drugs (salicylates or nonsteroidal antiinflammatory drugs), physical therapy, splinting, and adequate rest. Once erosive disease has appeared or significant extraarticular complications occur, suppressive therapy with gold salts, antimalarial drugs, or penicillamine is used; and, at times when severe complications occur or severe crippling is threatened, the judicious use of steroids or cytotoxic agents may be necessary.

In rheumatoid arthritis, as in all of the rheumatic diseases, the proper exercise program serves to maintain or increase the range of motion, strengthen muscle force, and improve physical fitness and endurance without worsening pain, inflammation, or deformity. In addition, special considerations must be given in rheumatoid patients to the ease of fatigability and the weakness that is characteristic of the disease. Histologic evidence for decreased number and size of Type II muscle fibers in muscle biopsies of rheumatoid patients correlates with their diminished endurance.[7,13,46] When evaluated by isometric strength, bicycle ergonometry, and walking time, rheumatoid patients have only 40–60 percent of the physical performance of age-matched controls.[14] Keeping these facts in mind, expectations for these patients must be tempered and compliance carefully monitored.

The patient's compliance with the exercise program and the effectiveness of the program can be greatly helped by taking advantage of the proper use of heat and/or cold applications to the involved joints. Heat may be applied to a single or a few specific joints by hot packs or a heating pad; or heat may be applied to all affected joints in a hot tub bath, whirlpool, or Hubbard tank. If there is significant difficulty getting the patient into and out of the tub, seating the patient in a chair in a stall shower with a bath sheet pinned around his/her neck to maintain maximal body contact with the hot water may also be very effective. Cold packs to acute or subacute joints after completing the set of exercises can be very effective in controlling post exercise pain and swelling. Please refer to Chapter 5 for a discussion of these modalities.

In designing exercise programs, the distinction between acute inflammation, subacute inflammation and stable disease is important.[55] Most patients present with acute inflammation and, if managed properly, will evolve to stable disease. This scheme is outlined in Table 2-1, with a summary of appropriate physical therapy intervention for each.

The acute phase of rheumatoid arthritis implies the presence of red, warm, swollen joints. In this first phase the purpose of a rehabilitation program is to prevent contraction deformities through immobilization of painful joints in splints whenever the patients rests or sleeps.[16] Exercises are directed at maintenance of full range of motion by means of range of motion exercises (see figs. 2-1 and 2-2). When pain is severe, passive motion by a therapist may be necessary, but as inflammation lessens, active, assisted exercises may be begun, progressing to active exercises. Aerobic and isometric exercises are less useful at

Table 2-1
Physical Therapy of Inflammatory Polyarthritis

Activity of disease	Therapy
Acute	Splinting
	Rest
	Passive ROM*
Subacute	Active assisted ROM exercises
	Hydrotherapy
	Isometric exercises
Stable	Isometric exercises
	Active ROM exercises
	Nontraumatic aerobic exercises
	(swimming)

*ROM = range of motion

this time because of the pain associated with their performance and the contribution they make towards worsening inflammation or joint injury.[2]

There is unequivocal evidence that in the acute phase of inflammation adequate rest (at times even hospitalization with complete bed rest) may be necessary for control of inflammatory polyarthritis.[41,51] Hydrotherapy may be especially useful in this phase if the patient can be assisted into and out of the pool without undue discomfort.

The subacute phase describes the time when the patient has progressed to the point when range of motion can be performed relatively painlessly and, while minor synovitis may be present, neither redness nor large effusions are present. At this point the patient may be instructed in various forms of isometric exercises for strengthening. Strengthening of the quadriceps and deltoids by this type exercise provides the patient with functional reserve.[38] If a pool is available, short periods of swimming may be encouraged as long as pain and excessive fatigue can be avoided.

When the disease process is stable, whether through remission or disease-suppression by pharmacologic means, the exercise program may be expanded to include nontraumatic, aerobic exercises including bicycle ergometry, swimming, and walking. Exercises such as jogging, dancing, and rope jumping should be avoided due to the trauma inflicted by them on the damaged joints. Aerobic fitness not only may contribute to improved strength and state of mind, but in some Scandanavian studies it has been suggested that disease activity may be modified by a regular program of such exercises.[15,45] During stable periods patients should continue their range of motion and isometric exercises.

It should be kept in mind that rheumatoid patients have a high incidence of cervical spine instability, and exercises requiring marked or rapid flexion or extension of the cervical spine may be injurious.

The exercise scheme outlined in this section may be applied to most other rheumatic diseases presenting with acute synovitis of peripheral joints (e.g. psoriatic arthritis, Reiter's Syndrome, and the connective tissue diseases). A number of these diseases (such as systemic lupus erythematosus, Reiter's disease, and crystalline induced arthritis) may present with a monarticular or polyarticular synovitis that will proceed through acute, subacute, and chronic stages, as described above.

EXERCISE AND MOBILIZATION TECHNIQUES IN THE SPONDYLOARTHROPATHIES

In the last 25 years a group of diseases known collectively as seronegative spondyloarthropathies have been recognized as being distinct from rheumatoid arthritis, with which they were previously frequently confused. Ankylosing spondylitis is the prototype of these diseases, but this group also includes Reiter's syndrome, and certain subsets of psoriatic arthritis and enteropathic arthritis. The common features of the spondyloarthropathies include negative tests for rheumatoid factor and radiologic sacroiliitis. There is significant clinical overlap within this group of diseases and a tendency to familial aggregation.[9] All of the seronegative spondyloarthropathies tend to affect the joints of the axial skeleton, including the sacroiliac joints, the spine, the hips, and the shoulders. There is a significantly higher incidence of the HLA B27 antigen in these patients than in the general population.[5]

These diseases are distinguished from each other by the presence of specific clinical features occurring in association with the common features of the seronegative spondyloarthropathies. In Reiter's Syndrome, one can identify the typical triad of conjunctivitis, urethritis, and arthritis. In psoriatic arthritis, psoriatic skin lesions or pitting of the nails are present. Enteropathic spondyloarthropathy is seen in association with chronic inflammatory bowel disease.

The management of these diseases is directed at the suppression of inflammation, the alleviation of pain, the prevention of deformity, the preservation of function, and the treatment of specific extraarticular manifestations such as iritis. In the case of the enteropathic spondyloarthropathies associated with inflammatory bowel disease, specific therapy against the bowel disease may not arrest the course of the spondylitis, but is necessary for patients' comfort and survival.[20]

The use of nonsteroidal antiinflammatory drugs, such as indomethicin, has been reported to be more effective than the use of aspirin in the treatment of these diseases.[19] Once a patient has gained adequate relief of pain and stiffness from a good program of nonsteroidal antiinflammatory medication, he should immediately be instructed in the basic exercise programs outlined in Figure 2-3. These exercises comprise the keystone of management and should be performed daily. They should be reviewed regularly with the patient by the physician or therapist. It has been recommended that patients perform postural and flexion exercises at midday, when stiffness has remitted and before fatigue sets in. Lunch time may be the patient's most motivated time of day.[52]

Few formal clinical studies have evaluated the effectiveness of these exercise techniques; however, in one British study confirmatory evidence was provided. In a prospective trial, marked improvement in cervical spine mobility was found in patients who continue a regular program of active mobilizing exercises.[47]

In addition to exercises, other measures to prevent deformities of the axial skelton are important in managing these diseases. The maintenance of an erect, upright posture is valuable in preventing kyphotic deformities. The use of a firm mattress and the use of no more than one pillow are also important in preventing cervical spine and thoracic spine deformities. Because of the frequent involvement of the costovertebral joints, deep inspiration exercises should be included in the patient's program to help preserve adequate respiratory excursion.

The patient should be instructed to avoid activity or exercise that places undue strain

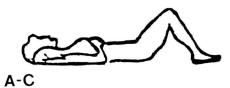

A-C

Fig. 2-3. Back Program Supine (with legs straight) (A) Quad sets: Tighten muscle above knee, hold for slow count of 5. Relax. Repeat ( ) times. (B) Gluteal Sets: Supine with legs straight tighten buttocks and hold for slow count of 5. Relax. Repeat ( ) times. (C) Pelvic tilt: Supine with knees bent, feet flat on surface, tighten abdominal and gluteal muscles forcing low back into surface. Relax. Repeat ( ) times.

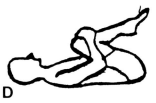

Fig. 2-3.(D) Double knee to Chest: Supine-bring both knees toward chest-Grasp knees with hands and gently stretch closer to chest-Maintain proper breathing pattern. Repeat ( ) times.

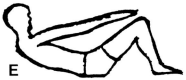

Fig. 2-3.(E) Modified curl-up: Supine with knees bent-feet flat without pillow with arms out-stretched, bring chin toward chest and attempt to sit up trying to touch knees with finger tips. Return slowly. Repeat ( ) times.

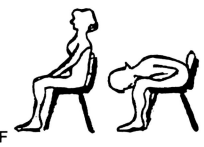

Fig. 2-3.(F) Sitting stretch: Sitting in chair, feet flat on floor spread about 2 feet apart. With arms crossed, bend forward allowing arms to pass between knees and gently stretch toward floor. Repeat ( ) times.

18

on back muscles, and to avoid activities and sports that produce physical trama, especially to the spine. Regular swimming has been suggested as the ideal activity for spondylitic patients.[52]

The occurrence of an inflammatory peripheral arthritis occurs in approximately 15–20 percent of patients with ankylosing spondylitis.[29] Likewise, peripheral arthritis, especially of the knee and small joints, are common findings in psoriatic arthritis, Reiter's Syndrome, and reactive arthritis.[8] These acutely inflamed joints should be treated in a manner similar to that discussed for the acute stage of rheumatoid arthritis. Joint splinting and heat or cold applications may be useful in controlling pain and inflammation. Range of motion exercises (passive, active assisted, or active, depending on the acuteness of the inflammation) will help to preserve function.

EXERCISE AND MOBILIZATION TECHNIQUES IN THE MANAGEMENT OF OSTEOARTHRITIS

Osteoarthritis is the most common of the rheumatic disorders. The disease is characterized by the degeneration of articular cartilage, with subsequent deformity and thickening of subchondral bone.[48] It may be distinguished from the inflammatory arthritides by the lack of synovial thickening on physical exam. Osteoarthritis is usually described as primary when there is no history of antecedent joint damage (fracture, infection, avascular necrosis), or associated metabolic diseases (ochronosis, hemochromatosis, Wilson's disease, or acromegaly), and secondary when there is a history of prior trauma or one of these disease processes is present.[35,42]

Virtually any joint in the body may be involved by osteoarthritis, but the most common sites are the joints of the wrist, the cervical and lumbar spine, the hips and the knees.[24] Following a discussion of the general management of osteoarthritis we will comment on these areas specifically.

Like many rheumatic diseases, the initial management of osteoarthritis begins with attempts to control pain by the use of aspirin or nonsteroidal antiinflammatory medications. Likewise, adequate rest, to prevent excess fatigue, and instruction in joint sparing techniques, to reduce trauma, are necessary. The next step is the outlining of an appropriate exercise program that will maximally preserve function. Adjunctive measures that benefit the patient include local joint injections, traction, and, at times, arthroplasty or joint replacement.[56]

The planning of an exercise program for a patient with osteoarthritis will include the previously discussed types of exercises, i.e. range of motion exercises, isometric strengthening exercises, and aerobic exercises that increase endurance (e.g. swimming). The patient's ability to perform the exercises will depend upon the success of previous interventions including pain relief, rest periods, and the amount of joint structural change. Generally it is better to start the patients on an easily managed program to avoid discouragement. Indications of excess exercise include postexercise pain that persists for greater than 30 minutes with rest, undue fatigue, increased weakness, decreased range of motion, and joint swelling.[56]

As in rheumatoid arthritis, if the joints are painful and show signs of inflammation (inflammatory osteoarthritis), passive range of motion exercise may be the only program indicated (see Table 2-1). Once a patient is tolerating an appropriate range of motion program, strengthening isometric exercises may be added. Isometric exercises are especially valuable in alleviating the symptoms of osteoarthritis of the knees and cervical spine.

The first carpometacarpal joint of the hand is the most common painfully involved of the small joints of the hand. Heberdene's nodes of distal interphalangeal joints and Bouchard's nodes of proximal interphalangeal joints are frequently cosmetic problems rather than a significant cause of pain or functional impairment. Therapy of carpometacarpal pain is best approached by use of a plastic working splint that holds the thumb in a few degrees of abduction. This usually allows pinching movements without painful joint motion. Active range of motion exercises for all the joints of the hand will help insure continued function.

Osteoarthritis of the cervical spine most commonly involves vertebrae C5-C6, with the most significant limitation of motion being in extension and lateral rotation. Range of motion exercises will help increase motion. These are demonstrated in Figure 2-2. This technique should be avoided in patients with radiculopathy or subluxation. A regime of isometric exercises of the cervical spine has been developed. The patient's head is turned toward one side as far as can be tolerated and, while holding both sides of the head, the therapist has the patient press his or her head against 1 hand for 6 seconds followed by 20 seconds of rest. This is repeated five to ten times. Isometric exercises are performed similarly, with pressure against first the forehead and then the occiput while the head is in a neutral position. This set of exercises should be performed twice daily. Again, precautions to prevent over-exercise must be taken.[18]

Adjunctive measures in the treatment of osteoarthritis of the cervical spine include the use of a neck pillow. This has been shown to be effective in approximately 70 percent of patients.[40] A soft cervical collar may help to prevent pain from muscle fatigue by providing extra support during activities such as working at a desk or riding in a car.

Osteoarthritis of the lumbosacral spine is often difficult to distinguish from idiopathic low back pain. Flexion and pelvic tilt exercises will benefit both these disorders. Hence, clear differentiation will not change therapy unless evidence of spinal stenosis or sciatica are present, suggesting possible benefit from surgical intervention.[31] See Figure 2-3 for spinal flexion exercises.

Osteoarthritis of the hip is a potentially crippling disorder, but with good management it may be well tolerated. Flexion contractures may be prevented by having the patient assume a prone position on a firm mattress for approximately 30 minutes twice a day.[44] Range of motion exercises may be done in a swimming pool or on a firm surface. The most functionally important exercises for the hip are flexion and abduction. For flexion the knee should be brought to the chest while lying in a supine position. The front of the knee is grasped to the chest, while the opposite knee is kept extended. This should be repeated 5 to 10 times. Abduction exercises are done in the same position by extending the legs one at a time as far away from the midline as possible, then returning to the midline. A piece of plywood placed on the foot of the bed, with the patient's foot resting on a skate board may be used to assist the patient in abducting the leg. This exercise should also be repeated 5 to 10 times. Rotation of the hip may be accomplished by lying supine with the feet separated 10 inches, and rotating the feet inward and outward as far as possible 5 to 10 times. Attempts to remove weight from the involved hip by means of a cane, crutch, or walker often decrease pain and preserve the ability to ambulate.[17] If hip pain progresses despite the use of adjunctive devices and exercise, then total hip replacement may yield excellent results provided the knees and feet are functioning well.

Osteoarthritis of the knees, like that of the hip, may be managed with adjunctive devices to relieve weight bearing, especially if the joint is unstable or locking and falls are a problem. Weight loss is a difficult but useful way of reducing trauma to all joints of the lower extremity.

The quadriceps muscle is of major importance in providing stability and support for the knee. Because quadriceps wasting is often an early finding in osteoarthritis of the knee, the use of isometric exercises is helpful for improving strength and function and preventing pain. Beginning with the leg in a very slightly flexed position the patient is instructed to contract both quadricep muscles maximally for 5 seconds, followed by 20 seconds rest. This may be repeated for 5 to 10 times in each set. Repeating this set 4 times a day quickly leads to normalization of quadriceps strength. The exercise may be done while lying in bed or before meals while sitting at the table. Range of motion exercises for the knees to preserve flexion and maintain full extension are also necessary and should be done daily (Fig. 2-2).

Osteoarthritis of the ankle and feet are common causes of foot pain. Range of motion exercises may benefit these conditions, but often these exercises must be combined with special orthotic footwear to best relieve symptoms.

The use of heat prior to exercise has been shown to diminish pain and to facilitate stretching.[36,44] Whether it is a hot shower, hot pack, hubbard tank, or paraffin bath for the hands, the use of such methods of heat application may greatly improve ease and effectiveness of the exercises.

EXERCISE AND MOBILIZATION TECHNIQUES IN THE MANAGEMENT OF IDIOPATHIC LOW BACK PAIN

Low back pain is a ubiquitous problem not only for rheumatologists and physiatrists, but also for orthopedic surgeons, primary care internists, and family practitioners. This problem has an enormous effect on the economy and the work place, causing much disability and absenteeism. The first burden of the physician is to diagnose structural causes of such pain, including intervertebral disc disease, renal disease, vertebral compression fractures, and abscesses or metastatic disease involving the spine or paravertebral structures. Once a specific diagnosis is clear appropriate treatment may be instituted. In a large majority of patients with low back complaints, the cause will be presumed to be idiopathic (i.e. due to muscle spasm, strain, or a combination of such with associated depression) because no cause will be identifiable on physical examination or laboratory and radiographic investigation. Since idiopathic low back pain is a diagnosis of exclusion, an alertness must be maintained to recognize other clues to a structural disease should they arise.

The treatment of functional low back pain is difficult. While there is no universally accepted approach to such patients, generally a balanced program of rest, pain relief, and exercise will produce good results. There are several studies demonstrating the effectiveness of flexion back exercises (William's Exercises) in these patients,[11,30,39,54] yet there has been criticism of study methods and findings.[11] In any case, we and many other rheumatologists and physiatrists feel that adherence to a regimen of flexion exercises benefits our patients' pain and helps prevent recurrent injuries. Nevertheless it must be kept in mind that many of these patients will improve no matter what type of intervention.

There are several reasons why exercise may be beneficial to these patients. First, there is evidence that the strength of the trunk extensors is often reduced in such patients with chronic low back pain.[1] Second, muscular insufficiency, in the form of decreased endurance, is a contributory factor in idiopathic low back pain.[3] Third, adequate strength of the trunk muscles is probably necessary for a full return to function. Therefore, a good exercise program should be maintained to increase both muscle strength and endurance.

A program of flexion exercises and toning exercises are illustrated in Figure 2-3. These exercises should be repeated as frequently as possible as long as pain does not develop or follow the completion of sets. Often appropriate weight loss will be necessary before the problem is well controlled. All patients with low back pain should be instructed in proper techniques for protecting the back while lifting and in proper posture for sitting, standing, and walking.

If pain is persistent despite adherence to appropriate rest, exercise, and antiinflammatory medication, then further referral to pain clinics or psychiatric counseling may be necessary. Please refer to Chapter 2 for a discussion of approaches to the control of chronic pain.

EXERCISE IN POLYMYOSITIS (INFLAMMATORY MUSCLE DISEASE)

Polymyositis and dermatomyositis both may be associated with synovitis, and this problem may be managed as the other types of acute synovitis discussed in this chapter (see Table 2-1). Special consideration must be given to the marked muscle weakness often seen in the acute phases of this disease, during which bed rest is desirable. Passive and assisted exercise should be undertaken only as strength returns. Care must be taken not to over-stretch weak and inflamed muscles. During this acute phase it is important that the limbs be maintained in functional position, and the use of splints may be necessary to avoid contractures. As strength improves and the level of muscle enzymes fall, a more active physical therapy program may be gradually introduced.[4] However, care must be taken even after all signs of active inflammation have ceased in order to prevent over stressing the muscles and producing decompensation. This requires very careful monitoring of the patient and his or her exercise program to gauge the onset of fatigue and to carefully evaluate muscle strength at intervals in order to detect early muscle decompensation.

REFERENCES

1. Addison R, Schultz A: Trunk strengths in patients seeking hospitalization for chronic low back disorders. Spine 5:539–544, 1980
2. Agudelo CA, Schumacher HR, Phelps PL: Effect of exercise on urate crystal-induced inflammation in canine joints. Arth Rheum 15:609–616, 1972
3. Alston W, Carlson KE, Feldman DJ, et al: A quantitative study of muscle factors in the chronic low back pain syndrome. J Amer Geriat Soc 14:1041–1047, 1966
4. Ansell BA: Management of polymyositis and dermatomyositis. Clin Rheum Dis 10:205–213, 1984
5. Arnett FC: HLA and the spondyloarthropathies, in Calin A (ed.): Spondyloarthropathies. Orlando, Grune & Stratton, 1984, pp. 297–322

6. Bluestone R, Bacon PA: Extra-articular manifestations of rheumatoid arthritis. Clin Rheum Dis 3:385–401, 1977

7. Brooke M, Kaplan J: Muscle pathology in rheumatoid arthritis, polymyalgia rheumatica and polymyositis. Arch Pathol 94:101–118, 1972

8. Calin A: Reiter's disease. Med Clin North Am 61:365–376, 1977

9. Calin A: Spondyloarthropathies: An Overview, in Calin A (ed.): Spondyloarthropathies. Orlando, Grune & Stratton, 1984, pp. 1–8

10. Clements PJ, Furst DE, Campion, DS, et al: Muscle disease in progressive systemic sclerosis. Diagnostic and therapeutic considerations. Arth Rheum 21:62–71, 1978

11. Davies JE, Gibson R, Tester L: The value of exercises in the treatment of low back pain. Rheumatol Rehabil 18:243–247, 1979

12. DeAndrade JR, Grant C, Dixon AS: Joint distension and reflex muscle inhibition in the knee. Bone Joint Surg 47A:313–322, 1965

13. Edstrom L, Nordemar R: Differential changes in type I and type II muscle fibers in rheumatoid arthritis. Scand J Rheumatol 3:155–160, 1974

14. Ekblom B, Lorgren O, Alderin M, et al: Physical performance in patients with rheumatoid arthritis. Scand J Rheumatol 3:121–125, 1974

15. Ekblom B, Lövgren O, Alderin M, et al: Effect of short-term physical training on patients with rheumatoid arthritis. Scand J Rheumatol 4:87–91, 1975

16. Gault SJ, Spyker JM: Beneficial effect of immobilization of joints in rheumatoid and related arthritides: a splint study using sequential analysis. Arth Rheum 12:34–44, 1969

17. Gerber LH: Aids and appliances, in Wright V (ed.): Arthritis in the Elderly. Edinburgh, Churchill Livingston, 1983, pp. 256–274

18. Gerber LH, Hicks JE: Rehabilitation in the management of patients with osteoarthritis, in Moskowitz RW, Howell DS, Goldberg VM, et al (eds.): Osteoarthritis; Diagnosis and Management, New York, W.B. Saunders, 1984, pp. 287–315

19. Godfrey RG, Calabro JJ, Mills D, et al: A double blind crossover trial of aspirin, indomethacin and phenylbutazone in ankylosing spondylitis. Arth Rheum 15:110, 1972

20. Greenstein AJ, Janowitz HD, Sachar DB: The extraintestinal complications of Crohn's disease and ulcerative colitis: A study of 700 patients. Medicine 55:401–412, 1976

21. Hague BV: Diaphragmatic movement and spirometric volume in patients with ankylosing spondylitis. Scand J Resp Dis 54:38–44, 1973

22. Halla J, Koopman WJ, Falahi S, et al: Rheumatoid Myositis Clinical and Histologic Features and Possible Pathogenesis. Arth Rheum 27:737–743, 1984

23. Harris ED: Rheumatoid Arthritis, in Cohen AS (ed.): Rheumatology and Immunology. New York, Grune & Stratton, 1979, pp. 168–187

24. Hoaglund F: Clinical manifestations of osteoarthritis. Clinica in the Rheumatic Diseases. 2:543–556, 1976

25. Isenber DA, Smith ML: Muscle disease in systemic lupus erythrmatosus a study of its nature, frequency and cause. J Rheumatol 8:917–924, 1981

26. Jackson CP, Brown MD: Is there a role for exercise in the treatment of patients with low back pain? Clin Orthop 179:39–45, 1983

27. Jayson MV, Dixon ASJ: Intra-articular pressure in Rheumatoid arthritis of the knee; pressure changes during exercise. Ann Rheum Dis 29:401–408, 1970

28. Johnson PM, Faulk WP: Rheumatoid factor: Its nature, specificity and production in rheumatoid arthritis. Clin Immunol Immunopathol 6:414–430, 1976

29. Kahn MS: Ankylosing spondylitis, in Calin A (ed.): Spondyloarthropathies. Grune & Stratton, 1984, pp. 143–161

30. Kendell PH, Jenkins JM: Exercises for backache: A double-blind controlled trial. Physiotherapy 54:154–157, 1968

31. Kirkaldy-Willis WJ, Paine KWE, Cauchoix J, et al: Lumbar spinal stenosis. Clin Orthop 99:30–50, 1974

32. Kottke F: The effects of limitation of activity upon the human body. JAMA 196:449–462, 1970

33. Lawrence MS, Meyer HR, Matthews NL: Comparative increase in muscle strength in the Quadriceps Femoris by isometric and isotonic exercise, and effects of the contralateral muscle. J Am Phys Ther Assoc 42:15–20, 1962

34. Leach RE, Stryker WS, Zohn DA: A comparative study of isometric and isotonic quadriceps exercise programs. J Bone Joint Surg 47A:1421–1426, 1965

35. Lee P, Rooney PJ, Sturrock RD, et al: The etiology and pathogenesis of osteoarthritis: A review. Semin Arthritis Rheum 3:189–209, 1974

36. Lehmann JF, Masock AJ, Warren CG, et al: Effect of therapeutic temperatures on tendon distensibility. Arch Phys Med Rehabil 51:481–487, 1970

37. Liberson WT, Asa MM: Further studies of brief isometric exercises. Arch Phys Med Rehabil 40:330–336, 1959

38. Machover S, Sapecky AJ: Effect of isometric exercise of the quadriceps muscle in patients

with rheumatoid arthritis. Arch Phys Med Rehabil 47:737–741, 1966

39. McKenzie RA: Prophylaxis in recurrent low back pain. N Zealand Med J 89:22–23, 1979

40. Melvin JL: Effectiveness of a cervical pillow for management of neck pain: a survey of patient use. (abstract) Arth Rheum 27:S133 (p. 133 inclusive)

41. Mills JA, Pinals RS, Ropes MW, et al: Value of bed rest in patients with rheumatoid arthritis. N Engl J Med 284:453–458, 1971

42. Moskowitz RW: Introduction to osteoarthritis, in Moskowitz RW, Howell DS, Goldberg VM, et al (eds.): Osteoarthritis Diagnosis and Management. New York, W.B. Saunders Company, 1984, pp. 1–7

43. Muller EA: Influence of training and inactivity on muscle strength. Arch Phys Med Rehabil 51:449–462, 1970

44. Nichols PJR: Osteoarthritis, in Rehabilitation Medicine. London, Butterworth and Co. 1980, Chapter 7. pp. 149–160

45. Nordemar R, Ekblom B, Zachrisson L, et al: Physical training in rheumatoid arthritis: a controlled long-term study. Scand J Rheumatol 10:17–23, 1981

46. Nordemar R, Edstrom C, Ekblom B: Changes in muscle fibre size and physical performance in patients with rheumatoid arthritis after short-term physical training. Scand J Rheumatol 5:70–76, 1976

47. O'Driscoll SL, Jayson MIV, Braddeley H: Neck movements in ankylosing spondylitis and their responses to physiotherapy. Ann Rheum Dis 37:64–66, 1978

48. Radin EL, Paul IL, and Tolkoff, MJ: Subchondral bone changes in patients with early degenerative joint disease. Arth Rheum 13:400–405, 1970

49. Rose DL, Radzyminski SF, Beatty RR: Effects of brief maximal exercise on the strength of the Quadriceps Femoris. Arch Phys Med Rehabil 38:157–164, 1957

50. Sharp GC: Mixed connective tissue disease. Bull Rheum Dis 25:828–831, 1975

51. Smith RD, Polley HF: Rest therapy for rheumatoid arthritis. Mayo Clin Proc 53:141–145, 1978

52. Smythe H: Therapy of spondyloarthropathies. Clin Orthop 143:84–89, 1979

53. Stevens JC, Cartlidge NEF, Saunders M, et al: Atlantoaoaxial subluxation and cervical myelopathy in rheumatoid arthritis. J Med 40:391–408, 1971

54. Wagner CJ: Williams flexion regime in the treatment of low back pain. J Int Coll Surg 18:69–76, 1952

55. Wilson CH: Exercise in Arthritis, in Basmajian JV (ed.): Therapeutic Exercise, 4th Edition. Baltimore, Williams & Wilkins, 1984, pp. 529–545

56. Wilson CH: Exercise in arthritis, in Basmajian, JV (ed.): Therapeutic Exercises, 4th edition. Baltimore, Williams and Wilkins, 1984, pp. 529–545

57. Woo SL, Matthews JV, Akeson WH, et al: Connective tissue response to immobility. Arth Rheum 18:257–264, 1975

Barbara J. de Lateur
Justus F. Lehmann

3

Strengthening Exercise

DEFINITIONS

Strength.   Strength may be defined as the maximum force that can be exerted by a muscle. Since this force varies with the speed and direction of contraction and with the mechanical conditions of contraction (leverage), the definition must be qualified. Practically, strength is often defined by its means of measurement.

Isometric strength.   Isometric strength is the maximum force that can be exerted against a relatively immovable object. The slight deformation that occurs is quantified by a strain gage.

Isotonic strength.   The term, isotonic strength, is a misnomer, since the force ("tone") exerted by the muscle changes constantly throughout the range of motion, due to changes of leverage of the muscle and of the weight lifted. However, the term is firmly entrenched in the language and is usually defined as the one repetition maximum or the ten repetition maximum.

One repetition maximum (1RM).   The largest weight that can be lifted against gravity through the full range of motion of the joint one time only.

Ten repetition maximum (10RM).   The largest weight that can be lifted against gravity through the full range of motion ten times only.

Isokinetic strength.   The maximum torque that can be developed at any given velocity of contraction. The measurement of this torque requires a rate-limiting device such as the Cybex II (Cybex Division of Lumex Inc., 2100 Smithtown Ave, Ronkonkoma, NY 11779).

Concentric contraction.   A contraction in which the overall length of the muscle decreases. A shortening contraction.

PRINCIPLES OF PHYSICAL MEDICINE AND REHABILITATION   ©1986 Grune & Stratton, Inc.
IN THE MUSCULOSKELETAL DISEASES   ISBN 0-8089-1773-0 All rights reserved.

Eccentric contraction. A contraction in which the overall length of the muscle increases—a lengthening contraction. Although "lengthening contraction" would seem to be a contradiction in terms, this usage is well established and refers to a paying out of the muscle against resistance. An example would be the action of the quadriceps as one descends stairs.

Dynamic contraction. One in which the levers (bones) move in relation to each other and the overall muscle length changes. Dynamic strength would include all of the types of strength listed above except isometric.

Static contraction. One in which the levers do not move in relation to each other and the overall length of the muscle does not change. Static strength is used interchangeably with isometric strength.

Kinesiology. The study of (human) movement. Originally defined as the explanation of human movement in terms of Newtonian physics, kinesiology has come to include physiologic aspects as well as mechanics of movement. The types of movement described serve different kinesiologic functions: shortening contractions accelerate the limb or body; static contractions stabilize the limb or the body in relation to the limb; and lengthening contractions decelerate the body, i.e., serve as shock absorbers.

When all motor units in a muscle are recruited and firing maximally, the force that can be developed in each of these types of contractions differs from the others in a predictable way.[2] Figure 3-1 shows this relationship. Thus, the greatest force is developed

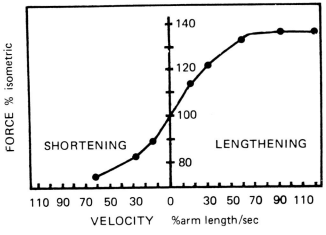

Fig. 3-1. Relationship of maximal force of human elbow flexor muscles to velocity of contraction. Velocity on abscissa is designated as percent of arm length per second. (From Knuttgen HG: Development of muscular strength and endurance, in Knuttgen HG (ed): Neuromuscular Mechanisms for Therapeutic and Conditioning Exercises. Baltimore, University Park Press, 1976. Redrawn from Asmussen E, Hansen O, Lammert O: The relation between isometric and dynamic muscle strength in man. Comm Dan Nat Assoc Inf Paral 20:11, 1965. With permission.)

with a rapidly lengthening contraction, somewhat less force with a slower lengthening contraction, and the least force with a rapid shortening contraction. The maximal isometric force is at the inflection point of this sigmoidal curve. Before there were readily available methods to measure the force of a lengthening contraction, the maximal isometric contraction was termed the maximal voluntary contraction (MVC), and this term is still used, even though it is not the maximum force that can be developed.[24]

Length-tension relationship. It is widely known that a muscle can develop its greatest tension at its resting length. What is not so widely known is the definition of resting length, since the muscle can rest, i.e. be electrically silent, at virtually any length in the intact human subject. To define, precisely, the resting length of a muscle, one must go to the experimental animal model. If, as in curve C, Figure 3-2, one detaches the muscle from its insertion in the anesthetized animal and places it at very short length, no tension is recorded in the muscle. If one gradually begins drawing the muscle out, it will, at some point, register minimal tension. That point (the x-intercept) is defined as the resting length. Further increases in length will result in more tension, all passive. If the muscle is then returned to the very short length, and a tetanizing volley of electrical stimuli is sent down the motor nerve of that muscle, tension will be developed, as shown in curve A. Since the total tension is a combination of the active and passive tension, at all lengths less than

Length – Tension Diagrams of Total and Passive Tension

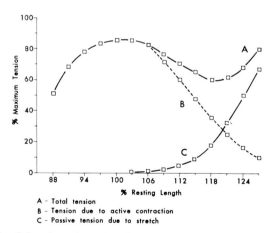

A - Total tension
B - Tension due to active contraction
C - Passive tension due to stretch

Fig. 3-2. Length-tension diagram for passive stretch of an unstimulated muscle is shown in lower Curve C. Curve A, showing total isometric tension when the muscle was stimulated at various lengths from maximal stretch through moderate shortening, represents the summation of active contraction plus passive tension due to the stretch. Active tension due solely to muscular contraction is obtained by subtracting passive tension, C, from total tension, A, and is represented by Curve B. Normal resting length is 100 percent. (Redrawn from Schottelius BA, Senay LC: Effect of stimulation-length sequence on shape of length-tension diagram. Am J Physiol 186:127–130, 1956. With permission.)

the resting length the total tension is equal to the active tension alone, because the passive tension is zero. It is obviously impossible to go through this type of maneuver in the intact human subject. A reasonable approach is to place the joint in at least mid-position, or with the muscle even longer, in order to arrive at an advantageous position on the length-tension diagram.

Torque.   What is measured in the intact human subject is not usually tension (although this can be done by such special devices as a Lissner clamp on the tendon of insertion) but torque, which is the effectiveness of a force in producing rotation of a limb around its axis (joint) and is the product of the muscle force and the perpendicular distance of the tendon of insertion from the axis of motion (see Fig. 3-3).[6]

Leverage.   Thus, in determining the torque, or effective rotatory force of a muscle, one must consider not only the length of the muscle but also its leverage. The distance of the tendon of insertion from the axis of motion (joint) is anatomically fixed for any given muscle, but the perpendicular distance will vary for that muscle throughout the range of motion of that joint. A leverage curve can be developed in isolation from the length-tension relationship.[5] Such a family of leverage curves for the various elbow flexors is given in Figure 3-4. One cannot infer from these curves that the brachioradialis is the "strongest" of the elbow flexors but that it does have the best leverage.

For a muscle of any given strength, with motor units recruited maximally, the torque that can be developed at any point in the joint range will be the net effect of leverage (mechanical factor), length of the muscle, and velocity of contraction. Samples of such curves, measured isometrically, are shown in Figures 3-5, 3-6 and 3-7.[3] The advent of the isokinetic dynamometer, a device that allows one to preset the limiting range of concentric contraction and to measure the torque developed throughout the range of motion, permits the clinician as well as the researcher to measure families of torque curves of various muscles. The torque developed by one of the authors (BJdL) while flexing and extending the knee at 3 rpm, 10 rpm, and 30 rpm is shown in Figure 3-8. These curves also illustrate the torque-velocity relationship, with decreasing torque at increasing rates of (shortening) contraction.

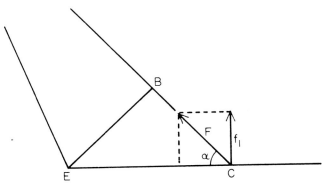

Fig. 3-3.   Two methods of computing torque. Torque equals f_1 × EC or F × EB. (From Brunnstrom S: Clinical Kinesiology, second edition. Philadelphia, FA Davis, 1966. With permission.)

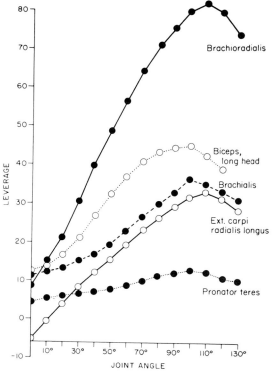

Fig. 3-4. Leverage curves of elbow flexors. Zero degrees—elbow extended. (From Brunnstrom S: Clinical Kinesiology, second edition. Philadelphia, FA Davis, 1966; plotted from data of Braune W, Fischer O: Die Rotationsmomente der Beugemuskeln am Ellbogengelenk des Menschen. Abhandl d K S Gesellsch d Wissensch 26:245–310, 1890)

DETERMINANTS OF STRENGTH

Concept of "Absolute" Muscle Strength

This relates the force that a muscle can develop to the cross-sectional area. Although there is some disparity of the values found for this, there is best agreement on the value of 3.6 kgm/cm^2 of physiologic cross-sectional area.[1,41] In order to understand what is meant by "physiologic cross-sectional area" one must contrast parallel muscles with pennate muscles (see Figs. 3-9 and 3-10). As the name suggests, parallel muscles have long fibers that stretch essentially from one end of the muscle to the other. The long parallel fibers adapt this type of muscle to speed of contraction (i.e. the contraction of the muscle results in a large excursion of the joint). The physiologic cross section is the cross section of the belly of the muscle. Pennate muscles, in contrast, are adapted to short, but forceful, excursions of the joint. They have numerous short fibers packed at an angle to the tendon of insertion. The physiologic cross section is found by taking multiple cross sections at right angles to the muscle fibers until all fibers have been included.

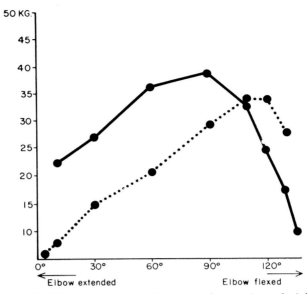

Fig. 3-5. Torque curves for flexion and extension of right elbow, from determinations on four male subjects. Solid curve: elbow flexion. Dotted curve: elbow extension. (From Brunnstrom S: Clinical Kinesiology, second edition, Philadelphia, FA Davis, 1966; redrawn from Bethe A, Franke F: Beiträge zum Problem der willkürlich beweglichen Armprothesen. IV. Die Kraftkurven der indirekten natürlichen Energiequellen. Münch Med Wochenschr 66:201–205, 1919. With permission.)

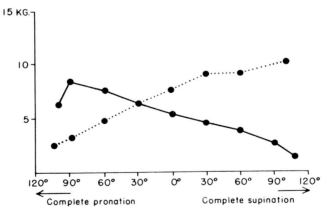

Fig. 3-6. Torque curves for pronation and supination of right elbow, derived from determinations on four male subjects. Elbow at 90 degrees of flexion. Solid curve: supination. Dotted curve: pronation. Zero: thumb upward. (From Brunnstrom S: Clinical Kinesiology, second edition, Philadelphia, FA Davis, 1966; redrawn from Bethe A, Franke F: Beiträge zum Problem der willkürlich beweglichen Armprothesen. IV. Die Kraftkurven der indirekten natürlichen Energiequellen. Münch Med Wochenschr 66:201–205, 1919. With permission.)

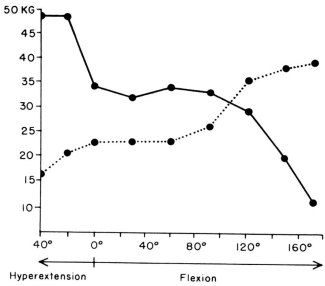

Fig. 3-7. Torque curves for flexion and extension of right shoulder, derived from determinations on four male subjects. Solid curve: flexion. Dotted curve: extension. (From Brunnstrom S: Clinical Kinesiology, second edition, Philadelphia, FA Davis, 1966; redrawn from Bethe A, Franke F: Beiträge zum Problem der willkürlich beweglichen Armprothesen. IV. Die Kraftkurven der indirekten natürlichen Energiequellen. Münch Med Wochenschr 66:201–205, 1919. With permission.)

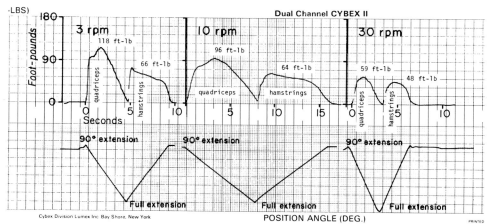

Fig. 3-8. Torque curves of quadriceps and hamstrings throughout 90 degree range of motion and at various isokinetic speeds. Note the greater strength of the quadriceps versus the hamstrings. With the subject seated, gravity hinders the quadriceps and helps the hamstrings progressively more at higher speeds. (From de Lateur BJ: Therapeutic exercise to develop strength and endurance, in Kottke FJ, Stillwell GK, Lehmann JF (eds): Krusen's Handbook of Physical Medicine and Rehabilitation, third edition. Philadelphia, WB Saunders Company, 1982. With permission.)

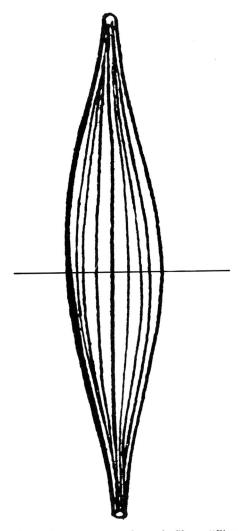

Fig. 3-9. Parallel arrangement of muscle fibers. "Physiologic" cross section is equal to cross section of muscle belly. (From Brunnstrom S: Clinical Kinesiology, second edition. Philadelphia, FA Davis, 1966. With permission.)

Recruitment Patterns ("Neural Factors")

The ability to exert brief, high-force contractions relates not only to the cross-sectional area of the muscle but also to the ability to "fire" the motor units rapidly and synchronously. Moritani and DeVries[29] studied the relationship of integrated electrical activity of muscle (IEMG) to isometric force and the change of that relationship with time and training. If care is taken to place the pickup electrode on the same place of the same muscle, then the IEMG will bear a linear relationship to the force developed by the muscle. Figure 3-11A shows that linear relationship, before training, in the solid line. The authors define (electrical) efficiency as the amount of IEMG required for a given force.

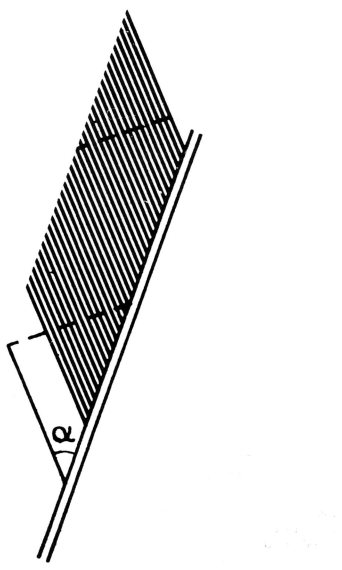

Fig. 3-10. In pennate muscle the physiologic cross section is determined by multiple sections at right angles to the fibers until all are included. (From Brunnstrom S: Clinical Kinesiology, second edition, Philadelphia, FA Davis, 1966. With permission.)

Figure 3-11A also illustrates one type of response to training: the broken line is merely an extension of the pre training line. There is increased activation, a form of learning, but no change in the ratio of electrical activity to force (E/F), i.e. no increase in efficiency. In contrast, Figure 3-11B shows a response to training in which there is no increase in activation, but an improvement in the E/F ratio, which would be seen with muscle hypertrophy. Figure 3-11C illustrates how the relative contributions of learning and hypertrophy

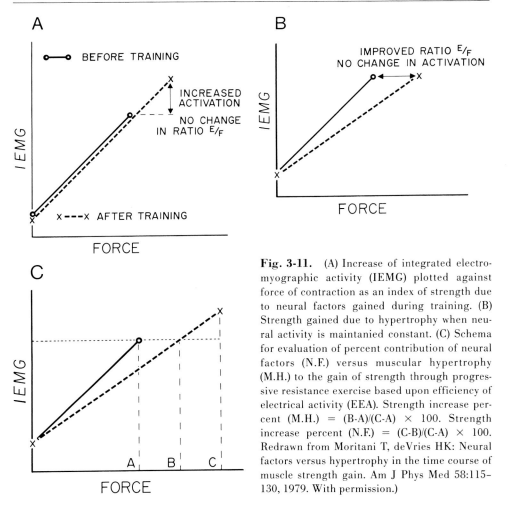

Fig. 3-11. (A) Increase of integrated electro-myographic activity (IEMG) plotted against force of contraction as an index of strength due to neural factors gained during training. (B) Strength gained due to hypertrophy when neural activity is mantanied constant. (C) Schema for evaluation of percent contribution of neural factors (N.F.) versus muscular hypertrophy (M.H.) to the gain of strength through progressive resistance exercise based upon efficiency of electrical activity (EEA). Strength increase percent (M.H.) = (B-A)/(C-A) × 100. Strength increase percent (N.F.) = (C-B)/(C-A) × 100. Redrawn from Moritani T, deVries HK: Neural factors versus hypertrophy in the time course of muscle strength gain. Am J Phys Med 58:115–130, 1979. With permission.)

could be determined. Figure 3-12A presents data from a female subject whose arm increased in isometric strength in response to a training program. At the end of two weeks of training, the ability to generate electrical activity has increased, resulting in increased force, but the E/F ratio has not changed. In subsequent weeks, the electrical activation increased only slightly, but the E/F ratio improved markedly. Thus, it may be inferred that in the early part of strength training, learning is responsible for the rapid improvement that is seen and that hypertrophy comes only later, requiring at least 3–4 weeks training for any significant (but still not maximal) effect. Figure 3-12B sheds considerable light on the controversy of cross-training. Can the homologous muscle of the nontrained limb benefit from training of the opposite limb? The untrained limb of this subject shows increased ability to generate electrical activity and a proportionate increase in force, but no change in the efficiency of that electrical activity (no decrease in E/F). Thus, the learning acquired by the subject can be applied to the untrained limb, but hypertrophy does not occur. Hypertrophy would only take place in an "untrained" limb if that limb were used in stabilization during training and thus inadvertently actually trained.

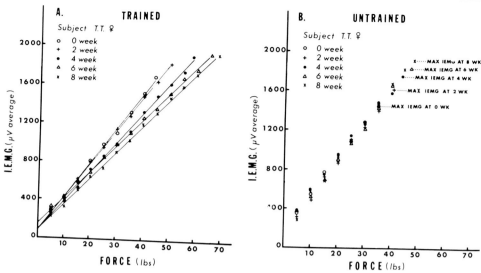

Fig. 3-12. Data plotted to show typical changes in the trained arm (A) as compared to the untrained arm (B) Both arms gained in strength but only the trained arm showed significant changes in the E/F ratio (hypertrophy). (From Moritani T, deVries HK: Neural factors versus hypertrophy in the time course of muscle strength gain. Am J Phys Med 58:115–130, 1979. With permission.)

Synchrony

Some inkling of what is going on in the process of learning is given by the work of Milner-Brown, Stein, and Lee.[25] They used a technique in which the firing of a single motor unit action potential (MUAP) in the first dorsal interosseous muscle of the hand triggered the sweep of the electrical averager. The mean rectified surface EMG could then be examined for clustering of activity at the time of firing of the single motor unit, a measure of synchronicity of motor unit activity. They found that weight lifters, as well as those persons who used their hands in frequent, brief, high-force activities in their work (such as bus drivers) had higher synchronization ratios than controls. Figure 3-13 compares the synchronization ratios of weight lifters and controls. They found that if the control subjects were placed on a weight training program, their synchronization ratios increased; if they dropped the training program, their ratios reverted gradually to control levels.

Muscle Types

Specialization of muscle in some animal species has long been recognized, not only by the biologist, but also by anyone who has carved or eaten the Thanksgiving turkey. The red, or dark, meat is rich in myoglobin and has a high local metabolic (aerobic) capacity. In man, muscle is generally a mosaic, not easily classifiable into red or white colors upon gross inspection. Local metabolic capability is unstable, changing with level of training and thus not suitable for primary classification. A highly stable characteristic of muscle, and the one now generally used for primary classification, is the rapidity of twitch (and relaxation). On this basis, motor units are classified as Type I (slow twitch) and Type II

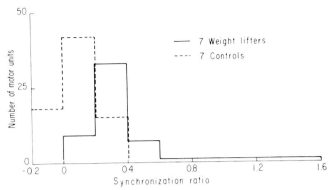

Fig. 3-13. Synchronization ratios for a number of motor units from weight lifters and controls. A value greater than 0.2 was assumed to represent a significant degree of synchronization. These values were rarely observed in control subjects, but were generally found in weight lifters. (From Milner-Brown HS, Stein RB, Lee RG: Synchronization of human motor units: possible roles of exercise and supraspinal reflexes. EEG Clin Neurophysiol 38:245–254, 1975. With permission.)

(fast twitch). The Type I muscle fibers are referred to as "slow oxidative" (SO; ST). Based upon their metabolic capacity, the Type II fibers are subdivided into at least two: "fast twitch oxidative-glycolotic" (FOG; FTa) and "fast twitch glycolytic" (FG;FTb). The twitch properties are shown diagrammatically in Figure 3-14. This twitch contraction speed is under the control of the nerve supply, and it appears that it can only be changed by changing the nerve supply, as in cross innervation experiments. Twitch times, and, in particular, differential twitch times, are not conveniently studied in the intact human subject. However, the activity of the enzyme myofibrillar ATPase does correlate with the fiber type and can be studied with relative ease after needle biopsy. After preincubation at a pH of 9.4 or 10.2, the FT fibers stain darkly for myofibrillar ATPase, as shown in Figure 3-15 (left). Adjacent serial sections can then be stained for glycogen or for enzymes that reflect the local aerobic capacity, such as succinic dehydrogenase (SDH) or reduced nicotinamide adenine dinucleotide diaphorase (NADH diaphorase), formerly called diphosphopyridine nucleotide diaphorase (DPNH diaphorase) (see Fig. 3-15, right). Semi-quantitative changes in these enzymes or in glycogen in response to training or acute activity studies can be made differentially in the fiber types and subtypes. Quantitative assays of enzyme activity can be made only in the muscle sample as a whole, with chemical, rather than histochemical, techniques. Histochemistry, photography, and planimetry can be combined to give changes in relative (ST:FT) and absolute fiber areas in response to training.[23]

Gollnick et al[16] used needle biopsy, chemical and histochemical techniques in the study of upper and lower extremity muscles of trained and untrained men. Those men who participated in such endurance activities as distance running and swimming had a relatively high percentage of slow twitch fiber areas (as high as 84 percent). The local aerobic capacity of the muscles of these athletes, reflected in their SDH activity, was much higher than that of the weight lifters or the untrained men. It was particularly high in the muscles used in their sport, such as the deltoids of canoeists and the vastus lateralis of bicyclists. The fiber areas (both Type I and Type II) were particularly large in those respective

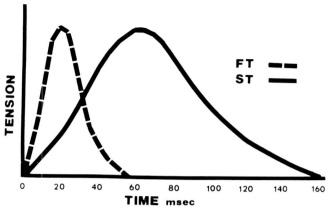

Fig. 3-14. Twitch characteristics (contraction relaxation curves) of slow twitch (Type I) and fast twitch (Type II) muscles. (From Ianuzzo CD: The cellular composition of human skeletal muscle. In: Knuttgen HG (ed): Neuromuscular Mechanisms for Therapeutic and Conditioning Exercise. Baltimore, University Park Press, 1976. With permission.)

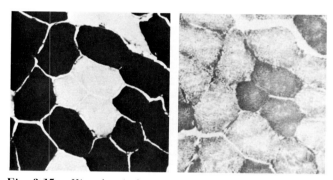

Fig. 3-15. Histochemical micrograph illustrating the fast twitch (FT) and slow twitch (ST) muscle fibers in human skeletal muscle. The micrograph on the left has been stained for myofibrillar ATPase. The light and dark stained cells are ST and FT fibers, respectively. The micrograph at the right is from a serial section of the muscle and has been stained for DPNH-diaphorase, which indicates the aerobic potential of the fibers. These micrographs illustrate that in human skeletal muscle ST fibers have a relatively high aerobic capacity, while FT fibers have a low capacity. (From Ianuzzo CD: The cellular composition of human skeletal muscle. In: Knuttgen HG (ed), Neuromuscular Mechanisms for Strengthening and Conditioning Exercise. Baltimore, University Park Press, 1976. With permission.)

muscles. In a weight lifter only the Type II fibers were particularly large. However, in another (former) weight lifter the largest diameters of all were found, both in the fast twitch and slow twitch muscle fibers. This vertical sample could represent selection of a sport by athletes who are particularly well suited to that sport, rather than response to training. In another study, Gollnick et al[15] carried out such assays before and after a five-month training program consisting of pedalling a bicycle ergometer one hour per day, four days per week, at 75–90 percent of maximal aerobic power. The ratio of slow twitch to fast twitch (ST:FT) fiber areas increased from 0.82 to 1.11 (p < 0.01). The local oxidative capacity was greatly enhanced in both fiber types. Glycolytic (anaerobic) capacity increased only in the Type II fibers.

Size Principle

There is a remarkable anatomic and physiologic orderliness in the neuromuscular apparatus. Larger motor units have larger cell bodies and axons; they have more muscle fibers and exert larger forces; the amplitude of their motor unit action potentials is also greater than that of the smaller motor units. The threshold of the small units is lower; that is, the small motor units are recruited at lower force levels and can be recruited without the larger units, although the larger units cannot be recruited without the smaller ones. All of these observations are referred to as the size principle, as articulated by Henneman.[19-21] Milner-Brown and coworkers have shown a linear relationship (within the limits of their technique) between force of a motor unit and level of recruitment in an isometric contraction: the higher the force, the later its recruitment.[26,27] During ballistic, i.e. extremely rapid, shortening contractions, the force of the fast-twitch fibers may be developed prior to that of the slow-twitch fibers, but it appears that they are not (electrically) recruited without the Type Is.

Consider once again the force-velocity curve (Fig. 3-1). It shows that, at full recruitment, less force can be developed with a rapid shortening contraction than with a slow one; less force with a slow shortening contraction than with an isometric; and less force with an isometric contraction than with a lengthening one. It also implies that, at any given submaximal load, more units will be recruited with a shortening contraction than with an isometric; more units will be recruited with a fast shortening contraction than with a slow one. These data underly the progressive rate training technique of Hellebrandt (see "Progressive Rate Training").

The Overload Principle

This term conjures the image of a subject hoisting a Herculean weight, but, in its broadest terms, the overload principle states only that in order to increase strength, muscle must be taxed beyond its ordinary daily activities.

Intensity Versus Endurance

When strength, or intensity of activity, is related to the maximum of which the individual is capable, there is a neat mathematical relationship between intensity of an activity and endurance at that level. Figure 3-16 shows this relationship for isometric force and endurance. If one exerts 100 percent of his force, he will be able to hold it for only a very short time (one second for the true peak force; about six seconds for a slightly lower force). This curve describes relative endurance. No matter how strong the subject is, 100 percent is still 100 percent, and he will hold it only one second. If, on the other hand, one has a maximum strength of 20 pounds, and if, by training, he increases his strength to 40

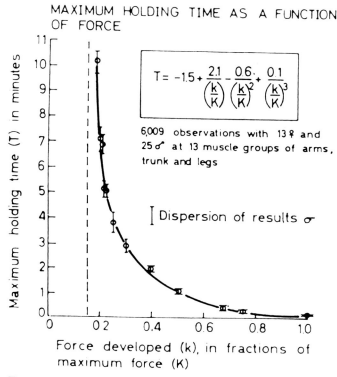

MAXIMUM HOLDING TIME AS A FUNCTION OF FORCE

$$T = -1.5 + \frac{2.1}{\left(\frac{k}{K}\right)} - \frac{0.6}{\left(\frac{k}{K}\right)^2} + \frac{0.1}{\left(\frac{k}{K}\right)^3}$$

6,009 observations with 13 ♀ and 25 ♂ at 13 muscle groups of arms, trunk and legs

$\mathbf{I}$ Dispersion of results σ

Fig. 3-16. Endurance and intensity of work. Static work: tension at fractions of maximum strength. (From Simonson E: Recovery and fatigue, in Simonson E (ed): Physiology of Work Capacity and Fatigue. Springfield, Charles C Thomas, 1971. Redrawn from Rohmert W: Ermittlung von Erholungspausen für statische Arbeit des Menschen. Int Z angew Physiol 18:123–164, 1960. With permission.)

pounds, his endurance at 20 pounds will go from one second to about 60 seconds. This endurance at a specified load is referred to as absolute endurance. The shape of the curve is similar for dynamic contractions as may be seen in Figure 3-17.

Fatigue

Entire symposia have been devoted to the definition and discussion of the physiologic mechanism of fatigue.[7] The authors have found the following operational definition of fatigue to be useful in studies involving human subjects: the inability or unwillingness of the subject to continue the prescribed task under the conditions of reinforcement in effect and known to the subject. Bigland-Ritchie[4] defines neuromuscular fatigue as any reduction in the force generating capacity of the total neuromuscular system regardless of the force required in any given situation. In that context, one may see the evidence of fatigue in Figure 3-18. Here the subject attempts to hold his or her maximal hand grip for five seconds. The force drops below 100 percent in less than a second and continues gradually to decline over the remaining four seconds. After two minutes of rest, the subject performs

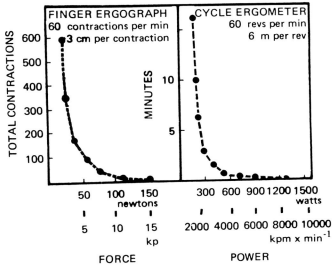

Fig. 3-17. Left panel: Relationship of endurance (as total contractions) of repeated flexion of third digit to effective force of contraction. Right panel: Relationship of endurance (as minutes to fatigue) of cycle ergometer exercise to external power production. In both panels, the intercept with the abscissa represents the exercise intensity for which the maneuver could be performed only once (and, therefore, the strength of the concentric movement). In both panels, endurance could be presented as either total contractions or minutes to fatigue, and, as the contraction rate and velocity are designated, either abscissa could be designated as force (per individual repetition) or power (work per unit time). (From Knuttgen HG: Development of muscular strength and endurance, in Knuttgen HG (ed): Neuromuscular Mechanisms for Therapeutic and Conditioning Exercises. Baltimore, University Park Press, 1976. With permission.)

a series of one second contractions at only 5 percent of the MVC for a period of ten minutes, following which he or she again attempts to exert a maximal contraction. The subject's new "maximum" is considerably less than the initial maximum. Thus, it can be seen that fatigue has a short-term decremental effect upon performance. It is axiomatic that one must not have an athlete attempt maximal performance two days in a row. The long-term effect of fatigue in training is another matter, as will be seen below.

Effects of Training

Fatigue Versus Mechanical Works

A two-phase, double-shift, transfer-of-training study was designed[10] to assess the relative effects of muscle fatigue in training versus the amount of mechanical work accomplished. In the first phase, the mechanical work was the same, but fatigue differed. Healthy young men were selected, and the right or left quadriceps randomly assigned to

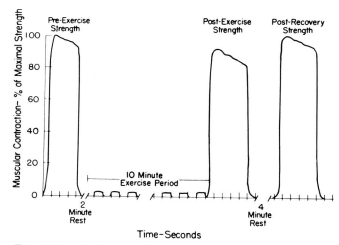

Fig. 3-18. Maximal tension can be maintained during a voluntary maximal contraction of hand grip for less than one second before evidence of fatigue appears as the available supply of ATP is exhausted. Fatigue (unavailability of ATP) increases in proportion to the intensity of activity, but can be demonstrated following ten minutes of intermittent contractions at 5 percent of maximal. (From Mundale MO: The relationship of intermittent isometric exercise to fatigue of hand grip. Arch Phys Med Rehabil 51:532–539, 1970. With permission.)

the fatigue task. The subject then lifted the weighted ankle (45 lbs) to full extension of the knee on the metronome count of one (metronome set at 60/min), held it in full extension through beat six, brought it down on beat seven, and up again on the next one. Subjects were paid per repetition of the fatigue side. The nonfatigue side was required to do the same number of repetitions, but with one full seven-second cycle rest between contractions. There were 30 training sessions. At the end there were five test trials where both sides went to fatigue and were paid independently. Four subsequent groups of (fresh) subjects carried out a similar protocol, but with a progressively shorter duty cycle for both sides and progressively more rest cycles for the nonfatigue side (2, 3, 4, and 5 cycles respectively). The summary of the test results for all five groups, fatigue and nonfatigue sides, is shown in Figure 3-19. It can be seen that the side that fatigued in training did much better in the test period.

In phase two (fresh subjects), both sides went to fatigue in training and were paid independently, but one side did so with a rest cycle and one side without. The side with a rest cycle could do far more repetitions (more mechanical work) than the side without. The results are shown in Figure 3-20. It is clear that the side that did more mechanical work did better in the test period, but not in proportion to the time spent. If curves 1 and 2 are compared, one sees that side one did 91 percent better in the test period, but spent 567 percent more time in training. Sides 3 and 4 are even more striking. Side 3 did 21 percent better in the test period but spent 917 percent more time in training. Thus, if motivation and time are essentially unlimited, pacing may result in somewhat better ultimate performance, as long as one eventually fatigues the muscle.

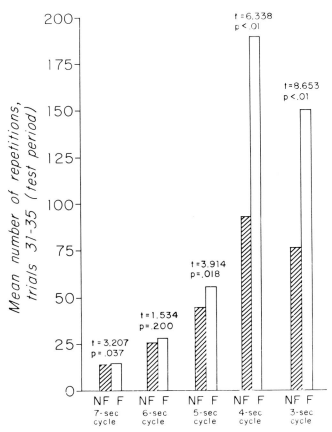

Fig. 3-19. Comparison of exercise performance at days 31 to 35 of nonfatigued versus fatigued quadriceps exercised according to schedule of Phase I. Both muscles performed the same amount of work each day during the first 30 days of training. NF = nonfatigued quadriceps; F = quadriceps exercised to fatigue. (From de Lateur BJ, Lehmann JF, Giaconi R: Mechanical work and fatigue: their roles in the development of muscle work capacity. Arch Phys Med Rehabil 57:319–324, 1976. With permission.)

Low Weights Versus High Weights

The DeLorme Axiom states that high-intensity, low-repetition exercises build strength; low-intensity, high-repetition exercises build endurance; and that each of these types of exercise is wholly distinct and wholly incapable of producing the results obtained by the other. In the extreme, this axiom must be true, but it is of interest and of practical importance to see to what extent it does *not* apply, i.e., to see if there is a range of training intensity that will give equal results under certain conditions. A double-shift, transfer-of-training study was designed to test this question.[9] Healthy young adult men were randomly assigned to one of four groups: two high weight groups and two low weight groups. The task for the quadriceps (unilateral) of each man was the same except for the amount of weight lifted: 55 pounds for the high weight group and 26 pounds for the low weight

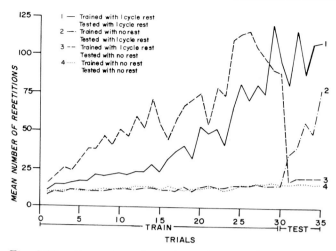

Fig. 3-20. Comparison of exercise performance during training of quadriceps muscles with and without rest periods and during double-shift testing at days 31 to 35. Both rested and nonrested muscles were exercised to fatigue each day. (From de Lateur BJ, Lehmann JF, Giaconi R: Mechanical work and fatigue: their roles in the development of muscle work capacity. Arch Phys Med Rehabil 57:319–324, 1976. With permission.)

group. At the first metronome beat, the subjects lifted the weighted foot to full extension of the knee, held it in full extension through the beat of 6, lowered the foot on 7 and raised it again on 1. Subjects were paid per repetition: 20 cents for the high weight and 5 cents for the low weight. The latter made more money than the high weight group (on the average), because they could do far more repetitions, particularly in the later stages of training. In order to maximize the money he earned, each man did the most repetitions of which he was capable, and pushed his own quadriceps to fatigue. At the completion of 15 training sessions, one group of high weight subjects shifted to the low weight task and one group of low weight subjects shifted to the high weight task and continued for four additional sessions, each man doing his appointed task to fatigue. On a final day a power test was carried out, in which each man was given 30 seconds to lift an intermediate weight as many times as possible. The results are shown in Figure 3-21. It can be seen that the positive transfer-of-training was immediate and complete; that is, the high intensity trained did as well on the low intensity task as those who had trained on the low intensity task, and the low-intensity trained did as well on the high intensity task as those who had trained on the high intensity task. All groups, on the average, did equally well on the power test. The equalizing factor in training and in testing was muscle fatigue as an endpoint, not some specified amount of mechanical work. Since all groups did equally well (were equally effective) it can be said that the high weight training was far more efficient, because much less time was spent in training.

Isometric Versus Isotonic

In the previous study there was interchangeability of tasks at a relative intensity of approximately 90–100 percent of maximal for the high weight group and about 40 percent of maximal for the low weight group as long as subjects went to the point of fatigue. It

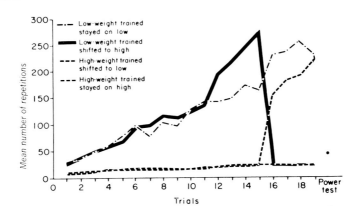

Fig. 3-21. Mean scores for each of the four groups for each of 15 training trials and each of 4 test trials. The mean score for each of the four groups on the power test is also shown. (From de Lateur BJ, Lehmann JF, Fordyce WE: A test of the DeLorme axiom. Arch Phys Med Rehabil 49:245–248, 1968. With permission.)

should be noted that the task was qualitatively identical for all groups; only the amount of weight lifted differed. It was then considered of interest to determine the effect of training to fatigue with a common weight, 50 pounds, but with a qualitatively different task, isometric versus isotonic. To keep the task pure, the experimenters[11] lifted the weight for the isometric subjects, who had only to hold the weight in full extension of the knee and were paid per second held. The isotonic groups had a pure dynamic task, with a lift to full extension but no hold. They were paid per lift. Results are shown in Figure 3-22. In contrast to the results seen with high and low weights, there was very little transfer of training. For those starting the opposite task, it was as though their training time had been wasted, since their performance was little better than the opposite group at the beginning of training. The isometric-trained group that shifted to the isotonic task showed some tendency to catch up to the latter (delayed transfer) but had not done so by the fourth test day. The group that trained isotonically and shifted to the isometric task showed no tendency to catch up (no delayed transfer).

Slow Versus Fast Shortening Contractions

Using the Cybex isokinetic dynamometer, Moffroid and Whipple[28] studied the effects, upon the torque-velocity curve, of training at 6 rpm versus training at 18 rpm. The results can be seen in Figures 3-23 and 3-24. Those who trained at 6 rpm showed improvement in torque at 6 rpm, and, to a somewhat lesser extent, at 3 and 0 rpm (0=isometric). In contrast, those who trained at 18 rpm showed a relatively uniform improvement at 18 rpm and those speeds below as well.

Interference?

Hickson[22] designed a study in which three groups trained either for strength (lower extremity weight training) or endurance (cycle ergometer or continuous running) or both (both programs at the same intensities, with at least two hours rest between the programs). As can be seen in Figure 3-25, there is a suggestion that combining the two programs interfered with improvement of strength development in the upper ranges. All of these studies point out the importance of keeping the training task as close as possible to the test task for qualitatively dissimilar tasks or for extreme quantitative differences. In contrast, the DeLorme Axiom study indicates good transfer of training between 40 and 100 percent of maximal for qualitatively identical tasks, as long as the subjects go to fatigue in training. The glycogen depletion studies of Gollnick et al[17] indirectly suggest this range may be as wide as 20–100 percent.

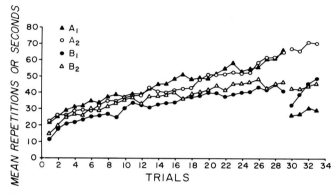

Fig. 3-22. Results of the isotonic-isometric comparison. Groups A_1 and A_2 were isotonically trained. Groups B_1 and B_2 were isometrically trained. Group A_1 shifted to the isometric task on day 30. Group B_1 shifted to the isotonic task on day 30. (From de Lateur BJ, Lehmann J, Stonebridge J, et al: Isotonic versus isometric exercises: a double-shift, transfer-of-training study. Arch Phys Med Rehabil 53:212–217, 1972. With permission.)

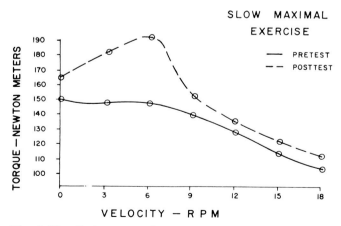

Fig. 3-23. Peak torques of quadriceps plotted against velocity of contraction before (solid line) and after (dotted line) a maximal exercise regime at 6 rpm. (From Moffroid MT, Whipple RH: Specificity of speed of exercise. Phys Ther 50:1692–1700, 1970. With permission.)

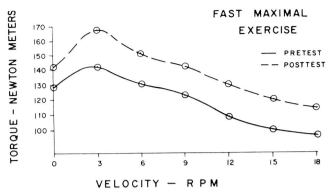

Fig. 3-24. Peak torques of the quadriceps plotted against velocity of contraction before (solid line) and after (dotted line) a maximal exercise regime at 18 rpm. (From Moffroid MT, Whipple RH: Specificity of speed of exercise. Phys Ther 50:1692–1700, 1970. With permission.)

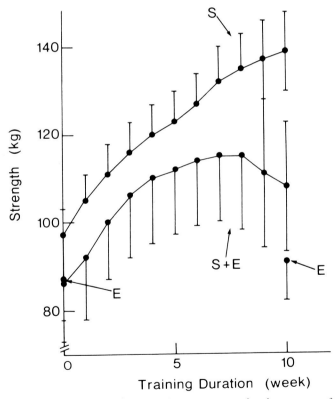

Fig. 3-25. Strength changes in response to the three types of training. Measurements were made on a weekly basis in the strength (S) and strength and endurance (S and E) groups. The endurance (E) group was tested before and after 10 weeks of training. (From Hickson RC: Interference of strength development by simultaneously training for strength and endurance. Eur J Appl Physiol 45:255–263, 1980. With permission.)

STRENGTH TRAINING PROGRAMS

Progressive Resistive Exercise (PRE)

As the name implies, this type of exercise overloads the muscle by increasing the weight lifted, while keeping the contraction number and rate of contraction constant. The prototypical PRE was described by DeLorme.[12,13] Once a week the 10-repetition maximum (10RM) is determined for the muscle to be trained. During the daily training session, the subject begins with 10 contractions at 50 percent of 10RM, then does 10 contractions at 75 percent of 10RM, and finishes up with 10 contractions at 100 percent of the 10RM. This technique has much to recommend itself, since it begins with a relatively low level of activity, which constitutes a warm-up, and pushes the muscle maximally, with subjects often unable to complete the 10 repetitions of the 100 percent 10RM.

The "Oxford" Technique

The inability to complete the final 10 repetitions at 100 percent of the 10RM load owing to fatigue was considered by some to be a fault of the DeLorme technique (although it is considered a virtue by the authors of this chapter). For this reason a reverse protocol was developed and dubbed the "Oxford" technique.[42] It is in all respects similar to the DeLorme technique, except that the subject begins with 10 contractions at 100 percent of the 10RM and takes off weight for the subsequent two sets of 10 contractions. This protocol lacks the warm-up and also is less demanding of the muscle overall. It is probably somewhat less effective than the DeLorme technique, although the definitive comparison study has yet to be done. Nevertheless, its use is very widespread; one is likely to receive this protocol if PREs are requested.

Progressive Rate Training

The force-velocity curve implies, and Hellebrandt has demonstrated, that muscle performance can be improved with a constant load, if the rate of contraction is gradually increased.[18] In addition to a set of weights, a metronome is required. A moderate, submaximal load is applied and the metronome is set at its lowest setting (about 40/minute). The load is raised on one beat and lowered on the next, giving 20 repetitions per minute on the first day. A fixed number of contractions may be done (such as 20 each day). The muscle is progressively "overloaded," not by increasing the load or the repetitions, but by increasing the metronome setting each day or every other day. It is an advantage of this technique that less time is required for the exercise with each increase in metronome setting. A possible disadvantage is the sound of the metronome, which might be annoying to therapists if they had to listen to it for multiple patients each day. Some metronomes have a flashing light and a means of turning off the sound, which would solve that problem. Nevertheless, this technique is not widely used.

The University of Washington (UW) Technique

A very simple technique is used at the hospitals of the authors (University of Washington, Seattle WA). A relatively high weight, one that can be lifted some 3–9 times, is selected. The patient then lifts this weight as many times as he or she can each day, and the repetitions are counted. When the patient reaches some fixed number, such as 20 (or 30), the weight is increased. When one considers the number of muscles that often need to be strengthened, this simple protocol often adds up to a large savings of therapist and patient time.

Brief Isometric Techniques

Müller[31] has shown that brief (1 second and 6 seconds), high force (65 percent and 100 percent MVC) isometric contractions rapidly increase isometric strength, and at least in his normal subjects, the more the better, within the range studied (see Fig. 3-26). Stoboy et al[39] (see Fig. 3-27) has shown that isometric strength can be improved in some disorders, such as disuse atrophy and old polio, but not in tabes dorsalis, presumably due to lack of proprioceptive feedback. On the other hand, most functional tasks have a dynamic component, and we have seen earlier that there is very little transfer of isometric training to an isotonic task. Also, isometric training is generally considered to be mild and suitable for patients with arthritis. This is true only if the isometric task itself is mild (low force); one of the authors has seen effusions develop in normal knees after prolonged, vigorous isometric exercise.

Equipment

When using any of the above protocols to strengthen the quadriceps, a shoe-plate with crossbar and weights, as shown in Figure 3-28 may be used. This is called a "quadriceps boot," or sometimes a "DeLorme boot." The advent of Velcro® has made possible the very versatile ankle and wrist self-adhering weights as well. Special exercise tables, which adapt to the positioning and leverage needs of the quadriceps, hamstrings, hip

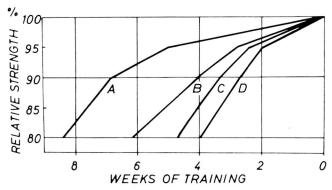

Fig. 3-26. Weeks needed to reach limiting strength from an initial relative strength of 80 percent; (A) by submaximal training (one daily contraction at 65 percent of maximum for one second); (B) by standard training (one daily maximal contraction for one second); (C) by daily maximal contraction for six seconds; (D) by multiple daily maximal contractions totaling 30 seconds in duration. (From Müller EA: Influence of training and of inactivity on muscle strength. Arch Phys Med Rehabil 51:449–463, 1970. With permission.)

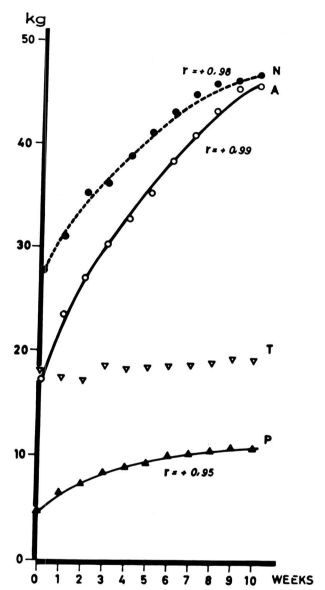

Fig. 3-27. Changes of maximum strength in the normal (•••), the atrophied (o-o-o), the tabetic (△ △ △) and the poliomyelitic (▲.▲.▲) groups due to isometric training. (From Stoboy H, Friedebold G, Strand FL: Evaluation of the effect of isometric training in functional and organic muscle atrophy. Arch Phys Med Rehabil 49:508–514, 1968. With permission.)

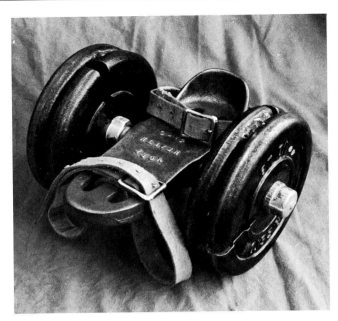

Fig. 3-28. Quadriceps boot with crossbar and weights. (From de Lateur BJ: Therapeutic exercise to develop strength and endurance, in Kottke FJ, Stillwell GK, Lehmann JF (eds): Krusen's Handbook of Physical Medicine and Rehabilitation, third edition. Philadelphia, WB Saunders Company 1982. With permission.)

adductors, and hip extensors are shown in Figures 3-29, 3-30, 3-31, and 3-32. The Elgin table has two particular advantages. It allows the hip adductors and extensors to be exercised throughout the full range of motion, which would not be practical without a counterbalancing device. In addition, the latter device permits controlled amounts of gravity-assistance, which is useful in the very weak muscles often seen with arthritic patients.

An old-fashioned, simple, inexpensive, and very useful device is shown in Figure 3-33. This is called a "fracture board" or "quadriceps board" and permits exercise of the quadriceps in the last few degrees of knee extension (terminal knee extension exercises or "TKEs"), when exercise throughout the full range of motion is contraindicated (see below).

Some Newer Equipment

It was shown earlier (Figs. 3-5 to 3-8) that the torque that a muscle or functional muscle group can produce varies throughout the range of motion of the joint. Thus, if one lifts a constant weight, the muscle may be underloaded at some points of the range.

Nautilus

In the attempt to match the torque curve of the muscle, the Nautilus® uses a special cam (the ribbed version of which resembles a cross section of the sea creature) to vary the load on the muscle. Special machines are available to isolate the various muscles of the

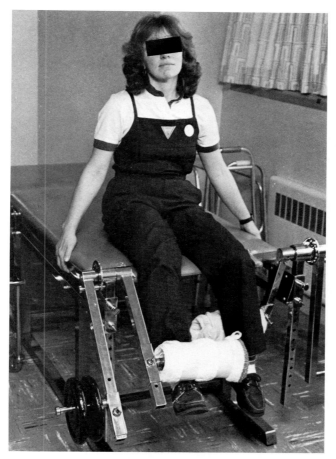

Fig. 3-29. N-K table with the angle between the load and lever arm set at 0 degrees. (From de Lateur BJ: Therapeutic exercise to develop strength and endurance, in Kottke FJ, Stillwell GK, Lehmann JF (eds): Krusen's Handbook of Physical Medicine and Rehabilitation, third edition. Philadelphia, WB Saunders Company, 1982. With permission.)

upper and lower limbs, neck, and trunk. Since the same muscles are used to raise (concentric contraction) and lower (eccentric contraction) the weights, the onset of fatigue is rapid, and this is an efficient exercise. Care must be taken in the use of this equipment, as in the use of free weights, if there is a painful portion of the range of motion (undue stress on the joint could occur). In contrast to free weights, however, pain inhibition and dropping of the weight are unlikely to produce injury with the Nautilus equipment.

Cybex II

This device allows one to preset the maximum speed of rotation. If one attempts to accelerate the lever arm of the machine, the device will accommodate the torque developed. This machine is shown in Figure 3-34. As one sets the maximum higher, less torque

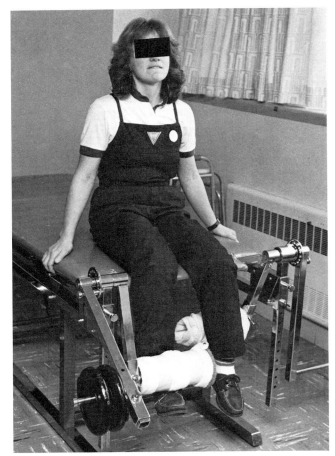

Fig. 3-30. N-K table with the angle between load and lever arm set at 45 degrees. (From de Lateur BJ: Therapeutic exercise to develop strength and endurance, in Kottke FJ, Stillwell GK, Lehmann JF (eds): Krusen's Handbook of Physical Medicine and Rehabilitation, third edition. Philadelphia, WB Saunders Company, 1982. With permission.)

will be developed, as seen previously in Figure 3-8. In contrast to the Nautilus devices, which use a cam to vary the load to match the torque curve that the average person can develop, the Cybex accommodates the torque that any given person actually does develop. This may be very high, such as 200 foot-pounds, or it may be minimal. As long as one does not attempt to accelerate the lever beyond the preset limit, one may push the lever through the range with one finger. This accommodation makes the device particularly well suited to the exercise of muscle that crosses painful or diseased joints (assuming the joint is not so acutely inflamed that all forceful exercise is contraindicated). Sudden pain inhibition does not result in any injury, since there is no weight to drop, other than the lever arm itself.

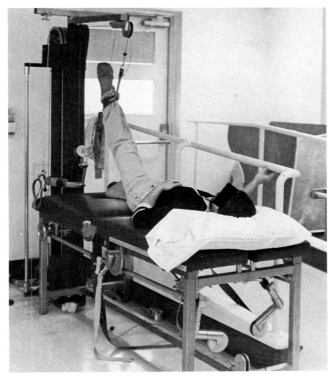

Fig. 3-31. Exercising hip extension on an Elgin table. (From de Lateur BJ: Therapeutic exercise to develop strength and endurance, in Kottke FJ, Stillwell GK, Lehmann JF (eds): Krusen's Handbook of Physical Medicine and Rehabilitation, third edition. Philadelphia, WB Saunders Company 1982. With permission.)

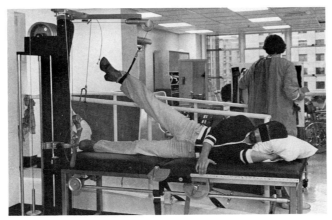

Fig. 3-32. Exercising hip adduction on an Elgin table. (From de Lateur BJ: Therapeutic exercise to develop strength and endurance, in Kottke FJ, Stillwell GK, Lehmann JF (eds): Krusen's Handbook of Physical Medicine and Rehabilitation, third edition. Philadelphia, WB Saunders Company, 1982. With permission.)

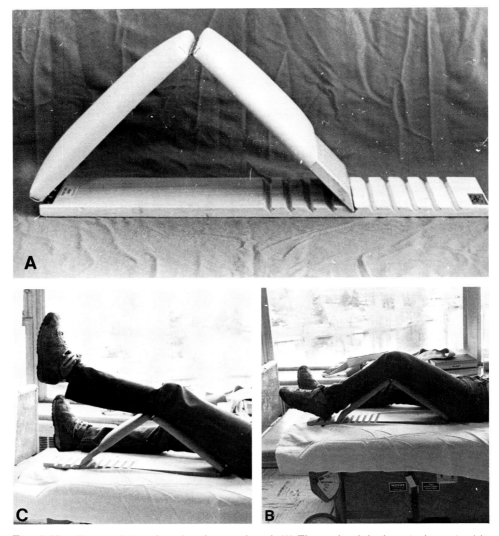

Fig. 3-33. The quadriceps board or fracture board. (A) The angle of the knee is determined by the slot in which the distal portion of the board is placed. (B) Subject using fracture board, knee flexed. (C) Subject using fracture board, knee extended.

Some Special Considerations in Arthritis

Why would one want to strengthen muscles in arthritis? Some reasons are readily apparent, such as improved mobility and self care or even the simple restoration of the lost bulk and strength. Another, less obvious, reason is extremely important in the long run. It has previously been pointed out that the kinesiologic function of lengthening contractions is shock absorption. With every step, these lengthening contractions take place at the hip, knee, and ankle. In an article that has become a classic, Saunders, Inman, and Eberhart[35] describe the major determinants of normal and pathologic gait. Among these are controlled dropping of the pelvis and knee flexion in stance phase of gait as well as controlled

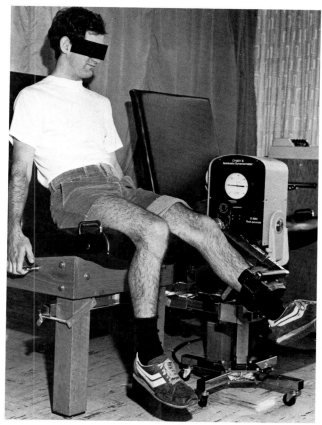

Fig. 3-34. The Cybex isokinetic exerciser.

plantarflexion at the ankle immediately after heelstrike (see Figs. 3-35 and 3-36). The authors discuss these determinants in terms of conservation of energy by reducing the amplitude and abruptness of the displacement of the center of gravity. Of equal importance is the shock absorption produced in these motions by lengthening contractions of the hip abductors, quadriceps, and ankle dorsiflexors. If these muscles are insufficient in their strength, the shock will be absorbed in the joints themselves (rather than by the muscles) and degenerative changes will accelerate.

Age and Muscle Hypertrophy

Moritani and DeVries[29,30] applied their technique, described earlier, to the development of strength by young (mean age 21.8 years) and aged (mean 69.6 years) subjects over an eight-week training period. Although both groups showed comparable increases in strength, they appeared to have done so by different mechanisms. After four weeks, the strength increases in the young men were mainly due to hypertrophy. In contrast, the older men showed almost no evidence of hypertrophy, and relied upon neural factors throughout the eight weeks. It would be of interest to follow such older subjects for 12 weeks or even longer periods of training to see if hypertrophy subsequently occurred. It is important to note, however, that strength increases did occur, even if hypertrophy did not.

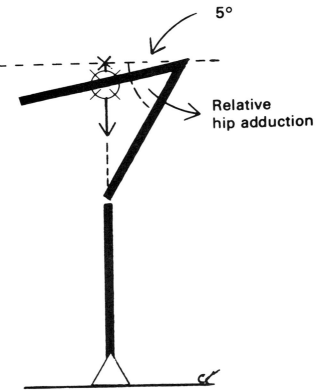

Fig. 3-35. Controlled dropping of the center of gravity (pelvis) in stance phase. (From Stolov WC: Normal and pathologic gait, in Rosse C, Clawson DK (eds): The Musculoskeletal System in Health and Disease. Hagerstown, Harper & Row, 1980. With permission.)

Osteoarthritis and Muscular Atrophy

Sirca and Susec-Michieli[38] studied the fiber types and areas of the gluteus maximus, gluteus medius, and tensor fasciae latae muscles in men and women who were undergoing surgery for osteoarthritis of the hip, and in previously healthy persons of various ages who had died suddenly. They found that the diameter of both Type I and Type II fibers decreased with progressive age, as did the relative percentage of Type II fibers. In osteoarthritis, however, there was selective loss of Type II fibers beyond what could be attributed to age. All these changes were considered due to disuse, as there was no evidence of neurogenic lesions.

Patellofemoral Joint Disease

The objective of any strengthening program in arthritis is to gain as much muscle training with as little joint stress as possible. This has been studied particularly well for the patellofemoral joint.[14,33] Deep knee bends are an example of an undesirable exercise. Figure 3-37 shows that the quadriceps muscle force goes up with progressive knee flexion in a deep knee bend; unfortunately, the patellofemoral joint reaction goes up even more. Figures 3-38 and 3-39 show that terminal knee extension exercises (TKEs; exercise in the

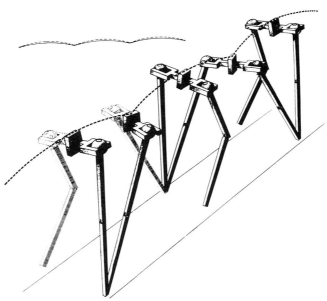

Fig. 3-36. The quadriceps controls knee flexion and the anterior tibial controls plantar flexion after heelstrike. (From Saunders JBDecM, Inman VT, Eberhart HD: The major determinants in normal and pathological gait. J Bone Joint Surg 35A:543–558, 1953. With permission.)

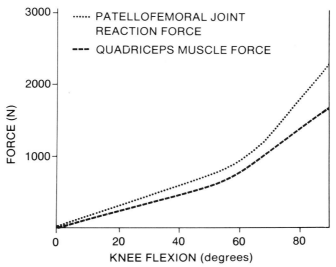

Fig. 3-37. Patellofemoral joint reaction force and quadriceps muscle force during knee bend to 90 degrees (three subjects). (Adapted from Reilly DT, Martens M: Experimental analysis of the quadriceps muscle force and patello-femoral joint reaction force for various activities. Acta Orthop Scand 43:126–137, 1972 by Frankel VH, Nordin M: Basic Biomechanics of the Skeletal System. Philadelphia, Lea & Febiger, 1980)

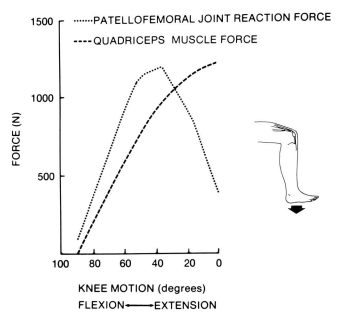

Fig. 3-38. Patellofemoral joint reaction force and quadriceps muscle force during knee extension against resistance provided by a 9-kg weight boot with the subject sitting and the lower leg free-hanging (three subjects). (Adapted from Reilly DT, Martens M: Experimental analysis of the quadriceps muscle force and patellofemoral joint reaction force for various activities. Acta Orthop Scand 43:126–137, 1972 by Frankel VH, Nordin M: Basic Biomechanics of the Skeletal System. Philadelphia, Lea & Febiger, 1980)

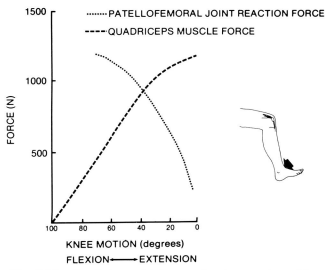

Fig. 3-39. Patellofemoral joint reaction force and quadriceps force during knee extension with resistance provided at a right angle to the long axis of the lower limb throughout knee extension. (From Frankel VH, Nordin M: Basic Biomechanics of the Skeletal System. Philadelphia, Lea & Febiger, 1980. With permission.)

last 0–15 degrees of extension) provide maximum quadriceps load with minimal patello-femoral joint reaction force, especially if the load is applied at right angles to the shin. This is the rationale for the use of the quadriceps or fracture board.

Anklyosing Spondylitis

In this disorder, it is particularly important to strengthen some muscles and to give little time to others. Without intervention, there is progressive flexion of the spine and progressive protraction of the shoulders. Therefore situps and pushups should be avoided and attention given to the spinal extensors and shoulder retractors. Spinal extensor exercises may have to be done as close to isometrically as possible, as active extension will irritate the facet joints of the spine, producing pain and the desire to relieve it by going into even more flexion. Strengthening the oblique abdominals isometrically will also help support the spine.

The Home Program

The need to perform these exercises correctly is apparent and justifies the initiation of these programs in the hospital, under the direction of an experienced physician and therapist. The need is also to develop a lifelong habit of exercise. After the exercise program is well established in the clinic, and progress begins to level off (usually in about 12 weeks), it is important to adapt the program to the equipment that is available at home, or to exercises that can be done without equipment. These should be tailored to the individual needs of the patient by the therapist, who, with the physician, should recheck the patient at progressively longer intervals, for encouragement and to be sure the exercises are still being done correctly.

ACKNOWLEDGMENT

This chapter is based in part on research which was supported by research grant G008300076 from the National Institute of Handicapped Research, Department of Education, Washington, DC 20202.

REFERENCES

1. Arkin M: Absolute muscle power. The internal kinesiology of muscle. Research Seminar Notes, Department of Orthopedic Surgery, State University of Iowa. 12D:123, 1938
2. Asmussen E, Hansen O, Lammert O: The relation between isometric and dynamic muscle strength in man. Comm Dan Nat Assoc Inf Paral 20:11, 1965
3. Bethe A, Franke F: Beiträge zum Problem der willkürlich beweglichen Armprothesen. IV. Die Kraftkurven der indirekten naturlichen Energiequellen. Münich Med Wochenschr 66:201–205, 1919
4. Bigland-Ritchie B, Woods JJ: Changes in muscle contractile properties and neural control during human muscular fatigue. Muscle and Nerve 7:691–699, 1984
5. Braune W, Fischer O: Die Rotationsmomente der Beugemuskeln am Ellbogengelenk des Menschen. Abhandl d K S Gesellsch d Wissensch 26:245–310, 1890
6. Brunnstrom S: Clinical Kinesiology, second edition. Philadelphia, FA Davis, 1966
7. Ciba Symposium 82: Human Muscle Fatigue: Physiological Mechanisms. London, Pitman Medical, 1981
8. de Lateur BJ: Therapeutic exercise to develop strength and endurance, in Kottke FJ, Stillwell GK, Lehmann JF (eds): Krusen's Handbook of Physical Medicine and Rehabilitation, third edition. Philadelphia, WB Saunders Company, 1982
9. de Lateur BJ, Lehmann JF, Fordyce WE: A test of the DeLorme axiom. Arch Phys Med Rehabil 49:245–248, 1968

10. de Lateur BJ, Lehmann JF, Giaconi R: Mechanical work and fatigue: their roles in the development of muscle work capacity. Arch Phys Med Rehabil 57:319–324, 1976

11. de Lateur BJ, Lehmann J, Stonebridge J, et al: Isotonic versus isometric exercises: a double-shift transfer-of-training study. Arch Phys Med Rehabil 53:212–217, 1972

12. DeLorme TL: Restoration of muscle power by heavy-resistance exercises. J Bone Joint Surg 27:645–667, 1945

13. DeLorme TL, Watkins AL: Progressive Resistance Exercise. New York, Appleton-Century Crofts Inc, 1951

14. Frankel VH, Nordin M: Basic Biomechanics of the Skeletal System. Philadelphia, Lea & Febiger, 1980

15. Gollnick PD, Armstrong RB, Saltin B, et al: Effect of training on enzyme activity and fiber composition of human skeletal muscle. J Appl Physiol 34:107–111, 1973

16. Gollnick PD, Armstrong RB, Saubert CW IV, et al: Enzyme activity and fiber composition in skeletal muscle of untrained and trained men. J Appl Physiol 33:312–319, 1972

17. Gollnick PD, Armstrong RB, Saubert CW IV, et al: Glycogen depletion patterns in human skeletal muscle fibers during prolonged work. Pflügers Arch 344:1–12, 1973

18. Hellebrandt FA, Houtz SJ: Methods of muscle training: the influence of pacing. Phys Ther Rev 38:319–322, 1958

19. Henneman E: Peripheral mechanisms involved in the control of muscle, in Mountcastle VB (ed): Medical Physiology, thirteenth edition. Saint Louis, The CV Mosby Co, 1974

20. Henneman E, Clamann HP, Gillies JD, et al: Rank order of motoneurons within a pool: law of combination. J Neurophysiol 37:1338–1349, 1974

21. Henneman E, Somjen G, Carpenter DO: Functional significance of cell size in spinal motoneurons. J Neurophysiol 28:560–580, 1965

22. Hickson RC: Interference of strength development by simultaneously training for strength and endurance. Eur J Appl Physiol 45:255–263, 1980

23. Ianuzzo CD: The cellular composition of human skeletal muscle, in Knuttgen HG (ed): Neuromuscular Mechanisms for Therapeutic and Conditioning Exercise. Baltimore, University Park Press, 1976

24. Knuttgen HG: Development of muscular strength and endurance, in Knuttgen HG (ed): Neuromuscular Mechanisms for Therapeutic and Conditioning Exercises. Baltimore, University Park Press, 1976

25. Milner-Brown HS, Stein RB, Lee RG: Synchronization of human motor units: possible roles of exercise and supraspinal reflexes. EEG Clin Neurophysiol 38:245–254, 1975

26. Milner-Brown HS, Stein RB, Yemm R: The contractile properties of human motor units during voluntary isometric contractions. J Physiol 228:285–306, 1973

27. Milner-Brown HS, Stein RB, Yemm R: The orderly recruitment of human motor units during voluntary isometric contractions. J Physiol 230:359–370, 1973

28. Moffroid MT, Whipple RH: Specificity of speed of exercise. Phys Ther 50:1692–1700, 1970

29. Moritani T, deVries HA: Neural factors versus hypertrophy in the time course of muscle strength gain. Am J Phys Med 58:115–130, 1979

30. Moritani T, deVries HA: Potential for gross muscle hypertrophy in older men. J Gerontol 35:672–682, 1980

31. Müller EA: Influence of training and of inactivity on muscle strength. Arch Phys Med Rehabil 51:449–462, 1970

32. Mundale MO: The relationship of intermittent isometric exercise to fatigue of hand grip. Arch Phys Med Rehabil 51:532–539, 1970

33. Reilly DT, Martens M: Experimental analysis of the quadriceps muscle force and patello-femoral joint reaction force for various activities. Acta Orthop Scand 43:126–137, 1972

34. Rohmert W: Ermittlung von Erholungspausen für statische Arbeit des Menschen. Int Z angew Physiol einschl Arbeitsphysiol 18:123–164, 1960

35. Saunders JBDecM, Inman VT, Eberhart HD: The major determinants in normal and pathological gait. J Bone Joint Surg 35A:543–558, 1953

36. Schottelius BA, Senay LC Jr: Effect of stimulation-length sequence on shape of length-tension diagram. Am J Physiol 186:127–130, 1956

37. Simonson E: Recovery and fatigue, in Simonson E (ed): Physiology of Work Capacity and Fatigue. Springfield, Charles C Thomas, 1971

38. Sirca A, Susec-Michieli M: Selective type II fibre muscular atrophy in patients with osteoarthritis of the hip. J Neurol Sci 44:149–159, 1980

39. Stoboy H, Friedebold G, Strand FL: Evaluation of the effect of isometric training in functional and organic muscle atrophy. Arch Phys Med Rehabil 49:508–514, 1968

40. Stolov WC: Normal and pathologic gait, in Rosse C, Clawson DK (eds): The Musculoskeletal System in Health and Disease. Hagerstown, Harper & Row, 1980

41. Von Recklinghausen H: Gliedermechanik und Lahmungsprothesen. Berlin, J. Springer, 1920

42. Zinovieff AN: Heavy-resistance exercises: the "Oxford technique." Br J Phys Med 14:129–132, 1951

Justus F. Lehmann
Barbara J. de Lateur

4

Therapeutic Heat and Cold, Hydrotherapy

One of the oldest forms of therapy is the application of heat or cold to alleviate the symptoms of musculoskeletal disease. Only recently, however, have the indications for such therapy been based on the knowledge of physiologic effects, and the efficacy verified or supported by clinical observation. These modalities are a valuable adjunct to other therapy; however, heat or cold applied by itself does not produce a cure in any of the indications.

PHYSIOLOGIC EFFECTS OF HEAT

Extensibility of collagen tissues. Heat increases the extensibility of collagen tissues (Fig. 4-1). At therapeutic temperatures the viscous properties of the collagen tissues become more dominant, whereas at normal tissue temperatures the elastic properties of the tissues are largely responsible for its mechanical behavior.[121] When these tissues are heated, they can be stretched with less force and with less likelihood of mechanical damage than when they are stretched at normal tissue temperature.[77] This effect on extensibility is clinically used for the treatment of joint contractures. In this context it is interesting to note that Vanharanta et al[116] found experimentally that ultrasound treatment with one watt/cm² (W/cm²) to the knee of the rabbit for five days produced an increase in the glycosaminoglycans.

Joint stiffness. Heat measurably decreases joint stiffness (Fig. 4-2),[3,49,125,126] an effect that could also be produced by steroid therapy.[125] This change may be used to relieve such symptoms as morning stiffness in rheumatoid patients. On the other hand, cold measurably increases the joint stiffness.

Pain. Heat application produces pain relief. The use of heat for this symptom is widespread and empirically based. It is likely that heat acts as a "counterirritant," that is, the thermal stimulus may decrease the perception of pain, consistent with the gate theory

PRINCIPLES OF PHYSICAL MEDICINE AND REHABILITATION
IN THE MUSCULOSKELETAL DISEASES

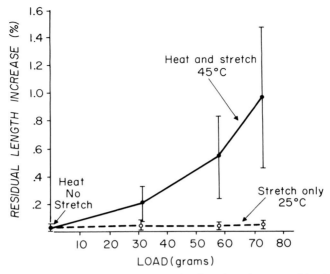

Fig. 4-1. Percent increase in tendon length as function of load in grams at 45°C (heat and stretch) and at 25°C (stretch only). (From Lehmann JF et al: Effect of therapeutic temperatures on tendon extensibility. Arch Phys Med Rehabil 51:481–487, 1970. With permission.)

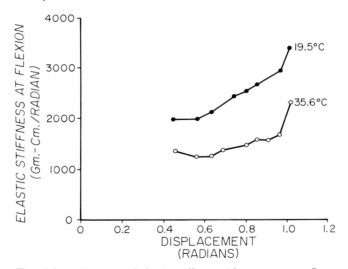

Fig. 4-2. Alteration of elastic stiffness with temperature. Open circles: Elastic stiffness at full flexion at different amplitudes of rotation, skin temperature 35.6°C. Closed circles: Same experiment with joint cooled with skin temperature 19.5°C. Stiffness was clearly increased. (From Wright V et al: Physical factors concerned with the stiffness of normal and diseased joint. Bull Johns Hopkins Hosp 106:215–231, 1960. With permission.)

of Melzack and Wall.[65,88,119] It could perhaps also be explained through the action of endorphins. There is some evidence that pain may be relieved by the temperature rise around the pain-sensing fibers.[61] In addition, if heat reduces muscle spasms, it may relieve the associated pain. In tension syndromes heat may relieve the sustained isometric muscular contraction and the associated ischemia, reducing discomfort and pain.

Muscle spasms.   Muscle spasms secondary to skeletal or joint pathology are clinically often relieved by heat application.[42,122] Mense[89] found that in a prestretched muscle at a tension of 100 ponds (one pond equals the force or weight of one gram on earth) the rate of firing of the IA afferents was increased by heating and depressed by cooling of the muscle, whereas those secondary afferents which had a low initial discharge rate showed an activation by cooling and a depression or cessation of firing by warming (Fig. 4-3). Therefore, the hypothesis can be advanced that if muscle spasm is a static rather than a dynamic phenomenon, this response of the secondary afferents to changes of muscle temperature may be the explanation for the clinical observation of relief from muscle spasm. There is also some evidence that stimulation of the exteroceptors of the skin in the neck decreases gamma fiber activity resulting in a decreased spindle excitability.[31] This may explain why superficial heating devices may also decrease muscle spasms.

Joint inflammation.   The effect on inflammatory conditions of joints is not clear. Clinically, heating of a joint and its inflamed synovium is considered to be contraindicated since vigorous heating may produce by itself an inflammatory reaction that is then superimposed upon the existing synovitis. No clear evidence, however, exists for this

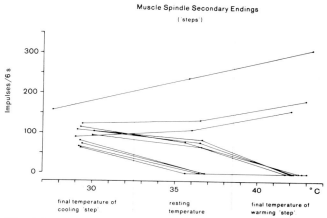

Fig. 4-3.   Impulse activity of 11 secondary spindle ending afferents under resting conditions and following temperature "steps." In each curve the three measuring points indicate the activity at the end of a cooling "step" (left), under resting conditions (35 to 37°C, muscle prestretched to 100 p) (middle), and at the end of a warming "step" (right). Note that in the cooled muscle all the secondary endings were active whereas in the warmed muscle the majority of the units was silent. (From Mense S: Effects of temperature on the discharges of muscle spindles and tendon organs. Pflugers Arch 374:159–166, 1978. With permission.)

assumption. Harris and McCroskery[40] and Harris and Krane[39] found that the activity of destructive enzymes such as collagenase is increased in vitro when the temperature is raised from 30 to 36°C. However, their experiments included only temperatures below the therapeutic range (41–45°C). On the other hand, Castor and Yaron[15] found that other enzyme systems may stop functioning within the therapeutic temperature range. Harris[41] showed that the inflamed synovium does not behave in response to heat applied with shortwave diathermy in the same fashion as the normal synovium. He observed the clearance of radioactive sodium injected into the knee joint. In the normal joint the clearance was markedly accelerated after heating, whereas in the presence of synovitis the initially high clearance rate before heating was reduced. The values obtained after short-wave application were similar in these cases to those obtained in the normal joint. Controlled clinical studies are not available. Therefore no definite conclusions on the effectiveness of vigorous heating of the joint structures themselves in active rheumatoid arthritis are possible.

Minor trauma.   Heat has also been used as an adjunct in the resolution of minor trauma. Experimentally the hemorrhages have been produced by either controlled quantifiable mechanical trauma or by injection of a measured quantity of blood into these tissues. The resolution of this type of hemorrhage after some heat application was compared with that of controls. Fenn,[28] Hustler et al[50] and Lehmann et al[68] found a more rapid resolution of the hemorrhage with heat application. It is important to delay use of heat until after the bleeding has stopped. Brown[12] and Pasila et al[100] suggested that this type of therapy should be used after the acute phase of trauma. These effects seem to be closely related to the observation that elevating the temperature of the tissues markedly increases the blood flow.[1,2,106–108] The effect on edema alone is more controversial.[63,64,112]

SELECTION OF MODALITIES

Local versus Distant Heat

In order to produce a vigorous physiologic response it is necessary to heat locally at the site of the pathology to maximally tolerated temperature levels. Superficial heating agents therefore can produce vigorous responses only in the skin and subcutaneous tissues. Therapeutic physiologic responses elsewhere are produced by reflex phenomena and are much less pronounced than the corresponding response at the site of heating. These reflex responses are also limited as to where they occur since they are dependent on the availability of an appropriate neural pathway.[63,64] Thus, heating the skin over a limb may actually produce blood flow increases in the skin of the opposite extremity.[31] In contrast, it may produce a reduction in the blood flow of the muscle under the heated skin unless the temperature of the muscle itself is increased. This represents a fragment of the temperature regulatory mechanism reducing flow to the inactive organs and diverting the blood flow to the skin when the core temperature rise should be prevented. In this case, the reflex response is limited to the skin of the opposite extremity. On the other hand, if only the surface of the abdomen is heated, we find a reduction of acid production in the stomach and a reduction of blood flow to the mucous membranes of the gastrointestinal tract and a reduction in smooth muscle activity such as peristalsis.[7] In summary, these reflex responses to distant heating, ie, heating of the skin, are limited in location, type, and quantity of the response.

In short, with superficial heat, only limited and mild responses can be obtained at the depths of the tissues. Such treatment applied to an extremity would increase the skin blood flow but may reduce blood flow to the synovium of the joint.[48]

On the other hand, if the site of the pathology in the tissues is vigorously heated, numerous physiologic responses can be produced to any desirable or undesirable degree. As an example, development of hyperemia is dependent on the tissue temperature produced (Fig. 4-4) and it is also dependent on the duration of the effective tissue temperature elevation (Fig. 4-5). From such experiments it can be concluded that the therapeutic range begins at about 40° and ends at about 45°C. Temperatures of 45° can be tolerated only for a short period of time without tissue damage.[58]

In conclusion, if a vigorous response is desired it is necessary to attain the highest temperature at the site of the tissue pathology to be treated, to elevate this temperature close to the maximally tolerated level and to maintain it for an adequate period of time.

Vigorous versus Mild Heat (Factors Influencing Reaction)

In order to produce vigorous heating of a given area it is crucial that a modality be selected that produces a temperature distribution with its peak at the site of the pathology. This temperature then has to be brought to the maximally tolerated level. If this temperature were exceeded any other place in the tissues a burn would result. A schematic drawing of the selection of a vigorous heating modality for the joint structure is given in Figure 4-6. On the other hand, mild heating effects can be obtained in either of two ways: (1) by lowering the output of the heating modality to produce temperatures within the lower part of the therapeutic range at the site of the pathology; (2) by using a superficial heating agent, relying upon reflexly produced physiological changes in the depths of the tissues.[71] When one considers that the effective temperature range extends only over approximately

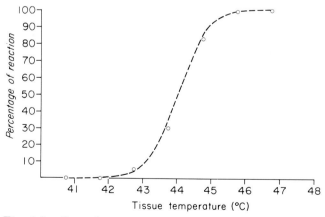

Fig. 4-4. Dependence of hyperemia on tissue temperature. (From Lehmann JF: The biophysical basis of biologic ultrasonic reactions with special reference to ultrasonic therapy. Arch Phys Med Rehabil 34:139–152, 1953. With permission.)

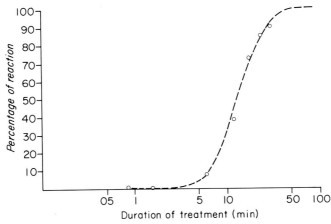

Fig. 4-5. Dependence of hyperemia on duration of treatment. (From Lehmann JF: in Krusen FH et al (eds): Handbook of Physical Medicine and Rehabilitation, first edition. WB Saunders, 1965, page 249. With permission.)

2°C (Fig. 4-4) the conclusion is that for proper control of vigorous heating or mild heating the therapist must master the technique of application to the point that he or she controls the temperature within ±1°C at the site of the pathology. In order to do that he or she must have adequate equipment. For vigorous effects, the tissue temperature must be kept in the upper part of the effective range. To obtain mild effects it must be maintained in the lower portion of the range.

It may be desirable to raise the temperature rapidly so that a greater portion of the time of application of the modality produces temperatures in the therapeutic and effective range. Rapid rise of temperature may also produce a greater reflex stimulation.

Selection of Modality

It is essential that the proper modality be selected for a given pathology and its site. The reason that there are so many heating modalities is largely due to the fact that while they all produce most of their effects by tissue temperature elevation, the location of the peak temperature throughout the distribution is unique for most modalities. This location, however, can be modified to a degree by change of technique of application.

Which Areas Are Selectively Heated?

Ultrasound

Definition. Ultrasound is an acoustic vibration. For therapeutic purposes the frequencies used are between 0.8 and 1.0 MHz with intensities up to 4 W/cm^2 and a total output of the applicator of 40 watts. The wavelength of ultrasound under those conditions in water or soft tissue is approximately 1.5 mm. Absorption is largely due to the protein content of the tissues.[14,103]

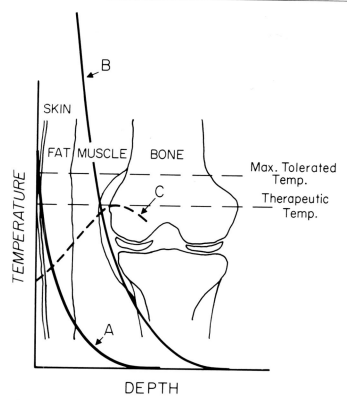

Fig. 4-6. Temperature distributions of superficial (A and B) and deep (C) heating agents. A: Temperatures stay within tolerance limits but joint capsule is not heated. B: Joint capsule is heated, but superficial temperatures exceed tolerance levels. C: Selective heating of joint capsule without exceeding tolerance levels. (From Lehmann JF et al: in Reid JM et al (eds): Interaction of Ultrasound and Biological Tissues, proceedings of a workshop held at Battelle Seattle Research Center 11/8/71 to 11/11/71, DHEW Pub (FDA) 73-8008. With permission.)

Mode of action. The main usefulness of ultrasound as a heating modality lies in the fact that it selectively heats tissue interfaces, that is, locations where the treatable pathology is often encountered. This selective rise of temperature is due to several factors. Tissues of different acoustic impedance produce reflection at the interface. The acoustic impedance is defined as the product of the sound velocity and density of a given tissue. The greater the mismatch of impedance the greater the amount of reflection. The reflected wave is superimposed upon the incoming wave and thus increases the energy available for absorption close to the interface. At an uneven interface scattering of the wave may occur, which increases the length of the wave pathway close to the interface. Therefore more energy is made available for absorption in that area. Further, the longitudinal compression waves of ultrasound, depending in part on the angle of incidence, are partially converted into transverse or shear waves. These are rapidly absorbed as they travel along the interface (Fig. 4-7).[16] Finally the superficial layer of a highly absorbing medium is also selectively heated, since attenuation of the ultrasound in that medium occurs rapidly. For instance, bone absorbs approximately ten times as much as skeletal muscle.[76] A typical pattern of relative heating, ie, the amount of energy absorbed at any given depth of the tissue and related to the value at the muscle-bone interface, is shown in Figure 4-8.[16] As a result of these biophysical considerations, selective heating can be expected at the following biological interfaces of therapeutic interest: the soft tissue-bone interface, especially joint capsule and synovium; scars within soft tissues; myofascial interfaces; nerve trunks; tendon and tendon sheaths.

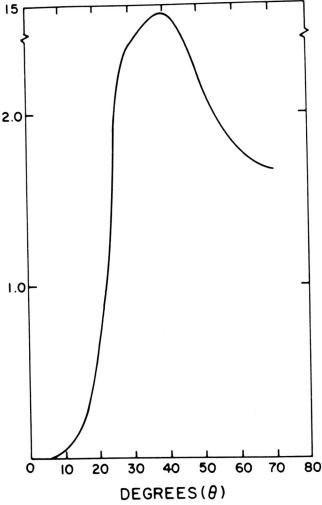

DEGREES(θ)

Fig. 4-7.   Ratio of heating due to shear wave to heating due to longitudinal wave versus the angle of incidence. (From Chan AK et al: Calculations of therapeutic heat generated by ultrasound in fat-muscle-bone layers. IEEE Trans Biomed Eng BME-21:280–284, 1973. With permission.)

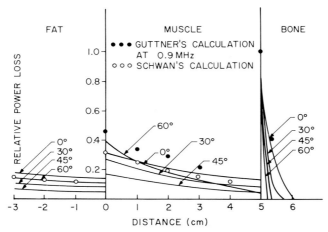

Fig. 4-8. Relative heating pattern in a three-layered system (fat-muscle-bone). Frequency: 1 MHz. Schwan et al's[104] and Güttner's[35] calculated values are superimposed, but these values are renormalized. (From Chan AK et al: Calculations of therapeutic heat generated by ultrasound in fat-muscle-bone layers. IEEE Trans Biomed Eng BME-21:280–284, 1973. With permission.)

Technique of application.   For a successful therapeutic application of this modality it is essential that adequate technique of application and adequate equipment be used. Adequate technique of application should consider the nonuniformity of the ultrasonic beam and the small diameter of the applicator's radiating surface. Therefore ultrasound application should be done with a moving applicator, covering, with overlapping strokes, a field 3 × 3 inches to 4 × 4 inches. This will lead to uniform exposure of the tissues and a relatively smooth, controlled rise of temperature into the therapeutic range. For vigorous heating it is essential that the temperature rise close to tolerance levels; that is, close to pain threshold. If deep pain occurs during application, the output of the applicator should be slightly reduced or the area treated slightly enlarged. If prickling pain occurs at the skin, this indicates inadequate coupling. For proper sound transmission from applicator to tissue, a coupling medium such as a commercial gel can be used. Mineral oil is equally effective and cheaper, but more messy.[120] These coupling media also lubricate for easy gliding of the applicator over the skin. It is important to avoid shaking air bubbles into the medium since this leads to a marked loss of transmission due to reflection. If treatment occurs with the limb submersed in water, one must prevent the collection of air bubbles on applicator and skin by periodically wiping both surfaces. The applicator should not touch the skin since water is a poor lubricant. The temperature of the applicator or coupling medium is important since higher temperatures lead to a selective rise of temperature at the skin and not at the desirable place in the depth of the tissues. Dipping of the applicator into tap water between applications would prevent excessive temperature rise within the applicator. If treatment occurs in the water bath the proper water temperature should be selected. If it is too high, surface heating will occur. If it is too low, the deep tissues may be cooled to the point that therapeutic heating is prevented.

For treatment of joints it is essential to realize that sound does not penetrate to the side of the joint opposite to the application because of reflection at the bone surface and the high rate of absorption in the bone.[76,80] Therefore a multiple field technique of application should be used, treating the joint, eg, the hip and shoulder, from all sides, anteriorly, laterally and posteriorly. It is important in such cases that each field should be exposed for five to ten minutes. This allows time for heat conduction from the superficial bone to the joint capsule and provides better capsular heating.[67] Ultrasound can be judiciously used in the presence of metal implants in spite of the reflection at the metal surface since the high thermal conductivity of the metal dissipates the heat fast enough to prevent localized burns.[59,60] On the other hand, materials used in joint replacement, such as high density polyethylene or methylmethacrylate should not be exposed to ultrasound, since at this time the available (unpublished) information shows that these materials rapidly absorb ultrasound and therefore may be selectively heated to destructive temperatures. Further experimental evidence is needed demonstrating that the exposure in situ would not endanger the implant. Such information is not available at this time. Barth and Bülow[4] showed that in growing dogs the epiphyseal lines could be treated with ultrasound of intensities in the therapeutic range below the pain threshold without any untoward effects, a finding confirmed by Vaughen and Bender.[117] It therefore can be assumed that therapeutic application to joints in children, if done within the proper doses below pain threshold, is acceptable.

Equipment. The criteria for therapeutically useful ultrasound equipment are as follows. The applicator should operate at a frequency of 0.8 to 1 MHz. It should contain a single crystal and not a mosaic of several crystals, to provide optimal uniformity of the field. The diameter of the physical size of the applicator should be close to the diameter of the radiating surface area. This allows skin contact and good coupling even over irregular surfaces of the body, whereas a physically large applicator may lose contact in the area of the radiating surface. The radiating surface area should be 7–13 cm². An applicator with a minimum of 5 cm² could be used for some of the indications. The equipment should have full wave rectification and filtering to prevent temporal peak outputs from exceeding destructive levels. The ratio of the peak intensity of the beam in the far field to average intensity should be close to 4:1 as a measure of uniformity of the output. A meter should indicate ultrasonic output transmitted into the tissues. The internal losses of an applicator should be kept to a minimum to avoid excess heating of the applicator and therefore of the skin surface.

Nonthermal effects. It has been shown in many experiments that most of the physiologically desired responses are due to temperature rise in the tissue. However, ultrasound is one modality that also can produce some effects via nonthermal reactions. These, however, are not proven to be of therapeutic usefulness. One nonthermal reaction, degassing or pseudocavitation, produces small highly destructive lesions around the gas bubbles formed in the tissues during the phase of rarefaction in the sound wave.[74,75] The occurrence of this phenomenon can be prevented by using proper equipment that does not produce excessive temporal or spatial peaks of intensity. Since the cavitation threshold is low in tissues with low cellular content and low viscosity of the fluid, exposure of the amniotic fluid, the fluid media of the eye, and other fluid accumulations in the body should be avoided. This applies only to therapeutic, and not diagnostic, intensities of ultrasound.

Summary. From the above discussion, the selection of ultrasound for clinical application is based on the selectivity of its heating effect, which has been borne out by clinical studies. Provided proper equipment and technique of application are used, this modality could be shown to be effective in such conditions as limitation of range of motion of joints due to tightness of periarticular structures or scar formation of the synovium irrespective of the initial cause of the condition, which may be prolonged immobilization, rheumatic processes, degenerative joint diseases, or trauma.

Shortwave

Definition. Shortwave diathermy is a form of high frequency current application at frequencies of 13.66 and 27.12 MHz, as allowed by the Federal Communications Commission.[17,18] The corresponding wavelengths are 22 and 11 meters respectively. The most commonly used frequency is 27.12 MHz with a wavelength of 11 meters.

Mode of action. Heating of the tissues depends on the current distribution. If there is a difference in current flow through different tissues, the tissue with the greatest current flow will be heated most as in tissues arranged in a parallel circuit. If the current flow is the same through all the tissues (as in tissues in series), the tissue with the greatest resistance will be heated most.[64] Two methods of application are used to obtain the current flow in the tissue. One uses induction coil applicators where the alternating magnetic field crosses the tissue and induces the current. The other uses condenser plates with the tissues between the plates, the alternating electric field inducing the current. With induction coil applicators the greatest current density is usually found in the superficial musculature. However, joints with very little cover of soft tissues such as knee and elbow or the small joints of the hands or feet may also be selectively heated.[118] As an example of tissues in parallel and in series circuit, the application of two condenser pads to the back is shown. The highest current density under the electrodes is found in the subcutaneous fat and between the electrodes in the superficial musculature (see Fig. 4-9).[57]

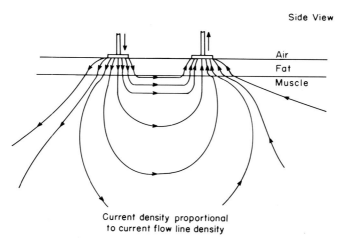

Fig. 4-9. Schematic drawing of current flow lines in uniform tissue layers when shortwaves are applied with capacitor plates in one plane to fat-muscle layers, side view. (From Lehmann JF: in Krusen FH et al (eds): Handbook of Physical Medicine and Rehabilitation, first edition. WB Saunders, 1965. With permission.)

Technique of application. For successful therapy, the use of proper techniques of application and proper equipment is essential. With both the condenser and induction coil applicators it is important that proper spacing of approximately 2 cm between the electrode and skin is maintained to assure that the tissues are exposed to a more uniform field. Close to the applicator, the field dilutes at a rapid rate with the highest intensities close to the applicator surface. Applicators that are covered with glass or plastic should not be applied directly to the skin since they grossly interfere with heat exchange and therefore selective heating of the skin would be the result (Fig. 4-10), whereas adequate heating can be produced with a 2 cm air space between the applicator and the skin (Fig. 4-11).[66]

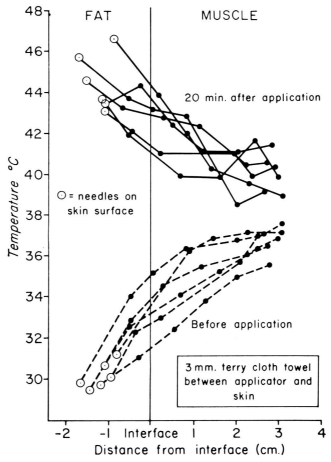

Fig. 4-10. Temperature distributions in six human thighs before and after the completion of 20 minutes exposure to short-wave diathermy (27.12 MHz) applied with the monode with 3 mm terry cloth inserted between applicator and skin. (Only five stars for needles appear because in two thighs the readings were identical.) (From Lehmann JF et al: Selective muscle heating by short-wave diathermy with helical coil. Arch Phys Med Rehabi 50: 117-123, 1969. With permission).

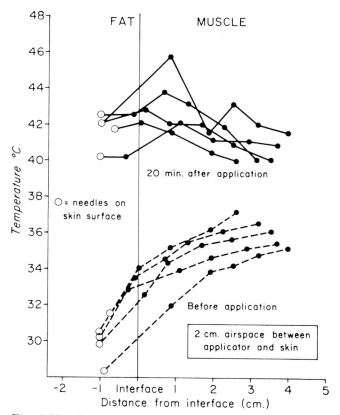

Fig. 4-11. Temperature distribution in five human thighs before and after the completion of 20 minutes of exposure to shortwave (27.12 MHz) applied with the monode with 2 cm air space between applicator and skin surface. (From Lehmann JF et al: Selective muscle heating by shortwave diathermy with a helical coil. Arch Phys Med Rehabil 50:117–123, 1969. With permission.)

Shortwave diathermy should not be applied in the presence of metal implants if the implant would be exposed to any appreciable amount of shortwave energy. The dangers involved are caused by shunting of currents through the metal implant with increasing current density surrounding the metal leading to burns. Until proven otherwise, intrauterine devices containing copper should not be exposed even though it is doubtful that any significant energy would reach them.[96] Contact lenses should also be removed before diathermy application in the vicinity of the eye. Excessive temperatures under the contact lens may occur when shortwave diathermy is applied.[105] It has been observed that shortwave diathermy may increase menstrual flow when applied just prior to, or during, menstruation.

Equipment. Exposure is usually for 20–30 minutes. Since shortwave diathermy is associated with large amounts of stray electromagnetic radiation, safety standards have become of increasing concern. The safety threshold for shortwave diathermy, in the absence of any evidence to the contrary, has been assumed to be the threshold for microwaves (5–10 mW/cm²). However, all information on current propagation and absorption suggests that actually the threshold should be considerably higher for shortwave diathermy. Commercial equipment often has inadequate output for vigorous heating. Therefore, it is important to select equipment that can raise the tissue temperature to tolerance limits. In addition, it is desirable that a variety of applicators be available to allow modification of technique of application and therefore modification of the tissue temperature distribution. Most of the modern equipment uses induction coil applicators with capacitive shielding; however, it has been shown that the ratio of specific absoption rate in fat to that in muscle varies according to design (Table 4-1).[78,79]

Summary.   In summary, when selecting shortwave diathermy for vigorous heating, it must be remembered that if two condenser applicators are used facing each other on either side of the tissue it is most likely that subcutaneous fat will be heated most. If two condenser plate applicators are used side by side parallel to the skin surface, the highest temperature will be obtained in the subcutaneous fat under the electrodes and in the superficial musculature between the electrodes. Induction coil applicators have a tendency to heat the superficial musculature selectively but can be used to heat the small joints of hands and feet and large joints such as elbow and knee covered by little soft tissue. It is essential to ascertain that the equipment has enough output to produce vigorous heating. Sufficient output is available if application with maximal output leads to discomfort levels in a short period of time.

Microwave

Definition.   Microwave diathermy is an electromagnetic radiation of frequencies of 915 and 2450 MHz, as approved for clinical use by the FCC.[17,18] The wavelength is of the order of 1 cm in tissue and 10 cm in air.

Table 4-1
Relative Heating Characteristics of Several
Diathermy Applicators at 27.12 MHz

Applicator	SAR Muscle/SAR Fat	
	Peak Value	Average Value
Siemens Monode*	1.47	1.23
IME** Round	1.83	1.75
IME** Pancake	2.15	2.29
IME** Square	2.27	2.67
IME** Magnatherm		
1000 Head	1.41	1.48
Enraf Circuplode	1.48	1.58
ElMed Magnode*	0.39	0.39

From Lehmann JF et al: Heating patterns produced by shortwave diathermy applicators in tissue substitute models. Arch Phys Med Rehabil 64:575–577, 1983. With permission.
 *Applicator is not electrostatically shielded
**IME: International Medical Electronics

Mode of action.   Propagation through the tissues, including reflection at interfaces and absorption characteristics of the tissues, will depend on their dielectric constants and conductivity values. In general, tissues with higher water content absorb more microwaves than drier tissues. The pattern of relative heating at 2456 MHz shows that due to interface reflection, too much energy is converted into heat in the subcutaneous fat and too little by comparison in the musculature; this defeats the purpose of deep heating unless there is very little subcutaneous fat cover (Fig. 4-12a).[72] This problem is virtually eliminated if a low frequency around 900 MHz is used (Fig. 4-12b). However, at both frequencies reflection at the bone interface may produce "hot spots" in front of the bone. Also because of the reflection, no significant amount of energy is available for absorption behind the bone.

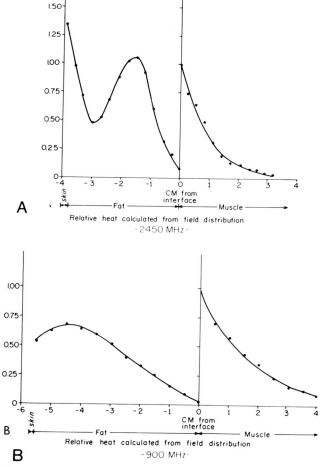

Fig. 4-12.   Pattern of relative heat calculated from field distribution at frequencies of 2450 (top) and 900 (bottom) MHz. (From Lehmann JF et al: Comparison of relative heating pattens produced in tissues by exposure to microwave energy at frequencies of 2,450 and 900 megacycles. Arch Phys Med Rehabil 43:69–76, 1962. With permission.)

Musculature, with a relatively high water content absorbs more than other soft tissue and bone. This applies even more to the situation of fluid-filled cavities, for instance the orb of the eye, or a joint with effusion.

Technique of application. Two types of applicators are available. One uses approximately 2 cm air spacing between applicator and skin. The other is in direct contact with the tissues. The applicators that are not in contact with the skin include the A, B, C, and E directors. The C and E directors have an antenna rod of ½ and one full wavelength dimension respectively, backed up by a reflector. The typical intensities of the distribution in the field are shown in Figures 4-13 and 4-14. The effective field size is close to the diameter of the reflector. However, since the antenna length is similar to the wavelength (12.2 cm) in air, the beam is very divergent and dilutes out rapidly with increasing distance from the applicator. Therefore these applicators should be applied at a distance of about 2 cm. These noncontact applicators have the disadvantage of much stray radiation. The direct contact applicators have less stray radiation and much better transmission into the tissues. Also, if desired, skin temperature can be controlled by air cooling through a radome. It is possible to develop meters that indicate the forward power entering the tissues, as required by a proposed Food and Drug Administration (FDA) standard.[29] Exposure time is usually 20–30 minutes.

In order to test the efficacy of deep heating of any one of the applicators, tissue substitute models have been developed that have the same electrical properties for a given

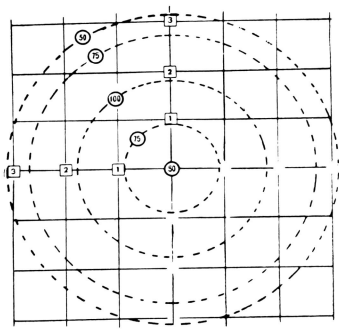

Fig. 4-13. Field pattern produced by "A" director at a distance of two inches in percent of maximal intensity (circles); distance from the center in inches (squares). (From Lehmann JF: in Krusen FH et al (eds): Handbook of Physical Medicine and Rehabilitation, first edition. WB Saunders, page 301, 1965. With permission.)

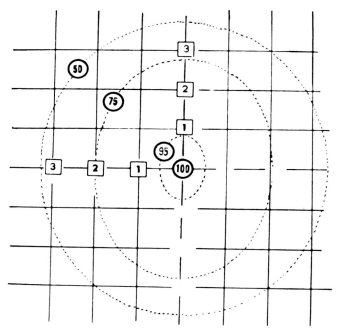

Fig. 4-14. Field pattern produced by "C" director at a distance of three inches in percent of maximal intensity (circles); distance from the center in inches (squares). (From Lehmann JF: in Krusen FH et al (eds): Handbook of Physical Medicine and Rehabilitation, first edition. WB Saunders, page 302, 1965. With permission.)

frequency as the human tissues. They can be shaped according to the anatomy to be exposed. These models can be scanned for infrared radiation after short-term microwave exposure and this information can be processed through a computer that may read out the isotherms of the temperature distribution (Fig. 4-15).[73]

Schematically, with known thermal properties of the tissue substitutes the initial linear transient (without heat conduction) allows the calculation of the specific absorption rate, not only for microwaves but also for shortwave diathermy in the human. These results obtained in the model have been verified in the human where the blood flow was eliminated with a tourniquet (Fig. 4-16). The temperature asymptote to the steady state with and without tourniquet shows the difference, which is due to blood flow cooling (Fig. 4-17). From the difference between these two temperature curves, the actual blood flow can be measured provided the thermal properties of the blood are known. It was found that at approximately 550 mW/cm^2 maximal power density of incident radiation, the specific absorption rate was as high in the human as approximately 170 W/kg in the muscle. The corresponding blood flow rate increase was marked, up to approximately 30 ml/100 g tissue/min.[73] With the direct contact applicators it was possible in the human to demonstrate uniform heating of the musculature throughout (Fig. 4-18).[20]

Concern about stray radiation has been emphasized lately for microwaves as well as for shortwave diathermy.[38,92] However, for relatively short term therapeutic exposure, in contrast to long-term occupational exposure, side effects are primarily thermal in nature. The cataract formation of the eye can be considered as a prototype. Figure 4-19 shows that

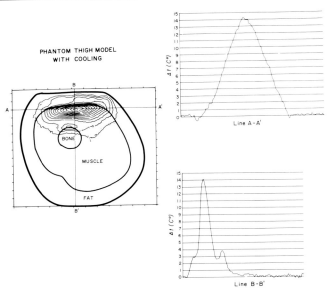

Fig. 4-15. Isotherms produced in phantom thigh model after exposure to a 13-cm square direct-contact microwave applicator operating at 915 HMz with radome and cooling. (From Lehmann JF et al: Evaluation of a therpeautic direct-contact 915-MHz microwave applicator for effective deep-tissue heating in humans. IEEE Trans Microwave Theory Tech MTT-26:556–563, 1978. With permission.)

power densities of less than 100 mW/cm^2 do not produce any cataracts even in long-term exposure.[36] On this basis it has been proposed that 10 mW/cm^2 or, more lately by the FDA, 5 mW/cm^2,[29] would be a safe exposure level for the patient's sensitive organs, such as brain, eye, testicles, and for the therapist applying the modality. It has been well documented that nonthermal effects exist, but under therapeutic conditions they represent neither a hazard nor do they seem to contribute to the therapeutic effectiveness. As mentioned, stray radiation is much more the problem with the applicators that do not have full contact with the skin than with any others. However, with all applicators one should avoid pointing the E (electric) field vector toward sensitive organs because in this direction there is always more stray radiation. For direct contact applicators it is recommended that if contact with the skin has to be lost it should not be in the direction of sensitive organs because maximal stray radiation occurs in the area of poor skin contact. With these precautions exposure of sensitive organs can be markedly reduced (Table 4-2).[82,83] Also the presence of metal implants in the microwave field represents a contraindication because excessive temperatures may develop in or surrounding the metal.

Equipment. Optimal applicator designs should meet the following criteria. The temperature should be higher in the musculature than in other tissues of the extremity exposed. The temperature distribution should be even throughout the musculature from subcutaneous fat to bone interface. The temperature throughout the field exposed should be even from edge to edge. The absorbed energy (Watts/kg) should be adequate to raise

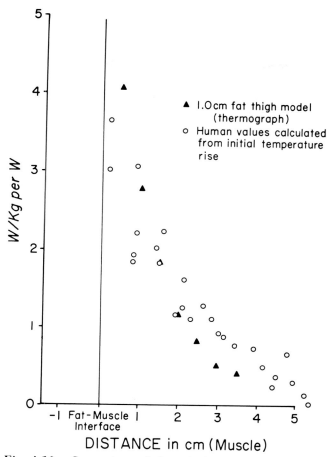

Fig. 4-16. Comparison of the calculations of the specific absorption rate (SAR) in thighs of human beings and models. (From Lehmann JF et al: Evaluation of a therpeautic direct-contact 915-MHz microwave applicator for effective deep-tissue heating in humans. IEEE Trans Microwave Theory MTT-26:556–563, 1978. With permission.)

tissue temperature to tolerance levels and therefore it should be approximately between 170 and 200 Watts/kg. At this level demonstrable physiological responses such as increased blood flow would be maximal. The stray radiation should be minimized, ie, at or below 5 mW/cm² at a distance of 5 cm from the edge of the direct contact applicator. The microwave generator should be equipped with a measuring device which indicates the forward power radiating into the tissues.

Summary. In summary, microwave should be looked upon as a modality to selectively heat tissues with high water content such as musculature. It is also capable of heating joints with little soft tissue cover such as the small joints of the hands and feet. If applied to any fluid-filled cavity such as a joint effusion, the output should be greatly reduced because of the high selectivity of absorption in this situation.

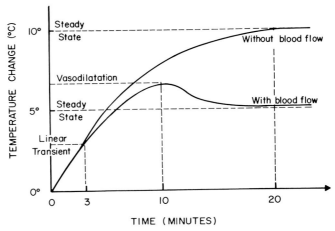

Fig. 4-17. Schematic representation of transient and steady-state temperatures for a typical tissue under diathermy exposure. (From Lehmann JF et al: Evaluation of a therpeautic direct-contact 915-MHz microwave applicator for effective deep-tissue heating in humans. IEEE Trans Microwave Theory Tech MTT-26:556–563, 1978. With permission.)

Superficial Heating Modalities

Definition and mode of action. Heating modalities are often divided into those that produce heating at the depth of the tissues and those which heat the superficial areas (Table 4-3).[64] Very often, superficial heat application is considered to be synonymous with mild heating; this is true only if one considers physiological responses in the depth of the tissues that are negotiated through reflexes. Depending on the temperature and duration of treatment, superficial heating agents may produce vigorous or mild effects locally within the superficial areas. It has been documented that hot packs, infrared and visible light produce essentially the same temperature distribution in the human irrespective of which part of the light spectrum is used (Figs. 4-20 and 4-21).[81] On the basis of more limited evidence, it can be concluded that paraffin, Fluidotherapy, and whirlpool application to a part of the body would produce the same temperature distribution.[64] In any one of those cases the most superficial tissues have the highest temperature.

Technique of application—Hydrocollator pack. The prototypical hot pack, the Hydrocollator pack, contains a silicate gel in a cotton bag that absorbs and holds a large amount of water, which in turn carries the calories needed for high heating capacity. These packs are heated by immersion into a thermostatically controlled water bath of 160 to 175° (71.1–79.4°C). Application is drip dry, for 20–30 minutes, on top of layers of terry cloth that slow the heat flow. Therefore some variation of dosage is possible by varying the thickness of terry cloth layers. It is essential that the terry cloth be kept dry; when wet or compacted it will conduct heat at a much more rapid rate and may lead to burns.

Technique of application—paraffin. Paraffin wax with a melting point of 125–130°F (51.7–54.4°C) is kept in a thermostatically controlled container. Application is

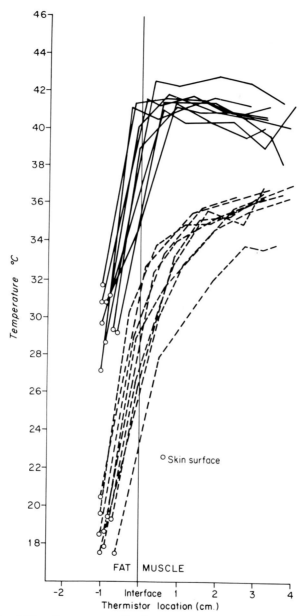

Fig. 4-18. Temperature distribution in nine volunteers with ≤ one cm of subcutaneous fat before (-----) and 20 minutes after after (————) microwave application. (From de Lateur BJ et al: Muscle heating in human subjects with 915 MHz. microwave contact applicator. Arch Phys Med Rehabil 51:147–151, 1970. With permission.)

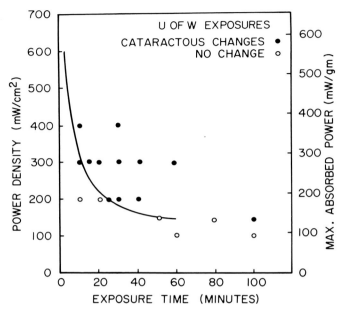

Fig. 4-19. Time and power-density threshold for cataractogenesis in rabbits exposed to near-zone 2450 MHz radiation. (From Guy AW et al: Effect of 2450-MHz radiation on the rabbit eye. IEEE Trans Microwave Theory & Tech MTT-23:492–498, 1975. With permission.)

Table 4-2

Stray Radiation Levels Produced at Sensitive Anatomic Sites

Site Irradiated	Site Measured	915 MHz Linearly Polarized Applicator	
		Parallel	Perpendicular
Thigh	Genitals	7	30
Anterior lateral aspect of shoulder	Eyes	20	2
Posterior lateral aspect of shoulder	Eyes	12	2
Trapezius	Eyes	2	2
Posterior neck	Eyes	1	13

Stray radiation levels in mW/cm^2, measured with E-field parallel and perpendicular to tissue axis. Input power normalized to 50 watts net for 915 MHz.

From Lehmann JF, et al: Microwave therapy: stray radiation, safety and effectiveness. Arch Phys Med Rehabil 60:578–584, 1979. With permission.

Table 4-3

Heating Modalities Subdivided According to Primary
Mode of Heat Transfer

Primary Mode of Heat Transfer	Modality	
Conduction	Hot packs	
	Paraffin bath	
Convection	Fluidotherapy	Superficial heat
	Hydrotherapy	
	Moist air	
Conversion	Radiant heat	
	Microwaves	
	Shortwaves	Deep heat
	Ultrasound	

From Lehmann JF, de Lateur BJ: Therapeutic heat, in Lehmann JF (Ed): Therapeutic Heat, third edition. Williams & Wilkins, p. 428 1982. With permission.

Comparison of Temperature Distribution in the Human
Thigh during Exposure to Infrared Radiation

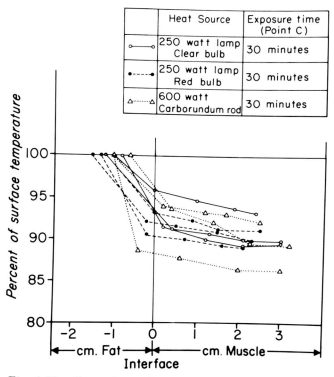

Fig. 4-20. Comparison of temperature distribution in the human thigh during exposure to infrared radiation in nine individuals using three modalities. (From Lehmann JF et al: Temperature distributions in the human thigh, produced by infrared, hot pack and microwave applications. Arch Phys Med Rehabil 47:291–299, 1966. With permission.)

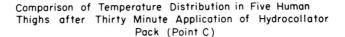

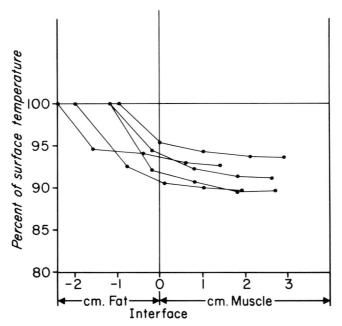

Fig. 4-21. Comparison of temperature distribution in five human thighs after 30-minute application of hydrocollator hot packs. (From Lehmann JF et al: Temperature distributions in the human thigh, produced by infrared, hot pack and microwave applications. Arch Phys Med Rehabil 47:291–299, 1966. With permission.)

usually only to small parts, ie, hands or feet. Two modes of application are used, the dip method and the submersion method. In the dip method, the part is repeatedly dipped into the paraffin until a thick glove of solidified paraffin has formed. A terry cloth wrap is applied for another 20 minutes. This method represents relatively mild heating since the specific heat of paraffin is low and therefore its heat carrying capacity is small. For vigorous heating, the part is submersed in the liquid paraffin for 20 minutes. Since paraffin solidifies at the relatively cool skin surface and since the solidified paraffin is a poor heat conductor it appropriately slows the heat transfer from the liquid paraffin to the part. This method, however, represents more vigorous heating than the dip method.

Technique of application—Fluidotherapy. The Fluidotherapy consists of a bed of finely divided solid, ie, glass beads with a diameter of 0.0165 in and a density of 155 lb/ft^3 or of ground cellulose particles, through which a thermostatically controlled air stream is blown. This produces a semifluid mixture in which the part is submersed. The physiological response can be modified by changing the temperature of the air flow. Contrary to some beliefs[9,10] there is no proof that this method is more effective in deep heating than in superficial heating methods. Temperatures in superficial joints achieved by

Fluidotherapy, paraffin bath, or whirlpool bath depend on the temperature of the medium and the method of application rather than on the modality itself. Application of this modality is again for 20–30 minutes.

Technique of application—hydrotherapy. Hydrotherapy is most often applied in the form of hot tub or whirlpool bath. For partial immersion, temperatures up to 113°F or 45°C may be applied without raising body temperature. For total body immersion in water over 100°F (37.8°C) body temperature should be monitored to prevent an inadvertent rise, since in these cases the normal heat regulatory mechanism is essentially disabled. Hydrotherapy has therapeutic effects in addition to those produced by heat. The whirlpool can be used to cleanse undermined skin sores, and the buoyancy of the water can be used for exercise with minimal stress on joints. Unless the total body temperature is raised, the highest temperatures are found again in the superficial tissues. Application is for up to 30 minutes.

Another form of hydrotherapy is the contrast bath that produces a maximal increase in blood flow and hyperemia in hands and feet. It has been used primarily to reduce stiffness in rheumatic diseases or degenerative joint disease.[86,124] The therapy starts with immersion into hot water at temperatures of 105–110°F (40.6–43.3°C) for 10 minutes followed by 1 minute of submersion in cold water (59–68°F, 15–20°C), which in turn is followed again by a cycle of 4 minutes hot water submersion and 1 minute cold application. The 4:1 cycle is repeated until the total application is finished after 30 minutes.

Technique of application—radiant heat. Radiant heat application with infrared or visible light is usually done with a heat lamp for 20–30 minutes. The quality of the lamp depends on its total output as measured by its electrical wattage. It also depends on the quality of the reflector, which assures an even heating pattern over a large area of the skin. Dosimetry is possible only by varying the distance from lamp element to skin. Since all the beams are somewhat divergent, increasing the distance reduces the incident intensity per cm^2. An alternative method to cover a larger area is the application of a single or double heat cradle. With radiant heat application the temperature regulatory mechanisms, including sweating, are still intact and therefore a body core temperature elevation usually does not occur.

Lasers

Definition. The characteristic difference between a laser beam and a beam of other light is, among others, its monochromaticity. The photons are all of the same wavelength. In other words, the laser is a columnated beam of photons of the same frequency with the waves in phase. It is possible to develop very well defined beams at very high intensities if desired. The divergence of such a beam is small and the beam can also be focused to pinpoint size. Measurement of the wavelength is usually in nanometers. The power densities are given in joules/cm^2 and the irradiance in Watts/cm^2.[34]

Mode of operation. Much of the biological effect of the laser is due to the characteristic properties of the photons. In most therapeutic applications the development of heat is a mode of producing the therapeutically desirable effects.

The best developed medical applications of lasers are surgical in nature. They have been used in ophthalmology for the treatment of glaucoma, bleeding retinal vessels, and retinal detachment. Lasers have been used in brain surgery because of their ability to make precise lesions with minimal bleeding. Lasers have also been used experimentally for arthroscopic knee surgery to evaporate loose foreign bodies such as torn menisci.

Attempts have been made to use laser therapy in rheumatoid arthritis. Goldman and associates,[33] used a Q switch neodymium laser at a wavelength of 1.06 nanometers with an output of 15 joules/cm^2 for 30 nanoseconds. Twenty-one patients received laser therapy to one hand and sham exposure to the other. The patients showed a subjective improvement in the joints of both hands, even in the hand where only a sham exposure was done. Objective laboratory findings did not show any changes in the titer of rheumatoid factor, nuclear antibodies, polyethylene glycol precipitates, or erythrocyte sedimentation rate. The only change that occurred was in the platelet aggregation measurements.

There is some experimental evidence that the rate of wound healing and repair of peripheral nerves may be increased after laser treatment.[37,91] Finally, laser has been used in chronic pain, possibly as a form of counterirritant. In summary, the use of laser as a therapeutic tool for arthritides should still be considered as experimental. Some of the applications should be evaluated against the efficacy of more conventional modes of treatment, such as light therapy and the use of counterirritant procedures.

CONTRAINDICATIONS TO HEAT

Heat should be applied with special precaution (if at all) over anesthetic areas or in an obtunded patient. Because of the absence of accurate dosimetry it is necessary in many cases to rely upon the patient's pain perception as a warning that injurious temperature thresholds are exceeded.

Ischemic tissue should not be heated because increased metabolic demand in the absence of an adequate vascular supply to increase the blood flow may result in an ischemic necrosis.

Since heat produces an increase in blood flow and hyperemia of the tissues, any bleeding tendency is increased. Therefore heat should not be applied in the presence of hermorrhagic diatheses.

Heat should not be applied to the gonads or the developing fetus. Congenital malformations are observed in increased numbers when uterine temperatures exceed 39°C, especially during the first six weeks of pregnancy.[21,22,24-26,32,44,46,90,93,95,111] Therefore, one should safeguard against general body temperature elevation and should not apply any modalities that are able to locally raise the uterine temperature. Other contraindications to general body temperature elevation include sensitive patients, ie, patients with steroid withdrawal where shock may be produced or multiple sclerosis patients where the symptomatology may be aggravated by temperature elevation. In spite of the currently extensive use of hyperthermia as an adjunct to other cancer therapy, heat applied in uncontrolled fashion may[45] increase the rate of tumor growth. Therefore one should avoid local heat application to such areas for other than controlled tumor therapy.

PHYSIOLOGIC EFFECTS OF COLD

Definition. Cryotherapy is the local application of cold for therapeutic purposes. Its use is based primarily on the understanding of some physiological responses considered to be of therapeutic significance. A number of these are confirmed by clinical observations, few by objective measurements or controlled studies. As in heat application, knowledge of the indications and selection of proper techniques of application are essential for success.

Mode of action.   Cold is indicated in the following conditions: (1) pain, (2) inflammation as it occurs in bursitis and arthritis, (3) muscle spasms secondary to joint and musculoskeletal pathology or nerve root irritation, and (4) minor trauma, in the early stages.

Pain.   Cryotherapy may reduce pain[6] by directly affecting the activity of pain nerve fibers and receptors, by alleviating painful muscle spasms, and by supplying a competing sensation as suggested by the gate theory of Melzack and Wall.[65,88,119] Experiments showed that cold applied with ethyl chloride spray, eg, to the web of the thumb, could easily increase the pain threshold at the tooth pulp (Fig. 4-22).[99]

Joint inflammation.   The effects of cold in inflammatory reactions such as in arthritides or in bursitis are produced through vasoconstriction reducing hyperemia; that is, heat and swelling. Cold application also reduces pain through the above-mentioned mechanisms. Cold probably also has an effect on the abnormal metabolic processes in the inflammatory reaction.[48] Specifically, for joints, it has been demonstrated by Harris and McCroskery[40] that destructive enzyme activity such as the activity of collagenase is significantly reduced at lower temperatures. The clinical implication has not been well documented as yet.

Muscle spasm.   Muscle spasms, as they occur secondary to joint or muscle pathology or nerve root irritation can be relieved by cold application. It has been shown that the

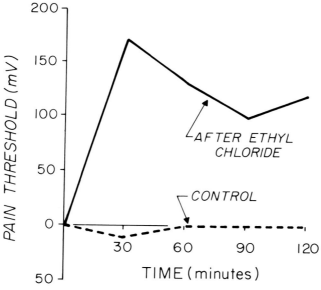

Fig. 4-22.   Effective of ethyl chloride spray on the pain threshold of normal human subjects. (From Parsons CM et al: Effect of induced pain on pain threshold. Proc Soc Exp Biol Med 60:327–329, 1945. With permission.)

temperature markedly affects the rate of firing from the IA afferents of the muscle spindle. Eldred et al[27] selectively cooled individual spindles and found that the rate of firing of the IA afferents decreased proportionately to the decrease in temperature (Fig. 4-23). This effect was thought to be produced by influencing the spindle receptors, rather than the spindle afferents.[53,84,98]

Lowering the temperature reduces the conduction velocity of all nerves. The nerve conduction velocities are reduced approximately 1.84 m/sec/C° between 36 and 23°C. Temperatures of approximately 4°C block nerve conduction.[19] Douglas and Malcolm[23] showed, in animal experiments, that there is a difference in susceptibility among nerve fibers. First affected are the small medullated, then large medullated fibers, and finally the unmedullated fibers. Specifically, cooling prolongs the recovery cycle of the smaller gamma fibers more than that of the larger alpha motor neuron fibers. This mechanism as well as the effect on the spindle may produce the decrease in muscle tone.

The neuromuscular junction and the muscle fibers themselves are much less sensitive to cold. Since cold is used to reduce muscle tone as in spasms, it is important that, if motor skill training occurs at the same time, one does not cool to the point that the sensory feedback loop is interrupted by affecting the large diameter sensory fibers. Also, cooling should not be limited just to the skin since this may facilitate alpha motor neuron discharge and therefore increase rather than relieve spasms.[43,53,115]

Minor trauma.   Local cold application produces a vasoconstriction that is negotiated through the sympathetics but also represents a direct effect of the lowered temperature on the blood vessel walls.[102] Cold is commonly used in acute minor trauma such as sports injuries and sprains of joint. The main therapeutic benefits are a reduction in bleeding, a reduction in edema formation, and a reduction in pain. Cold is commonly used in conjunction with compression.

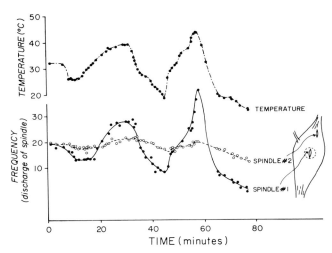

Fig. 4-23.   Effect of local change in temperature on discharge of spindle. Circle about side of spindle indicates area of contact by thermode. Spindle #2, 2 cm away was little affected. (From Eldred E et al: The effect of cooling on mammalian muscle spindles. Exp Neurol 2:144–157, 1960. With permission.)

TECHNIQUES OF COLD APPLICATION

Cold is most commonly applied with a pack containing melting ice and water with a temperature of 32°F or 0°C. An alternate method is the immersion of the portion of a limb in a mixture of ice and water. Also terry cloth dipped in water mixed with ice shavings has been used. After dipping, the cloth is rung out and applied rapidly. This type of packing has to be repeated frequently. It should be noted that when cooling muscle to relieve secondary spasms, adequate time should be allowed, since the cold has to penetrate through the insulating fat layer. Only in a very thin individual are ice applications for a period of 10 minutes effective. In other individuals with a thicker layer of subcutaneous fat, much longer exposure may be necessary.[62] Finally, ice massage has been used moving a block of ice over the surface to be cooled. This usually results in cooling of the skin and is therefore a method of choice for facilitation of alpha motor neuron discharge. This method produces muscle cooling only after a much longer period of time than ice packing. Also available are refrigeration units with temperature control. Chemical packs usually have a poor temperature control mechanism. The application of ethyl chloride or chloro-fluoromethanes in the form of a spray for surface cooling and pain relief is done from a distance of approximately one meter with stroking movements. In acute injuries it is essential not to cool longer than necessary to reduce bleeding, swelling, and pain. There is experimental evidence[85] that tissue repair is significantly delayed if healing occurs at lower temperatures of the tissues.

HEAT VERSUS COLD

From the discussion of heat and cold it is apparent that many effects can be produced both by heat and cold application. Muscle spasms seem to respond equally. Pain may be reduced by both modalities. On the other hand, blood flow, bleeding, and edema formation are accelerated by heat application and reduced by cooling. Joint stiffness is decreased by heat and increased by cold therapy.

ADVERSE EFFECTS OF COLD

There are four major cold hypersensitivity syndromes. They are relatively rare but the sequels may be very damaging. The first reaction is due to histamine release as a result of cold application, which produces headache, malaise, erythema, itching, urticaria, sweating and facial flush, and may lead to vascular shock with syncope.[51] There may be also puffiness around the eyes, laryngeal edema and gastrointestinal upset with hyperacidity and pain. The second group of reactions are due to cold hemolysins and agglutinins. Malaise, chills, and fever may be produced; paroxysmal hemoglobinuria may occur. The skin manifestations would include urticaria and Raynaud's phenomenon. The third group of hypersensitivity reactions occurs in the presence of cryoglobulins. In addition to the already described skin manifestations, ulceration necrosis as part of Raynaud's phenome-non and purpura are more common. There may be gastrointestinal bleeding with epistaxis and conjunctival hemorrhage may be observed. In the most severe cases the syndrome may produce blindness and deafness. General manifestations include chills and fever. Finally, an exaggerated vasopressor response in patients susceptible to hypertensive disease may be observed. These syndromes are most likely to occur in response to reduction of body core temperature or sumbersion of limbs in ice water. Especially vasoconstriction could lead to necrosis of the terminal parts such as fingers and toes as a result of angiospasm.

Most of these syndromes occur in association with skin manifestations. Ice application in a limited area, such as the skin of the thigh or lower back, may reveal the hypersensitivity of the patient prior to the application of more vigorous cryotherapy. Most important, a good medical history and examination may identify cold hypersensitivity.

USE OF HEAT AND COLD IN ARTHRITIDES AND RELATED SYNDROMES

For successful therapeutic application of these modalities, it is essential to remember that they are a valuable adjunct but not a cure. Therefore, the modality should be used in conjunction with other approaches. For successful therapy, it is most important that a diagnosis be made, identifying the pathology to be treated. On this basis a decision should be made whether heat or cold should be applied. A decision has to be made whether vigorous or mild heat effects should be produced. If a vigorous response is desired and heat is the modality of choice, the selection of the specific modality should be made on the basis of the temperature distribution this modality produces. The peak temperature should be produced at the site of the pathology to be treated. Finally, for beneficial results it is a basic prerequisite that adequate equipment and technique of application are used.

Muscle spasm secondary to joint and skeletal pathology. Muscle spasm is often associated with pain. Relaxation of painful muscle spasm can be achieved by either heat or ice application. Heat application can be done by using superficial heating agents such as Hydrocollator packs or the heat cradle for 20–30 minutes (daily or b.i.d.) Also shortwave induction coil applicators can be used for 20–30 minutes (daily or b.i.d.). Muscle spasm can be relaxed by cold application in the form of ice packs. Because the mechanism of spasm relaxation is thought to reduce spindle sensitivity, it is essential that muscle cooling occur. Applications usually should be for at least 10 minutes, often 20–30 minutes.

Back pathology. The therapeutic goal in patients with back pathology irrespective of the underlying cause is often to relieve the painful muscle spasm. Heat and cold application can be used as described above. Landen[56] compared the results of treatment with heat and cold in such cases (Figs. 4-24, 4-25 and 4-26) and found improvement that was essentially equal, irrespective of which modality was used. This is not surprising since the underlying physiologic mechanism is the same in ice and heat application. If short-wave diathermy is used, it is recommended that two induction coil applicators or a large applicator be used to cover the area of the back adequately. Two condenser pads applied side by side parallel to the surface of the skin would also be effective. Additional relief may be achieved by a deep, sedative massage.

Myofibrositic trigger points. So-called myofibrositic trigger points have been also treated with heat and cold, usually in conjunction with some frictional massage. Ultrasound in small dosage, for instance 0.5–1.0 Watts/cm^2, with a total output up to 5–10 watts has been used. Cold is frequently applied with an evaporative cooling spray.[8,30,54,55,109,110,114]

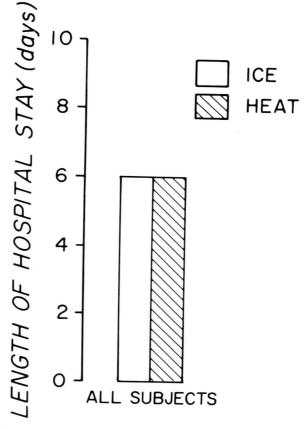

Fig. 4-24. Average days of hospitalization after heat and ice treatment of back pain syndromes. (From Landen BR: Heat or cold for the relief of low back pain? Phys Ther 47:1126–1128, 1967. With permission.)

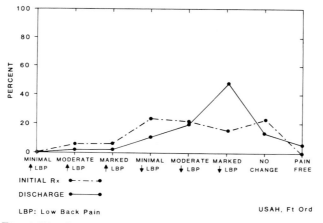

Fig. 4-25. Response of low back pain to treatment with ice. (From Landen BR: Heat or cold for the relief of low back pain? Phys Ther 47:1126–1128, 1967. With permission.)

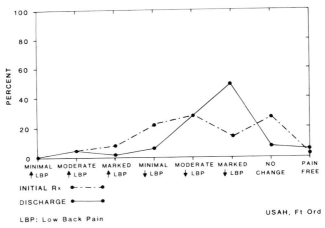

Fig. 4-26. Response of low back pain to treatment with heat.
(From Landen BR: Heat or cold for the relief of low back pain?
Phys Ther 47:1126–1128, 1967. With permission.)

Treatment of delayed muscle soreness as it occurs after vigorous exercise is not improved by ice massage. Yackzan et al[127] found that this symptom is actually aggravated if the treatment is delayed for 24 hours postexercise. A reduced range of motion was associated with this aggravation.

Joint contractures. The limitation of the range of motion may have various causes. It may be due to a burned-out rheumatic process, degenerative joint disease, trauma, or prolonged immobilization. Joint contractures are often due to a shortening of fibrous tissues resulting from scarring of the synovium, the joint capsule, the ligaments, and other periarticular structures. Immobilization may be a cause of limited joint range because connective tissue adapts to the length in which it is placed on a long-term basis. The objective of the treatment of this chronic condition is to selectively raise the temperature to maximally tolerated levels in the connective (collagen) tissues limiting the joint motion. The modality of choice for heating these structures selectively is ultrasound applied with stroking technique. Using multiple field application is necessary. The hip and the shoulder, as examples, are treated with three fields applied anteriorly, laterally, and posteriorly. Each field is exposed for about 5–10 minutes with ultrasonic intensities up to 3–4 Watts/cm^2 with a total output of approximately 30–40 watts.[60,61,80] Treatment should be in conjunction with stretching and other joint mobilization techniques. Mobilization techniques should be applied either during or immediately after the heating. There has been evidence that this procedure worked in a clinical controlled trial of elderly patients with hip fractures with surgical fixation with Richards screws. Both groups of patients received the same range of motion exercise program. The group that received radiant heat prior to this program served as a control for the ultrasonic group. The group treated with ultrasound had greater range of motion and ambulation capability (Table 4-4).[70]

Shortwave diathermy can be effectively used only in joints with little soft tissue cover. Elbows and knees can be heated by shortwave diathermy induction coil applicators if ultrasound is not available. Wakim et al[118] showed that the knee joint temperature could be elevated with shortwave diathermy application.

Table 4-4

Change in Range of Motion Produced by Ultrasound and Infrared Radiation after One Week of Treatment

	N	Ultrasound Mean Change	t*	P	N	Infrared Mean Change	t*	P
Hip								
Flexion	15	21.67	8.360	0.01	15	5.40	1.772	0.10
Extension	15	10.40	4.746	0.01	15	−3.20**	1.555	0.20
Abduction	15	6.33	3.201	0.01	15	−1.67**	1.116	0.30
Adduction	15	9.67	5.484	0.01	15	−1.20**	0.748	0.50
External rotation	14	12.86	5.872	0.01	15	0.20	0.094	0.99
Internal rotation	14	10.93	5.187	0.01	15	−1.60**	0.680	0.60
Knee								
Flexion	15	18.33	4.604	0.01	15	10.33	2.906	0.02
Extension	15	3.60	3.454	0.01	15	−3.47**	2.706	0.02

From Lehmann JF et al: Clinical evaluation of a new approach in the treatment of contracture associated with hip fracture after internal fixation. Arch Phys Med Rehabil 42:95–100, 1961. With permission.

*All t tests based on the differences between pre-treatment ROM and ROM after one week of treatment, using the matched pairs method.

**When the mean is expressed as a negative value, range of motion has been lost during treatment.

Degenerative joint disease (DJD). If joint contracture is due to degenerative changes where bony spurs interfere with motion, any form of heat therapy including ultrasound will be ineffective. Soft tissue contractures resulting from DJD should be treated as described above. In degenerative joint disease of the hands, as in Heberden's nodes, acute symptomatology should be treated with mild superficial heat such as radiant heat for 20 minutes or by using paraffin bath with the dip method, followed by deep sedative massage and mild range of motion exercises.

In the chronic phase, with stiffness as a leading symptom, contrast bath can be used in addition.

Rheumatoid arthritis. In the presence of acute or subacute inflammatory synovitis, vigorous heating of the joint and its synovium is contraindicated. However, superficial heat application with the heat lamp or heat cradle can help to relieve secondary muscle spasm and stiffness[3,125,126] and perhaps reflexly lower the elevated joint temperature.

Hydrotherapy in the form of Hubbard tank or whirlpool bath has the advantage of providing mild superficial heat, which reduces stiffness. In addition, the buoyancy of the water minimizes stress on the joints, and allows more comfortable range of motion exercises. Hand and foot stiffness, which is often encountered in chronic cases, can be alleviated by the contrast bath or by the mild paraffin wax application using the dip method. Fluidotherapy may also be helpful.

Ice application to acutely involved joints is controversial. There is a clinical impression that ice may relieve pain and therefore may make range of motion exercises more comfortable. Yet there is objective evidence that joint stiffness is increased.[3,125,126] Clinical studies supported by quantitative measurements and controls are not available.[101]

Ankylosing spondylitis. In ankylosing spondylitis, patients often complain of upper and lower back pain and stiffness. The motion of the spine and the costovertebral joints is often restricted leading to a reduced vital capacity. It has been shown that in the chronic stage, ultrasound applied to the facet joints of the vertebral column and to the costovertebral joints in combination with deep breathing exercises reduced pain and increased chest expansion and vital capacity.[47] This type of therapy is advantageous because it can be repeated frequently without any cumulative untoward side effects. It should not be used in the acute stages of the inflammatory process. It should be used in conjunction with a complete regimen including antiinflammatory agents, postural instructions, and exercise. Alternate methods are the hot tub bath or Hubbard tank; or the heat lamp or heat cradle, followed by deep sedative massage. The expectation is primarily a relief of pain. There is no evidence that the natural history of the process is significantly altered.

Periarthritis of the shoulder. The associated limitation of range of motion is the result of tightness of the joint capsule and periarticular structures. In the acute phase, when there is an extreme tenderness and a significant inflammatory component, ice packs or ice massage are the modality of choice.

After the resolution of the acute phase, mild superficial heat is an acceptable alternative. This type of treatment should be used in conjunction with antiinflammatory drugs and appropriate exercises, ie, Codman's exercises, at the early stages. At the later stages where the acute reaction has subsided but the painful shoulder with severe joint limitation persists, ultrasound is the modality of choice to selectively raise the temperature in the contracted capsular tissues. Three fields of application are used: anterior, lateral, and posterior. Stretch and joint mobilization techniques should be used at the same time[87] or at least immediately after the treatment. In a controlled study it was shown that ultrasound therapy is superior to other modalities if used in conjunction with the proper joint mobilization techniques.[69] Patients were assigned to two groups: one received ultrasound and the other received microwave. Both received the same type of exercise program. The duration from onset to treatment was the same in both groups, as was the age and sex distribution, and the range of shoulder rotation, flexion, and abduction. After treatment the gain in range of motion was significantly greater with ultrasound, which selectively heats the joint and periarticular structures, as compared with microwaves which heats only musculature and may relieve secondary muscle spasm (Table 4-5).

Reflex sympathetic dystrophy, shoulder-hand syndrome including Sudeck's atrophy. The pain and joint stiffness can be treated with the same method as described above for the management of joint contractures. If sympathetic blocks are used in con-

Table 4-5

Gain in Range of Motion after Ultrasonic and Microwave Treatment

	After treatment with			
Gain in	Ultrasound		Microwaves	
Forward flexion	27.4°	±2.3°*	16.1°	±1.5°*
Abduction	32.6°	±2.5°*	21.2°	±2.1°*
Rotation	45.4°	±2.8°*	17.3°	±4.0°*

From Lehmann JF et al: Comparison of ultrasonic and microwave diathermy in the physical treatment of periarthritis of the shoulder. Arch Phys Med Rehabil 35:627-634, 1954. With permission.
*Standard error of the mean.

junction with this type of therapy, it seems to be advantageous to apply the physical therapy while the stellate ganglion block is still effective.

Subacromial bursitis. In the acute stages of subacromial bursitis with an associated acute inflammatory reaction, ultrasound should not be used. The selective rise of temperature at the bursa would aggravate the inflammatory reaction and associated hyperemia and exudate acutely increasing the pain. The pain can be relieved by inserting a needle in the bursa and removing content that relieves the painful pressure. In addition, hydrocortisone, often in combination with a local anesthetic, is injected. Ice application is used as an adjunct. At the later stage, the condition would be best treated with mild heat application and a proper exercise program to prevent tightening of the capsule of the glenohumeral joint. The presence of calcium deposit in the bursa is not an indication for ultrasound since it spontaneously resolves at the same rate whether ultrasound is used or not. If the deposit is large, impinging upon the acromion and limiting motion, it should be surgically removed. Any associated stiffness of the shoulder joint should be treated as was described under periarthritis.

Bursitis. Bursitis in other locations such as over the greater trochanter of the femur, over the patella, or at the junction of the patellar tendon with the tibial tuberosity should be treated like the subacromial bursitis. In most of these cases, however, range of motion exercises are less crucial. In all bursitis, local therapy is commonly combined with local or systemic application of antiinflammatory agents.

Frozen shoulder. After surgical manipulation of a frozen shoulder it is most important that physical therapy in the form of ice packs and active assistive range of motion exercises be done shortly after the patient comes out of anesthesia. This is essential to maintain the gain of range of motion in the presence of the trauma caused by the manipulation. Ice is extremely helpful because it reduces pain, but medication should be used as well. Also during rest, positioning of the shoulder in different attitudes is important. As soon as the acute phase has subsided, mild superficial heat such as infrared should be used in conjunction with the exercise program, which now should include Codman's exercises. Ultrasound may be indicated later since there is a tendency of the capsule to bind down. Judgment has to be used as to how much stretch or to which degree joint mobilization techniques should be used in conjunction with this type of therapy.

Dupuytren's contractures. The disease is a contracture of the palmar fascia. The nonsurgical treatment of this fibrous contracture consists of ultrasound application. Ultrasound is the modality of choice to be used in combination with stretching since it selectively heats the contracted tissues. Intensities of 0.5–1.5 W/cm^2 with a total output of 5–15 watts are used with stroking technique. Vigorous heating should be achieved. Water at close to normal body temperature is used as a coupling medium. Stretch at the same time or immediately after sonation is used. It is essential to check on the success of the program by periodic measurements. More severe contractures of this type usually require first surgical excision.

Epicondylitis. This condition usually involves the common tendon of origin of the wrist and finger extensors at the lateral epicondyle of the humerus. There is an inflammatory reaction in the acute stage and therefore treatment should be primarily that of rest and splinting, combined with ice application. Also, antiinflammatory agents are used in conjunction with this therapy. It may include injection of local anesthetic and hydrocortisone. If pain persists in the subchronic stage, mild superficial heat application or mild shortwave diathermy administration could be tried. In the chronic stage or in case of frequent recurrences, ultrasound may be used since it selectively raises the temperature of the common tendon of origin and the extensor aponeurosis. Application should always be in small doses such as 0.5 W/cm^2 at a total output of about 5 watts with stroking technique for 5–10 minutes. Ultrasound is contraindicated in the acute stage.

Skin contractures.   These contractures as they occur in scleroderma frequently first involve the interphalangeal and metacarpohalangeal joints. They can be treated with ultrasound with subsequent joint mobilization techniques, range-of-motion exercises and stretching. The ultrasonic output should be relatively low starting with no more than 0.5 W/cm^2 with a total output of 5 watts. Application is usually done in the waterbath that is approximately body temperature. To assess success, as in all other therapies, it is essential to periodically measure the range of motion. In the absence of improvement, the management should be reviewed and if indicated therapy should be altered or discontinued. Clinical observation suggests that frequently even the sores or small necroses that develop at the tips of the fingers may heal under this regimen. The ultimate course of the disease is not altered. An alternate method of treatment of this condition is the use of paraffin bath with either dip or immersion method. Also treatment with shortwave diathermy or microwaves could be tried.

Raynaud's disease.   The digital arteries respond excessively to vasospastic stimuli in this condition and produce the characteristic bilateral symmetrical blanching and cyanosis of the skin of the digits followed by redness. The changes are usually precipitated by cold exposure and relieved by warmth. Abnormalities of the sympathetic nervous system seem to play a role. Ultrasound application has been advocated[13] locally and to the sympathetics in an attempt to reduce the manifestation of the disease. More controlled clinical investigations will be necessary. The treatment for Raynaud's phenomenon is similar.

Minor trauma.   The typical representative of this group of conditions is the ankle sprain. There is evidence that swelling is reduced if ice and compression are applied early.[94] Basur et al[5] found that the return to work occurred in a higher percentage of cases earlier after the injury (Fig. 4-27) when ice application and compression were used than when a compression bandage was used alone.[97] In practice, it is essential that ice and pressure be applied early to prevent bleeding and edema formation. Ice also reduces pain. It is important to realize that application of ice beyond the time when it is essential to prevent bleeding and edema formation retards healing as shown in experiments by Lundgren et al.[85] The measured tensile strength of an incision scar was significantly less if healing occurred at lower temperatures. Later when the primary goal is resolution and mobilization, superficial heat in conjunction with an active assistive range of motion exercise may be applied using a whirlpool bath or heat lamp. In case of later contractures, ultrasound can be used in the same fashion as described for periarthritis of the shoulder. Ice also reduces torsional laxity of the knee after exercise and running.[113] It is interesting to note that also ultrasound has the same measurable effect.[11]

Temporomandibular joint.   The causes of temporomandibular joint dysfunction and pain syndrome are multiple and may include arthritides, malocclusion, tooth infection,

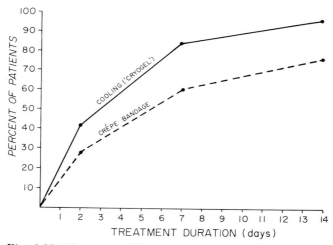

Fig. 4-27. Percentage of patients with ankle sprain returning to full activity, plotted against time from onset. (From Basur RL et al: A cooling method in the treatment of ankle sprains. Practitioner 216:708–711, 1976. With permission.)

and physiologic factors. Conditions such as malocclusion and tooth infection should be corrected first. In addition, ultrasound in relatively small dosage, ie, 0.5 W/cm²–1.5 W/cm² and a total output of 5–15 watts should be used in conjunction with range of motion, stretching, relaxation techniques and other physical therapy techniques.[52,123]

Summary statement. In summary, understanding of the physiological mechanism by which heat and cold therapy are effective allows the selection of the correct modality, the proper equipment and technique of application. A number of the indications thus evolved have also been confirmed by clinical studies. The preceding examples may serve as a guide for the appropriate use of these modalities which must be used in conjunction with other therapeutic approaches.

ACKNOWLEDGMENT

This chapter is in part based on research supported by research grant G008300076 from the National Institute of Handicapped Research, Department of Education, Washington, DC 20202.

REFERENCES

1. Abramson DI, Bell Y, Rejal H, et al: Changes in blood flow, oxygen uptake and tissue temperatures produced by therapeutic physical agents. II. Effect of short-wave diathermy. Am J Phys Med 39:87–95, 1960

2. Abramson DI, Bell Y, Tuck S Jr, et al: Changes in blood flow, oxygen uptake and tissue temperatures produced by therapeutic physical agents.

III. Effect of indirect or reflex vasodilatation. Am J Phys Med 40:5–13, 1961

3. Bäcklund L, Tiselius P: Objective measurement of joint stiffness in rheumatoid arthritis. Acta Rheum Scand 13:275–288, 1967

4. Barth G, Bülow HA: Zur Frage der Ultraschallschädigung jugendlicher Knochen. Strahlentherapie 79:271–280, 1949

5. Basur RL, Shephard E, Mouzas GL: A cooling method in the treatment of ankle sprains. Practitioner 216:707–711, 1976

6. Benson TB, Copp EP: The effects of therapeutic forms of heat and ice on the pain threshold of the normal shoulder. Rheumatol Rehab 13:101–104, 1974

7. Bisgard JD, Nye D: The influence of hot and cold application upon gastric and intestinal motor activity. Surg Gynecol Obstet 71:172–180, 1940

8. Bonica JJ: Management of myofascial pain syndromes in general practice. JAMA 164:732,1957

9. Borrell RM, Henley EJ, Ho P, et al: Fluidotherapy: evaluation of a new heat modality. Arch Phys Med Rehabil 58:69–71, 1977

10. Borrell RM, Parker R, Henley EJ, et al: Comparison of in vivo temperatures produced by hydrotherapy, paraffin wax treatment, and Fluidotherapy. Phys Ther 60:1273–1276, 1980

11. Brody DM: Running injuries. CIBA Clinical Symposia 32:1–36, 1980

12. Brown AM: Physical medicine in athletic rehabilitation. Maryland Med J 19:61–64, 1970

13. Buchtala V: The present state of ultrasonic therapy. Br J Phys Med 15:3–6 passim, 1952

14. Carstensen El, Li K, Schwan HP: Determination of the acoustic properties of blood and its components. J Acoust Soc Am 25:286–289, 1953

15. Castor CW, Yaron M: Connective tissue activation. VIII. The effects of temperature studied in vitro. Arch Phys Med Rehabil 57:5–9, 1976

16. Chan AK, Sigelmann RA, Guy AW: Calculations of therapeutic heat generated by ultrasound in fat-muscle-bone layers. IEEE Trans Biomed Eng BME-21:280–284, 1973

17. Code of Federal Regulations, Title 21—Food and Drugs, Chapter 1—Food and Drug Administration, Part 890—Physical medicine devices. U.S. Government Printing Office, Washington, D.C., 1984

18. Code of Federal Regulations, Title 27—Telecommunication, Chapter I—Federal Communications Commission, Part 2—Frequency allocations and radio treaty matters; general rules and regulations. U.S. Government Printing Office, Washington, D.C., 1984

19. de Jong RH, Hershey WN, Wagman IH: Nerve conduction velocity during hypothermia in man. Anesthesiology 27:805–810, 1966

20. de Lateur BJ, Lehmann JF, Stonebridge JB, et al: Muscle heating in human subjects with 915 MHz. microwave contact applicator. Arch Phys Med Rehabil 51:147–151, 1970

21. Dietzel F, Kern W: Kann hohes mütterliches Fieber Missbildungen beim Kind auslösen? Geburtshilfe und Frauenheilkund 31:1074–1079, 1971

22. Dietzel F, Kern W, Steckenmesser R: Missbildungen und intrauterines Absterben nach Kurzwellenbehandlung in der Frühschwangerschaft. Münch med Wochenschr 114:228–230, 1972

23. Douglas WW, Malcolm JL: The effect of localized cooling on conduction in cat nerves. J Physiol 130:53–71, 1955

24. Edwards MJ: Congenital defects in guinea pigs. Arch Path 84:42–48, 1967

25. Edwards MJ: Influenza, hyperthermia, and congenital malformation. Lancet 1:320–321, 1972

26. Edwards MJ, Mulley R, Ring S, et al: Mitotic cell death and delay of mitotic activity in guinea-pig embryos following brief maternal hyperthermia. J Embryol exp Morph 32:593–602, 1974

27. Eldred E, Lindsley DF, Buchwald JS: The effect of cooling on mammalian muscle spindles. Exp Neurol 2:144–157, 1960

28. Fenn JE: Effect of pulsed electromagnetic energy (Diapulse) on experimental hematomas. Canad Med Assoc J 100:251–254, 1969

29. Fine SD: Microwave diathermy equipment. Federal Register 40:23877–23878, 1975

30. Fischer AA: Diagnosis and management of chronic pain in physical medicine and rehabilitation, in Ruskin AP (ed): Current Therapy in Physiatry, Philadelphia, WB Saunders, pp 84–101, 1984

31. Fischer E, Solomon S: Physiological responses to heat and cold, in Licht S (ed): Therapeutic Heat and Cold, second ed., Baltimore, Waverly Press, pp 126–169, 1965

32. Ghietti A: Embriopatia da onde corte. Minerva Nipiologica 5:7–12, 1955

33. Goldman JA, Chiapella J, Casey H, et al: Laser therapy of rheumatoid arthritis. Lasers in Surg Med 1:93–101, 1980

34. Goldman L (ed): The Biological Laser: Technology and Clinical Applications, New York, Springer-Verlag, 1981

35. Güttner W: Die Energieverteilung im menschlichen Körper bei Ultraschall-Einstrahlung. Acustica 4:547–554, 1954

36. Guy AW, Lin JC, Kramar PO, et al: Effect of 2450-MHz radiation on the rabbit eye. IEEE Trans Microwave Theory & Tech MTT-23:492–498, 1975

37. Haina D, Brunner R, Landthaler M, et al: Animal experiments on light-induced woundhealing. Laser in Biomedical Research (IV) 22-1—22-3, 1977

38. Hamburger S, Logue JN, Silverman PM: Occupational exposure to non-ionizing radiation and an association with heart disease: an exploratory study. J Chronic Disease 36:791–802, 1983

39. Harris ED Jr, Krane SM: Cartilage collagen:

substrate in soluble and fibrillar form for rheumatoid collagenase. Trans Assoc Am Phys 86: 82–94, 1973

40. Harris ED Jr, McCroskery PA: The influence of temperature and fibril stability on degradation of cartilage collagen by rheumatoid synovial collagenase. N Engl J Med 290:1–6, 1974

41. Harris R: Effect of short wave diathermy on radio-sodium clearance from the knee joint in the normal and in rheumatoid arthritis. Arch Phys Med Rehabil 42:241–249, 1961

42. Harris R: Physical methods in the management of rheumatoid arthritis. Med Clin North Am 52:707–716, 1968

43. Hartviksen K: Ice therapy in spasticity. Acta neurol Scand 38 (suppl 3): 79–84, 1962

44. Harvey MAS, McRorie MM, Smith DW: Suggested limits to the use of the hot tub and sauna by pregnant women. Canad Med Assoc J 125:50–53, 1981

45. Hayashi S: Der Einfluss der u.S.W. bzw. u.u.K.W. auf den maligen Tumor. Japan J Med Sci, III. Biophysics 6:138*, 1940

46. Hendrickx AG, Stone GW, Henrickson RV, et al: Teratogenic effects of hyperthermia in the bonnet monkey (Macaca radiata). Teratology 19: 177–182, 1979

47. Hintzelmann U: Ultraschalltherapie rheumatischer Erkrankungen. Deutsch med Wochenschr 74:869–870, 1949

48. Horvath SM, Hollander JL: Intra-articular temperature as a measure of joint reaction. J Clin Invest 28:469–473, 1949

49. Hunter J, Kerr EH, Whillans MG: The relation between joint stiffness upon exposure to cold and the characteristics of synovial fluid. Canad J Med Sci 30:367–377, 1952

50. Hustler JE, Zarod AP, Williams AR: Ultrasonic modification of experimental bruising in the guinea-pig pinna. Ultrasonics 16:223–228, 1978

51. Juhlin L, Shelley WB: Role of mast cell and basophil in cold urticaria with associated systemic reactions. JAMA 177:371–377, 1961

52. Kessler RM, Hertling D: Management of Common Musculoskeletal Disorders. New York, Harper and Row, 1983

53. Knutsson E, Mattsson E: Effects of local cooling on monosynaptic reflexes in man. Scand J Rehabil Med 1:126–132, 1969

54. Kraus H: Clinical Treatment of Back and Neck Pain, New York, McGraw Hill, pp 112–126, 1970

55. Kraus H: Treatment of myofascial pain, in Ruskin AP (ed): Current Therapy in Physiatry, Philadelphia, WB Saunders, pp 143–161, 1984

56. Landen BR: Heat or cold for the relief of low back pain? Phys Ther 47:1126–1128, 1967

57. Lehmann JF: Diathermy, in Krusen FH, Kottke FJ, Ellwood PM Jr (eds): Handbook of Physical Medicine and Rehabilitation, Second Edition. Philadelphia, Saunders, pp 224–327, 1965

58. Lehmann JF: The biophysical basis of biologic ultrasonic reactions with special reference to ultrasonic therapy. Arch Phys Med Rehabil 34:139–152, 1953

59. Lehmann JF, Brunner GD, Martinis AJ, et al: Ultrasonic effect as demonstrated in live pigs with surgical metallic implants. Arch Phys Med Rehabil 40:483–488, 1959

60. Lehmann JF, Brunner GD, McMillan JA: Influence of surgical metal implants on the temperature distribution in thigh specimens exposed to ultrasound. Arch Phys Med Rehabil 39:692–695, 1958

61. Lehmann JF, Brunner GD, Stow RW: Pain threshold measurements after therapeutic application of ultrasound, microwaves and infrared. Arch Phys Med Rehabil 39:560–565, 1958

62. Lehmann JF, de Lateur BJ: Cryotherapy, in Lehmann JF (ed): Therapeutic Heat and Cold, third edition, Baltimore, Williams & Wilkins, pp 563–602, 1982

63. Lehmann JF, de Lateur BJ: Diathermy and superficial heat and cold therapy, in Kottke FJ, Stillwell GK, Lehmann JF (eds): Krusen's Handbook of Physical Medicine and Rehabilitation, third edition, Philadelphia, Saunders, pp 275–350, 1982

64. Lehmann JF, de Lateur BJ: Therapeutic heat, in Lehmann JF (ed): Therapeutic Heat and Cold, third edition, Baltimore, Williams & Wilkins, pp 404–562, 1982

65. Lehmann JF, de Lateur BJ: Ultrasound, short-wave, microwave: superficial heat and cold in the treatment of pain, in Wall PD, Melzack R (eds), Textbook of Pain, New York, Churchill Livingstone, pp 254–273, 1984

66. Lehmann JF, de Lateur BJ, Stonebridge JB: Selective muscle heating by shortwave diathermy with a helical coil. Arch Phys Med Rehabil 50:117–123, 1969

67. Lehmann JF, de Lateur BJ, Stonebridge JB, et al: Therapeutic temperature distribution produced by ultrasound as modified by dosage and volume of tissue exposed. Arch Phys Med Rehabil 48:662–666, 1967

68. Lehmann JF, Dundore DE, Esselman PC, et al: Microwave diathermy: effects on experimental muscle hematoma resolution. Arch Phys Med Rehabil 64:127–129, 1983

69. Lehmann JF, Erickson DJ, Martin GM, et al: Comparison of ultrasonic and microwave diathermy in the physical treatment of periarthritis of the shoulder. Arch Phys Med Rehabil 35:627–634, 1954

70. Lehmann JF, Fordyce WE, Rathbun LA, et al: Clinical evaluation of a new approach in the treatment of contracture associated with hip fracture after internal fixation. Arch Phys Med Rehabil 42:95–100, 1961

71. Lehmann JF, Guy AW: Ultrasound therapy, in Reid JM, Sikov MR (eds): Interaction of Ultrasound and Biological Tissues; proceedings of a workshop held at Battelle Seattle Research Center, Seattle, Washington, November 8–11, 1971, DHEW Publication (FDA) 73-8008

72. Lehmann JF, Guy AW, Johnston VC, et al: Comparison of relative heating patterns produced in tissues by exposure to microwave energy at frequencies of 2,450 and 900 megacycles. Arch Phys Med Rehabil 43:69–76, 1962

73. Lehmann JF, Guy AW, Stonebridge JB, et al: Evaluation of a therapeutic direct-contact 915-MHz microwave applicator for effective deep-tissue heating in humans. IEEE Trans Microwave Theory & Tech MTT-26:556–563, 1978

74. Lehmann JF, Herrick JF: Biologic reactions to cavitation, a consideration for ultrasonic therapy. Arch Phys Med Rehabil 34:86–98, 1953

75. Lehmann JF, Herrick JF, Krusen FH: The effects of ultrasound on chromosomes, nuclei and other structures of the cells in plant tissues. Arch Phys Med Rehabil 35:141–148, 1954

76. Lehmann JF, Johnson EW: Some factors influencing the temperature distribution in thighs exposed to ultrasound. Arch Phys Med Rehabil 39:347–356, 1958

77. Lehmann JF, Masock AJ, Warren CG, et al: Effect of therapeutic temperatures on tendon extensibility. Arch Phys Med Rehabil 51:481–487, 1970

78. Lehmann JF, McDougall JA, Guy AW, et al: Electrical discontinuity of tissue substitute models at 27.12 MHz. Bioelectromagnetics 4:257–265, 1983

79. Lehmann JF, McDougall JA, Guy AW, et al: Heating patterns produced by shortwave diathermy applicators in tissue substitute models. Arch Phys Med Rehabil 64:575–577, 1983

80. Lehmann JF, McMillan JA, Brunner GD, et al: Comparative study of the efficiency of shortwave, microwave and ultrasonic diathermy in heating the hip joint. Arch Phys Med Rehabil 40:510–512, 1959

81. Lehmann JF, Silverman DR, Baum BA, et al: Temperature distributions in the human thigh, produced by infrared, hot pack and microwave applications. Arch Phys Med Rehabil 47:291–299, 1966

82. Lehmann JF, Stonebridge JB, Guy AW: A comparison of patterns of stray radiation from therapeutic microwave applicators measured near tissue-substitute models and human subjects. Radio Science 14:271–283, 1979

83. Lehmann JF, Stonebridge JB, Wallace JE, et al: Microwave therapy: stray radiation, safety and effectiveness. Arch Phys Med Rehabil 60:578–584, 1979

84. Lippold OCJ, Nicholls JG, Redfearn JWT: A study of the afferent discharge produced by cooling a mammalian muscle spindle. J Physiol 153:218–231, 1960

85. Lundgren C, Muren A, Zederfeldt B: Effect of cold-vasoconstriction on wound healing in the rabbit. Acta chir scand 118:1–4, 1959

86. Martin GM, Roth GM, Elkins EC, et al: Cutaneous temperature of the extremities of normal subjects and of patients with rheumatoid arthritis. Arch Phys Med 27:665–682, 1946

87. McGee M, Freshman S: Ultrasound and stretch: a decreased range of motion. A slide-tape presentation. Health Sciences Learning Resources Center, University of Washington, 1978

88. Melzack R, Wall PD: Pain mechanisms: a new theory. Science 150:971–979, 1965

89. Mense S: Effects of temperature on the discharges of muscle spindles and tendon organs. Pflügers Arch 374:159–166, 1978

90. Menser M: Does hyperthermia affect the human fetus? Med J Australia 2:550, 1978

91. Mester E, Toth N, Mester A: The biostimulative effect of laserbeam. Laster in Biomed Res (IV) 22-4–22-7, 1977

92. Michaelson SM: Bioeffects of high frequency currents and electromagnetic radiation, in Lehmann JF (ed): Therapeutic Heat and Cold, third edition, Baltimore, Williams & Wilkins, pp 278–352, 1982

93. Moayer M: Die morphologischen Veränderunger der Plazenta unter dem Einfluss der Kurzwellendurchflutung. Tierexperimentelle Untersuchungen. Strahlentherapie 142:609–614, 1971

94. Moore CD, Cardea JA. Vascular changes in leg trauma. South Med J 70:1285–1286 passim, 1977

95. Mussa B: Embriopatie da cause fisiche. Mineva Nipiologica 5:69–72, 1955

96. Nielsen NC, Hansen R, Larsen T: Heat induction in copper-bearing IUD's during short-wave diathermy. Acta Obstet Gynecol Scand 58:495, 1979

97. Nilsson S: Sprains of the lateral ankle ligaments. Part II. A controlled trial of different forms of conservative treatment. J Oslo City Hosp 33:13–36, 1983

98. Ottoson D: The effects of temperature on the isolated muscle spindle. J Physiol 180:636–648, 1965

99. Parsons CM, Goetzl FR: Effect of induced pain on pain threshold. Proc Soc Exp Biol Med 60:327–329, 1945

100. Pasila M, Visuri T, Sundhold A: Pulsating shortwave diathermy: valuable in treatment of recent ankle and foot sprains. Arch Phys Med Rehabil 59:383–386, 1978

101. Pegg SMH, Littler TR, Littler EN: A trial of ice therapy and exercise in chronic arthritis. Physiotherapy 55:51–56, 1969

102. Perkins JF Jr, Li M-C, Hoffman F, et al: Sudden vasoconstriction in denervated or sympathectomized paws exposed to cold. Am J Physiol 155:165–178, 1948

103. Piersol GM, Schwan HP, Pennell RB, et al: Mechanism of absorption of ultrasonic energy in blood. Arch Phys Med 33:327–332, 1952

104. Schwan HP, Carstensen EL, Li K: Electric and ultrasonic deep heating diathermy. Electronics 27(March):172–175, 1954

105. Scott BO: Effects of contact lenses on shortwave field distribution. Br J Ophthal 40:696–697, 1956

106. Sekins KM, Dundore D, Emery AF, et al: Muscle blood flow changes in response to 915 MHz diathermy with surface cooling as measured by Xe^{133} clearance. Arch Phys Med Rehabil 61:105–113, 1980

107. Sekins KM, Emergy AF, Lehmann JF, et al: Determination of perfusion field during local hyperthermia with the aid of finite element thermal models. J Biomech Eng 104:272–279, 1982

108. Sekins KM, Lehmann JF, Esselman P, et al: Local muscle blood flow and temperature responses to 915 MHz diathermy as simultaneously measured and numerically predicted. Arch Phys Med Rehabil 65:1–7, 1984

109. Simons DG: Muscle pain syndromes—part I. Am J Phys Med 54:289–311, 1975

110. Simons DG: Muscle pain syndromes—part II. Am J Phys Med 55:15–42, 1976

111. Smith DW, Clarren SK, Harvey MAS: Hyperthermia as a possible teratogenic agent. J Pediatr 92:878–883, 1978

112. Stillwell GK: General principles of thermotherapy, in Licht S (ed): Therapeutic Heat and Cold, second edition. Baltimore, Waverly Press, pp 232–239, 1965

113. Stoller DW, Markolf KL, Zager SA, et al: The effects of exercise, ice and ultrasonography on torsional laxity of the knee. Clin Orth Rel Res (174):172–180, 1983

114. Travell J, Rinzler SH: Pain syndromes of the chest muscles: resemblance to effort angina and myocardial infarction, and relief by local block. Can Med Assoc J 59:333–338, 1948

115. Urbscheit N, Bishop B: Effects of cooling on the ankle jerk and H-response. Phys Ther 50:1041–1049, 1970

116. Vanharanta H, Eronen I, Videman T: Effect of ultrasound on glycosaminoglycan metabolism in the rabbit knee. Am J Phys Med 61:221–228, 1982

117. Vaughen JL, Bender LF: Effects of ultrasound on growing bone. Arch Phys Med Rehabil 40:158–160, 1959

118. Wakim KG, Porter AN, Krusen FH: Influence of physical agents and of certain drugs on intraarticular temperature. Arch Phys Med 32:714–721, 1951

119. Wall PD, Melzack R: Textbook of Pain, New York, Churchill Livingstone, 1984

120. Warren CG, Koblanski JN, Sigelmann RA: Ultrasound coupling media: their relative transmissivity. Arch Phys Med Rehabil 57:218–222, 1976

121. Warren CG, Lehmann JF, Koblanski JN: Elongation of rat tail tendon: effect of load and temperature. Arch Phys Med Rehabil 52: 465–475, 1971

122. Weidenbacker RA, Smith C: Does heat cause relaxation? Phys Ther Rev 40:261–265, 1960

123. Wienberg LA: The etiology, diagnosis, and treatment of TMJ dysfunction-pain syndrome. Part III: Treatment. J Prosth Dent 43:186–196, 1980

124. Woodmansey A, Collins DH, Ernst MM: Vascular reactions to the contrast bath in health and in rheumatoid arthritis. Lancet 2:1350–1353, 1938

125. Wright V, Johns RJ: Physical factors concerned with the stiffness of normal and diseased joints. Bull Johns Hopkins Hosp 106:215–231, 1960

126. Wright V, Johns RJ: Quantitative and qualtitative analysis of joint stiffness in normal subjects and in patients with connective tissue diseases. Ann rheum Dis 20:36–46, 1961

127. Yackzan L, Adams C, Francis KT: The effects of ice massage on delayed muscle soreness. Am J Sports Med 12:159–164, 1984

John B. Redford

5

Orthotics

Orthotics, a term describing the development, manufacture, and application of splints and braces, is a relatively new one but its practice is very old. Splints and braces have been used since antiquity for orthopedic conditions. What is new is the wide variety of materials available, the novel designs based on biomechanical principles, and the introduction of many more modular or prefabricated types.

An orthosis is generally considered a device that is attached or applied to an external surface of the body, but the field of orthotics also encompasses other equipment such as adaptive seating and provision of various assistive devices, which are described in another chapter. Therefore, the orthotist must work closely with the physician and therapist to meet the problems of the patient with musculoskeletal problems. Ideally, for more complex rehabilitation problems, the physician determines the need for the orthosis or appliance. The physician then discusses it with the patient, the orthotist, and the therapist or nurse. The orthotist makes recommendations about materials and manufacture and the nurse or therapist ensures the orthosis is worn and the patient is trained to use it. After the orthosis is supplied, the physician should review its effectiveness in meeting the problem. In rehabilitation units, therapists often determine the need for orthoses by evaluating functional problems, sometimes using temporary devices, then they can recommend to the physician the best devices to prescribe. In many cases, therapists may actually make the orthosis; for example, hand orthoses for arthritic patients and those recovering from hand surgery are more usually made by occupational therapists than orthotists.[13]

ORTHOSES: GENERAL CONSIDERATIONS

Indications for orthoses include one or more of the following: (1) relief of pain, (2) protection of weak or healing musculoskeletal segments, (3) prevention of correction of deformities, and (4) functional improvement. For musculoskeletal disorders, relief of pain is often a primary consideration; for example, reducing the motion aggravating a painful wrist by a rigid resting splint or unloading a painful joint in the lower extremity through an ischial weight bearing orthosis. Protection of weak or healing segments is well illus-

PRINCIPLES OF PHYSICAL MEDICINE AND REHABILITATION
IN THE MUSCULOSKELETAL DISEASES

103

trated by fracture bracing. Such braces are lighter than casts and lessen the chances of adjacent joints stiffening after fracture because they encourage mobility in the uninvolved segments. Prevention and correction of deformity is shown best in the use of orthotics in children. Lack of balanced muscle pull or uneven resistance to gravitational forces can deform the limb or the spine of a child more readily than in an adult. Orthopedics literally means "straightening the child" and that is exactly what many orthoses such as those used in scoliosis, like the Milwaukee brace, are designed to do. Close supervision of the forces involved and the compliance of the child when wearing such braces is essential for successful use. Family counseling and involvement is also absolutely necessary if such orthoses are to be used effectively.

Orthoses for prevention of deformity are much easier to design and use than those made for correction. Correction usually requires either applying dynamic force such as a spring or elastic band or serial casting used to reduce a knee flexion contracture.

In a sense, all orthoses are designed to improve function by reducing pain, relieving weight bearing, or correcting deformity. Some orthoses, however, have functional improvement as their primary purpose—for example, the balanced forearm orthosis or ball bearing feeder. This consists of a trough to support the forearm and a series of levers providing free elbow and shoulder motion so that with gravity assistance, the patient with a paralyzed shoulder and elbow can touch his face or reach a table (See Fig. 5-1).

Consistent terminology has been a serious problem for orthotics. Over the years, many orthoses have been named after the original creator; for example, the Taylor brace, a spinal orthosis; its name tells nothing about the function or location of the device. The approved method of naming orthoses today advocated by the American Orthotic and Prosthetic Association, is to label them by the joints they encompass. Thus, a brace for the lower limb enclosing the knee, ankle, and foot, become a knee-ankle-foot orthosis or KAFO instead of a "long leg brace." In the upper limb, a support splint for the wrist and hand is

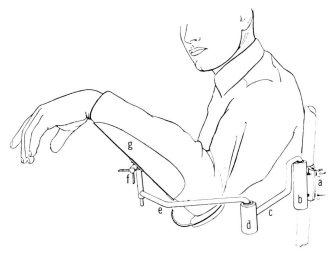

Fig. 5-1. Balanced forearm orthosis on wheelchair. (a) assembly; (b) proximal ball bearings; (c) proximal swivel arm; (d) distal ball bearings; (e) distal swivel arm; (f) rocker arm assembly; (g) trough (Reproduced from JB Redford: Orthotics Etcetera. Baltimore, Williams and Wilkins 1978. With permission.)

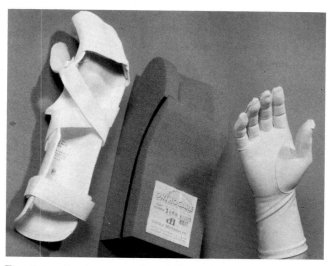

Fig. 5-2. Hand supports: from left to right: thermoplastic static resting hand orthosis, foam static resting wrist hand orthosis (Orthocare), stretch glove to control hand edema.

a wrist-hand-orthosis or WHO instead of a "cockup splint." A description of use of these recommended terms along with forms recommended for prescription appears in the Atlas of Orthotics.[1]

In addition to the anatomical terminology, labels describing orthoses by their expected function have been widely advocated, especially in hand orthotics. Generally there are three kinds of orthoses: (1) static or resting—those used exclusively for rest such as a resting WHO for painful hand and wrist (Fig. 5-2), (2) Functional—those used in some way to enhance function such as the wrist driven flexor-hinge tenodesis splint to provide pinch to quadriparetic patients; and (3) Dynamic—those with actively moving parts that provide more than static force, such as a hand orthosis with elastic bands and cuffs to increase metacarpophalangeal joint flexion (Fig. 5-3).

A good orthotic prescription, therefore, should consist of naming the joints to be enclosed and indicating the purpose or biomechanical function. Selection of materials

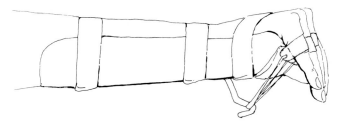

Fig. 5-3. Dynamic wrist-hand orthosis with elastic and leather loops to reduce MCP extension contracture. (Drawn from photograph and reproduced from J D'Astous: Orthotics and Prosthetics Digest. Ottawa, Edahl Productions Ltd., 1983. With permission.)

may also be added to the prescription. There is a wide variety of choice and new types of plastics for orthotics are being introduced every year.

Generally, for temporary devices, plaster or low temperature thermoplastics (those that can be directly molded to the skin without burning) are the most widely used because of their low cost and easy application. For permanent devices where strength is required such as in the spastic paralysis of the lower limb, stainless steel may be necessary but aluminum alloy and newer types of high temperature thermoplastics are often preferable. Selection of materials is best left to orthotists as they understand best not only the nature of the material but also its cost, and, more importantly, the labor involved. Whenever possible, the orthotist should advocate preformed and modular components over completely custom made orthoses as this saves considerable expense. Other considerations in materials include durability, tissue tolerance, resistance to deformation, hygiene, and cosmetics. The latter must always be considered; no matter how well an orthosis functions, a sensitive patient may refuse to wear it if it looks unsightly. For a complete discussion of materials, see Orthotics Etcetera.[14]

A basic biomechanical principle in fitting an orthosis is the "3-point pressure principle." Two pressure forces at either end of the orthosis are resisted by an opposite force in the middle. For example, to stablize a fracture of the lower thoracic spine, a pad applied over the sternum and another over the anterior pelvis is counterbalanced by a third pad over the thoracolumbar area as in the cruciform thoracolumbosacral orthosis, TLSO, for osteoporotic fractures (Fig. 5-4). Another example is the KAFO with the locked knee in which pressure from the pad anterior to the knee is counteracted by the pressure from the

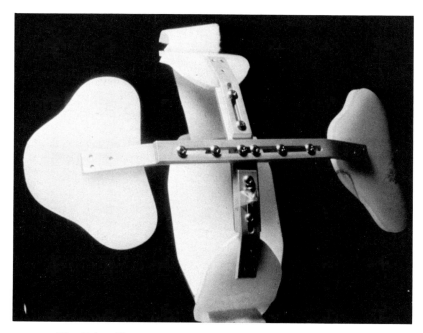

Fig. 5-4. Thoracolumbar orthosis of the cruciform type. The upper and lower triangular anterior pads are opposed by a posterior pad linked by a straps to the central horizontal bars.

posterior thigh and calf cuffs. An excellent discussion of the forces involved in lower extremity orthoses is detailed by Lehmann.[8]

Inappropriate alignment of these pressure forces may cause shear stresses. These can be transferred to the orthosis, producing an increase in wear and stress over the underlying tissues. More significantly, poor alignment may even result in increasing the deformity, especially in a growing child. This is an important reason why orthoses fitted to children should be regularly checked. In fact, all major orthoses that produce strong opposing forces should be checked for proper alignment.

Whenever possible, an orthosis should be designed to be applied, adjusted, or taken off by the patient without assistance. No constriction, edema, numbness, or skin blanching or irritation should be noticed by the wearer. The patient must be taught to look for and report any of these abnormal findings to physician or orthotist. He or she should also learn the principle of gradually breaking into wearing an orthosis by an increased number of hours of wear daily. Keeping all parts clean and in working order must also be stressed by the orthotist.

Although physicians and orthotists are often pleased with how cleverly an orthosis solves the problem, in the final analysis it is the patient's tolerance for appliances or gadgets that settle whether or not the orthoses will be used. If the patient complains of discomfort or interference with function, the orthosis should be modified or discarded, especially after a trial in a therapy department under good supervision. One proof of the effectiveness of the orthosis may be gained in the follow-up clinic; when the device shows significant evidence of wear, it is obviously being used. However, one must be wary of patients like those with back pain who become "addicted" to braces. One should carefully review whether the device is still serving its original purpose, especially if it might be the cause of atrophy or muscle weakness.

UPPER LIMB ORTHOSES

Hand and Wrist Orthoses

Hand orthoses play a crucial role in the management of arthritis and other musculoskeletal disorders affecting the hand and wrist. A new subspecialty of occupational therapy, hand rehabilitation, has developed around these orthoses. Since the introduction of low temperature thermoplastics that can be easily molded to the hand, treatment of many hand conditions, both before and after surgery, has become much easier. In fact, without carefully applied hand orthoses, many new hand surgical procedures would not have been successfully developed. However, use of hand orthoses must be supervised with care, and a sound understanding of biomechanics of hand function is absolutely necessary if fitting them is to be successful.

For the purpose of classification, hand orthoses can be most readily divided into static or dynamic types. Static orthoses vary considerably in design and are generally used to immobilize finger joints or increase function by holding digits in a more desirable position. In most applications, the static orthosis holds the hand and wrist in a position of function; that is, with the thumb abducted at right angles from the palm in a position of opposition to the index finger and the other metacarpophalangeal (MCP) joints, which are slightly flexed. The wrist should be slightly extended at about 15°. Static orthoses of this type are designed mainly to be used at night and with patients who have wrist and hand

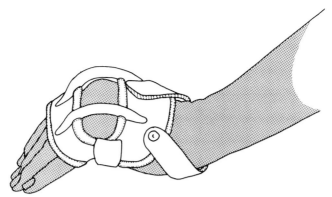

Fig. 5-5. Metacarpophalangeal orthosis to keep MCP joints flexed with "lumbrical bar" over proximal phalanges.

pain aggravated by motion such as those with rheumatoid arthritis. Static WHOs do not all have to be custom made as there are some good commercial ones available, generally in several sizes. The Futuro* splint has been very popular and a foam type is shown in Figure 2.[6] An elasticized glove is also shown in this figure. It can be worn with or without the orthosis and is used in controlling hand edema; for example, in rheumatoid arthritic patients—to combat morning stiffness.

Many hand orthoses are designed to hold joints in positions of flexion and overcome deforming forces such as unopposed action of the long extensor tendons in ulnar nerve palsy (Fig. 5-5). Dynamic finger orthoses are generally not well accepted by patients, but those that hold joints in a functional position and resemble rings have been quite successful (Fig. 5-6). Thumb orthoses are mainly designed to protect the carpometacarpal and metacarpophalangeal joints of the thumb. These joints are often painful in such conditions as rheumatoid arthritis and osteoarthritis. The thumb can still remain functional for "3 jaw chuck pinch" even if the CMC and first MCP joints are stablized as shown in Figure 5-7. This type of thumb orthosis is also indicated in inflammatory conditions of the long tendons of the thumb (DeQuervain's disease) or in thumb instability from rhematoid arthritis.

Dynamic orthoses generally utilize springs or elastics to add assisting forces (Figure 5-3). They thus control certain motions or provide a more constant and adjustable stretch than do static splints. In fitting dynamic orthoses, custom fitted plastic splints are generally preferable, although commercially available elastic and metal reinforced fabric splints such as those developed by Bunnell are often effective and less expensive.[3]

These commercially available splints are most useful for a short period of time, particularly after surgical procedures, but are unlikely to be worn on a long-term basis.

Burns frequently involve the hand; often only with dynamic orthoses, can contractures be prevented. For example, burns on the dorsum of the hand may cause hyperextension of the MCP joints. Such burns are initially treated with a static WHO that keeps the wrist at 10° of extension but holds the MCP joints fully flexed. Later, hooks may be glued to the fingernails and rubber bands attached to them and to a volar outrigger. This

---

*Futuro Wrist Splint, Futuro Co. Division of Jung Corp., Cincinnati, OH

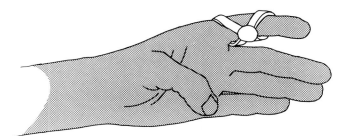

Fig. 5-6. Ring-type finger orthosis to prevent hyperextension of proximal interphalangeal joint.

dynamic splint will induce flexion of the MCP joints, preventing the hyperextension deformity that is commonly seen in unsplinted hands.

A wide range of other hand problems occur after burns and are treated with orthoses. Each case should be carefully analyzed and particular care taken to avoid excessive pressure over unhealed skin.

Prevention of MCP subluxation in ulnar drift in rheumatoid arthritis is a great challenge. The use of hand orthoses to prevent this deformity is controversial. By restricting MCP flexion and ulnar deviation it should be possible to counteract the deforming forces produced by the unbalanced pull of the flexor tendons causing this deformity.[5] The orthosis should prevent volar subluxation and ulnar drift at each MCP joint by supporting the proximal phalanges at their base. Although many arthritic patients have been provided with these orthoses, no convincing study has proven their value.

Perhaps this lack of proven results with ulnar drift is a good example of one of the major problems in hand orthotics. How do you convince the patient to wear an orthosis consistently? The device must be cosmetically acceptable and comfortable and not interfere with any desired hand function. When used in a limited way after surgery or burns, this may be acceptable. However if it is provided for chronic conditions such as rheumatoid arthritis, it must be worn for months to have any effect. Only the most compulsive patient may comply with such wear.

Few studies of compliance in use of hand orthotics are available.[12] We are starting to

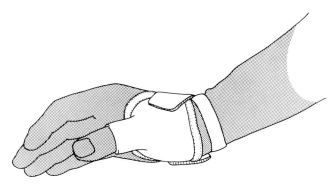

Fig. 5-7. Thumb orthosis to stabilize metacarpophalangeal and carpometacarpal joints of thumb.

study compliance with timing devices attached to orthoses that will record exactly how long they are worn over a given period. If this can be well documented, then we may learn more about the value of not only hand orthoses but all orthoses in preventing deformity. At the present time, descriptions are mostly subjective; only based on clinical impressions of preventive value.

Other Upper Limb Orthoses

Orthoses for the elbow and shoulder are rather limited in number and in function. Elbow orthoses are principally used to protect elbow flexors. For the latter, static orthoses have been used that have adjustable dial locks of adjustable turnbuckle bars that are gradually turned to force the elbow into extension and combined with active exercise programs where possible.

Although the shoulder is vital for reach and hand placement, its multiple axes of movement present very difficult problems to the orthotist. Generally, for controlled shoulder movement and support must be applied to the elbow so the humeral head will be retained in normal relationship to the glenoid. In practice, the most common shoulder orthoses are those used to support the paralyzed hemiplegic shoulder or immobilize fractures about the shoulders. For hemiplegia or spastic paralysis, many types of slings using bandages, webbing, and plastic devices have been recommended, but unless they are applied correctly the subluxation may still occur. Furthermore, these orthoses generally also interfere with the elbow and hand function so that, in effect, the whole arm is immobilized in an attempt to support one joint. This is vital, of course, in fracture healing but for paralysis it presents a difficult problem.

Recently, for paralyzed shoulders, we have been using a new concept in shoulder stablization, the Hemi-Hook Harness† (Fig. 5-8). This device consists of two cuffs wrapped around the upper arms and held together by a yoke. It allows both the affected an unaffected arm to be free for other movement. It is easily applied and adjusted but particularly in patients with flaccid hemiplegia. Recently we have tried it on patients with shoulder weakness secondary to trapezius paralysis following radical neck dissection with some success.

Other types of shoulder orthoses include the overhead sling with spring suspensions and the balanced mobile arm supports discussed earlier. These devices assist shoulder mobility by reducing gravity effect from the weakened extremity but can really only be used by patients confined to wheelchairs or in a sitting posture.

SPINAL ORTHOSES

The primary purposes of spinal orthoses are pain control, protection against further injury, and prevention of deformities. This is achieved through the biomechanical effects of supporting the trunk, reducing spinal loading, or altering motion and realignment of the spinal segments.

Prescription of spinal orthoses requires an accurate assessment by a physician who is familiar with the biomechanical changes associated with pathology in the spine. In gen-

---

†Orthopedic Equipment Co., Bourbon, IN

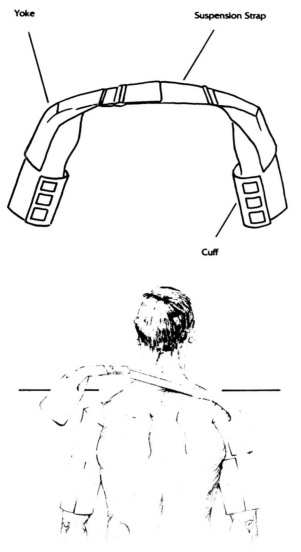

Fig. 5-8. Hemi-hook Harness. Velcro straps close cuffs around upper arms and Velcro attachments under the lateral pieces of the yoke grip to the outer surface of the arm cuffs. (Reproduced with permission from Biomet Incorporated, Warsaw, IN.)

eral, these devices tend to be overprescribed; the unwarranted effects of most of them need always be considered. Reliance on spinal orthoses may cause muscle atrophy by reducing muscle activity needed to provide trunk support. Furthermore, patients often become psychologically dependent on these orthoses. Therefore, whenever a subject wears a neck or back brace, he or she should be instructed to perform isometric exercises, unless of course this might aggravate an acute fracture of other serious injury.

Cervical Orthoses

In cervical spine, most orthoses control mainly flexion and extension and provide only limited control over rotation and lateral bending.[7] They are used primarily for painful traumatic and nontraumatic disorders to reduce motion and possibly unload the weight of the head from the body. As the cervical area has the greatest variety and degree of motion of the spine, it is impossible to completely immobilize it. Even the halo orthosis allows some slight motion. In this device, the head is fixed by screws through a metal halo around the skull and the halo is fixed to vertical bars attached to the molded body jacket or sometimes a pelvic band. It is used primarily to immobilized a cervical fracture or immobilize after a spinal fusion.

Less rigid than the halo are the "poster type" appliances such as the SOMI (sternal-occipital-mandibular-immobilizer). In these types, vertical struts or posts to hold molded pads under the chin and occiput are attached to a yoke covering the shoulders and sternal area. Patients have trouble wearing these devices; they are difficult to keep adjusted and to maintain unaltered support when shifting from lying to sitting posture.

A plastazote collar with anterior and posterior rigid plastic supports (the Philadelphia collar) provides almost as much support as the "poster" devices although more rotation is allowed and it is much more comfortable. Commonly used in the late healing phases of cervical fractures or in acute neck sprains, this cervical orthosis is probably the one most widely used today.[7]

The degree of immobilization from soft collars made of felt, foam, or polyethylene with padding around the borders is very limited. Collars serve mainly through sensory feedback to remind the subject to limit neck motion. Soft collars are also often helpful for night pain or patients with mild cervical spine disorders.

Thoracic and Lumbar Orthoses

For bracing the remainder of the spine, a wide variety of TLSOs (thoracolumbar-sacral-rothoses) and LSOs (lumbar-sacral-orthoses) are available, many with confusing eponyms (Knight, Williams, and Jewett braces). The best way to remember the different types is to consider the components and biomechanical functions. Does the orthosis have horizontal thoracic and pelvic bands? Are there medially or laterally located uprights? Where are the various pads placed? The purpose of the brace can generally be judged by the nature of these components. Obviously the more the hardware, the greater the stability of the brace but usually the more discomfort. Actually, if a great deal of rigidity is required in spinal support; for example, after surgical fusion, it is more popular today to use polyethylene or polypropylene molded jackets. Some of these, like the Boston braces,‡ come preformed and thus, only need further adjustments through heating and molding to achieve their purpose instead of the older techniques of molding over a custom-made cast.[4]

A TLSO usually used to provide hyperextension after lower thoracic or upper lumbar compression fractures, such as the Jewett brace, is somewhat differently designed from those like the "chair back" brace that control back pain using posterior uprights. It has two rigid bars that surround the trunk and a "3-point pressure" system achieved by pads over both the sternum and anterior pelvis and a third pad for counter pressure at a mid-

---

‡ Boston Brace, Physical Support Systems, Inc. Windham, N.H.

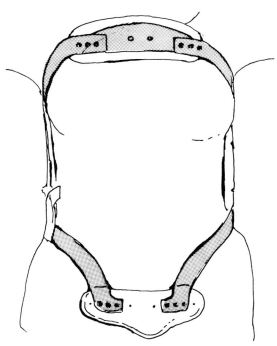

Fig. 5-9.   Thoracolumbar flexion control orthosis (Jewett brace) anterior view (posterior pad lies at thoracolumbar junction). (Drawn from a photograph and reproduced from J D'Astous: Orthotics and Prosthetics Digest. Ottawa, Edahl Productions, Ltd., 1983. With permission.)

point over the back (Fig. 5-9). This TLSO is reasonably well tolerated by younger subjects but very difficult or impossible to use in the elderly.

It has been demonstrated that the air and fluid-filled abdominal and thoracic cavities surrounded by the trunk muscles form a rigid tube to support the spine under stress.[11] When a tight corset is worn about the abdomen, an increase in the intra-abdominal and thoracic pressure results from the tightening of the corset. Therefore, spinal orthoses with pads surrounding the abdomen add outside support to this system and provide some stress relief on structures in the lower spine. It is this intrinsic or hydropneumatic weight bearing system that protects the lower back from much of the daily stress and strain. When the system is weakened by disuse or obesity, the spine is more readily injured. Why is a corset or abdominal binder sometimes just as effective in controlling chronic back pain as rigid metal or plastic orthoses? The explanation lies in the enhancement by a corset of this hydropneumatic intracavity system with its supporting effect like the stiffened walls of a giant football.

A useful device for moderate pain in the lumbosacral area, which fits more comfortably than the older "chair back" braces or lulmbosacral corsets, is the "Warm'n Form" brace.§ This consists of a wide, elasticized abdominal binder, closed in front with Velcro. To provide rigidity, it has a rectangular piece of thermoplastic molded to the contours of

_____

§ Warm'n Form, Jerome Medical, Mt. Laurel, NJ.

the lower back and inserted into a pouch at the back. It produces only slight restriction of lumbar spine movements, and probably acts mainly by augmenting the intrinsic support by the pneumatic weight bearing system just described.

Special orthoses have been designed to control idiopathic scoliosis and prevent its progression. Those for the thoracic spine can be truly described as CTLSO's (cervical-thoracolumbar-sacral-orthoses). They are designed to prevent spinal curves, partly through forcing the wearer to keep herself from loading the spine by relieving uncomfortable pressure from the rigid upper pad under the chin. In this way, there is forced extension of the spine combined with well placed external pressure pads to prevent the spine from collapsing further. To be really effective, an orthosis for scoliosis demands a high degree of skill in fitting with proper application and regular adjustment. Therefore, these orthoses should only be applied in special clinics or by a team consisting of an experienced physician, an orthotist, and a physical therapist working closely together.

Indications for bracing of the low back continue to be controversial. There seems to be no uniform agreement about the proper approach. Generally, however, it has been agreed that orthoses are generally prescribed for persistent low back pain, particularly when associated with spondylolisthesis, pseudoarthrosis, or as part of a trial of immobilization prior to considering spinal fusion. It has been demonstrated that no brace is capable of effectively immobilizing the lumbosacral region; in fact, spinal motion may be actually increased in segments adjacent to the upper and lower ends of a spinal brace or corset.[18] Therefore, it has been suggested that a spinal brace simply serves as a reminder to the patient to avoid excessive motions as these may cause discomfort along the margins of the brace. Thus, orthoses produce a form of immediate biofeedback to tell the patient that movement has exceeded the safety margins of his back; that is, orthoses serve as a kind of low back motion monitor.

LOWER LIMB ORTHOSES

Orthoses to relieve arthritic or musculoskeletal pain in the lower limbs have not been nearly as successful as those used for paralysis. In fact, since the advent of joint replacement surgery, they may be less frequently used, but when surgery is not feasible, alternatives must be considered. Another practical factor to consider before prescribing is ease of application. In severely involved arthritic patients, leg braces often cannot be applied without assistance. Therefore, long-handled shoe horns with Velcro straps, automatic locks, and other special features need incorporating in orthoses for such patients.

Lower limb orthoses for musculoskeletal disorders are of two basic types: those designed to reduce axial loading and those to improve joint stability or minimize deformity.

Orthoses to Reduce Axial Loading

Two examples of orthoses to reduce axial loading are the ischial weight bearing KAFO and the potellar tendon bearing AFO. Ischial weight bearing orthoses, using a Thomas ring, are obsolete. Today, such orthoses incorporate the principles of quadrilateral socket fitting developed for above knee amputees. The upper thigh portion is custom molded to the patient and has a high lateral wall, a high anterior portion with a prominent "Scarpa's triangle bulge," and lower medial and posterior walls to provide weight bearing on the ischial tuberosity. Lehmann has shown that such an orthosis with fixed or locked knee and patten bottom can completely unload the lower limb. Even without a patten, a patient who is trained not to push off vigorously can unload the lower limb up to 90 percent when provided with an orthosis with a locked knee and rocker bottom shoe.[8] Therefore, a KAFO fitted with an ischial weight bearing portion can be very useful in nonhealing fractures or painful inflammation or instability of lower limb joints when the clinical situation requires nonweight bearing.

The patellar tendon bearing (PTB) orthosis is an axial unloading AFO designed to transmit the forces from the knee through the patellar tendon area into the cuff and down through uprights through a shoe to the ground. To reduce stress at heel contact, a solid ankle type heel (SACH) can be fitted to the shoe and to reduce force at toe off, a rocker bottom sole can be added. The PTB cuff is bivalved and closure is accomplished by ski boot-type buckles as this cuff portion must grip the leg firmly to efficiently reduce weight bearing (Fig. 5-10). Unfortunately, this brace has not proved as comfortable as the ischial

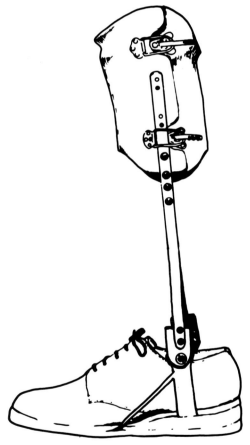

Fig. 5-10. Patellar tendon bearing orthosis with standard upright double stop ankle joint and sole plate extending to the matatarsal head area. (Reproduced from JB Redford: Orthotics Etcetera. Baltimore, Williams and Wilkins, 1980. With permission.)

weight bearing type even when very carefully fitted and aligned. However, it has been helpful in nonunion of fractures, painful ankles, and hind foot problems such as calcaneal fractures.[8]

If this PTB brace cannot be tolerated in a patient with a painful ankle, a molded plastic AFO has often been helpful to reduce ankle motion or stabilize a hind foot deformity (Fig. 5-11). The position of the ankle trim line determines the degree of control or flexibility at the ankle. Advancing this line anteriorly results in more stability; moving it posteriorly results in less.[9] These orthoses do not require a leather shoe with removable heel and sole. In fact, the better designed newer types of running shoes are often prescribed with these AFOs to reduce weight bearing stresses on the foot and ankle. Fracture orthoses incorporate the above principles of axial unloading for healing fractures in the lower limb. For further discussion of this important subject, see Sarmiento.[16]

Orthoses to Improve Joint Function

Lower limb orthoses to reduce joint instability or deformity can be considered according to the joints they are designed to protect. Thus, there are hip, knee, and ankle-foot-orthoses and these will be considered in sequence.

Few orthoses are really suitable to improve hip stability—that is best done with crutches. However, some orthoses have been designed to protect the hip and prevent deformities from untreated Legg-Calve'-Perthese disease or juvenile coxa plana. In cases of bilateral hip involvement, this orthosis holds the hips in abduction. It is fitted with the universal midline joint to allow reciprocal bipedal gait without crutches and ease in sitting (Fig. 5-12). For unilateral hip involvement an abduction orthosis has been designed that

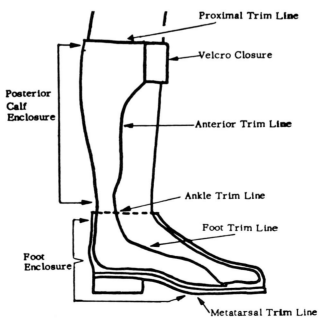

Fig. 5-11. A diagram of features of the standard plastic ankle foot orthosis.

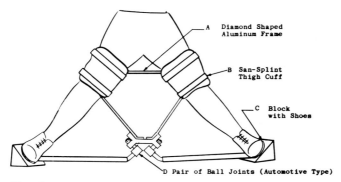

Fig. 5-12. Toronto Legge-Perthese orthosis (Reproduced from JB Reford: Orthotics Etcetera. Baltimore, Williams and Wilkins, 1980. With permission.)

holds the hip in 45° abduction and 20° of internal rotation. These bilateral or unilateral orthoses are worn to allow spherical ossification and regeneration to occur in the femoral head.

Effective bracing for the unstable knee has presented many problems, no doubt due to the peculiar functional structure of the knee, which is not simply a hinge joint. For the mildly inflamed or unstable knee, the elastic fabric knee splints or "cages" with or without reinforcing metal hinges, seem to provide some comfort and reduce knee joint stress during weight bearing. Probably they act through biofeedback mechanisms to warn of extra knee stress. If the subject tends to develop lower limb edema, below knee hose must be supplied, as well. These encircling knee "cages" also cannot be used in patients with vascular insufficiency.

A great improvement in knee orthoses has been the introduction of the Lenox-Hill brace. This custom designed knee orthosis has wrap around elastic, gum rubber, and fabric straps and a rigid light metal "cage" portion so that mediolateral and rotary stability of the knee is enhanced (Fig. 5-13) to varying degrees of allowance for flexion and

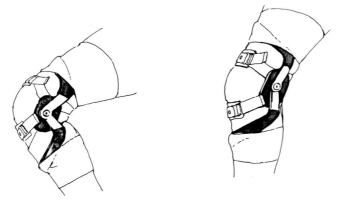

Fig. 5-13. Lenox-Hill knee orthosis (Drawn from a photograph and reproduced from J D'Astous. Orthotics and Prosthetics Digest. Ottowa, Edahl Productions., 1983. With permission.)

prevention of hyperextension can be built in to the brace. Thanks to this knee orthosis, many professional athletes with moderate knee instability have been able to continue their careers. Anterior posterior instability from ligamentous laxity is even more difficult to treat effectively but an original orthosis has been designed by Martin. It uses polypropylene rods in place of joints.[10] We expect more use of plastic joints. The Japanese have reported on a number of experimental types.[17] If plastic joints can be made really durable they obviously have advantages over metal. They are lightweight, noseless, corrosion free, and comfortable in use because of the coincidence with joint axes. In the presence of severe knee instability, particularly from rheumatoid arthritis, bracing using KOs may be very difficult. Sometimes, KAFOs with single metal uprights can be fitted. However, most cases require a full KAFO with standard metal uprights joined together by bands posteriorly above and below the knee, and with or without knee locks or controlled ankle joints. If there is a valgus deformity, a molded pressure pad may need to be applied to the medial side of the knee or better, a molded pretibial shell added anteriorly. This shell should extend from a few inches below the knee to above the patella to assure good knee alignment.[8]

Foot and Ankle Orthoses

Ankle and posterior foot pain and deformity have already been discussed briefly in connection with PTB orthoses. The degree of bracing required will depend largely on the degree of deformity. Some mild foot problems and leg pain may simply be corrected by realignment of the posterior foot in the shoe using a heel cup (Fig. 5-14), available at most sporting goods stores.[4]

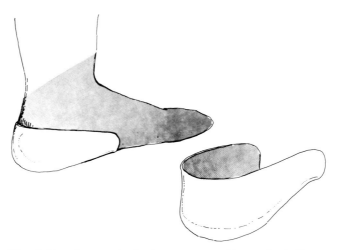

Fig. 5-14. A corrective heel cup—a type of foot orthosis (Drawn from a photograph and reproduced from J D'Astous. Orthotics and Prosthetics Digest. Ottowa, Edahl Productions Ltd., 1983. With permission.)

In any orthosis, the type of shoe worn, of course, greatly affects the performance. As previously noted, the new plastic molded AFOs enable the wearer to use jogging shoes or any rubber soled shoes as long as the heel height is kept the same when the shoes are changed. However, if metal uprights must be attached by a caliper, the shoe has to be made of leather with a removable sole. There must be a rigid, preferably steel arch, extending from the heel to the metatarsophalangeal joint line to support the longitudinal arch. A firm well-fitting heel counter must hold the heel in optimal alignment and prevent the foot from sliding up and down in the shoe. The toe box must be able to accommodate deformities and prevent any abnormal pressure on the foot. The shoe should not be the slip-on type but rather have laces or Velcro closures to allow varying distribution of supporting forces over the top of the foot. The extra depth shoe, which has ¼ inch more depth from top to sole than standard oxfords, has greatly improved the ability to fit deformed feet and insert molded plastic AFOs to patients with toe deformities. Because foot problems and their corrections will be discussed in another chapter, further discussion of shoes will not be given here. But it should be remembered that a shoe is a type of orthosis and as much attention must be paid to fitting shoes to disabled persons as is given to fitting other orthoses. Rubin et al have given complete and helpful review of selection of shoes for orthoses.[15]

CONCLUSION

This chapter has provided a summary of orthotic principles and some of the devices available. For further details, the reader is referred to some textbooks.[1,4,8,13] For a rapid appreciation of the appearance and types of orthoses, we would particularly recommend Orthotics and Prosthetics Digest.[4]

Orthoses should always be prescribed with the expectation that the patient will wear them. In most cases, it is essential to check the fit and wear of the orthosis in follow-up visits or the value of the device will be lost. For all types of orthoses, it is important that the wearer can put on and take off the appliance whenever possible by himself. Orthoses should conserve time and energy, not increase energy consumption and they should be as simple and durable as possible since frequent need for repair will certainly result in poor utilization. Patients should be taught the simple maintenance of their orthoses such as cleaning the rubber or plastic and oiling of joints, when necessary.[13]

As prefabrication of orthoses has been steadily increasing, there are more varieties and types of commercially available orthoses than ever before. Unfortunately, fitting is always a problem unless the device is custom made; thus, use of prefabricated orthoses is often confined to temporary conditions.

Concern continues to be expressed by many patients and physicians over the cost of orthoses. One possibility for reducing cost is more central fabrication. In the United States, there are now many major geographic distribution centers that stock premade or multiple components for orthotic devices that can be mailed overnight to local orthotic facilities. If measurements are made directly on patients and then to a fabrication center, a custom-made orthosis will be returned. Then, the completed orthosis needs only to be fitted and modified for the individual patient at less overall expense. Because cost control has become such a major issue in providing adequate medical care, we expect in the future to have more development of central fabrication facilities.

REFERENCES

1. American Academy of Orthopedic Surgeons; Atlas of Orthotics. St. Louis CV Mosby, 1975

2. Bobechko WP, McLauren CA, Motloch WM: Toronto Orthoses for Legg-Perthes disease. Artificial limbs, 12:2, 1968

3. Bunnell, S: Bunnell's Surgery of the Hand, Ed. Boyes, JH (editor) 4, Philadelphia, JB Lippincott, 1964

4. D'Astous J (ed): Orthotics and Prosthetics Digest Ed. 2. Ottawa, Edahl Productions, 1983

5. Flatt AE: Ulnar Drift, in Care of the Rheumatoid Hand Ed. 3. St. Louis, CV Mosby, 1974, p. 249

6. Gumpel JM, Cannon S: A Crossover Comparison of Ready Made Fabric Wrist Splints in Rheumatoid Arthritis. Rheumatology and Rehabilitation. Vol. 20, 1983, pp. 113–115

7. Johnson RM, Hart DL, Simmons, EF, et al: Cervical Orthoses: A Study Comparing Their Effectiveness in Restricting Cervical Motion in Normal Subjects. J Bone Joint Surg 59A:332–339, 1977

8. Lehmann JF: Lower Extremity Orthotics, Kottke F. (ed): in Krusen's Handbook of Physical Medicine and Rehabilitation. Philadelphia, W.B. Saunders, 1982, pp. 539–574

9. Lehmann JF, Esselman PC, Ko, MJ, et al: Plastic Ankle Foot Orthoses: Evaluation of Function. Arch Phys Med Rehabil. 64:402–407, 1983

10. Martin TA: An External Cruciate Ligament Orthosis, in Mastro BA (ed): A Review of Orthotics and Prosthetics. The American Orthotic and Prosthetic Association. Washington, D.C., 1980

11. Morris JM, Lucas DB, Bresler B: Role of the Trunk in Stability of the Spine. J Bone Joint Surg 43A:327, 1961

12. Rapoff MA, Lindsley CB, Christopherson ER: Improving Compliance with Medical Regimens: Case Study With Juvenile Rheumatoid Arthritis. 65:267–269, 1984

13. Redford JB (ed): Principles of Orthotic Devices, in J.B. Redford (ed): Orthotics Etcetera (Ed. 2). Baltimore, Williams and Wilkins, pp. 1–21

14. Redford JB, Licht S: Materials for Orthotics, in J. B. Redford (ed): Orthotics Etcetera (Ed. 2). Baltimore, Williams and Wilkins, pp. 53–79, 1978

15. Rubin G, Bonnarrigo D: The Shoe As A Component of the Orthosis, in Mastro BA (ed): Selected Reading: A Review of Orthotics and Prosthetics. The American Orthotic and Prosthetic Association. Washington, D.C., 1980

16. Sarmiento A, Sinclair WF: Fracture Orthoses, in Atlas of Orthotics: American Academy of Orthopedic Surgeons. St. Louis, CV Mosby, 1975, pp. 245–254

17. Watanabe H, Kutsuna T, Morinaga H. et al: New Plastic Joints for Plastic Orthoses. Prosthetics and Orthotics Int'l. 6:21–23, 1982

18. Waters RL, Morris JM: Effects of Spinal Supports on the Electrical Activity of the Muscles of the Trunk. J Bone Joint Surg 52A:51, 1970

Sam C. Colachis, Jr.

6

Traction

HISTORICAL BACKGROUND

Traction is the process of pulling an object across a surface. In medicine, it is a technique of applying a force to a part of a human body to stretch tissues, separate joint surfaces or bony parts, relieve dislocations, and treat fractures. Traction and manipulation were practiced by Hippocrates in the Fifth Century B.C.[1] Descriptions of levers and pulleys of Archimedes were used in Alexandrian orthopedics.[4] Galen discussed the subject in the Second Century. Avicenna, near the year 1000, taught Hippocrates' methods, and Pare, in the Sixteenth Century, demonstrated illustrations and manipulative techniques.[23] Patients have been strapped to a ladder, head or feet down, and raised with a winch only to be dropped on a hard surface imparting a strong distraction to spinal joints to supposedly straighten a deformity.[1] Traction has been given at the shoulder and pelvic area, simultaneously, to a person in the prone position, while a third person jumps on the dorsal spine to correct a kyphosis or scoliosis. This form of therapy at times, has been disasterous, but nevertheless has contributed to the historical background in the treatment of back disorders. Hippocrates disapproved of the former method of using a dropped ladder to reduce dislocated vertebrae. He referred to this as an outmoded technique and preferred the latter method of traction, cephalad and caudad, while applying a steady pressure of the palm to the involved area.[70]

For the past few hundred years, traction has been the modality of treatment of painful disorders and care of spinal deformities.[5] Balanced suspension splints were introduced in the early Nineteenth Century; later came the use of skin traction for fractures in the lower extremities and then a new experience of a variety of skeletal methods were introduced.[45,62] In this chapter, traction will be confined to the clinical use in conservative treatment of painful conditions of the neck and lower back.

PRINCIPLES OF PHYSICAL MEDICINE AND REHABILITATION IN THE MUSCULOSKELETAL DISEASES

PRINCIPLES OF TRACTION

Traction has been prescribed for many clinical entities, including symptoms arising from pressure of nerve roots, from degenerative joint disease, and spinal injuries.[61] The objectives of traction are: (1) stretch posterior spine region, (2) widen disc spaces, (3) separate apophyseal joints, (4) enlarge interspaces at the intervertebral foramina, (5) stretch muscles and ligaments, and (6) relieve spinal discomfort. It is the author's opinion that few controlled experiments have been done and traction has been considered an empirical form of treatment. The methods of application used have contributed to the confusion. Traction can be applied manually, continuously, intermittently and intermittently pulsed, in a vertical or horizontal direction, inclined plane; either supine or prone, or an inverted position of the body.

Various factors alter the evaluation of treatment. There are interrelationships of type of halter, halter placement, proper positioning, pulley system or mechanical device, angle of rope pull, tractive force, duration of the force, and length of time of traction. The frictional or surface resistance to traction, resistance of the muscle and soft tissue stretch, spasms or tightness of the tissues, and pain factors all contribute to the results of treatment. Gravity may resist or assist traction. The degree of spinal lordosis will influence the amount of traction necessary and various factors need to be considered, to find the least effective force to provide separation of the vertebrae. Clinically, the ability of the patient to accept traction, without discomfort, will vary with one's tolerance and response to stretching. Stretching may cause some temporary discomfort, but a painful experience is not to be tolerated.

ANATOMY AND MOTION OF THE CERVICAL SPINE

Development of the human spine occurs in three overlapping stages: Blastemal, chondrogenous, and that of ossification. The cervical curve is convex anteriorly and begins at the apex of the odontoid process and ends at the middle of the second thoracic vertebrae.[38] This lordosis results from the greater depth of the intervertebral discs anteriorly than that posteriorly. The cervical spine consists of five segments having "common" motions and two transitional vertebrae, C_1 and C_7. The atlas, C_1, functions principally with the occiput and the seventh cervical vertebrae, C_7, functions similarly with the thoracic vertebrae, with less motion than the other cervical vertebrae.[7]

The principal motion at the atlanto-occipital joint is flexion-extension in the saggital plane. Because of the differential radii of the condyles, movement is similar to the knee joint, with the joint tightening in hyperextension and loosening in flexion. Motion at the atlanto-axial joint is primarily about the transverse plane, although both flexion-hyperextension and lateral bending can occur to some degree. The articulation is the most mobile joint in the spinal column.[29,50]

The typical joints of the cervical spine, below the atlanto-axial articulation are different from those anywhere else in the spinal column. The anatomy and clinical significance of these joints have been reviewed elsewhere.[7]

The range-of-motion of the cervical spine is dependent on the flexibility of the intervertebral discs, the shape and inclination of the articular processes, the laxity of ligaments, the integrity of the capsular structures, and the thickness and length of the neck. Besides the normal voluntary movement of the cervical spine, there are also involuntary movements that have been described in detail; the relationship to the therapeutic approach in certain disease entities is clinically apparent.[69]

Fielding has noted by cineradiographic techniques, that during flexion and extension of the cervical spine, the vertebral bodies shift anteriorly and posteriorly, respectively, with a comminant change in the shape of the intervertebral discs. The reverse occurs in hyperextension. In flexion, the foramina enlarge and in hyperextension they narrow.[29]

The central cervical segments, C_2 to C_6, may be functionally divided into upper C_2 and C_3, middle C_4 and C_5, and lower C_6 segments. In the normal adult, the most active region is the mid-cervical segment. Using cineradiography, Jones[50] noted motion between the fourth and fifth cervical vertebrae, including the disc between C_5-C_6, is greater than other positions of the cervical spine.

At the present time, anatomic visualization by cineradiography is far from ideal and it is virtually impossible to measure separation of the vertebral bodies accurately or to note angle changes except in a gross manner.

According to Jackson,[49] the point of greatest stress and strain occurs at the level of the fourth and fifth articulation, C_4-C_5, in hyperextension and between the fifth and sixth, C_5-C_6, cervical vertebrae in flexion. Two separate parallel lines were drawn from the posterior surface of C_2 and C_7, respectively, noting the point of intersection. Limitation of motion of the cervical spine will alter the point of greater stress and strain, depending upon the degree and level of motion in the area of fixation.

Recording movements at the various segmental levels have been shown by Kottke and Mundale,[55] who measured angles formed by intersecting lines from adjacent vertebrae in flexion and hyperextension. They found that 50 degrees of flexion and 45 degrees of extension occurred between the atlas and the seventh cervical vertebrae, C_1-C_7. The greatest amount of flexion-extension occurred in the interspace between the fifth and sixth, C_5-C_6, although there was almost as much motion at the C_4-C_5 and the C_6-C_7 interspaces.

Colachis and Strohm[13] measured motion of the cervical spine in ten normal male subjects by transferring measurements of the vertebral bodies to each successive radiograph and recording intervertebral distances during cervical spine motion. The anterior apex of T_1 was chosen as a pivot point for the line representing the shortest distance between C_2 and T_1. The angle of displacement of the cervical spine was measured by superimposing the radiographs, demonstrating flexion and hyperextension on radiographs showing the neutral position. The results of this study showed greater motion of the cervical spine in flexion than in hyperextension in all subjects. This was substantiated by the measurements both of the intervertebral spaces and angles of displacement. The total intervertebral motion of the cervical spine anteriorly as compared to posteriorly was found to be in a ratio of 2:1 as the neck moved from hyperextension to the flexed position. There is a ratio of 1.5:1 anterior compression to posterior elongation of the intervertebral disc of the spine, as the spine is flexed from the neutral position, whereas, a ratio of 2.5:1 anterior elongation to posterior compression occurs as the spine is hyperextended from the neutral position. The greatest compression anteriorly and elongation posteriorly occurred at the C_5-C_6 interspace as the cervical spine was flexed. As the cervical spine was hyperextended, the elongation anteriorly and compression posteriorly occurred at the same intervertebral level. The greatest total motion anteriorly and posteriorly occurred at the C_5-C_6 interspace, followed by the C_4-C_5 interspace and the C_6-C_7 interspace, respectively. The least total motion, both anteriorly and posteriorly occurred C_7-T_1 interspace. The individuals with long slender necks showed a greater degree of flexion and extension than those with short necks.

In the neutral position, the mean intervertebral disc height was found to be 31 mm anteriorly and 21.5 mm posteriorly. The mean anterior total body depth was 79.5 mm and the posterior body depth was 85 mm, showing a difference of 5.5 mm. However, there was almost a 10 mm difference in the intervertebral heights and, therefore, this is the primary reason for the curve of the cervical spine and as the difference becomes greater, the lordotic curve in the neutral position increases.

REVIEW OF THE LITERATURE

McFarland and Krusen,[67] in 1943, took lateral radiographs of nine persons before and during traction; in this group six were normal and three had osterarthritis of the cervical spine. They drew a line across the base of C_7 and another line at the top of the atlas, or at the base of the occiput. Measurements were made (1) along the tips of the posterior spinous processes, (2) at the posterior margins of the bodies of the cervical vertebrae, and (3) at the anterior margins of the bodies of the cervical vertebrae. They used a Sayre's halter that was described in 1877 for the use of traction in Pott's disease. Traction of 45–100 pounds was given to adults ages 55–65 years. The average increase in distance along the tips of the spinous processes, the posterior margins, and the anterior margins of the vertebrae was 10.9 mm, 6.5 mm, and 2.8 mm, respectively. In one normal individual who received 85 pounds of traction, the cervical curve straightened and the average increase in the distance between the vertebral arches of the foramina from C_3 to C_7 was found to be 1.5 mm. The exact procedures for making the measurements were not clearly defined and no statistics outlined. A technique of radiant heat for 30 minutes, effleurage, and traction of 70–80 pounds applied slowly, was given and when the force desired was reached, the head was rotated gently to the right or to the left and traction slowly released. Now this is to our knowledge, the first study noted in which cervical traction on normal persons was mentioned.

DeSèze and Levernieux,[26] in 1951, described the work of Ranier regarding the effects of traction on the fibrous tissue of the spine. The vertebral column was isolated, osseous tissue removed, and fibrous tissue remained consisting of annulus fibrosis of the disc and posterior and anterior vertebral ligaments. Gradual traction was given to the specimens. In the cervical region, an elongation of 10.0 mm occurred with 88 pounds; a rupture in the C_5-C_6 area resulted with 121 pounds. In the thoracic area, an elongation of 11.0 mm occurred with 88 pounds and a rupture of D_5-D_6 occurred with 352 pounds. The elongation of 15 mm occurred between D_8 and the sacrum with 264 pounds and a rupture occurred at D_{11}-D_{12} with 440 pounds. The resistance of the ligaments was much greater with a slow and gradual traction.

Prepared specimen segments of vertebral arches and ligamenta flava only, showed elongation of 2.8 cms for the cervical column at 15 pounds; 4.0 cms in the thoracic column with 20 pounds, and 4.5 cms in the lumbar area with 29 pounds. Only 26 pounds of traction will detach the ligamenta flava between C_1 and C_2. These cadavers, however, were kept for several months and even years so that one could surmise that in the normal individual, the ligamenta flava, due to it's elasticity, could be stretched easily without detachment under greater forces.

DeSèze and Levernieux used comparative studies of X-rays taken before and during cervical traction and noted that traction first produced straightening of the normal curvature in the vertebral segments. The intervertebral spaces widened mainly in the posterior segment and the lamina and spine apophyseal joints separated. The tractive force of 260

pounds was required to obtain a total separation of 2 mm between the cervical vertebrae C_5–C_6 and C_6–C_7. This was measured in the lateral radiographic view. On one patient, they found that a tractive force of 440 pounds was necessary to obtain a 10 mm separation between the top surface of C_4 and the top surface of T_1. This, however, was measured in the anterior-posterior view of the cervical spine.

In cervical radiculopathy, (140 patients) good results (disappearance of pain and the return of normal activity) were noted in 77 percent and the earlier the treatment, the better the results. If the conditions lasted over 2 months, the percentage of good results dropped to 65 percent. They particularly noted the fact that it was difficult to state in advance which patients would benefit specifically from traction.

Judovich,[52] in 1952, evaluated over 60 patients who presented signs and symptoms of a laterally displaced cervical disc; shoulder girdle pain with radiation to the arm and hand or pain in the neck and scapular and precordial area, some numbness and tingling in 1, 2, or 5 fingers. There was discomfort in the interscapular area with the presence of poor grip and pain was worse in the recumbent position, awakening from sleep. Hyperextension or rotation to the painful side aggravated the condition and appeared to be intensified on downward compression of the cervical spine. He used a vertical head halter with forces from 5 to 50 pounds and 50 percent had received relief at the upper poundage. He applied vertical traction to seven patients who presented signs of the laterally displaced cervical disc. Lateral radiographs were taken at successive forces of 5, 10, 15, 20, 25, 30, 35, 40, and 45 pounds of traction. He noted that the earliest measurable change occurred with the use of 25 pounds of traction. It was his impression that this was the minimal level of adequate traction that should be used in the average cases of intractable pain resulting from a herniated disc. In some patients, pain was increased with forces up to 25 pounds, but relieved somewhat at 25–30 pounds of pull. At 45 pounds of pull, maximum, "stretch" was 14 mm and a minimum "stretch" of 3 mm with an average of 5 mm. The measurements were made from the inferior surface of C_2 to the superior surface of C_7. In six of the seven patients, a small widening was noted at the apophyseal joint. The technique of measurement was not reported. It was Judovich's impression that the curve of the cervical spine straightened with 20–25 pounds of traction. He concluded that early separation of the vertebrae coincides with the relief of signs and symptoms in his patients.

Jackson[49] had studied the cervical spine cineradiographically in several patients during treatment with an intermittent traction device. She noted that ten pounds of traction lifted the weight of the head, but produced no visible distraction of the vertebrae. Visible distraction was produced with 20–25 pounds of pull, concomittantly with an increase in the size of the intervertebral foramina, as demonstrated in the oblique position. The normal lordotic curve was completely straightened with a pull of 35 pounds and separation of the vertebrae were even more apparent. No specific measurements were made, however. Jackson thought that the method of application of a tractive force and duration of intermittent traction were quite important. A greater tractive force could be applied to a patient if he or she experienced a minimum of discomfort to the chin and the temporomandibular joints.

Using myelograms in cadavers, Taylor,[82] in 1953, found that when the neck was hyperextended, the ligamenta flava were compressed between the adjacent laminae to form bulges that projected forward into the spinal canal. This is of minor importance in normal people in whom the spinal cord can move forward toward the anterior wall. If there is a protrusion on the anterior wall or if there are osteophytic growths, compression of the cord may occur.

Stoddard,[81] in 1954, was critical of vertical traction, because his patients experienced

difficulty in relaxing in this condition. The patient's head was also hyperextended by this method. He had noted that extension of the head decreased the size of the intervertebral foramina and flexion increased the size of the intervertebral foramina. He mentioned that neck flexion to 30 degrees was the best possible condition to facilitate relaxation and seemed to open the foramina to maximal extent. He also cited articles by Taylor on the problem of extension of the spine. Sustained traction had the disadvantage of confining the person to bed as well as making relaxation difficult if sustained more than a few minutes. He preferred intermittent traction, because he thought rhythmic movements might stimulate circulation, since there are no valves in the spinal veins and holding the head stationary might retard venous flow. His treatment consisted of manipulation if traction did not assist the patient after six to eight treatments and then he reverted to traction once again. He would generally commence gradually holding the traction for 30-60 seconds and then release slowly.

Shenkin,[78] in 1954, studied 27 patients suffering from pain in the neck and upper extremity as a result of disturbances of the cervical spine causing root compression. His impression was that all suffered enough pain to be surgically explored. Of the 27 patients, 2 were involved in rear-end collisions, 8 had sudden abrupt turning of the head or turning in bed when the supporting muscles of the head were relaxed, and 17 had no specific trauma recalled by the patients other than recurrent stiff necks over a period of years. There had been a loss of the normal curve in all patients by X-ray and acute reversal of the curve in nine patients. The complaints varied four to six weeks in the majority of the patients and one to five years in a few of the patients. The ages of the patients were from 20 to 60, with an average age of 40. Myelography was done on 11 patients, 5 prior to surgery and in the other 6 there had been contemplation of surgery. Four of the patients with abnormal myelograms did not respond to traction and were found to have a herniated disc. There was a clear evidence of herniation in 8 of the 11 patients on myelography and 3 of them were normal. They were given the type of intermittent traction suggested by Judovich, 50 pounds for 5 seconds and then released for a 5 second period. There was partial restoration of the cervical lordosis in 17 of the 27 patients following the use of traction. Twenty-two of the patients that were not operated on showed 16 completely relieved and 6 discharged with a neck support. There was a follow-up of 6 months to 2½ years.

Martin and Corbin,[68] in 1954, described improvement in 61 patients for radicular pain, of duration 4 days to several years. There were 42 males and 19 females in the group. Traction of 30-100 pounds was given depending upon their tolerance, with the average pull of approximately 60 pounds. An overhead Sayre's head sling was used with traction of one to three minutes, twice a day. The number of treatments varied from 1 to 42 with an average of approximately 8. At the end of the initial treatment, there was 67 percent improvement with no change in 33 percent. Later results showed approximately 77 percent improvement with 3 percent no change and 20 percent that had surgical intervention. The impression was that intensive vertical traction for short periods of time was more effective than horizontal traction with less tractive force.

Krusen,[56] in 1955, studied over 800 cases of individuals that complained of pain in the neck and shoulders, associated with headaches and classified as "cervical syndromes." His experience proved herniation of the nucleus pulposus in the neck comprised a very small percentage of the cervical problems. Forty-one percent of the 800 individuals had a history in injury from auto accidents, severe injuries to the head, falls and indirect injuries to the neck area; 17 percent of those had fractures whereas, 59 percent (472) had no history of

injury. Of this latter group, about 18 percent had cervical fibrositis and over 2/3 or 67 percent had tension neck problems, involving environmental factors producing tension. There was a small percentage of advanced cervical osteoarthritis and some with the scalenus syndrome, with 24 individuals having a herniation of a disc with weakness and atrophy and some sensory changes. Fifty-seven percent of the patients were in the 30-40 age group and 60 percent were female and 40 percent were males. Seventy percent of the females were in the noninjury group and 45 percent in the injury group. Among the tension group, the females outnumbered the males 3 to 1. Therapy, in the form of either short wave or microwave diathermy, was given for a period of 30 minutes, with massage followed by vertical traction with a Sayre's sling, according to the method of Hanflig.[11] Traction was given one to three minutes, with gentle manual rotation, starting with 30 pounds of traction. There were supervised active exercises, with rotation and lateral bending, but no extension exercises and a tetanizing current of low voltage was given for relaxation of the muscles. The evaluation was rated according to good, which was marked to complete relief; moderate, which was subjective relief with some definite changes in subjective findings; and no improvement. The treatment time varied from 3 days up to 1 year, with an average of 4-5 weeks in the injury group; 3 days to 34 weeks, with an average of 3-4 weeks in the noninjury group; and 1 to 29 treatments with an average of 8 treatments in the fibrositic group. His conclusion was that the length of time elapsing from the onset of the complaints until the start of therapy had minimal effect on the degree of improvement. The effective duration of treatment, on the degree of improvement, was not significant and there was no optimal treatment time and the injury often precipitated tension, aggravating the situation. A mention had been made that the non-injury group were patients that provided their own financial means.

Erickson,[28] in 1956, had used similar treatment with diathermy or baker, 30 minutes prior to the use of cervical traction. His method used the Sayre's head sling with traction varying from 30 to 90 pounds, depending upon the tolerance, with an average of approximately 60 pounds. There was assistance in rotation of the head slowly to the maximum range-of-motion during traction. Traction of the cervical portion of the spinal column, in many cases, gave prompt relief. He thought that X-ray examination of the cervical portion of the column in the presence of a protruded disc, usually would disclose the loss of the normal curve, with narrowing of the intervertebral spaces. It was his impression that intensive vertical traction, for short periods of time, was more effective than cervical traction applied with the patient in bed in the supine position.

Various methods of traction have been available with techniques of vertical traction as applied in clinical practice were described by Hanflig. Garland,[33] who gave an excellent review of spinal traction in 1957, quoted Krusen has having listed the following advantages of vertical over horizontal traction: (1) the convenience of application, (2) the elimination of friction, (3) the accuracy of measurement, (4) the facilitation of certain types of manipulation. However, he felt that there was a place for both horizontal and vertical traction.

Cyriax claimed that during manual traction, which he estimated at a maximum of 300 pounds, he could double to total cervical interspace distance.[23] Radiography was carried out before and during the heavy traction. He then superimposed radiographs and he claimed that the distance between the upper surface of T_1 and the upper surface of C_4 increased 10 mm, with an average of 2.5 mm at each intervertebral level. This was demonstrated in the anterior/posterior radiographic view. It is extremely difficult to measure accurately, the intervertebral space in this view.

Crue,[21] in 1957, studied the cases of 20 patients whose past history showed little or no relief from cervical traction in the supine position. With the neck flexed at 20-30 degrees, however, 19 of the 20 patients had moderate to complete relief. He advocated the pull at the occiput to cause flexion of the neck. One of the diagnostic signs in cervical radiculopathy was radiating pain on hyperextension of the neck. Flexion caused pain due to tightness, but usually there was no radicular pain. He noted in the cervical skeleton, that the spinal foramina were anterior to the mid-line of the spinal canal and, therefore, the fulcrum was not at the facet joints. The articulating surfaces slide upon one another, the most fixed point being anterior to the vertebral body; thus in flexing the spine, the long diameter of the foramen was increased showing an enlargement. In a 31-year-old normal subject, he found that the vertical diameter of the C_5-C_6 intervertebral foramina increased 1.5 mm when the neck moved from 10 degrees extension to 20 degrees of flexion. In a 35-year-old patient with cervical radiculitis of 9 years duration and spurring at several foramina, he noted a change of 2 mm in the vertical diameter of the intervertebral foramina, C_5-C_6 after the patient was given 5 pounds of traction at 20 degrees flexion for 24 hours.

Wramner,[93] in 1957, studied 63 patients with various cervical complaints. He took radiographs of three patients before and after ten minutes of traction, with the patients in the same posture and found that the cervical spine extended 1.8-2.0 mm. The specific method of measurement was not reported.

Lawson and Godfrey,[59] in 1958, were unable to duplicate Judovich's findings. They took radiographs of 22 patients, before and during cervical traction. Overhead cervical traction was used in the experiments. For most of the patients, 40-60 pounds of traction were given for 20 minutes and then radiographs were taken. In a few cases, 100 pounds of traction was applied for 1 minute with a follow-up radiograph. In 2 patients, one was given 6 pounds of traction for 8 hours and the other was given 16 pounds for 8 hours. Cervical traction produced an increase in the arch length of 1-2 mm. Measurements were made through the mid-point of each successive cervical body from the tip of the odontoid process of C_2 to the inferior border of the body of C_7. A change of less than 2 mm was not considered significant. There was no significant separation of the cervical vertebrae, although there was an overall increase in the height, 3.4 mm, at the end of each treatment. The subjects returned to the pretreatment state after a few hours. In their report, there is no reference regarding the age or the type of patients treated.

Rowe,[77] in 1963, treated patients with chronic symptoms of fatigue and discomfort from cervical osteoarthritis with short periods of overhead traction, followed by active exercises, consisting of rotating the head to the extreme right and left, in flexion and extension. Traction was to be applied with the cervical spine at 20-25 degrees of forward flexion. He thought 8 pounds of weight was sufficient if given for 15-20 minutes. If traction was given in bed, the head of the bed needed to be elevated 40-45 degrees to give a forward lift to the neck of 20-25 degrees. No radiological studies were done nor specific measurements made.

Bard and Jones,[3] in 1964, studied the effects of intermittent and static traction with cineradiography. The study included 26 individuals with, and 4 without, symptoms referable from the neck. The ages varied from 25 to 66 years, and the study included 24 women and 6 men. No attempt was made to evaluate the therapeutic value of traction. Each person had a chin-occiput head halter and was seated receiving 30 pounds of traction. The head and neck were pulled forward to produce ten degrees of flexion at the mid-cervical spine. This traction was noted primarily at the C_4-C_5 and at the C_5-C_6 levels. Evidence of

unilateral facet separation occurred and both unilateral and bilateral increase in the foramina was noted in the oblique position. No differences, grossly, were noted in comparison of static or intermittent traction. However, voluntary muscle contraction could overcome the effect of 30–55 pounds of traction.

Colachis and Strohm,[13] in 1965, noted that flexion of the neck without traction, could separate the cervical vertebrae posteriorly. They postulated that less tractive force, applied with the neck in a flexed position, might accomplish the same separation of the vertebrae as a greater force applied in the neutral position.

Ten subjects, aged 22–33 years, volunteered for the study,[15] none having a previous history of neck trauma nor cervical complaints. Without previous preparation, such as the use of a heat modality or several minutes of traction "warm up," each subject was placed on a table in the supine position, with the vertex of the skull six inches from the end of the traction table. A 1 piece cervical halter was placed around the chin and occiput and side straps were attached to a 12 inch steel bar, connected to a pulley, which connected to a platform at the end of the table in a manner that the angle of the platform could be varied between 0 and 35 degrees from the horizontal (Fig. 6-1). However, the angle of rope pull did not coincide with the platform angle and this was found to be 6, 15, 20, and 24 degrees. A minimal force of 30 pounds was used in the experiment. Since this was a minimal single tractive force for a duration of only 7 seconds, an additional 20 pounds, or a total of 50 pounds, at a force of 24 degrees was given. Fifty pounds of tractive force was well tolerated at 24 degrees, but there was some discomfort at 6 degrees.

Radiographs were taken before, during, and at the end of the application of tractive force. Eight positions were used in the study and forces varied between 0 and 50 pounds at 6, 15, 20, and 24 degrees. Before any tractive force was applied, a slack in the system was removed and this was found to be approximately five pounds and constant throughout. The vertebral bodies were labeled and the anterior and posterior segments defined. The specific detailed measurements were made, both anteriorly and posteriorly, from the lower

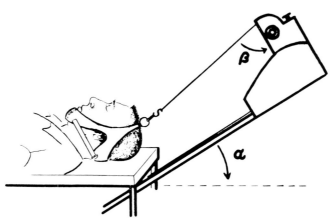

Fig. 6-1. Line drawing showing technic of applying tractive force and relationship of rope angle B to platform angle. (Reprinted from Colachis SC Jr, Strohm BR: A study of tractive forces and angle of pull on vertebral interspaces in the cervical spine. Arch Phys Med Rehabil 46:820–830, 1965. With permission.)

surface of C_2 to the top surface of T_1. There was a total of 208–232 radiographic measurements for each subject. "The angle of displacement" or total movement of the cervical spine was recorded for each change in tractive force and angle of rope pull.[13]

The results of this study indicated that there was a definite relationship between the separation of the vertebral bodies and the amount of tractive force and angle of rope pull. The amount of intervertebral separation posteriorly increased as the neck was flexed and the separation increased as the tractive force was increased. In all subjects, there was an increase in the vertebral separation posteriorly with a tractive force of 30 pounds at each change of angle of rope pull compared to 0 pounds of tractive force. The changes that occurred anteriorly were less specific; some subjects showed compression and others elongation at the lower angles of rope pull, but the mean values were negative (compression) as the angle of rope pull exceeded 15 degrees. Compression of the vertebrae anteriorly appeared to be a function of neck flexion alone, since the tractive force of 30 pounds at 20 degrees and tractive forces of 30 and 50 pounds at 24 degrees did not produce a significant difference.

The mean angle of displacement of the cervical spine increased to a greater extent with the tractive force than with the angle of rope pull. Since the normal cervical spine is moderately elastic, anterior compression with concomitant separation of the vertebrae posteriorly appeared as one flexed the neck. The total intervertebral motion of the cervical spine, anteriorly and posteriorly, from hyperextended to the fully flexed position, was noted to be in a ratio of 2:1.[13] Flexion of the neck, therefore, caused twice the anterior compression as posterior elongation. Traction, in this present study, produced elongation posteriorly, but negligible changes anteriorly. A tractive force of 30 pounds for a duration of 7 seconds could produce separation of the cervical vertebrae and the greater separation occurred at an angle of rope pull of 24 degrees; and 50 pounds of traction produced greater separation than 30 pounds.

The 10 same subjects, aged 23–34, volunteered for a follow-up study.[14] Without previous use of a heat modality or trial session of traction, the subjects, again, were placed on the same traction table and head halter applied. The amount of tractive forces was 30 pounds, given at a specific angle of 24 degrees for 7, 30, and 60 seconds, and also a tractive force of 50 pounds was given at the same angle of rope pull for 7, 30, and 60 seconds, respectively. Radiographs were taken at 7, 30, and 60 seconds. The traction was then discontinued, a radiograph was taken again when the slack in the system was removed. A time interval of 90 seconds intervened. Successive radiographs were taken at 7, 30, and 60 seconds, with 50 pounds of tractive force.

The results of the study show that there was a positive relationship of intervertebral separation both anteriorly and posteriorly to the tractive force. The amount of intervertebral separation does not vary significantly with the duration of 7, 30, or 60 seconds of tractive force. All subjects showed a posterior elongation with each change in duration and change in tractive force. The ratio of mean anterior elongation to posterior elongation was 0.5 mm to 2.5 mm or 1:5 for a 30 pound tractive force, and the ratio was 0.7 mm per 3.5 mm or 1:5 for a 50 pound tractive force (Fig. 6-2). The posterior vertebral surface separated five times more than the anterior surfaces. This substantiates a previous study, which showed a relationship of 1:5 for both 30 and 50 pounds of tractive force for a duration of seven seconds at an angle of 24 degrees of rope pull.[15]

Flexion of the normal neck, from the hyperextended to a fully flexed position, produced twice the anterior compression as posterior elongation.[13] Traction, however, produced posterior elongation as well as anterior elongation. It is apparent that only traction

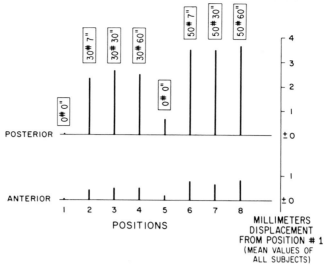

Fig. 6-2. Mean values of intervertebral differences anteriorly and posteriorly of all subjects. There is an average anterior elongation of 0.5 mm and a posterior elongation of 2.5 mm with a tractive force of 30 pounds. There is an average anterior elongation of 0.7 mm and a posterior elongation of 3.5 mm with a tractive force of 50 pounds. The tractive force is, therefore, not related to time. (Reprinted from Colachis SC Jr, Strohm BR: Cervical traction: relationship of traction time to varied tractive force with constant angle of pull. Arch Phys Med Rehabil 46:815–819, 1965. With permission.)

can produce the effect of a reversed ratio of 1:5 in comparison to the normal spine motion of a ratio of 2:1.

The tractive force of 30 pounds or 50 pounds produced elongation regardless of the duration of traction, although there was little difference noted posteriorly, when the duration was 7, 30, or 60 seconds. Posterior elongation was significantly greater with 50 pounds of tractive force compared to 30 pounds.

Colachis and Strohm,[16] in 1966, studied 10 normal subjects, 22–29 years of age, with a mean age of 25 years. These subjects gave no history of neck trauma nor surgical complaints, and their lateral radiographs, in the neutral, fully flexed, and hyperextended position, were normal. Traction was applied to the subjects in the supine position at an angle of 24 degrees of rope pull. A tractive force of 30 pounds was applied for seven seconds, with a rest period of 5 seconds between each tractive force and the total time of intermittent traction was 25 minutes. Radiographs were initially taken without the use of any heat modality, not "trial" session of traction, and the slack in the system was removed. Radiographs were taken during the application of traction at 5, 10, 15, 20, and 25 minutes. The traction was then discontinued and the subjects remained on the traction table for an additional 20 minutes. Radiographs were taken at 5, 10, and 20 minutes after traction ceased to note any residual effects. The time devoted to each subject, including traction and the taking of radiographs, was approximately 45 minutes.

The results of this study showed that in all subjects, the mean total separation of the vertebrae, both anteriorly and posteriorly, increased as the time of intermittent traction was increased. The maximal mean vertebral separation occurred at 25 minutes, showing a 4.6 mm posterior elongation and a 3.0 mm anterior elongation. (Fig. 6-3) The vertebral separation, both anteriorly and posteriorly, was significant to a 5 percent level at the end of 20 minutes of traction and to the 1 percent level at the end of 25 minutes of traction as compared to the results at the end of 5 minutes. At the end of 20 minutes, the residual effects, posteriorly were no longer evident (0.5 mm) but the vertebral separation anteriorly was 1.7 mm. The greatest vertebral separation anteriorly occurred at the C_4-C_5 segmental level and reached a maximum in 25 minutes, of approximately 1.0 mm (Table 6-1). The greatest separation posteriorly, occurred at the C_6-C_7 segmental level, and increased during the application of traction to a maximum at 25 minutes of approximately 1.5 mm. The least amount of vertebral separation was noted at the C_2-C_3 and the C_7-T_1 interspaces, where less than 0.5 mm was noted. In the period after traction ceased, the greatest residual vertebral separation at 5, 10, and 20 minutes was present at the C_5-C_6 interspace anteriorly, where less than 0.5 mm was present and the C_6-C_7 space, posteriorly. The least residual during the period after traction ceased, occurred at the C_7-T_1 interspace. Anterior and posterior separation, after five minutes of intermittent traction, was 1.7 mm and 3.4 mm respectively, or a ratio of 1:2. At the end of 25 minutes of intermittent traction, the anterior and posterior separation was 3 mm and 4.6 mm respectively, or ratio of 1:1.5. The lower ratio in this study is due to the relative greater separation anteriorly. During the period after cessation of traction, the ratio of anterior to posterior separation was approximately 1:1, 2:1, and 3:1 at 5, 10, and 20 minutes, respectively. This compares well with the normal spine ratio of 1.5:1 that exists in the erect sitting position.[13]

The mean angle of displacement of four degrees was comparable to the value of 4.4 degrees found in a previous study,[13] in which 30 pounds of tractive force was given at 24 degrees of rope pull at 7, 30, and 60 seconds. Since the angle of displacement represents the total movement of the cervical spine from a specified initial position, it would suggest that 24 degrees angle of rope pull would approximate the maximal angle of rope pull, which would be desired to demonstrate the optimal straightening of the cervical spine

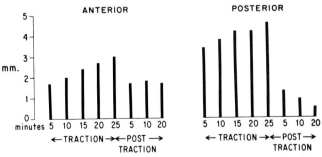

Fig. 6-3. Mean total vertebral separation (C_2-T_1) in all subjects during and after traction. (Reprinted from Colachis SC Jr, Strohm BR: Effect of duration of intermittent cervical traction on vertebral separation. Arch Phys Med Rehabil 47:353–359, 1966. With permission.)

Table 6-1

Mean Vertebral Separation at Each Segmental Level During and Following Traction

	Traction						Post-traction	
Duration (minutes)	5		15		25		20	
Segmental Level	A	P	A	P	A	P	A	P
C_2-C_3	0.15	0.15	0.25	0.45	0.35	0.45	0.30	0.25
C_3-C_4	0.20	0.50	0.50	0.50	0.50	0.60	0.20	−0.05
C_4-C_5	0.40	0.50	0.55	0.55	0.85	0.55	0.20	0.05
C_5-C_6	0.35	0.70	0.50	1.05	0.55	1.15	0.50	0.00
C_6-C_7	0.25	1.30	0.20	1.30	0.45	1.45	0.25	0.25
C_7-T_1	0.35	0.20	0.35	0.30	0.25	0.35	0.20	0.00
Mean total	1.70	3.35	2.35	4.15	2.95	4.55	1.65	0.50

without producing the reverse lordosis. (Figs. 6-4 and 6-5) The negative value of −1.3 degrees mean angle of displacement noted at 20 minutes after cessation of traction, would indicate that the total height of the anterior intervertebral disc from the second cervical vertebrae (C_2) to the first thoracic vertebrae (T_1), did not return to the initial position; in fact, it is noted that a residual of 1.7 mm was present anteriorly, whereas, no posterior residual was noted. This would tend to produce an increase in the cervical lordosis, which might be of significant clinical value since it might be possible to reverse any preexisting "straightening of the spine" with the use of traction, as was noted by Shenkin.[78]

Previous studies in the movement of the cervical spine in flexion and hyperextension revealed that the greatest movement, both anteriorly and posteriorly, occurred at the C_5–C_6 interspace.[13] Kottke and Mundale noted the greatest amount of flexion and extension occurred at the interspace between C_5 and C_6 cervical vertebrae, although, there was almost as much movement at C_4–C_5 and at the C_6–C_7 interspaces. From the results of these latter studies, one might expect to find the greatest vertebral separation at the C_5 and C_6 interspace during traction. From the present study, however, the greatest motion anteriorly was at the C_4–C_5 segmental level and greatest separation at the posterior level and the C_6–C_7 segmental level. DeSèze and Levernieux noted that a total separation of 2 mm between the cervical vertebrae of C_5–C_6 and C_6–C_7 occurred with a tractive force of 260 pounds. Crue[21] found that the greatest separation of the vertebrae, as measured by the vertical diameter of the foramina, occurred at the C_5–C_6 intervertebral foramina during traction.

The results of the most recent studies showed that a tractive force of 30 pounds, if applied for a duration of seven seconds, with a rest period of five seconds, at an angle of 24 degrees of rope pull, could produce a proportional increase in the mean separation of vertebrae in all subjects during 25 minutes of traction. The greatest separation posteriorly occurred at the C_6–C_7 segmental level and anteriorly at the C_4–C_5 segmental level with the least amount of vertebral separation at the C_7–T_1 level. Twenty minutes after cessation of traction, no posterior residual was present, but anterior residual was minimally noted.

Laurin,[58] in 1966, discussed cervical traction as a useful, simple therapeutic procedure to be used in the home. He noted some indications in which it was beneficial: (1) cervical disc disease, with or without nerve root irritation, unless there is a gross neurological deficit; (2) facet osteoarthritis; (3) acceleration extension injuries without unstable post-traumatic lesions. He felt that cervical traction was rarely dangerous, but nonetheless, some contraindications should be observed: (1) inadequate investigation in that cervical

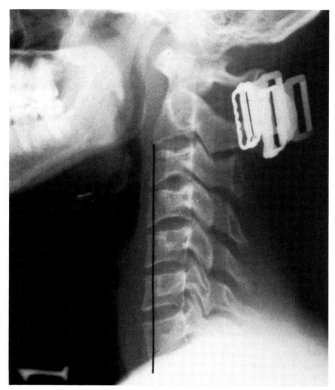

Fig. 6-4. Initial position in which no traction was applied. The slack in the system was removed. Angle of displacement is 0 degrees. (Reprinted from Colachis SC Jr, Strohm BR: Effect of duration of intermittent cervical traction on vertebral separation. Arch Phys Med Rehabil 47:353–359, 1966. With permission.)

traction should not be prescribed without a thorough neurologic and orthopedic or radiologic examination; (2) neoplastic disease; (3) unstable post-traumatic lesions of the cervical spine; (4) cervical brachial pain associated with important neurologic deficits.

Patients suffering from neck pain usually exhibited cervical spasm with a decrease in cervical lordosis, which was confirmed radiographically. He had noted that pain was invariably aggravated by forceful extension of the cervical spine, whereas flexion was less painful, although it could be limited. He felt that the antalgic muscle spasms could cause the patient to unconsciously flex his cervical spine in an attempt to relieve the pain. The object of cervical traction was to assist the patient in these pain relieving maneuvers, but if applied in the position of cervical extension, it would restore the pain producing situation and would cancel any benefits that the traction could achieve. This had been noted previously by Bard and Jones[3] in regard to any muscle tension opposing the effects of traction. He had taken cervical radiographs during the application of traction and had noted cervical lordosis present. While traction was given in a slight position of extension, the increased disc height was not striking and seemed to be more noticeable in the upper disc spaces. The posterior displacement of C_5 on C_6 appeared to have been aggravated and the facet subluxation at that level increased. There was no pain relief. He then applied

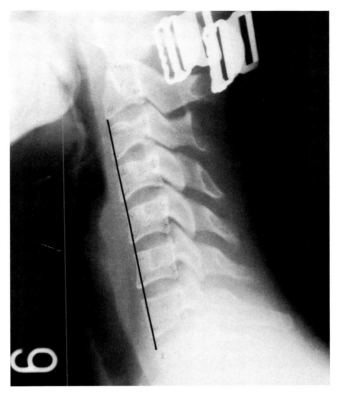

Fig. 6-5. Same subject. Twenty-five minutes of traction. Anterior and posterior elongations are 1.5 mm and 6 mm respectively. Angle of displacement is 8 degrees. (Reprinted from Colachis SC Jr, Strohm BR: Effect of duration of intermittent cervical traction on vertebral separation. Arch Phys Med Rehabil 47:353–359, 1966. With permission.)

traction, but in a position of flexion, and the patient was apparently facing the door instead of turning his back to the door while obtaining traction through a pulley mechanism over the door. Pain relief was gradual and definite. The displacement of C_4 on C_5 as well as C_5 on C_6 had been corrected. If more flexion was applied to the head, then the relief appeared to be complete. He had noted that cervical traction was used to treat symptoms and not a disease, and therefore, was an empirical form of treatment and the actual mechanism by which it relieved pain was not precisely known. He had suggested a technique in which a patient could be given home traction by using a rope mechanism to a pulley system over a hanger of a door and then affix the rope to the handle of a door, by winding it 10–15 times around the shaft of the door knob. The important aspect was to face the door rather than have the back to the door where hyperextension would be produced. He also placed two large books, usually telephone books, approximately 2–3 inches in thickness, in the seat of the chair in which the individual was sitting. As the fixed traction was applied, in a few moments if there was no pain relief, even after modifying the direction of traction, he would remove a book so that the traction would be increased in the neck by a fraction of the body weight. By moving away from the door, cervical flexion would be increased and usually the relief was achieved in a short period of time. Specific instructions should be given with respect to the direction of traction, strength of traction, duration of traction, and frequency of treatments.[58]

Valtonen, Moller, and Wiljasalo,[85] in 1968, studied intermittent and continuous cervical traction for a period of 25 minutes in 21 patients suffering from cervical complaints. Continuous traction was thought to relieve muscle spasm and pain and intermittent traction had a massage-like effect upon muscles and ligamentous capsular structures. It relieved muscle spasm, decreased swelling and produced better circulation. Twenty-one patients, age 24–68 years, with a mean of 49 years of age, were studied. There were 10 males and 11 females, who gave a history of neck and head pain with radiation to the shoulders, arm, or fingers, suggesting a root irritation. Traction was applied to the subjects in the supine position, with motorized traction machines (Fig. 6-6) (Tru-trac by Tru-Eze Mfg. Co., Temecula, California) at an angle of 24 degrees of rope pull. Each patient was treated with both intermittent and continuous traction given on separate days. The neck muscles were warmed with short-wave diathermy and slightly massaged. A tractive force between 20 and 25 pounds was applied. The duration of pull was seven seconds. The rest period was five seconds. Radiographs were taken during the phase of pull. The same tractive force was used in both intermittent and continuous traction in each patient. The distance between the X-ray unit and the patient was approximately 50 inches. The lateral radiographs were taken of the cervical spine before traction was begun and at 5, 15, and 25 minutes after the beginning of traction. Traction was discontinued for an additional 20 minutes, and radiographs were taken at 5 and 20 minutes after the cessation of traction to note residual effects. The study appeared to be very similar to those of Colachis and Strohm.

The results of the study revealed an elongation of the cervical spine to be approximately twice as great when intermittent traction was utilized as compared to continuous traction. However, the absolute changes of total cervical spine distraction was 0.64 mm. The greatest elongation was 2.5 mm and, in most cases, the elongation was between 0.5

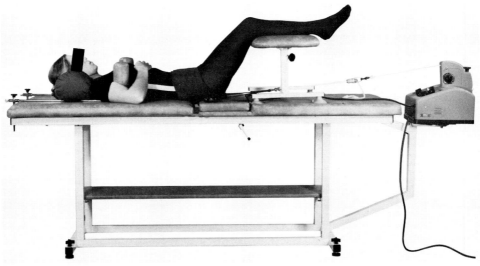

Fig. 6-6.   Courtesy of TRU-EZE MFG. CO. INC., Temecula, Calif.

mm and 1 mm. The difference in the two studies was striking. The authors noted that the average mean of subjects (medical students) used by Colachis and Strohm was 25 years of age, compared to the mean age of 49 in this study. The latter group had various cervical complaints with clear roentgenological changes in the cervical spine. A force of 20–25 pounds was used in the latter study as compared to 30 pounds used in the study of Colachis and Strohm. They measured distance from C_2 to the top of the C_7 vertebra, as opposed to C_2 to the top of T_1, but, the amount of movement between C_7 and T_1 was minimal. They felt that the difference was in the quality between the materials used in these two studies as a major reason for the difference in the result. In both studies, a separation of the vertebrae were proportionately increased to a maximum in 25 minutes.

Differences could be accounted for by the method of measurement between the vertebrae to note exact differences, as outlined in the previous study[16] in which 232 individual measurements were made. It was also noted that the vertebral traction of 24 degrees of rope pull, in the study of Valtonen,[85] showed the individual's head being lifted up with the use of pillows that would decrease the angle of flexion. The distance from the end of the table, which was not specified, would also change the angle at which traction was given. One other additional factor was the distance of the head from the X-ray unit. This was approximately 50 inches and there is a magnification factor at a distance less than 72 inches, which was the distance in the study of Colachis and Strohm. The distance of 72 inches was chosen to decrease the effective parallax. A correction factor would be needed if the subject was too close to the X-ray machine. Results of the present study indicated that intermittent traction was suggested over continuous traction.

Valtonen and Kiuru,[84] in 1970, treated 212 patients suffering from a variety of symptoms related to the cervical spine syndrome. These were divided into six groups: (1) pain and tingling radiating down the hands and digits; (2) pain radiating to the anterior chest wall; (3) pain radiating to other regions, for example, the head, shoulder, occiput, and interscapular region; (4) headaches over the frontal and temporal region; (5) vertigo; and (6) clear neurological findings of weakness and atrophy in the muscles in addition to the symptoms in group 1. Most of the patients were in group 1. The results of the study showed that 40 percent of the patients had suffered from their symptoms over 12 months and 35 percent of the patients had symptoms less that 4 months, with 25 percent between 4 and 12 months. The roentgenological findings showed that 90 percent of the patients had narrowing of the disc spaces as well as foramina narrowing. Gross degenerative changes were present. Only 4 percent had normal roentgenogram findings and 20 percent had anomalies suggesting an old fracture, blocked vertebrae, or marked postural changes. The changes most frequently found were at the C_5–C_6 and next at the C_6–C_7 interspace and, thirdly, at the interspace of C_4–C_5. The patients were treated with short wave diathermy in most cases, the next in frequency was infrared and occasionally microwave or ultrasound. After the application of the heat, manual massage was applied for relaxation for 10–15 minutes. The patient was given exercises and then cervical traction was applied in all cases. Most of this was done by continuous traction in the supine position, with a simple collar, rope, pulley, and weight system. A few were given the intermittent motorized traction, as described in their previous paper,[85] and some were given continuous traction with the patient seated. Direction of pull was usually chosen to produce a slight flexion of the cervical spine; the tractive force used was between 7 and 29 pounds, according to the weight and position of the patient, and treatment was given 3 times a week with an average of 11 treatments over a 4 week period. The results of the treatments showed a complete cure in 19 percent (complete disappearance of the main symptoms), marked improvement in 42 percent (nearly complete disappearance of the main symptoms of the patient), slight improvement in 23 percent (clear decrease in the patient's subjective distress), and no improvement in 16 percent. The highest percentage (cured or markedly improved) of 68 percent was in group 1 and the lowest percentage of 47 percent in the group complaining of headaches; the next group with the least amount of assistance at 55 percent for those that had suffered from vertigo. It was also noted that 31 percent of all patients had been treated previously with cervical traction varying from 4–13 months. In the present study, there was no correlation between the duration of symptoms and the results of treatment. There appeared to be an indication of continuous need of repeated courses of treatment required by the patients suffering from the cervical syndrome. Because of the variety of methods of treatment with the various modalities and not being consistent in the choice, there is some question of the results other than showing a variation in the response to multiple procedures. A previous study had shown that intermittent traction was more effective than continuous traction, but in this study, there was a mixture of these two types of traction and also the weight involved was less than previously used.

Yates,[94] in 1972, noted that traction had been applied, apparently, for many years and appeared to be effective in some cases. He questioned whether any improvement during traction might not be due to spontaneous recovery. Because of the uncertainty, the indications and contraindications must consist of folklore, personal experience, and a small element of applying scientific fact. Traction could be expected to distract intervertebral and apophyseal joints and enlarging intervertebral foramina. A patient with root pain and a past history of malignant disease should not receive traction unless malignant involvement of the spine is excluded. Sustained traction of sufficient force might be effective in patients with brachialgia, especially with neurological findings. Yates did not believe that traction for uncomplicated cervical spondylosis would be any more helpful than traction to a knee or hip with degenerative joint disease and distraction of a degenerative apophyseal joint would only give temporary relief during traction. He believed traction contraindicated in rheumatoid arthritis (atlantoid-axial subluxation), psoriatic arthritis, or ankylosing spondylitis. Atheromatous obstruction of the carotid or vertebral arteries could be exacerbated by neck pressure. Traction was contraindicated in vertebral disease, osteoporosis, sepsis, and malignancy.

Richardson,[76] in 1972, noted that traction was helpful to patients with radicular symptoms in upper extremities, where numbness, tingling, and pain were present. Symptoms were usually unilateral and associated occipital headache could be due to irritability of the upper cervical roots. Complaints do occur, with and without significant X-ray evidence of degenerative joint disease or spondylosis. He believed the effectiveness of cervical traction was variable because of poor technique. This was due to the improper instruction given to the patient regarding the use of traction, insufficient tractive force, improper angle of pull, and infrequent sessions. He suggested treatment twice a day initially for 15–20 minutes, pressure of a halter on the occiput and chin, and the patient sitting, facing a door with a bracket fitted over the door top, with suspension of a rope with a weight on one end and a halter on the other. The head should be pulled in a slight flexion. Traction can be interrupted if tiring. The weight can be started at 15 pounds and increased daily 2–3 pounds, up to 35 pounds or more, for relief of symptoms. Traction can be reduced to once daily in 10–14 days; then reduced to 3 times a week for 2 more weeks, and, if asymptomatic, to continue traction twice a week for 2 months. A word of caution was noted by the author in that most manufacturers of home traction devices depict a picture of the apparatus viewing the patient sitting with his back towards the door, producing extension of the neck, which might aggravate the symptoms. He further advised a firm mattress with sufficient thickness of a pillow to keep the neck in straight alignment, especially when side lying. Because of the susceptability to cervical trauma from rear-end collisions, the car head rest should be properly adjusted.

Varma et al,[86] in 1973, suggested the use of traction as one of the major modalities in the treatment of cervical spondylosis. Traction was applied to 8 patients with spondylosis with a force of 30 pounds at a 24 degree angle of rope pull for a period of 2 minutes. Lateral radiographs at 36 inches were taken before, at the last stage of traction, and 5 minutes after cessation of traction. The results showed intervertebral separation of 2.3 mm and 3.0 mm in the anterior and posterior components, respectively, between C_2 and T_1. The greatest separation was noted at the C_6–C_7 interspace followed by the C_5–C_6 level. It was mentioned that patients with discogenic changes at the C_6–C_7 level associated with radicular changes, responded well to cervical traction. There was no mention as to the cervical level of involvement in these patients nor the duration, frequency, or length of treatments.

Weinberger,[91] in 1976, questioned the role of intermittent traction in the treatment of soft tissue injuries. Neurophysiology did not provide a satisfactory theory that explained the phenomenon of muscular "spasms," which were said to be present following an injury to the neck. He questioned whether long continued intermittent traction, ranging from ten pounds to total body weight pull, was, in fact, therapeutic or traumatic. Nevertheless, such treatments were prescribed in physiotherapy departments and at home for many months. In the author's opinion, treatment was believed to be nonphysiological and irrational. Long continued treatment and litigation resulting from the effects of an injury were over and above the effects of the traumatic experience and may be largely responsible for the prolonged physical complaints noted following an automobile collision in which soft tissues were noted to be injured. Nevertheless, the employment of strong intermittent traction could easily be challenged on the basis that it is irrational, counterproductive, nonphysiologic, and traumatic. Its manner of use, at many times, might even be said to verge on the sadistic. A sprained neck was thought to heal best if movements were restricted until the pain disappeared. The use of a Crutchfield tongs, however, was highly effective in terms of realignment of cervical vertebrae displacement and it would be unacceptable to use tongs in nonskeletal injuries. Intermittent traction offered a form of therapy in various departments, as well as being valued by plaintiff attorneys, because it dramatized the client's injuries. There was a question of traction relieving muscle spasm and pain. It was not questioned that extreme painful conditions, called "spasm," did occur, following a joint or nerve injury, in which the muscle groups were difficult to stretch. One notes, also, an apparent shortening or listing that occurs in the spine following trauma. However, many times no one may be aware of precisely what condition is being treated or what tissue is designated as a target for treatment. If spasm and involuntary contraction of muscle or a reflex contraction is due to nociceptive stimuli, it is highly unclear as to what spasm is and whether or not this is truly a condition following a soft tissue injury. Intensive experiments to reproduce spasm have failed. Muscles that are thought to be in spasm are electrically silent.[42] Muscles adjacent to spanning a fracture of long bones, where the phenomenon of spasm is noted, shows electrically silent muscles. The spasm of poliomyelitis is also electrically silent. Common leg cramps do show some spontaneous electrical activity of contractions. If one stretches a muscle severe enough, a strain will result or a sprain within the ligamentous tissue.

It was his belief that many complaints of sore muscles by patients for a day or two after each session of intermittent traction would, therefore, be due to the fact that the traction would aggravate the condition being treated. The author also felt that the term fibromyositis or fasciitis was to be termed as mythical, with the belief that existence held by many clinicians might be irrational in view of the fact that muscle pathologists have never identified such a condition. Minor trauma resulting in sprain or strain would not initiate a self-perpetuating inflammation and any painful disorder that had an "itis" should not be further traumatized. The time-certified treatment of articular injuries, including spinal joints, should be rest until the healing occurs and also the resolution of any associated hemorrhage. Only when healing is complete, should motion be started. It did not make sense that collars be given to immobilize the neck at the same time that intermittent traction be administered to stretch out "spasm" and distract joints. Any effort to pull the foramen apart would also pull strongly on both the joint capsules and the annular ligaments. Intermittent traction, many times, is started early and it would appear that this would be obviously traumatic to a normal disc, as well as to a disc that might be aged with some evidence of laminar splitting or annular fraying. One might believe that likely changes could be accelerated by intermittent traction, and that the late X-ray alterations that possibly would be ascribed to an accident might well be induced by the therapeutic meddling of persistent intermittent traction. The advanced degenerative joint diseases, such as rheumatoid arthritis, ankylosis, spondylitis, and osteoporosis, may be traumatized by iatrogenic treatment. What the author felt was needed was a study of effects of intermittent traction, as well as some basic assumptions. It appeared that repeated cervical trauma may have perpetuated and aggravated an already skeletal abnormality. Some authors have written on the subject of "whiplash" and have felt that the best treatment was perhaps the least treatment. Traction that was carried on for months and through hundreds of sessions was not treatment, but a succession of calculated traumas.

The author did point out the inadequacy of our knowledge regarding the cause and relationships to pain and spasms and, also, many times, the ineffectiveness of the various forms of treatment that are available. There also may be a lack of hard data that intermittent heavy traction is physiological sound treatment. One should reevaluate therapy for soft tissue injuries by promotion of research on the subject.

Goldie and Reichmann,[34] in 1977, studied 15 individuals. Five of these, ages 21–29, were females who did not have neck pain. Ten others, 5 female and 5 males, ages 36–58, showed discogenic changes in the lower cervical spine. Traction of 30 pounds was given for 10 seconds at a 45 degree angle from the underlying surface. This was done slowly, five to ten times each. Simultaneous tomography was used with seven films, which represented sections of the cervical spine. The difference in change was measured at the center of the disc, between individual segments and not in the spine as a whole. Traction, as a treatment of neck pain, was not evaluated. Widening occurred in 7 of the 54 segments, but, was less than 1 mm and estimated to be 0.4–0.7 mm.

Deets, Hands, and Hopp,[25] in 1977, compared cervical traction in the sitting and supine positions. Eight female subjects received 30 and 40 pounds of traction at a 45 degree angle of rope pull. Intermittent traction, for seven seconds hold and seven seconds release, was used. A warm-up period of five pulls was used before lateral radiographs were taken. The results of their studies showed increased posterior intervertebral separation, in the supine compared to the sitting position, as measured between the C_4-C_7 vertebrae. The measurements, on an individual basis, were quite variable and inconsistent, in comparing 30 and 40 pounds in the sitting and supine positions. This may have been the results of poor relaxation, poor muscle guarding, and discomfort in the sitting position.

Effectiveness of traction is very dependent on contraction of neck muscles, as noted previously.[3]

Harris,[43] in 1977, reviewed the literature and treatment guidelines. Two main objectives were stretching the posterior cervical region and enlargement of the intervertebral foramina. He emphasized that most investigators agreed that neck flexion was important in the application of cervical traction and, generally, it was agreed that the supine position was mechanically desirable and more relaxing. The relaxed, modified long-sitting position, described by Cailliet,[7] had merit, especially for home use.

Ching,[11] in 1979, did note the debate in logic of cervical traction, but relates his experience as a successful modality of treatment. If aggravation of the condition occurs, then it would be useless, no matter what position of the head or neck. He did not use overhead or intermittent traction, because greater forces than 12–15 pounds would be needed to overcome the head alone. The problem of discomfort of the TMJ is more common and he utilized the supine position with lighter weights, using the greatest weight that was comfortable. He felt effectiveness of traction might be due to the tiring of the muscles, then relaxing, allowing traction on the ligamentous structures. He questioned the ability of many practitioners in the proper use of cervical traction and the importance of thorough evaluation of the patient clinically.

Shore, Schaefer, and Hoppenfeld,[79] in 1979, recognized iatrogenic TMJ difficulty in patients treated with cervical traction for cervical spine pain syndromes. The force on the chin subjects the temporomandibular joint (TMJ) to become weight bearing rather than the usual minor loads due to muscle tension, although, bruxism can produce severe forces at the joint. In patients with normal dental occlusion, the force of the chin piece is transmitted to the maxillary bones, via the teeth, and partially to the temporomandibular joint. If malocclusion is present because of the absence of the posterior teeth, however, then stresses are placed on the temporomandibular joints and the TMJ symptomatology may be evident. It may be necessary to prescribe occlusal splints to relieve the pressure. One must be aware of a similar problem following a hyperextension-flexion injury to the neck, allowing the jaw to open and then suddenly close, via the mental reflex, producing sudden pressures at the TMJ area, resulting in synovitis.

Grieve,[39] in 1982, concluded the purpose and value of traction. He described the association of traction and manipulation treatment in spine joint disorders in relation to the phenomenon of restoring presumable shifted disc material to its "proper" place by sustained pull. He mentioned that Bourdillon stated "there appears no evidence to suggest actual disc protrusion can be reduced by this means." This would be in counter distinction with the views of Cyriax.[22,23]

There appears to be no doubt that traction could produce measurable separation of the vertebrae and effects on surrounding tissues.[15,16,84,85] Questions as to why procedures relieve symptoms arose. Pain produced in joint structures is not fully understood and are muscle "spasm" and pain interdependent?[35] Although cervical spondylosis may be a predisposing factor in nerve root symptoms, one notes great surprise in conditions that a nerve root may be compressed and altered slowly from an osteophytic lesion, without clinical evidence of irritation or dysfunction. Sudden pressure to nerve roots are something quite different and quickly apparent clinically. One questions whether traction can also reverse serial tissue changes in the cervical syndrome and perhaps the use of an anti-inflammatory agent would be of greater value.

Caution is suggested in cases of developmental stenosis where the cord may be exposed to trauma and traction would not be advised due to decreased vascularity.[31]

Traction and flexion may cause problems in cervical myelopathy. Traction is one way of utilizing mobilization to treat conditions of painful movement. It must be controlled, assessed carefully, and results properly recorded.

Waylonis et al,[88] in 1982, described a new pneumatic home cervical traction device to provide relief of symptoms of cervical radiculopathy associated with osteoarthritis, so often present in clinical medicine. The counter weight system usually available has some distinct disadvantages: (1) lack of patient compliance, (2) difficulty in application in the elderly and debilitated, (3) tensing of the cervical paraspinal and upper extremity muscles during adjustments of the apparatus, and (4) discomfort while using the device. The pneumatic device (prototype I) exerts a distractive force through a pneumatic cylinder, mounted on a bracket, above the patient's head. The patient has a standard head halter attached to the cylinder piston. The activation of the pneumatic cylinder was performed by a foot pump connected by tubes into the air cylinder. The tractive force exerted by the differential pressure in the cylinder varied from 0 to 40 pounds, but, 25 pounds was used in the study and the neck was flexed facing the door. A second, (prototype II) cooperation with Jobst Company, Toledo, used a similar pneumatic cylinder activated by a hand pump or automatically cycling electric air pumps. The traction cycle was adjustable, as well as the length of treatment, and corrected automatically for any loss of tractive force due to shifts of the patient's position or the loss of cylinder pressure.

Cervical traction (prototype I) was given to 17 patients with a diagnosis of osteoarthritis and cervical radiculopathy. The mean age was 48 (25–67 years) and all had experience with the home counterweight units. Traction of 25 pounds was applied. This was self-applied, intermittently, for 25 minutes. This was done with cycles of one minute "on" and 30 seconds "off." Of the 17 patients, 14 preferred the pneumatic to the conventional method: less work, less cumbersome, more relaxing, and even traction were noted. The disadvantages included: more cumbersome and loss of pressure with the shift of the neck. The counterweight system, on the other hand, was faster and simpler in application, but, was jerky, relaxation was less cumbersome. Slightly less energy was noted in the pneumatic device.

Using the prototype II, 36 patients, who were presently on a home counterweight program using traction 7–10 years, 1 to 3 times daily, were studied. The mean age was 55 (37–75 years) in the group composed of 25 men and 11 women. The traction force varied from 10 to 50 pounds and was the same force used previously at home. Of the 36 patients, 29 (81 percent) preferred the pneumatic to the conventional weight system. The device was easy to use, "workable," and gave a steady and progressive onset of traction. The disadvantage was minor air pressure losses and the complexity of the unit. Those who used the conventional method preferred the compactness for storage and travel.

It was felt that the older and weaker persons would benefit from this type of traction with greater compliance. It might be used for long periods of conservative treatment for chronic cervical syndromes. A suggestion for prescribing pneumatic devices (depending on availability) would be as an adjunct to a program initially started using the counter-weight system.

In a study in 1963, vertebral angiography was performed on consecutive autopsies.[6] The arteries were catherized below the C_5 vertebra and opacified with a barium suspension, given at a level so that the constant head pressure was equivalent to the subjects systolic pressure a few months prior to death. Radiographs were obtained in 41 cadavers, whose average age was 64 years, in the following positions: head and neck neutral, in full extension, full extension and rotation 90 degrees to the right and then left, and finally with the return to the neutral. Complete occlusion of one vertebral artery was noted in 5 of 41 subjects (12 percent) on positioning alone and this always occurred in extension and rotation of the head to one side with complete occlusion of the vertebral artery on the opposite side to which the head was rotated. Continuous traction to the head in the long axis of the body was given to the same subjects with the tractive force of 50 percent of body weight. During traction, complete occlusion occurred on 27 of 41 (66 percent) subjects, 17 of whom had occlusion occur on the opposite side of rotation. All occlusions were at or above the C_2 level, noting 80 percent or 26 of 32 at the atlanto-axial joint. In this series, no complete occlusions occurred adjacent to osteophytes or other projections in the mid and lower spine.

The authors were not sure whether a temporary, complete occlusion of the vertebral artery might have an effect on a person during daily life, and if vertebral insufficiency did indeed exist, the importance of adequate anastomoses with the carotid system became evident. Insufficiency of the vertebral arteries usually occurs in persons over 50 years of age with complaints of dizziness or vertigo, diplopia or other visual changes, transient weakness of the extremities, or brief loss of consciousness. The tractive forces used, however, in these experiments were 50 percent of body weight, which far exceeds what is given conventionally in physical medicine.

Rath,[75] in 1984, discussed in detail, the various types of traction, from the simple manual traction to the turkish towel under the occiput to the more complicated mechanical methods and home traction devices. Supine position was advantageous for patient relaxation. He noted the importance of sound, physiological approach to treatment, and response of the patient to treatment would guide his choice of the position of tractive force to relieve the patient's complaints. He discussed posture and the importance of position, sleeping with adequate support to the neck in the supine position and lateral support in the sidelying position, to maintain a neutral position of the neck. All patients need instructions in posture, position, and biomechanical considerations to insure their active participation in recovery.

Jackson has used traction for neck injuries for many years. She felt that conventional methods of continued traction by head halter was not well tolerated because of the discomfort to the chin and lower jaw. Five or ten pounds of traction did little more than partially lift the weight of the head from the neck and kept the patient still. Fifteen to 20 pounds of traction was required to produce any distraction of the vertebrae. With 35 pounds of pull, the cervical spine became straightened, radiographically, and there was visable distraction of the vertebrae. The use of motorized intermittent traction appeared to supplant other forms of traction application. (Fig. 6-7) It was felt that intermittent traction relieved muscle spasm, with a massage-like effect on the muscles and ligamentous and capsular structures. This prevented formation of adhesion between the dural sleeves of the nerve roots and adjacent capsular structures. The main advantage of intermittent traction was that it could be controlled in the amount and the duration, which gives the maximum amount of traction with a minimum amount of discomfort to the patient's chin and jaw. Patients with postinjury and degenerative changes in the cervical spine appear to show very little distraction of the involved vertebrae. This was due, according to Jackson, to the thickness and the fibrosis of ligamentous and capsular structures.

Treatment could begin with low poundage of 15-20 pounds of traction and could be gradually increased to 25-40 pounds. Some patients that had very thick muscles in the neck might need as much as 50 pounds of traction. She also recommended 30 minute daily intermittent traction treatments for 3-6 days, followed by treatments 3 times a week for 1-

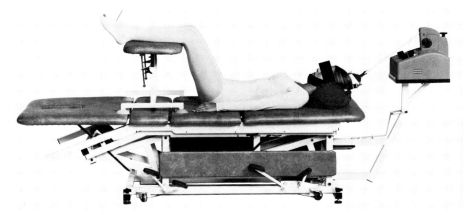

Fig. 6-7.   Courtesy of TRU-EZE MFG. CO. INC., Temecula, Calif.

2 weeks. Thereafter, one or two treatments each week might be necessary for a period of two to three weeks. In many cases, however, no more than five to six treatments were needed.

The patient could be placed in a chair beneath the pulley or a hook in the ceiling with a head halter applied with a spreader bar and then weights attached to the ends of the rope for home or office traction. It was suggested that a scale be placed between the patient and the pulley to record the amount of force, since it might be less than the weight applied to the rope and halter. It was not advisable to use more than 20 pounds of weight with this type of traction. It has been found that 50 pounds of weight can cause severe ligamentous damage.

A contour donor chair[87] has been described as useful in applying intermittent overhead traction. The head and trunk are well supported and the arm rests provide adequate relaxation. The chair can position the body in a reclined or upright position.

LUMBAR TRACTION

The main reason for applying lumbar traction is to produce a distractive force to the bony and soft tissue structures in hope of separating them. The smallest force necessary to produce a therapeutic effect should be used. The question then arises as to whether the goal of vertebral separation, if achieved, will produce relief of the clinical symptoms. Will distraction of tissues, alone, affect the structures to which the pain is attributed? In acute situations of trauma resulting in strains, sprains, tears, hemorrhage, or subsequent inflammation, it may be without reason to treat these conditions by forcible stretching.

Few controlled experiments have been undertaken and the methods used in these experiments have precipitated some confusion.[17] The massive tractive forces used in some studies are not of practical value. The lack of proper positioning of the patient during application of traction has led to further conflicting reports. Traction can be applied manually, by gravity in an upright or inverted position, continuously, or intermittently and in a horizontal or vertical direction.[65]

Anatomy and Clinical Application

Differences in anatomy of the lumbar spine area as compared to other areas of the spinal column have been described in detail from the anatomical, functional, and clinical viewpoints.[8,9,38,69,74] A thorough study has been made of the cineradiographic features of the cervical spine; however, the depth and density of the tissue in the low back region, together with the length of the lumbar spine, make comparison with the cervical spine inappropriate.

The lumbar spine has five vertebrae and produces a normal curve of lordosis or "sway back" in the erect position. The weight bearing portion of the spine is composed of functional units containing two vertebral bodies separated by the intervertebral disc. The extensions of the vertebral body are the pedicles and lamina and two posterior facet joints. These latter joints are aligned vertically in the lumbar spine to allow forward and backward bending, but, prevent or restrict twisting or lateral bending. During flexion of the spine, the protection that the facets afford to the disc's annular fibers is lessened because of the facet separation. In a twisting maneuver, the lack of protection of the facet joints places stress on the annular fibers. Twisting of the disc is the only motion that can tear annular fibers. Ligaments encase the disc, reinforcing the annulus; anteriorly by the anterior longitudinal ligament and posteriorly by the posterior longitudinal ligament. Potential pathological significance is the fact that the posterior longitudinal ligament is, in fact, present throughout the entire vertebral column until its caudal approach at the lumbar area. It starts to narrow progressively from L_1 to L_5–S_1 interspace where it is one-half of its original width. Its inherent structural weakness occurs at a level of greatest static stress and kinetic strain.[7]

The nucleus is under great pressure and if the annular fibers tear, the pressure within produces an escape to the periphery. This results in irritation of the contained tissues producing pain and disability.[9]

Lumbar traction has been prescribed for many clinical entities, primarily those with symptoms arising from pressure on nerve roots; from degenerative joint disease and from low back pain resulting from various types of trauma.[12,20,22,74] Its successful use by physicians, physical therapists, and layman, has earned for it a reputation as a dependable, therapeutic specificity in cases of ruptured intervertebral discs.

Review of the Literature

Traction, for the reduction of a pulpy disc protrusion, was suggested by Cyriax,[23] in 1950. His first approach to a displaced fragment of cartilage was manipulative reduction, whereas, nuclear protrusion requires immediate reduction by traction unless some contraindication is present. A person subject to a "click" in the back, followed by severe lumbar pain fixing him in flexion, has a cartilaginous displacement suited to manipulation. Nuclear protrusions do not occur in the elderly, since the nucleus pulposus ceases to exist by age 60. The smaller cartilaginous displacement may cause lumbar, gluteal, or sciatic symptoms. Primarily postero-lateral protrusions, producing sciatica, are almost never reducible by manipulation. The symptoms of pain usually begin in the calf or thigh, without previous backache, because of unlikely pressure on the dura. By contrast, the secondary postero-lateral protrusion, with a backache, followed by root pain, may be suitable to manipulation unless neurological weakness is present or gross lumbar deviation exists. Properly applied traction, according to Cyriax, produces three effects at the affected joint: (1) increasing the interval between the vertebral bodies, thus enlarging the space into which the protrusion must recede; (2) tautening the posterior longitudinal ligament exerting a centrepital force at the back of the joint; and (3) suction.

DeSèze and Levernieux,[26] in 1951, gradually applied traction to segments of the spine in which muscle had been removed from normal and pathological postmortem specimens, and studied total resistance of the whole disco-ligamentary formation of the vertebral column. This was done under radiological control a few hours after death. A force of 11 pounds straightened the lordosis in a spinal segment T_9–L_5; 20 pounds produced a 9.5 mm total elongation and 5 minutes after traction, the elongation was 4 mm. There was a 1.5 mm separation between the lumbar vertebrae L_3–L_4. A tractive force of 88 pounds produced a 16 mm elongation with a 3–4 mm stretch in the lower lumbar segments.

Muscular elasticity demonstrates a special resistance to traction. The stretched muscle, once released, shortens itself less than it has been elongated and does not return to its same dimensions prior to stretching. If repeated, the stretched muscle becomes longer after each traction.[5] A muscle supposedly at rest is already contracted with a specific tonus. A muscle pulled by a minimal force will behave as an elastic body, and as the force increases the elongation of the muscle will be limited by a reacting contraction called stretch reflex.[32] Under the effect of traction, the muscle opposes a resistance due to its visco-elasticity and that of its contraction. As a result, larger tractive forces are necessary in the living body to produce real separation of the vertebrae. DeSèze and Levernieux estimated that a tractive force of 726 pounds was necessary to obtain a separation of 1.5 mm at the L_4–L_5 vertebral level, and 805 pounds was required to obtain a separation of 2 mm at the L_3–L_4 level. Almost 385 pounds was required to overcome the mechanical resistance of their apparatus and 20 pounds to overcome the visco-ligamentary formation.

DeSèze and Levernieux attempted to study the effect of an opaque liquid injected into the dural sac, to note any change in the disc under traction. They were unable to see any transformation of disc rupture under traction as the opaque fluid divided into fragments during elongation. However, vertebral radiography under traction did reveal an air space in the interior of the disc. This phenomena occurs when articular surfaces are separated. This may be explained by the release of gas due to the evaporation of synovial liquid in a cavity, submitted to strong depression. This has occurred in finger joints and the shoulder joints under prolonged traction of the arm. Some have felt the air bubble pathognomonic of degeneration of the nucleus pulposus in the center of an intact annulus fibrosus, where an imaginary space is produced. During stretching and elongation, the cavity is apparent and disappears after stretching ceases. Although traction enlarges intervertebral spaces, the question still arose as to the usefullness of this modality. They felt that the results of a 4 year study of 1200 patients, receiving 12,000 tractions, justified the value of traction. Mechanical traction with a hydraulic jack was used and the force applied slowly and regularly. The patient was kept for ten minutes under maximal traction and then the traction was released. In acute problems, daily sessions were given. In chronic pain, the sessions occurred on alternate days and continued. As improvement occurred, the frequency was given every fifth and tenth day. If no improvement occurred after six sessions, the traction was discontinued. The treatment was controlled by a physician at each session, who judged the quality of results and determined the need and frequency of further treatment. Following the traction, the patient was placed in the bed and given a massage or electrical stimulation.

Of the treated cases, 50 percent had sciatica, 22 percent had lumbar pain primarily, 8 percent dorsal pain, 5 percent cervical pain, and 15 percent cervical radiculopathy. There were 70 percent good results (complete recovery with disappearance of pain, and return to normal activity), doubtful results in 7 percent (those improved but not sufficient control in follow-up treatment), and 23 percent negative, in which no substantial improvement occurred in the first 6 sessions and traction was abandoned.

The patients with sciatica were in the age group of 17–75 and maximal frequency of pain was in the age group 30–35. Those over 60 years of age improved less rapidly. Good results were obtained in 93 percent (29 cases) within 1 month; 71 percent (129 cases) with 1–3 months; 62 percent (162 cases) within 3–12 months and 60 percent (64 cases) over 1 year. The results showed that traction cured a great number of patients with sciatica, but failed in a third of the cases.

Judovich,[51] in 1954, used live subjects and one cadaver, sectioning the latter transversely through the L_3–L_4 interspace, separating it into upper and lower segments. A hospital bed with a firm mattress was used for the traction studies. Traction was applied separately to each of the segments of the specimen. Leg and pelvic traction was given. The hip and knee joints were disarticulated, weighed, and traction was then applied to all disarticulated segments separately. Results of the study showed that the average surface traction resistance of the body was approximately 54 percent of the total body weight. The lower body segment, distal to the L_3–L_4 interspace, weighs 48 percent of the total body weight, and 54 percent of the weight of the lower segment is also required to overcome its surface resistance. This is, therefore, equal to 26 percent of the total body weight. This was designated as *dissipated force factor*. It is evident that a force in excess of 26 percent of body weight is necessary to have any stretch effect on the lumbar spine. Traction, as routinely practiced clinically today, may act as a placebo, allowing the patient to rest in bed, but does not exert any tractive force in the lumbar vertebral spaces.

Judovich[53] used pelvic motorized intermittent traction and utilized 75–90 pounds to his patients. Elevation of the legs in a sling, during traction, would eliminate one-third of the loss due to surface resistance and also keep the lumbar spine in flexion. Elevating the foot of the bed six inches during traction in the Trendelenburg position would yield only a five percent increase in counter traction.[54] He favored the use of a split traction table to allow the decrease in resistance in the lower body segment. He mentioned that patients who suffered trauma, strain, hemorrhage, and metabolic disturbances of muscle and inflammation (intrinsic) would be aggravated by traction, but in spastic conditions, eg, torticollis, due to basal ganglion disease, patients did not complain of pain during traction, but of tightness and a pulling sensation.[53]

Hirsch and Nachemson,[46] in 1954, performed some disc compression studies on fresh lumbar spines taken from autopsy. They were concerned about the causes of lumbago and whether or not the presence of rupture in a disc was so severe that the disc no longer offered resistance to any mechanical strain. The second and fourth lumbar discs, and in exceptional cases others, were tested. All musculature was removed from the spine, while skeletal and ligamentous parts were carefully preserved intact. A disc with half of the upper and half of the lower vertebral body, together with the intervertebral joints, had been sawed off. A special type of strain gauge was used to adequately measure both static and dynamic deformations of the disc. The deformation of the disc would take place rapidly during the first few seconds and then the elastic curve would approach a certain equilibrium and sometimes this might take several hours. The compressibility of healthy discs was greater in the fourth than the second lumbar vertebrae. They had noted that an 88 pound load would cause changes of approximately 1 mm. For a person weighing between 155 and 175 pounds, approximately 88 pounds was the weight that the vertebral column bears when the patient is in the upright position. The load of 220 pounds, however, would increase the compression to approximately 1.4 mm. It was surprising to note how small changes of form that arose with loads of 220 pounds, of how the disc appeared to be so constructed to carry these loads. In cases of the healthy disc, neither a hemilaminec-tomy nor a total laminectomy would lead to any appreciable disturbance in the behavior of the intervertebral discs. They could not support the idea that factors other than the disc themselves could play any part in carrying the loads applied vertically to a cross-section through the vertebral column. The degenerative discs were more easily compressed than healthy discs and were more sensitive to increasing loads. At 88 pounds, about the same value was obtained as in healthy discs, but at 200 pounds, there was approximately a 2 mm change as compared to a 1.5 mm change for healthy discs.

They attempted to transmit force to the intervertebral discs in a very short period of time by a method of "dealing blows" by allowing weights to fall from various heights. They noted that 220 pounds would give a compression in a normal disc of about 1.4 mm and an expansion of 0.75 mm. In a degenerative disc, ie, when the annulus fibers were ruptured, then a compression of 2 mm was the effect of a 220 pound load. The mechanical behavior of the disc depended on how fast the stress was placed upon it. If a disc was subjected to a short rapid acting force, it started to oscillate; these oscillations, irrespec-tive of the strength of the blow, were of short lived intensity. The more frequently the strains occurred the higher the frequency of oscillations.

There appeared to be no difference in the bearing capacity, whether the arches were intact if hemilaminectomy or total laminectomy had been performed. This tended to support the idea that the discs themselves, by far, play the most important role in carrying loads. The discs have the power of adaptation to mechanical stresses and the greater the load applied, the less would be the capacity for shock absorbing.

The intervertebral disc has a certain elastic quality that has been confirmed. It also has the capacity statically to adjust itself to different mechanical demands and represents a dynamic system in which the disc mass is constantly in motion. The smallest trauma can produce great stress in a low back if the force acts rapidly. The changes in shape of the disc are of such intensity and frequency that it is very difficult to believe that muscular reactions can stabilize and protect a back from these variations in form.

Frazer,[30] in 1954, referred to the work of DeSèze and Levernieux, who were then recognized as the most prolific writers on traction. He considered the amounts of traction used by these authors as excessive and recommended traction of 300–400 pounds for 4–5 minutes as sufficient with an increase of force applied gradually. He did not feel that lengthy periods of traction were necessary. He questioned the use of horizontal traction because of the surface resistance encountered. The advantage of vertical traction was that one could utilize the patient's body weight. He emphasized that ligamentous and muscular resistance must be overcome during traction. The thoracic corset was attached to an overhead self-locking hoist and the pelvic corset was connected to an attachment to the floor.

He noted only 6 of 25,000 cases as contraindications for traction; dislocation of an apophyseal articulation, cardiovascular reaction to mitral stenosis, paresis of the leg after disappearance of sciatica and three cases of hyperallergic reactions.

Cyriax[24] advocated 100–200 pounds of traction for 2–3 periods of 20 minutes each with a 5 minute rest period in pulpy herniations. Daily tractions were given for 7–14 days and stopped if no improvement occurred after 12 sessions. Traction was given for a period of 1–4 weeks. According to the reference of R.A. Young of the analysis of cases having a laminectomy, 56 percent protrusions were cartilaginous and 44 percent were pulpy. Since manipulation is instantly effective, this is tried first and if it fails then traction is started. Manipulation is sure to fail if two or more neurological signs are present, eg, ankle jerks, weak muscles, or cutaneous analgesia.

Cyriax felt that disc protrusions were common in practice and that maintenance of lumbar lordosis provided the main safeguard against protrusion; that a reasonable degree of lordosis in childhood would be a safeguard against later life problems. He advocated epidural anesthesia on an out-patient basis with introduction intrathecally, via the sciatic hiatus, of 50 ml of 0.5 percent Procaine solution. The pain reduced in 1–2 hours and the lesion may reduce itself. Only 1 percent failures in the introduction of the needle occurred and he had performed this in over 10,000 cases prior to 1950.

Crisp,[20] in 1955, thought 40–80 pounds to be sufficient if applied 15–20 minutes continuously. He felt that it was important that the correct posture of the patient be observed. The patient would be lying prone. It was essential that the lumbar spine would be flattened or neutral position. This was done by placing a pillow, of suitable size, under the abdomen in an attempt to stretch the capsule of the posterior joints and the intervertebral ligaments. It was his opinion that spinal traction had not completely fulfilled his original hopes. It did prove a valuable modality in many painful conditions of the neck and back, provided the right case was selected and right technique employed. The usual cause of pain in the back was felt to be a disc protrusion and, therefore, spinal traction should be possible to reduce the prolapse and that one or more treatments would help reduction. However, he referred to this as wishful thinking, for the nucleus is retained in the annulus under considerable pressure; therefore, traction might temporarily reduce the prolapse and certainly would tend to recur if traction was released. He also felt that traction sometimes gave relief in cases of a contused disc with impending protrusion. This would be in cases of a rupture of a few annular fibers with little or no bulge being present. He felt that the one type of disc lesion that spinal traction is unlikely to benefit is a complete nuclear protrusion in the lumbar region and still moreso if it had progressed to extrusion. Degeneration of a disc was a slow process and it would take a number of years before it would give rise to pain. When it did, the pain frequently would arise in posterior joints rather than the disc area. A degeneration and narrowing of the disc affected the normal relationship of the facet joints, which would lead to erosion of the cartilage, osteoarthritis, and capsulitis and the last condition being a source of chronic pain. He thought in terms of intervertebral derangement rather than disc lesions as being more common. He then began to feel that traction or manipulations so frequently did relieve, but on occasion failed or even aggravated the situation. Thus, it became evident to him that the incidence of true disc protrusions or extrusions were less then generally believed. Traction frequently would relieve pain by perhaps releasing a nick in the synovial membrane or partial subluxation stretching the tight and painful capsular ligament or freeing an adherent nerve root. He found it difficult to imagine traction as permanently reducing a nuclear protrusion unless the annular lesion was small. The use of traction might temporarily increase the pain in case of a true protrusion, but seldom aggravated the lesion. If there was aggravation, then he advised rest and occasionally the use of an epidural injection, although, he was not convinced of the efficacy of that method. There are cases when there is temporary relief when a patient is receiving traction, but the problem may start when the traction is reduced and the pain returns with increased intensity. In the treatment, however, of older age groups with chronic low back pain, he felt that lumbar traction had its greatest value. When discs became narrowed, they produce secondary changes in the posterior joints where thickened and sensitive capsules give rise to chronic backache. It is the patient whose lumbar pain is relieved by activity who derives such remarkable relief from several treatments on the traction table. He used the analogy of a sprained ankle that would stiffen when rested, loosened when exercised, and fully completely cured by manipulation.

Masturzo,[66] in 1955, devised a method to permit variations in disc elasticity. He had noted from previous investigators that a minimum of 660 to a maximum of 1100 pounds was necessary to rupture an annulus, allowing the nucleus to protrude. He submitted a disc to compression and traction tests and carried out selecto-elastodiscograms. This was carried out in patients in the standing position, initially. The traction in such a case was obtained by a system of cephalic suspension and the compression was affected by allowing the patient to wear a special jacket provided with various weights. By means of this technique, traction and compression were effected by weights attached to straps, which rolled on pulleys and were fixed to the patient. The traction was effected by placing the straps in a centrifugal direction and compression by placing them in the contripetal direction. The method permitted a force of traction and compression up to 440 pounds without any suffering on the part of the patient. However, during the course of the compression tests, there were a few that had an increase in pain. It was noted that the normal area of intervertebral space between L_4–L_5 vertebrae was calculated to be 600 mm^2 and at the L_5–S_1 area at 400 mm^2. He noted, that in his experience, that any variation exceeding one-tenth of this area by the effect of traction or compression would be an expression of a pathological condition of the disc. In the case of an annular protrusion, variations of the intervertebral space during the compression test were about the same as those revealed by the traction test. However, in the second stage of disc disease, represented by rupture of the annulus, variations caused by the compression seemed to be greater than that by traction. They had noted a decrease in the intervertebral space during compression was more pronounced than the increase in the same space during traction.

The behavior of the ruptured disc, he felt, was in accordance with the observations of Hirsch and Nachemson.[46] He had noted that the use of the selecto-elastodiscogram showed very little increase in the widening of the intervertebral space during traction, but, a rather remarkable decrease during compression. The full treatment consisted of 12 applications but treatment could be repeated several times during an interval from a few days to several weeks. It was also noted that during the treatment period, it was recommended that the patient lie down in bed for a few hours after any attempt at vertebral traction.

A method was used to apply traction with the use of an inclined plane. It had been effected by means of a thoracic corset, fixing the patient to the upper part of a sloping plane and the weight of the inferior part of the body did produce the traction with the inclination at 45°. Sixty patients suffering from sciatica were given this therapy; 15 presented clear signs of nuclear herniation; 30 had annular protrusions revealed by the elasto-discography; 10 had symptoms of vertebral arthrosis with osteophytes; and 5 showed no radiological symptoms, but, a slight alteration in the elasticity of the disc as detected by the elasto-discogram. Of the 15 patients suffering from disc herniation, 12 were failures and only 3 had some improvement. Of the 30 cases of protrusion, 25 had remarkable improvement that lasted by wearing a corset, and in the other 5 cases, no appreciable success was achieved. In the case of vertebral arthrosis and osteophytes, there were eight of ten failures with two showing transitory improvement and in the last group there was lasting improvement in all five.

It was his conclusion that there were definite advantages in using the incline method of traction and could be substituted for other methods of vertebral distraction. It was advisable to treat patients in the second stage in which there was annular protrusion without severe herniation and that those present with osteophytes did not respond to treatment and, therefore, treatment might be contraindicated. Elastodiscography was of value in establishing the existence of the alteration of the disc. He also noted that lumbago, occurring under industrial conditions, might also be regarded as a result of discopathy and suggested the use of vertebral traction for the prevention of lumbago and sciatica in industry.

Lawson and Godfrey,[59] in 1958, applied traction to six subjects to whom pelvis girdles were anchored and traction applied to the thoracic cage. They also constructed a machine to measure height of the individuals accurately with a standard error $\pm$ 1 mm. Tractive forces of 150 pounds showed an increase in the arch (curvature) from the superior border of L_1 to the superior border of S_1 of 1–4 mm. Arbitrarily, it was felt that variations in measurement less than 2.0 mm were not significant. They felt that measurements of individual vertebral distances would not be an accurate guide to the overall lengthening and shortening of a region of the spine to be measured in any individual case. Although they concluded that no separation of the vertebrae had actually taken place, the average height of 36 patients treated with at least 10 trials was increased by 3.43 mm per treatment. Over a four week period, two patients showed an increase in height of 8 mm, but their height returned to normal within a few hours. No reference was made as to the age or type of patient studied.

Lehmann and Brunner,[60] in 1958, applied vertical traction with a hydraulic hoist, serially administering forces of 100, 200, and 300 pounds in 19 healthy students. Radiographs were taken at rest, before and during traction. In another series of 19 volunteers, traction of 300 pounds was applied for 5 minutes with a build-up and release in less than 30 seconds. X-rays were taken at rest, during traction, and 30 minutes after traction. Lines were drawn from the top surface of one vertebrae, and the bottom surface of the vertebrae above. The distance between the two lines was measured in the center of the interspace. Measurements were also taken of the width of the intervertebral space, both anteriorly and posteriorly. They showed a midvertebral separation of 2.6 mm at the L_5–S_1, interspace; 1.4 mm at the L_4–L_5 interspace; and 1.3 mm at the L_3–L_4 interspace during 300 pounds of traction. The chest harness was designed similar to that as described by Frazer. The posterior widening was statistically significant whereas the anterior separation was not. It was concluded that this type of traction produced an efficient stretch of the lumbar musculature as well as intervertebral separation. The most difficult complication was that with obese persons, there appeared to be a tendency to faint under heavy traction. This was explained on the basis of pressure being applied at the chest and abdomen and possibly a decrease in venous return, which made breathing difficult. However, none of the volunteers actually did faint, since the hydraulic device permitted a very fast release and smooth action.

This latter study was the first attempt to measure accurately the intervertebral changes that take place both anteriorly and posteriorly. This is of extreme importance since elongation posteriorly is "relative" when anterior compression occurs. Posterior elongation is of consequence only when anterior elongation or minimal compression occurs. If this is not the case, then traction cannot produce effective vertebral distraction,[15,16] and no other claim than simple mechanical stretching of tissues can be made.[8]

Worden and Humphrey,[92] in 1964, described 21 experiments in which 5 "normal" subjects received traction up to 132 pounds, while in the supine position, for periods of approximately 60 minutes. The traction was given in the cephalic direction as well as the caudal direction. The standing height was measured with the subjects before and after traction in the "normal" or relaxed position and in the "tall" position, in which the subject deeply inhaled, attempting to stand as tall as possible, straightening the spine especially in the lumbar area. Height increases were recorded after all stretching periods and these ranged between 1 mm and 30 mm. The average increase in the "normal" standing position was 8 mm and in the "tall" position was 11.5 mm. There appeared to be some retention of the height after several days of repeated traction on two subjects. They apparently lost their increased height at the rate of about 4 mm/hour.

Gray,[36] in 1967, theorized that if traction alone, or manipulation alone, could relieve some of the symptoms attributable to a disc protrusion, then the combination of the two could perhaps provide even a more effective means of treatment. He procured the services of an expert anesthetist because of the unusual positions involved. The patient was anesthetized on a maneuverable table in which a cuffed endotracheal tube was inserted. The patient was then converted to the prone position and advanced at the head end so that the anterior superior-iliac spine were at the level of the end of the table. Padding was applied at the end of the operating table for which the body hung. The knees were fully flexed and the limbs and head maintained in a position of hanging down over the edge. A selected muscle relaxant was given intravenously and then the position for traction and manipulation was achieved by pumping up the table, tilting the head upwards so that the angle of the table was approximately 25–30°. The upper half of the upper body then hung vertically to the floor, fully relaxed with a slight degree of lumbar flexion. After five minutes of gravity traction, manipulation was performed in which the operator faced the back of the patient, grasped the torso and the upper part of the thorax, and twisted steadily and strongly in one direction and then the other. This was described in principle as being likened to the application of torsion force to the head of a screw in using a screwdriver. Lateral flexion could be applied, but it was probably not effective. There was some complication that had to be avoided and they would take precautions to prevent dislodgement of the endotracheal tube, and it was considered advisable to spray the larynx with a 4 percent anesthetic solution. There was need also for increased ventilation in the hanging position, which was maintained for some seven minutes. Of the ten cases recorded by this method, there was failure in 50 percent of the cases and success of varying degrees in the other 5 subjects. The author felt that radiographic proof of the significant degree of distraction of the lumbar spine would perhaps support the adoption of this type of treatment in refractory cases of lumbar disc protrusion.

Hood and Chrisman,[48] in 1968, treated 40 patients, ranging in age from 22 to 63 years with a mean of 40 years, by means of intermittent motorized pelvic traction. There were 12 women and 28 men. The patients had a diagnosis of a ruptured intervertebral disc with both leg and back pain, except for one that had muscular atrophy and weakness with a sensory deficit. All except two had a positive straight-leg-raising test. Treatment consisted of heat in the form of hydrocolator or ultrasound followed by intermittent pelvic traction on a Tru-trac (Tru-Eze, Temecula, California) table. The knees and hips were flexed attempting to flatten the lumbar spine and a split table was used. The slack in the system was taken up and traction for a period of 20 minutes was given daily with a tractive force of 65–70 pounds. Twenty-one (53 percent) of the 40 patients diagnosed as having a ruptured disc showed good improvement with pelvic traction. Of the other 19 patients who were in the same condition or worse, 18 had surgery. It was noted that in 16, the disc protrusions were lying below or medial to the nerve root.

Smyth and Wright[80] had noted from experimental evidence that pressure on spinal nerves from a herniated intervertebral disc irritated the nerve causing it to become hypersensitive. They tied a loop of nylon thread around the involved nerve roots during surgery, bringing the thread up through the body surface, so that when pulled upon it would come against the same area where the disc had pressed. A second loop was brought up through the dura mater, or placed around additional nerve root and a third loop through the ligamentum flavum, interspinous ligament, and annulus fibrosus. In no instance was traction exerted on the nerve root. In all of the cases, the patients who went to surgery were relieved by their symptoms from the operation. In the postoperative experiment, the touching of the nerve root by pulling on the nylon thread, simulated the preoperative pain. The patients were insensitive to stimulation or pull of the dura mater, ligamentum flavum, the interspinous ligament, and the annulus fibrosus. It was concluded that pain had been caused by irritation of the nerve root by the herniated disc. It was found that nerves subjected to prolonged irritation by a disc protrusion were much more sensitive than the unaffected ones. The author suggested that irritation of this hypersensitive nerve by postsurgical fibrosis might account for sciatica in some cases.

Chrisman and Associates had demonstrated at surgery a separation of the laminae by manipulation, stretching the ligamentum flavum and the joint capsule. They postulated that a stretch provided more room for the spinal nerve and accounted for the relief of symptoms in 51 percent of the patients that they had manipulated. In a controlled group of patients, given the same conservative treatment as the manipulation group, poor results were noted at 73 percent.

The present study, with the ruptured intervertebral disc, showed that 53 percent improved with intermittent pelvic traction and they felt that this was due to stretching of the ligaments of the posterior intervertebral foramen providing additional space for the nerve, to relieve the pressure from the encroaching disc material. They felt that, in review of the literature, little separation between the vertebral bodies was accomplished with tractive forces that were difficult to tolerate by the patient and, therefore, treatment aimed at restoring the disc to its normal status was unrealistic. In the surgical reports, in 16 of the 18 cases that went to surgery, it was noted that the discs that were lying in the nerve root axillla, 1 had adhesions and 1 report was not specific as to the disc location. It was their conclusion that the traction was as good as manipulation without the necessary problems of anesthesia. The major benefits from this treatment was stretching the posterior ligaments of the intervertebral foramen, thus increasing the space available for the nerve root.

Mathews,[63] in 1968, studied the effects of lumbar traction by epidurography in three patients, who had sciatica with limited straight-leg-raising. Traction was applied with the patient in the prone position on a conventional couch with a thoracic corset in the upper trunk and a pelvic harness attached to a low gear winding mechanism. One patient, age 20 and with a 1 year history of lumbar pain with right sciatica, but no disc prolapse, was used as the control. Traction of 115 pounds was supplied. Lateral radiographs were taken before and 29 minutes later. There was a slight lessening of the normal undulation of the posterior longitudinal ligament joint at L_2–L_3–L_4–L_5. Thirty minutes post traction showed a slight return toward the original ligamentous contour. No vertebral distraction was noted on superimposition of the radiographs.

A second patient, age 46, with a history of back pain and sciatica with no motor deficit, but a decrease in sensation in the leg, showed disc protrusions between L_1–L_2, L_2–L_3 and L_3–L_4, noting a filling defect. Undulations were noted from protrusions against the anterior wall of the dural sac. Traction of 120 pounds was given for 38 minutes. At the end of traction, there were no signs of a disc prolapse and undulations disappeared. Fourteen minutes after cessation of traction, the filling defects reappeared. Superimposition of the radiographs before and during traction demonstrated a vertebral distraction of 2 mm per disc space. After 20 days, symptoms recurred and a contrast epidural study revealed similar disc prolapses as noted initially.

A third patient, age 67, had a 3 month history of back pain and sciatica to the lateral foot and decreased straight-leg-raising to $50°$. A disc protrusion was noted at L_3–L_4 and traction was applied at 120 pounds. A reduction of the protrusion was noted after four minutes. After 20 minutes, the protrusion was less and traction was continued for an additional ten minutes, for a total of 30 minutes of traction. Ten minutes after traction ceased, the L_3–L_4 protrusion returned to two-thirds of its original size. Superimposition of the radiographs before and 20 minutes after traction, showed a vertebral separation of 2 mm per disc.

The results of the study demonstrates that traction can indeed reduce a lumbar disc prolapse and suction force is suggested. Separation of the lumbar vertebrae at 2 mm per space was noted, but this was only significant when a prolapse was present.

Gray,[37] in 1969, described a method in which a tractive force is provided by body weight acting on a polished incline plane (an angle of $12°$ to the horizontal) with the lower limbs being unrestricted. A series of 40 cases of only those patients whose symptom complex included sciatica, and purposely excluded patients treated for low back pain only. The patient should have pain of greater or lesser sciatic distribution; that is, pain involving part of the whole length of one or both limbs from the buttocks to the toes, located postero-laterally in the proximal part of the limb and generally postero-laterally or anterior in the distal part. In some cases, the symptom was the first attack and in other cases a recurrence. All patients were adults with the predominance of males. All patients had been given various forms of treatment prior to the referral.

In making the diagnosis, the onset of symptoms was usually associated with a sudden back strain, especially in forward flexion; aggravation of pain by coughing or during spinal flexion-extension; positive straight-leg-raising and Lasègue test; weakness, wasting or impaired tendon reflexes; and relief of pain by a maneuver calculated to decompress the lumbar disc. This would be a type of (1) trial by traction by suspension from a door, (2) trial by traction in lumbar extension with the back of the individual against the back of the observer who is applying the traction or, (3) trial by traction in lumbar flexion in which the individual faces the back of the observer who is applying the traction.

In less severe cases, manipulation was generally tried before traction. Time was allowed to insure the absence of substantial benefit. Traction was given for two hours or less, three times a day. In a minority of cases, the patient may have continued his employment and traction was given two to three hours each evening and three times a day on the weekends, combined with rest. The body weight traction was provided on a polished surface of an apparatus inclined at an angle of approximately $12°$ to the horizontal. Traction could be given in the hospital or in the patient's home under the supervision of the author. As soon as improvement permitted, a gradual routine of spinal exercises was incorporated including lateral flexion and rotation in the standing position and "windmill" type of exercises with forward flexion and rotation. All extension exercises in the prone position were intentionally avoided.

Of 14 cases, in which there were no signs of neurological abnormality (exclusive of the sciatic, femoral nerve stretch test), there was effectiveness in various degrees of nine people and failure in five, showing a ratio of 2:1. Of the 26 cases that neurological abnormality, effective relief varying in degree, was noted in 17 cases and failure in 9. According to the author, the outcome of its use was unfortunately unpredictable, but, he had mentioned this is true with various forms of treatment. In some cases, it produced complete resolution of the symptom complex and was recommended for trial not only in cases of discogenic sciatica, but in cases of incapacitating low back pain. It should be appreciated, according to the author, that progressive assessment usually demonstrated the likely outcome within a few days.

Colachis and Strohm,[17] in 1969, studied the effects of intermittent traction on separation of the lumbar vertebrae. Ten medical students, age 22–25 years of age, volunteered for the study. None had a previous history of back trauma nor lumbar spine complaints. Their body weights ranged from 125 to 180 pounds with a mean of 148 pounds. Without previous preparation, such as the use of a heat modality or trial in traction, each subject was placed on a split traction table in the supine position (True-Eze Manufacturing Company, Temecula, California, Fig. 6-6). The lower gluteal area was placed over the distal split segment and the legs were supported on a stool for maximum comfort of each subject with the legs parallel to the table. The pelvic-femoral angle ranged between 65° and 70°. The angle of rope pull in all subjects was approximately 18° (Fig. 6-8).

Tractive forces of 50 and 100 pounds were applied for 15 minutes intermittently with a tractive force applied for 10 seconds and a rest period of 5 seconds. Traction was discontinued for a period of 10 minutes between the force of 50 and 100 pounds. In 5 of the subjects, 100 pounds of tractive force was applied continuously for 5 minutes after a complete rest of 5 minutes following the application of 100 pounds of intermittent traction.

Three lateral photographs were taken on each subject in the supine, Thomas, and curl (both thighs and legs completely flexed) positions prior to traction. Lateral radiographs were then taken during traction in the following sequence; initial (Fig. 6-9); after 15 minutes of intermittent traction at 50 pounds; after a 10-minute rest; after 15 minutes of intermittent traction at 100 pounds; after 5 minutes of continuous traction (after a 5-minute rest period, Fig. 6-10); and 10 minutes posttraction. A total of nine radiographs

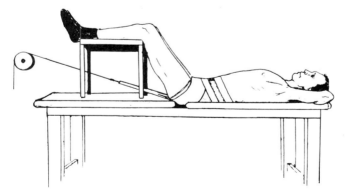

Fig. 6-8. Position for pelvic traction, the legs are parallel to the split table with the thighs at 70 degrees and the angle of rope pull, 18 degrees. (Reprinted from Colachis SC Jr, Strohm BR: Effects of intermittent traction on separation of lumbar vertebrae. Arch Phys Med Rehabil 50:251–258, 1969. With permission.)

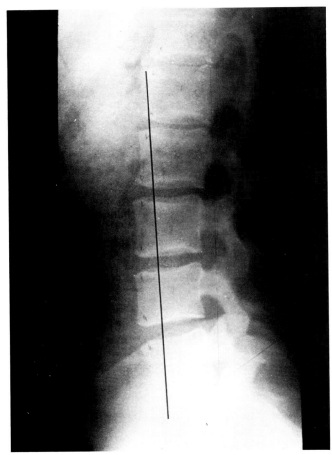

Fig. 6-9. Initial position of traction with no tractive force applied. Angle of displacement 9 degrees. (Reprinted from Colachis SC Jr, Strohm BR: Effects of intermittent traction on separation of lumbar vertebrae. Arch Phys Med Rehabil 50:251–258, 1969. With permission.)

were taken at an object distance of 60 inches and correction was applied for parallax. The vertebral bodies were labeled and the anterior and posterior borders defined on the radiographs. Engineering fine point dividers were used in the measurements. The heights of the vertebrae, anteriorly and posteriorly, were measured initially and transferred to each successful radiograph, and the magnification factor was corrected.

The results of this study showed that in all subjects the mean total posterior separation of the lumbar vertebrae increased as the tractive force increased. The mean total anterior separation decreased minimally during traction. The mean change in vertebral separation at each segmental level, before, during, and following traction are noted in Table 6-2. This is a summary of 960 individual measurements in all subjects. There was a statistically significant difference in posterior vertebral separation with 50 pounds of tractive force. When 100 pounds of tractive force was applied, there was anterior and posterior vertebral separation that was statistically significant whether the tractive force

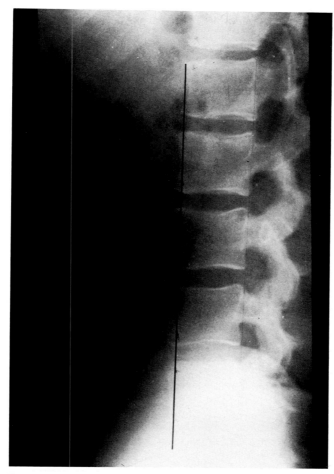

Fig. 6-10. Lateral radiograph after 5 minutes continuous traction of 100 pounds. Angle of displacement 15 degrees. (Reprinted from Colachis SC Jr, Strohm BR: Effects of intermittent traction on separation of lumbar vertebrae. Arch Phys Med Rehabil 50:251–258, 1969. With permission.)

Table 6-2

Mean Vertebral Separation (mm) at Each Segmental Level in All Subjects

| Traction Force | 50 | | 100 | | 100 | | Post | |
| Duration (in min.) | 15 | | 15 | | 5 (cont.) | | Traction | |
Segmental Level	A	P	A	P	A	P	A	P
L_1–L_2	0.60	0.30	0.60	0.40	0.85	0.55	0.40	0.30
L_2–L_3	−0.80	0.60	−0.75	1.50	−0.80	1.25	−0.35	0.50
L_3–L_4	−0.50	0.90	−0.65	1.40	−0.55	1.30	−0.05	0.40
L_4–L_5	−0.20	0.60	−0.45	1.55	−0.90	1.85	0.25	0.60
L_5–S_1	−0.05	0.35	0.15	0.10	−0.40	0.30	−0.05	−0.05
Mean total	−0.85	2.75	−1.10	4.95	−1.80	5.25	0.20	1.75

was intermittent or continuous. Some posterior residual separation was noted ten minutes after traction. The greatest separation during traction occurred at the L_1–L_5 segmental level.

The mean weight of all subjects was 148 pounds, which according to Judovich,[51] would indicate that 38 pounds of tractive force is required to remove frictional resistance alone. Since the legs were elevated and the split table was used in the experiment, the frictional resistance was minimal and the 50–100 pounds of intermittent force could be utilized more effectively. When traction was applied, the ratio of anterior to posterior movement was 1:3 with 50 pounds of intermittent force; a ratio of 1:4.5 with 100 pounds of intermittent force; and a ratio of 1:3 when 100 pounds of continuous force, was used. Therefore, it becomes clear that traction reverses the normal relationship of vertebral movement. When 100 pounds of intermittent traction was applied in the lumbar spine, the ratio was 1:4.5 anterior to posterior movement: traction alone can produce this reversed ratio.

In this experiment, the greatest movement of the lumbar spine during traction did not occur at the L_5–S_1 interspace. Since the lumbar spine was partially flattened, prior to the application of traction (Fig. 6-9), little separation might be expected. Normal movement of the lumbar spine from extension to the fully flexed position, revealed the greatest movement at the L_4–L_5 interspace with essentially equal movement at the L_3–L_4 and L_5–S_1 segmental level.

The mean total vertebral separation from the first lumbar vertebrae (L_1) to the first sacral segment (S_1) in all subjects (mm) before, during, and after traction, is shown in Figure 6-11. The mean heights of lumbar intervertebral discs and vertebral bodies in the initial position of lumbar lordosis was 55.5 mm anteriorly and 25.5 mm posteriorly, and 139.5 mm anteriorly and 145.5 mm posteriorly, respectively. This difference of 6 mm (L_1–

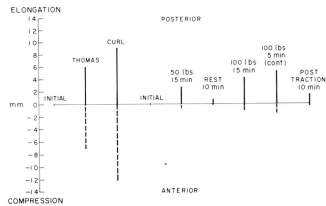

Fig. 6-11. Mean total vertebral separation form L_1–S_1. (mm) in 10 normal male adults before, during and after lumbar traction. Solid lines indicate increase in separation (elongation) while dotted lines indicate compression. (Reprinted from Colachis SC Jr, Strohm BR: Effects of intermittent traction on separation of lumbar vertebrae. Arch Phys Med Rehabil 50:251–258, 1969. With permission.)

S_1) in the vertebrae compared to 30 mm in the intervertebral discs, accounts for the normal lordosis in the lumbar spine.

Other investigators[20,21,23,30,60] have found it necessary to use several hundred pounds of tractive force to note even minimal vertebral separation. High tractive forces used in the lumbar region are neither practical nor without discomfort. Special mechanized equipment for each investigator does not allow the practicing physician the opportunity to participate in using this modality. If forces greater than 100 pounds are used, the tolerance of the patient is dependant upon the thoracic compression, since stabilization is necessary. For this reason, the authors attempted to use practical tractive forces that would not cause discomfort to subjects. If 50 pounds, or preferably 100 pounds of force can be used effectively to produce vertebral separation, then it would seem reasonable to employ these lesser forces for comfort and ease of application.

Nachemson and Elfstrom,[71] in 1970, performed intravital discometry in two normal subjects in vertical traction. The nucleus in normal and slightly degenerated discs behaved hydrostatically and the pressure was 50 percent greater than the outer applied load per unit area. This is due to the elastic resistance of the annulus fibrosus. Therefore, the normal disc is thought to be a simulated tire with a relatively high internal pressure.

A new pressure sensitive needle was inserted into the L_3–L_4 disc space and discometry performed in the supine, prone, and vertical traction position. Dynamic measurements were made during common motions; eg, walking, jumping, laughing, coughing, straining, and "doing back strengthening" exercises, and discal pressures were measured by a subminiature pressure transducer.

Traction of 72 pounds was applied in the supine position to two individuals for three seconds, with five second intervals, between three to five times. Traction applied vertically in the standing position decreased the pressure to a moderate extent. Traction with 60 percent of body weight was needed to reduce the standing pressure by 25 percent. According to the results, traction will produce a decrease in the intradiscal pressure best applied in the supine position.

Straining, coughing, and laughing, while in the standing position, increased the load by approximately 40 percent (coughing) and 50 percent (straining) compared to the normal standing position. Slow walking increased the pressure 15 percent. Side bending and twisting increased the pressure 25 percent and jumping increased the pressure 40 percent. Lifting, with bending of the back and the knees straight, increased the pressure almost 300 percent. Pressures in the supine and prone position were 50 percent of those in the standing position. Isometric abdominal muscle exercises in the "crook-lying" position and hyperextension back exercises, gave lower pressures than the customary sit-up type exercises.

Yates,[94] in 1972, noted forces in excess of 70 pounds would be required to produce effective lumbar vertebral distraction; therefore, manual methods appeared to be impractical and continuous traction could not be tolerated. Recumbent traction with small weights probably achieved little more than keeping the patient in bed. Sometimes, daily traction treatment benefited some patients that had intermittent or continuous sciatica. Cases that obtained relief by lying down often seemed to get worthwhile benefits from the use of traction. Patients with recurrent or intractable back pain, frequently would get agonizing pain when being relieved of traction. In such a situation, it might be necessary to release the traction very slowly. Most elderly patients tolerated traction poorly, but fortunately, their sciatica usually responded to short periods of rest. He felt that the agonizing sciatica or root interruption would be relieved best by epidural injection of a local anesthetic. Longstanding sciatica, present for more than six months, was often resistent to traction. A large central disc could produce bilateral sciatica that might respond to traction. In such a case, however, the risk of bilateral compression of the third and fourth sacral roots might interfere with the bladder function. Traction was obviously contraindicated in vertebral disease such as Paget's, osteoporosis, osteomalacia, spondylitis, sepsis, and malignant deposits. He stated that clinical experience indicated that the traction appeared to produce worthwhile relief of pain in root problems in a number of cases.

Weber,[90] in 1973, described the only controlled study of lumbar traction in the management of low back pain. Eighty-six patients were studied, who had radiating pain with neurological signs corresponding to a lesion of the L_5–S_1 root, as well as a positive radiculogram showing indentation of the dural sac and/or widened or shortened root pocket. However, 14 dropped out in the course of the treatment because of aggravation of symptoms. There were two groups: one consisting of 37 patients who received actual traction and referred to as "treated group" and 35 other patients that received stimulated traction referred to as the "controlled group." There were 42 men and 30 women; 85 percent of the patients were between 30 and 60 years of age. Nothing was mentioned as to the random sampling of these patients. Group 1 was given a tractive force corresponding to an equivalent of one-third of body weight. In Group 2, a force of approximately 15 pounds, which was to have the effect of merely tightening the harness. The force was intermittently exerted and was evenly increased and decreased, interrupted by five second pauses. Traction, consisting of a bench and a Tru-trac motor, was administered for 20 minutes, once a day for 5–7 days. In order to prevent serious complications during traction treatment to patients with a disc prolapse, the treatment was carried out with a force that was in the lower end of the effective range. The following variable factors were examined before and after traction therapy: the mobility of the lumbar spine in the sagittal and frontal plane, Lasègues test (actually straight-leg-raising), Achilles' reflex, motility, sensory function, the need for analgesics, and the patient's feeling of pain in the back and in the legs. In addition, the physiotherapist's impression of the patient's condition was recorded.

The reported improvement in the back and in the legs appeared to be the same in both groups. The physiotherapists reported their impressions of the conditions of the patient on the basis of clinical judgement before and after the treatment. The impressions were based, mainly, on the patient's ability to perform physical activity. The question of whether or not the therapist knew who received real traction or simulated traction was not stated, but they were probably adjusting the traction for the patients. In three patients, there was an improvement that appeared to be marked and these patients did receive traction, but the group was too small for any significance. It was noted that intermittent traction was used since this appeared to be best tolerated by the patients, but the treatment was discontinued as soon as the patient reported any aggravation of his pains. The tendency for spontaneous improvement of sciatica was noted so that comparable control material might be required in order to be able to draw conclusions from the study. In the present study, it appeared that the treatment had no effect. A comparison with the result from the controlled group did not show any difference. It was their conclusion that traction therapy in the group suffering from sciatica due to a prolapsed disc, had little effect apart from the psychological. Comparison between the treated group and controlled group failed to show any significant differences in terms of pain, mobility of the lumbar spine, or neurological signs.

There is some question as to the conclusion of the study on the basis that there was no evidence of separation of the vertebrae since no X-rays were taken during the traction. One noted, also, that from the work of Judovich,[51] 26 percent of the body weight is necessary to overcome merely the frictional resistance of the surface. In this case, 30 percent of the body weight was used in the treated group. One wonders whether there was sufficient time to evaluate the effects of traction for 5–7 days, when many of the studies in the literature have revealed much heavier forces for several days or weeks to relieve sciatic symptoms.

Chahal,[10] in 1975, used continuous lumbar traction for 8–10 weeks in the treatment of acute dorso-lumbar injuries associated with paraplegia. He used 22 pounds of weight on either side of a padded pelvic belt connected to the pelvis. Continuous lumbar traction, in seven cases, gave excellent recovery of motor power; sensation and bladder control in six and good recovery with residual bilateral foot drop in one. By conservative treatment, only three patients had excellent recovery, five had good recovery, and seven remained paraplegic. There was complete recovery of the bladder in 6 out of 7 cases treated by traction as compared to 3 out of 15 treated by a conservative regime and operative technique. It was his feeling that continuous lumbar traction was a safe and rewarding method in fresh dorso-lumbar spinal injuries associated with paralysis. He did mention, however, that these were primarily of the cauda equina type injuries where traction was helping. Where the cord was damaged, he felt that no amount of traction was going to be of any benefit. Where the nerve roots were damaged, he felt that better alignment occurred, given a better chance for the roots to recover immediately if only partially damaged, or possibly to regrow. He also mentioned a simple counter traction effort by lifting the foot of the bed 9–12 inches so that the body weight of 140–150 pounds would act as a counter traction.

Mathews and Hickling,[64] in 1975, did what was described as a double blind study, in that neither patient nor assessor was aware of the amount of traction given. Patients were admitted to the trial or study if they had sciatica, of at least three weeks duration, with or without back pain. Sciatica was taken to be severe and well delineated pain, posterior in the leg and radiating down to the knee. Patients of either sex, age 20–60, were not excluded from the trial even if they had been treated previously by manipulation or if there was evidence of spondylolysis, significant spondylolithesis, or spina bifida occulta. All patients had a radiograph of the lumbar spine. Patients were examined before starting the trial and at three weeks, six weeks, and three months from the start. Those patients that were designated "controlled" for the first three weeks, were offered "treatment" for the subsequent three weeks. Straight-leg-raising was estimated not to be more than a 5° error. All patients were asked to judge by what percentage pain had changed, assuming the level upon entry to the trial to be 100 percent. Reproducibility of measurements were only established for the straight-leg-raising test and it was decided to rely for assessment on this measurement and to the patient's own assessment of alteration of pain. Patients were randomly allotted to either treatment or controlled groups. Treatment consisted of traction on a couch using a force of at least 80 pounds applied via a pelvic harness. The trunk was restrained with a thoracic harness. The maximum traction was 135 pounds and given for 30 minutes daily, 5 days a week for 3 consecutive weeks. The treatment could be varied at the discretion of the therapist, the patient's position being altered or traction increased. Between treatments, patients were not specifically restricted from any activity. The controlled group underwent the exact same routine except a traction force of 20 pounds was applied.

This study used traction that had previously been demonstrated to be capable of reducing the size of a disc bulge and had applied it more frequently and for a longer period, as well as using a double blind controlled technique. The lack of statistical significance, however, may result from the small size of the group. As one might expect, at the time of three month follow-up, there was such a wide variety of fates that had overtaken the patients, there was no comparison between any of the groups that could be made.

Gupta and Ramarao,[10] in 1978, described the use of epidurography in lumbar disc prolapse while applying traction. The patients had sciatica or low back pain severe enough to interfere with their work and positive limited straight-leg-raising or femoral nerve stretch test with or without neurological deficit. They had not been relieved by initial bed rest for 7–10 days and plain roentgenograms of the spine were normal. The pretraction epidurograms showed a definite defect confirming and correlating with the clinical diagnosis. Fourteen cases received epidurography with a water soluable contrast media. The patient was placed on a couch and bilateral skin traction, with adhesive plaster, was applied to both thighs with 60–80 pounds of weight, while the foot end of the bed was raised 9–12 inches. The weights were removed intermittently when the patient was uncomfortable, usually with a rest period of about 15–20 minutes after 3 or 4 hours. Ten to 15 days of continued traction was given and clinical examination and epidurography were repeated at the end of that time. The results of 10–15 days of heavy traction showed that 10 cases were described as good (a marked improvement in clinical condition and the effects on the epidurograms disappeared), fair in 2 (definite improvement in clinical conditions, but posttraction epidurograms revealed persistence of the defect though reduced in size), and poor in two (neither improvement in clinical condition nor in the defect on epidurograms). Superimposition of both sets of lateral epidurograms (pre- and posttraction) showed an average vertebral distraction of 0.5 mm per disc space, but the exact lumbar spaces were not identified.

Abnormal myelograms are common in the general population.[17] Myelographic abnormalities were noted in 300 patients who were studied for posterior fossa myelography to establish a diagnosis in acoustic tumor. Myelograms of the spinal axis were obtained even though the patients had no symptoms of cervical or lumbar nerve root compression at the time of examination. If an abnormality was noted in the contrast column on fluroscopic examination, additional views were obtained to delineate the defect. If there was any history suggesting radicular syndrome due to degenerative disc disease, the patient was excluded from the study. The results from the study showed that 37 percent of the individuals examined had a disc abnormality on myelogram. The defect was single in 19 percent and multiple in 18 percent. The lumbar abnormality was 24 percent and the cervical abnormality was 21 percent. Defects were found in both the lumbar and cervical areas in 8 percent.

Oudenhoven,[72] in 1978, administered gravitational lumbar traction in an attempt to overcome friction between the body and hospital bed and to produce lumbar distraction. A harness was applied to the lower chest and traction began on a tilt table at 35° extending up to as much as 85° of tilt. Treatment intervals were approximately 30 minutes to 1 hour in duration, 6–8 times daily, depending upon the tolerance. When the pain was relieved, the patient was continued at that angle of tilt for a duration of three days. The results of the study of 121 patients showed that 87 percent of the patients, without a true disc herniation and no previous operative treatment, were no longer occupationally disabled. Forty-five percent of those that had one or more back operations, not including fusion, reported good pain relief. Those that had had a spinal fusion, had no relief. It was his conclusion that gravitational traction was ineffective in all who had an extruded disc; such treatment was also ineffective in patients having had a spinal fusion. It was postulated that relief of chronic pain and extremity pain was due to distraction of the lumbar vertebrae and resolution of the inflammatory response to the posterior longitutional ligaments and anterior dura (sinuvertebral nerve). It was further postulated that failures may be due to postoperative fibrosis or ankylosis of the root and the sinuvertebral nerve at multiple levels. The studies did not intend to assess forms of conservative treatment other than gravitational traction, and absolute bed rest remained the simplest most effective treatment for the acute back and extreme pain of musculoskeletal origin. It was emphasized that pelvic traction may do no more than keep the patient at strict bed rest.

Coxhead et al,[19] in 1981, studied four types of treatment for sciatic symptoms: traction, exercises, manipulation, and the use of corsets. Treatments were assessed in a random controlled trial of 322 out-patients. The design was factorial. There were 16 treatment groups, enabling a comparison of the combination of methods as well as individual methods. The treatment lasted for 4 weeks and patients were reviewed at the end of this period and at the end of 4 and 16 months after entry into the trial.

Traction was with a motor-driven "Tru-trac" apparatus giving intermittent traction at preset forces and time intervals; exercises were based on a group of exercises showing all ranges of motion and muscle groups; manipulation by the technique of Maitland and a corset that was a ready-made fabric available in three sizes for lumbar support. All patients received short wave diathermy and a half hour of "back school" lectures for which the subject matter was standardized. The duration of each treatment and its intensity (tractive or manipulative force applied and the grade of exercises given) were at the physiotherapists' discretion. Treatment was discontinued if the patient became free of symptoms. Progress was assessed by comparison of whether a patient felt better or worse after four weeks of treatment; by asking the patient to assess his or her improvement or deterioration at the completion of the treatment; on the basis of return to work to normal activities at the end of four weeks' treatment and at 4 months after entry; and by a postal questionnaire 16 months after entry into the trial on the presence or absence of pain in the back or legs and any further treatment during the intervening year. There were some patients that dropped out during the first month and some that were lost in the follow-up. In all, 292 patients (91 percent) were assessed at the end of the treatment, 250 (78 percent) were assessed at 4 months after entry, and 258 (80 percent) replied to the questionnaire at 16 months. At 4 weeks, 78 percent of all patients said they had improved whether or not they had received a particular treatment. Those having traction or manipulation may have done better than those that did not receive it, but there were no differences in the case of exercises or corset use. The effect may have been due to the number of types of treatments and not to a specific treatment used in combination. The fewer the types of treatment received during the trial, the higher the proportion of patients who had further treatment in the next three months. There was a lack of any consistency, at four months, for those having particular treatment to have done better than those who did not receive treatment.

The trial confirmed a high rate of spontaneous recovery reported by others. Seventy-eight percent of the patients reported improvement, irrespective of specific treatment. There was no conclusive evidence that any of the four individual treatments were effective, but it was possible that each confirmed some benefit, particularly manipulation. The trial had three main limitations; (1) there was no satisfactory way of measuring progress as they relied mainly on subjective assessment of the patients themselves; (2) it was possible that some treatments were more effective in certain types of patients than in others, as this had been suggested in the case of manipulation, so the characteristics of those thought especially likely to benefit have not been objectively defined; and (3) the trial was neither single blind or double blind. The main difference between this and other trials was the use of combinations of different treatments. There were no beneficial effects of treatments detectable at 4 or 16 months. In the short term, active physical therapy with several treatments appeared to be of value in the out-patient management of patients with sciatic symptoms, but it did not seem to confirm any long term benefit.

Anderson, Schultz, and Nachemson,[2] in 1983, studied the in vivo effects of active (subject induced) and passive body traction on the pressure within the lumbar intervertebral disc. The pressure within the nucleus of the L_3 disc was measured in four volunteers, three women and one man. Their ages ranged from 19 to 23, with a mean of 22 years. Their mean weight was 138 pounds. They were all in good health and none had a history of back injury or significant back pain. No abnormalities were found on routine clinical orthopedic examination.

Intradiscal pressure was measured by means of a subminiature pressure transducer built into the tip of a needle.[71] Traction was applied in two ways: active and passive. In active traction, the subject's pelvis was fitted with a harness attached to a spring force scale and in turn was attached to a frame at the foot of the traction table. This autotraction table had been previously used. The subjects were lying on their left side to avoid interference with the needle. They were asked to pull slowly with increasing force up to 100 pounds on the spring scale and to maintain that force for 2 minutes. When passive traction was applied, the patient was again lying on the same table. Two investigators, one pulling at the pelvis and the other under the arms, administered traction for 30 seconds. All tests were repeated once.

The results revealed that during traction (auto traction) this pressure increased considerably and in relation to the tractive force. These increased pressures were sustained over a two minute period. During passive traction, pressures generally remained at the resting levels, but sometimes were increased, other times were reduced. Active traction increased disc pressure considerably and passive traction had little effect. The main factor that would raise disc compression force, and therefore disc pressure, is the contraction of the trunk muscles crossing the levels of the motion segment. Active traction, in this study, increased disc pressure, presumably because it was accompanied by strong contractions of the trunk muscles.

The purpose of spinal traction is to reduce pressure within the discs and to open up the disc spaces; therefore, traction has to be administered in a manner that will allow trunk muscles to relax. Biofeedback or passive traction, perhaps, may accomplish this. Active traction seemed less likely to do so. Clinically, it remains to be determined when, in whom, and what kind of traction therapy may be beneficial.

Ancient history has recorded that treatment of back disorders[1] by traction were thought to be less likely to be benefited by the head downward because the weight of the head and the top of the shoulders, when allowed to hang downward, is small; such cases are more likely to be made straight when traction was applied with the feet hanging down since the inclination downward was greater.

More recently, there has been a great interest in the "inversion therapy" for treatment of back pain. One hangs upside down, like a bat, for 10–15 minutes by a ankle-holder or gravity boots. These were developed in 1965 by Robert Martin.[73] This may not have any effect on the back problems permanently, but tends to provide symptomatic relief temporarily. There were no radiographic studies to indicate any separation of the vertebrae nor controlled studies to date regarding this form of subjective relief.

Traction of this type is based upon the principle of body weight using gravity to stretch tissues of the spine, eg, the muscles, ligaments, fascia, and possible discs. The person may simply hang or perform exercises while in traction.[9] One must be cautious in this type of therapy, as blood pressure can increase producing hemorrhage in the eyes and vascular insult to the brain. Yoga exercises have been done in patients accustomed to gradual inversion over many years, so precautions must be adhered and gradual changes in position must be observed.

Gianakopoulos, Waylonis, Grant, et al,[89] in 1985, evaluated the use of inversion devices as a means of producing lumbar distraction. They used three gravity traction devices: (1) the Backtrac, (2) Back-On-Trac (Lossing Orthopedics), and (3) Gravitational Lumbar Traction System (Camp). The latter device had the subjects suspended in the upright position with a corset-like vest worn around the rib cage, whereas, the other two were involved with inversion. Twenty subjects with chronic low back pain, ages 23–66, composed of 12 men and 8 women, volunteered for the study. Periods of inversion were up to 20 minutes. Lateral lumbar spine radiographs were taken in the standing position and after 5–15 minutes of inversion. Measurements were carried out at the anterior and posterior aspects of the intervertebral space and also the center of the interspace and these were averaged.

The results of the study showed that 13 of the 16 symptomatic patients felt improved after inversion. One subject experienced marked increase of discomfort and two subjects had a dramatic improvement up to three hours of symptomatic relief. The pain relief gradually increased in duration as inversion was used on a regular basis. The most significant changes involved the cardiovascular system. All subjects demonstrated elevation in both systolic and diastolic pressure. The average increase in blood pressure was 17 mm systolic and 16 mm diastolic while in the inverted position. The heart rate slowed 16 beats/minute on an average. Distraction of the lower lumbar spine intervertebral spaces occurred with inverted traction in all cases with the range of 0.3–4.0 mm with a mean average of 1.5 mm at the L_3–L_4 interspace, 1.6 mm at the L_4–L_5 interspace, and 2.0 mm at the L_5–S_1 interspace. The side effects included periorbital and pharyngeal petechiae, persistent headache, persistent blurred vision, conjuctival injection, and contact lens discomfort in one patient. Nasal stuffiness was noted by most patients. It was suggested that individuals with any medical problems, potentially exacerbated by elevation in blood pressure, intercranial pressure, or mechanical stress of the inverted position, should be considered contraindications to inversion therapy. Other potential contraindications might include cardiopulmonary disease, glaucoma, chronic headache, GI reflux, artificial hip replacements, motion sickness, and chronic sinusitis.

Deyo,[27] in 1983, discussed conservative treatment of low back pain describing the expense, work loss, and risk of side effects. Common problems were related to failure of randomized subjects in experimental designs, use of "blind" observers, compliance, inadequate description of technique, patient and relevant outcomes. Studies may not clearly support the results, validity, or application of treatment in low back pain. Better methods for insuring blind therapy, measuring compliance, and assessing outcomes are needed.

SOME INDICATIONS AND CONTRAINDICATIONS
FOR TRACTION

Some of the indications for traction are: (1) intervertebral disc disease, with or without root irritation; (2) disc protrusion; (3) facet osteoarthritis; (4) some soft tissue injuries; and (5) to stretch muscles and ligaments.

The contraindications[45] are: (1) acute soft tissue injuries; (2) neoplastic diseases[57]; (3) unstable post-traumatic lesions; (4) some cases of sciatica with neurological deficit; (5) inadequate investigation; (6) cord compression[31]; (7) infectious disease of the spine; (8) osteoporosis; (9) rheumatoid arthritis with ligamentous instability or subluxation in the upper cervical spine; and (10) late pregnancy.

SUMMARY

Conflicting evidence of the benefits of traction appear in the literature. Clinicians differ regarding the advantages of traction.[83] Traction can produce separation of the vertebrae and facets, increase the foraminal space, relieve acute and chronic symptoms, but clear scientific evidence may be lacking the therapeutic value, other than immediate relief. In some cases, traction may actually increase the discomfort.

Traction should not be used in the acute phase of neck injuries because the muscles are tender and there may be some hemorrhaging in the neck muscles, including the posterior part of the pharynx.[18] Trying to pull against these muscles will simply counteract the natural splinting tendency. It is preferable to wait two or three weeks. If there is any sign of nerve involvement in that period, either a positive electromyogram or weakness on clinical examination, then traction may be helpful. To find out if a patient can tolerate traction, the clinician should grasp the base of the skull with one hand, the chin with the other, and move the head in flexion while applying traction. If he can do this without eliciting pain, the patient can probably tolerate cervical traction, in the flexed position with the head brought forward. Intermittent traction is generally more effective than steady traction because it allows greater tractive forces to be applied over prolonged periods of time with less discomfort. Some patients may need 35–45 pounds of traction, intermittently, over a 25 minute period to obtain relief. Seldom can a patient tolerate 20–25 pounds of continuous traction for a period of 10–15 minutes. Frequently, the patient is given home traction of 8–12 pounds for 15–20 minutes. This amount of traction is generally ineffective. Flexion of the neck, facing the door, is the appropriate method of application (Fig. 6-12).

There is no effective device for home traction—other than a conventional traction table device—to the lumbar spine, because of the amount of tractive force necessary to produce the desired effect; therefore, almost all equipment is designed for the upper spine.

There is no one halter device that is satisfactory. The ideal halter allows the greatest pull at the occiput with minimal force at the chin-piece to avoid pressure at the temporomandibular joints. One type of halter used by the author is illustrated in Figures 6-12 and 6-13. The advantage is that it is so constructed that during traction the jaw is slightly opened, and thus, avoids the pressure at the temporomandibular joints. Unfortunately, the large side pieces cause undo pressure on the ears if the tractive force exceeds 25 pounds.

Ideally, the pull should come from the occiput with minimal or no force at the chin,

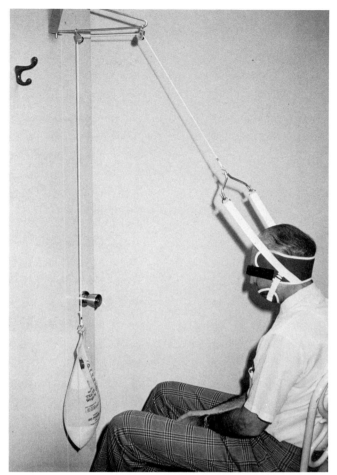

Fig. 6-12. Home cervical traction unit with patient facing the door in relaxed position and the neck flexed.

but this may require a forehead band. Some types of polyaxial traction have been described with the patient giving a counter force by the feet via a pulley system and straightening the knee, to provide pull to the halter. A simple method of traction utilizes a turkish towel applied at the occiput and crossed over the forehead and pulled by the physician or therapist. This can be repeated several times, but does demand energy on the part of the evaluator. In clinical practice, the use of a Saunders Cervical Traction Device does not contact the chin or apply force to the temporomandibular joints. It is a V-shaped device attached to a shaft connected to a traction source of a commercial traction table (Fig. 6-14). It is comfortable during traction in some patients, but the disadvantage is that the size does not vary to the shape of the head and does not fit a heavy necked individual.

In the author's experience, the greatest benefit from cervical traction occurs in the case of discogenic disease with acute symptoms of nerve root involvement. The response can be dramatic and, combined with nonsteroidal antiinflammatory drugs (NSAI) the

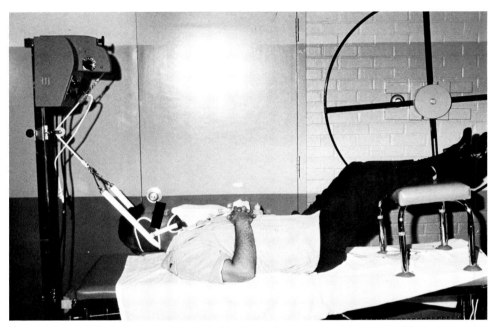

Fig. 6-13. Cervical traction being applied in the supine position with the neck lifted off the table surface and the lower extremities relaxed.

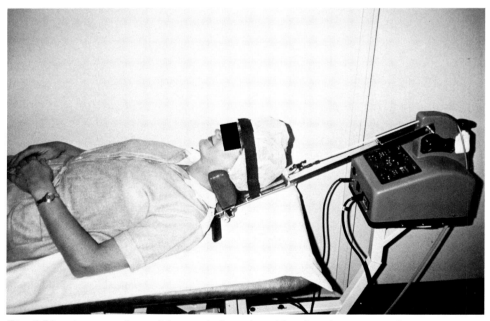

Fig. 6-14. Apparatus for applying cervical traction with pull at the occiput and none at the chin. Traction unit (Courtesy of Saunders Cervical Traction Device and TRU-EZE MFG. CO. INC.)

relief may be quickly apparent. Unfortunately, many patients need long term traction to control the complaints of recurrent neck pain with radicular symptoms.

There are patients that do not tolerate horizontal traction as well as vertical. The author has noted cases in which "clicking" of the neck is noted on rotation of the head and may occur in hyperextension-flexion injuries of the spine. These cases have been helped with higher traction forces of 45–60 pounds, for a duration of 60 seconds and rest periods of 15–30 seconds, repeated several times. It appears that patients can tolerate these large forces for short periods and may have relief in cases that have not been assisted in the horizontal position. The neck needs to be flexed and not extended if rotation is added[6] and an adjustable chair seems to serve the purpose. (Fig. 6-15)

The author has found benefit with the use of heavy pelvic traction of 85–100 pounds in only 50 percent of the cases referred for nerve root irritation with or without muscle weakness and reduced or loss of reflexes. It does appear that there is a greater percentage of relief and recovery with traction in those cases having nerve irritation in the L_4–L_5

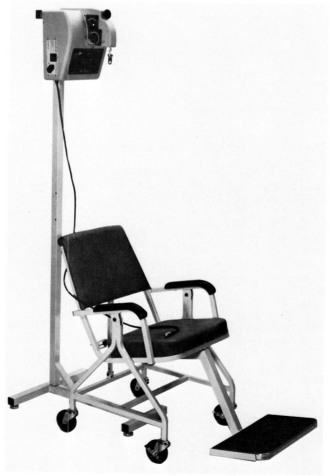

Fig. 6-15. Courtesy of the TRU-EZE MFG CO. INC., Temecula, California

rather than L_5–S_1 distribution. This may be due to the greater movement in the vertebrae noted previously.[17] If there is any increase in discomfort with traction, it is discontinued. Traction in bed, while in a hospital, has not been effective other than allowing the patient to remain still. It is uncomfortable to prescribe this modality for several hours, particularly at night, as it does not allow the patient to change into more comfortable positions. Frequently, traction is ordered in bed for long periods of homeopathic tractive forces with no regard to the position of the pelvis or lower extremities.

Traction should be administered only after careful history, physical examination and work-up. Diagnostic radiography, thermography, electrodiagnostic and laboratory tests assist the physician in his armamentarium so that a diagnosis has been formulated and indications for traction are established. Traction may be given with some form of heat and massage. The use of selective exercises and manipulation can prove most helpful in many cases. When properly administered with specific indications, traction can provide surprising relief of pain and discomfort.

REFERENCES

1. Adams F: The Genuine Works of Hippocrates, Vol 1. New York, William Wood and Company, 1886, pp 105–123

2. Anderson GBJ, Schultz HB, Nachemson AL: Intervertebral disc pressures during traction. Scand Rehab Med (Supp) 9:88–91, 1983

3. Bard G, Jones MD: Cineradiographic recording of traction of the cervical spine. Arch Phys Med Rehabil 45:403–406, 1964

4. Bettmann OL: A Pictorial History of Medicine. Springfield, Charles C Thomas, 1962, pp 30–31

5. Bouckaert JP: Les propriéte mécaniques du muscle. Compte rendu du 1er congrès international de biologic appliquée al éducation physique et aux sports. Bruxelles, 1939, pp 75–101

6. Brown B St J, Tissington Tatlow WF: Radiographic studies of the vertebral arteries in cadavers (effects of position and traction of the head). Radiology 81:80–88, 1963

7. Cailliet R: Neck and Arm Pain (ed 2). Philadelphia, F A Davis Co, 1981, pp 1–20, 124–131

8. Cailliet R: Low Back Pain Syndrome (ed 3). Philadelphia, F A Davis Co, 1981, pp 90–94

9. Cailliet R: Understand Your Backache. Philadelphia, F A Davis Co, 1984, pp 131–136

10. Chahal AS: Results of continuous lumbar traction in acute dorso-lumbar spinal injuries with paraplegia. Paraplegia 13:1–10, 1975

11. Ching C: In defense of cervical traction. Resident and Staff Physician 8:89–93, 1979

12. Christie BGB: Discussion on the treatment of backache by traction. Proc R Soc Med (Section of Physical Medicine) 48:811–814, 1955

13. Colachis SC Jr, Strohm BR: Radiographic studies of cervical spine motion in normal subjects: flexion and hypertension. Arch Phys Med Rehabil 46:753–760, 1965

14. Colachis SC Jr, Strohm BR: Cervical traction: relationship of traction time to varied tractive force with constant angle of pull. Arch Phys Med Rehabil 46:815–819, 1965

15. Colachis SC Jr, Strohm BR: A study of tractive forces and angle of pull on vertebral interspaces in the cervical spine. Arch Phys Med Rehabil 46:820–830, 1965

16. Colachis SC Jr, Strohm BR: Effect of duration of intermittent cervical traction on vertebral separation. Arch Phys Med Rehabil 47:353–359, 1966

17. Colachis SC Jr, Strohm BR: Effects of intermittent traction on separation of lumbar vertebrae. Arch Phys Med Rehabil 50:251–258, 1969

18. Colachis SC Jr: Diagnosis and management of whiplash injuries. Current Concepts on Pain and Analgesia 4:1–2, 1977

19. Coxhead CE, Meade TW, Inskip H, et al: Multicentre trial of physiotherapy in management of sciatic symptoms. Lancet 1:1065–1068, 1981

20. Crisp EJ: Discussion on the treatment of backache by traction. Proc R Soc Med (Section of Physical Medicine) 48:805–808, 1955

21. Crue BL: Importance of flexion in cervical traction for radiculitis. USAF Med J 8:374–380, 1957

22. Cyriax J: Trial by traction (letter). Br Med J 1:522–523, 1976

23. Cyriax JH: Textbook of Orthopaedic Medicine, Diagnosis of Soft Tissue Lesion. (ed 7) Vol 1, Baillière Tindall, London, pp 160–168, 493–499

24. Cyriax J: The treatment of lumbar disc lesions. Brit M J 2:1434–1438, 1950

25. Deets D, Hands KL, Hopp SS: Cervical traction:

A comparison of sitting and supine positions. Phy Ther 57:255–261, 1977

26. DeSèze S, Levernieux J: Les tractions vertébrales: premières études expérimentales et résultats thérapeutiques d'apres une expérience de quatre années. Sem Hop Paris 27:2085–2104, 1951

27. Deyo RA: Conservative therapy for low back pain. JAMA 250:1057–1062, 1983

28. Erickson DL: Cervical traction and other physical therapeutic procedures for pain about the neck and shoulders. Minn Med 373–377, 1956

29. Fielding JW: Cineroetgenography of the normal cervical spine. J Bone Joint Surg 39:1280–1288, 1957

30. Frazer EH: The use of traction in backache. Med J Aust 41:694–697, 1954

31. Fried LC: Cervical spinal cord injury during skeletal traction. JAMA 229:181–183, 1974

32. Fulton JF: Physiologie du système nerven. Vigot, éditeurs, 1947

33. Gartland GJ: A survey of spinal traction. Brit J Phys Med 20:253–258, 1957

34. Goldie IF, Reichmann S: The biomechanical influence of traction on the cervical spine. Scand J Rehav Med 9:31–34, 1977

35. Goldie I, Landquist A: Evaluation of the effects of different forms of physiotherapy in cervical pain. Scand J Rehab Med 2–3:117–121, 1970

36. Gray FJ: Combination of traction and manipulation for the lumbar disc syndrome. Med J Aust 54:958–961, 1967

37. Gray FJ: An assessment of body-weight traction on a polished incline plane in the treatment of discogenic sciatica. Med J Aust 2: 545–549, 1969

38. Gray's Anatomy (British Ed) Warwick R, Williams PL. (eds) Philadelphia, W B Saunders Company, 1973, pp 411–414

39. Grieve GP: Neck traction. Physiotherapy 68:260–265, 1982

40. Gupta RC, Ramarao SV: Epidurography in reduction of lumbar disc prolapse by traction. Arch Phys Med Rehabil 59:322–327, 1978

41. Hanflig SS: Pain in the shoulder girdle, arm and precordium due to foraminal compression of nerve roots. Arch Surgery 46:652–663, 1943

42. Harrell A, Mead S, Mueller E: The problems of spasm in skeletal muscles JAMA 143:640–644, 1950

43. Harris PR: Cervical traction: Review of the literature and treatment guidelines. Physical Therapy 57:910–914, 1977

44. Hickling J: Spinal traction techniques. Physiotherapy 58(2):58–63, 1972

45. Hinterbuchner C: Traction, in Rogoff J (ed): Manipulation, Traction and Massage. Baltimore, Williams & Wilkins, 1980, pp 184–210

46. Hirsch C, Nachemson A: New observations on mechanical behavior of lumbar discs. Acta Orthop Scand 23:254–283, 1954

47. Hitselberger WE, Witten RM: Abnormal myelograms in asymptomatic patients. J Neurosurg (L.A.) 28:204–206, 1968

48. Hood LB, Chrisman D: Intermittent pelvic traction in treatment of the ruptured intervertebral disc. Phys Ther 48:21–30, 1968

49. Jackson R: The Cervical Syndrome (ed 3). Springfield, IL, Charles C Thomas, 1971, pp 245–261

50. Jones MD: Cineradiographic studies of the normal cervical spine. California Med 93:293–296, 1960

51. Judovich BD: Lumbar traction therapy and dissipated force factors. The Journal—Lancet 74:411–414, 1954

52. Judovich BD: Herniated cervical disc; a new form of traction therapy. Am J Surg 84:646–656, 1952

53. Judovich BD, Nobel GR: Traction therapy; a study of resistance forces. Am J Surg 93:108–114, 1957

54. Judovich BD: Lumbar traction therapy; elimination of physical factors that prevent lumbar stretch. JAMA 159:549–550, 1955

55. Kottke FJ, Mundale MO: Range of mobility of the cervical spine. Arch Phys Med Rehabil 40:379–382, 1959

56. Krusen EM: Pain in the neck and shoulder; common causes and response to therapy. JAMA 159:1282–1285, 1955

57. La Ban MM, Meerschaert JR: Quadriplegia following cervical traction in patients with occult epidural prostatic metastasis. Arch Phys Med Rehabil 56:455–458, 1975

58. Laurin CA: General practice: Cervical traction in the home. Canad Med Asso J 94:36–39, 1966

59. Lawson GA, Godfrey CM: A report on studies of spinal traction. Med Serv J Can 14:762–771, 1958

60. Lehmann JF, Brunner GD: A device for the application of heavy lumbar traction: its mechanical effects. Arch Phys Med Rehabil 39:696–700, 1958

61. Licht S: Massage, Manipulation and Traction (ed 1) New Haven, E Licht, 1960, pp 220–258

62. Loeser JD: History of skeletal traction in the treatment of cervical spine injuries. J Neurosurg 33:54–59, 1970

63. Mathews JA: Dynamic discography; a study of lumbar traction. Ann Phys Med 9:275–279, 1968

64. Mathews JA, Hickling J: Lumbar traction; a double-blind controlled study for sciatica. Rheumatol Rehabil 14:222–225, 1975

65. Mathews JA: Effects of spinal traction. Physiotherapy 58:64–66, 1972

66. Masturzo A: Vertebral traction for treatment of sciatica. Rheumatism 11:62–67, 1955

67. McFarland JW, Krusen FH: Use of the Sayre head sling in osteoarthritis of cervical portion of spinal column. Arch Phys Med Rehabil 24:263–269, 1943

68. Martin GM, Corbin KB: An evaluation of conservative treatment for patients with cervical disc syndrome. Proc Staff Meet Mayo Clinic 29:324–326, 1954

69. Mennell J Mc M: Back Pain Diagnosis and Treatment Using Manipulative Techniques. Boston, Little Brown and Company, 1960, pp 56–79, 94–108

70. Mettler CC: History of Medicine, Mettler FA, (ed.): Philadelphia, Blakiston, 1947, pp 798–802

71. Nachemson A, Elfstrom G: Intravital dynamic pressure measurements in lumbar discs. A study of common movements, maneuvers and exercises. Scand J Rehabil Med Supp 1:5–40, 1970

72. Oudenhoven RC: Gravitational lumbar traction. Arch Phys Med Rehabil 59:510–512, 1978

73. Paris EL: The upside-down cure. Forbes 122 (Sept) 1983

74. Quinet RJ, Hadler NM: Diagnosis and treatment of backache. Seminars in arthritis and rheumatism 8:261–287, 1979

75. Rath WW: Cervical traction, a clinical perspective. Ortho Rev 13:29–48, 1984

76. Richardson PF: Traction in cervical arthritis. Maryland State Med J 21:19–21, 1972

77. Rowe CR: Current concepts in therapy. Cervical osteoarthritis. N Engl J Med 268:1178–1179, 1351–1353, 1963

78. Shenkin HA: Motorized intermittent traction for treatment of herniated disc. JAMA 156:1067–1070, 1954

79. Shore NA, Schaefer MG, Hoppenfeld S: Introgenic TMJ difficulty: Cervical traction may be the etiology. J Pros Dent 41:541–542, 1979

80. Smyth MJ, Wright V: Sciatica and the intervertebral disc. J Bone Joint Surg 40A:1401–1417, 1958

81. Stoddard A: Traction for cervical nerve root irritation, Physiotherapy 40:48–49, 1954

82. Taylor AR: Mechanism and treatment of spinal cord disorders associated with cervical spondylosis. Lancet 1:717–720, 1953

83. Traction for neck and low back disorders. Med Lett Drugs Ther 17:16, 1975

84. Valtonen EJ, Kiuru E: Cervical traction as a therapeutic tool. Scand J Rehabil Med 2(1):29–36, 1970

85. Valtonen EJ, Moller K, Wiljasalo M: Comparative radiographic study of the effect of intermittent and continuous traction in elongation of the cervical spine. Ann Med Int Fenn 57:143–146, 1968

86. Varma SK, Gulatia R, Mukherjee A, et al: The role of traction in cervical spondylosis. Physiotherapy (London) 59:248–249, 1973

87. Vasudevan SV, Thielen PL, Melvin JL: Contour donor chair: device to maximize effects of overhead cervical traction. Arch Phys Med Rehabil 64:285, 1983

88. Waylonis GW, Denhart C, Grattan MM, et al: Home cervical traction: evaluation of alternate equipment. Arch Phys Med Rehabil 63:388–391, 1982

89. Waylonis GW, Gianakopoulos G, Grant PA, et al: Inversion devices: Their role in producing lumbar distraction. Arch Phys Med Rehab 66:100–102, 1985

90. Weber H: Traction therapy in sciatica due to disc prolapse. J Oslo City Hosp 23:167–176, 1973

91. Weinberger LM: Trauma or treatment? The role of intermittent traction in the treatment of cervical soft tissue injuries. J Trauma 16:377–382, 1976

92. Worden RE, Humphrey TL: Effect of spinal traction on the length of the body. Arch Phys Med Rehabil 45:318–320, 1964

93. Wramner T: Observations on the symptoms and diagnosis of cervical rhizopathia and experience with vertebral traction. Acta Rheumatol Scand 3:108–114, 1957

94. Yates DAAH: Indications and contra-indications for spinal traction. Physiotherapy 54:55–57, 1972

John B. Redford

7

Assistive Devices

Pain, on joint motion or on joint stress, is the major complaint that distinguishes patients with musculoskeletal disorders, particularly arthritics, from those with most other chronic disabling conditions. The primary purpose of any appliance or orthosis in such patients is therefore to reduce stress on joints to protect them against further injury. The second major purpose in the use of self-help aids in such patients is to decrease energy consumption. Most arthritic patients complain of fatigue, especially those with systemic conditions such as rheumatoid arthritis. Therefore, a balance between rest and exercise forms a cornerstone of any treatment regimen for rheumatoid arthritis. Only by conserving energy can the body fight the debilitating inflammatory effects of systemic forms or musculo-skeletal diseases.

Reducing energy consumption may be essential for the disabled person to function effectively. For example, it does little good to teach a seriously disabled arthritic patient to dress independently if, by the end of the task, he or she is so exhausted that performing other functional activities efficiently is impossible. Patients fatigued or weakened by misguided attempts to ensure total independence of self care can be vulnerable to more accidents and further stresses on arthritic joints. Fortunately, today with many automatic devices and conveniences in the modern home or work place, it is easy to provide energy conservation programs for patients. This takes careful planning and should be part of the rehabilitation program for any patient with a serious musculoskeletal disorder.

Prescription of any assistive device or self help aid appears deceptively simple. Nevertheless, in many instances, proper understanding of kinesiology and the biomechanics of the device is essential if it is to be effective. In many instances, therefore, patients need professional guidance regarding the best choice for their functional problems. A self-help aid enables the user to perform a personal task that would either be impossible without other help or in a shorter time with less energy. Whatever its purpose, the device must be an acceptable alternative for other possibilities. Therefore, selection and use of devices should be an integral part of the rehabilitation process either during training or following discharge.

Unfortunately, in our gadget-minded society, along with the proliferation of self-help

PRINCIPLES OF PHYSICAL MEDICINE AND REHABILITATION
IN THE MUSCULOSKELETAL DISEASES

aids and assistive devices, there has been a proliferation of sales people, all too eager to sell the public many expensive self-help appliances. Often these are either unnecessary or much more costly than simpler ones that could be made at home. Physicians and others who are concerned about needs of the disabled should be aware of this and advise patients accordingly. On the other hand, a large number of items, readily available from such sources as the Sears catalog, do not require any referral to a rehabilitation facility or patient training. A number of sources for devices and equipment are given in a list at the end of the chapter.

ASSISTIVE DEVICES FOR MUSCULOSKELETAL DISEASE: GENERAL CONSIDERATIONS

In considering assistive devices for patients with arthritis and other musculoskeletal disabilities, two basic principles must be observed: small joints need more protection than large ones with bigger muscles and, whenever possible, activities should be done with gravity stresses minimized. This former principle applies particularly in carrying or lifting; for example, using a sling over the shoulder to carry heavy bag rather than a small hand grip. An example of the second principle is to slide or use rollers for heavy objects rather than trying to lift them.[11]

Cordery, an occupational therapist, in a classical review of joint protection,[1] further elaborated on these principles with three recommendations: (1) "reduce the force necessary to accomplish the activity"; for example, use built-up handles for tools to reduce the need for tight grip, (2) "change the method, sometimes choose the lesser of two evils"; for example, squeeze wet sponges by pressing down with the palm rather than by grasping or when standing up from an armchair, push up with the forearms rather than the wrists, (3) "use equipment, if necessary," for example, most rheumatoid arthritics should use electric can openers instead of manual ones.

For many arthritic patients, choosing the methods and equipment to protect joints is difficult, and some patients are not even aware of the need to spare their joints. How many times have we listened to stoical patients who think they can fight their arthritis by "walking it away." Although physicians and others can be helpful in guiding patients, occupational therapists play a major role in advising arthritic patients on joint protection and energy conservation. As most patients have no appreciation of efficient body mechanics, they must be taught good posture and proper seating to minimize joint stress. Unfortunately, too many designers of appliances and furniture for every day use also have no appreciation of body mechanics and posture. Consider, for example, the low, soft, over-stuffed sofas in most living rooms. Such common hazards around the home must be pointed out.

Not only can occupational therapists guide patients in choosing devices and modifying home environments, such as the kitchen, but also, they can emphasize scheduling and pacing of activities to avoid fatigue and reduce pain. A time tested rule covering a specific activity for an arthritic patient is that the activity should not cause pain; in the exercise area, any pain induced should subside within two or three hours and should not be present in the area on the following day. Physicians and therapists can teach patients to observe this rule by providing sound advice on proper methods for performing otherwise stressful activities, such as effective use of equipment and proper scheduling of activities.

A patient, severely disabled with a musculoskeletal disorder and needing special assistive devices, requires a full rehabilitation assessment to integrate these devices into a total rehabilitation program. Such patients are best treated at rehabilitation centers where a full rehabilitation team can evaluate equipment needs and training and assess the home environment. In fact, before prescribing any permanent equipment, careful attention must be given to the proposed living arrangements; they must relate to the degree of functional disability or supplying equipment may be worthless.

Patients who are less disabled often do not need such an elaborate assessment. Sometimes equipment can be rented or even borrowed from a rehabilitation department on a trial basis before purchase, thus saving expense. For most patients, cost is always a consideration; thus, simple aids are generally better than complex ones. All persons giving advice regarding self-help aids should be aware of costs, especially when any third party carrier is reluctant to pay for equipment that is considered a "comfort" and not a "medical necessity." Unfortunately, this is a rather arbitrary decision for assistive aids for many disabled patients. If a functional aid will restore potential for reemployment, cost should be of secondary importance, particularly if the patient receives encouragement from his employer or other associates to return to work. The importance of this must be stressed to third party payers who may be reluctant to provide expensive equipment.

The patient's emotional response to assistive devices must always be considered. If he or she can function reasonably well without the aid or has not yet accepted a certain degree of irreversible impairment, the equipment may never be used. In addition, if much education is needed to use an appliance, it will be discarded unless training is readily available. The less conspicuous the self-help aid, the more acceptable it may be. Cognitive ability also must be considered. Providing a device is useless if the subject cannot understand its purpose or learn how to use it.

Assistive aids have been classified into seven major categories: mobility, eating, dressing, hygiene, communication, recreation, and miscellaneous. The last category will not be reviewed in this chapter; it includes specific devices for maintenance of body functions such as respirators and specialized adaptations for certain vocational pursuits. Using this classification, the United States Veterans Administration has recently published an excellent comprehensive "Directory of Living Aids for Disabled Persons," and it includes names and addresses of most rehabilitation equipment vendors in the United States.[12]

Mobility Aids

Most patients with painful joints and weakness of the lower limbs benefit from hand-held walking aids. Up to 25 percent of body weight can be transferred away from the lower limbs with a cane; crutches and walkers can reduce weight bearing by 50 percent and provide more stability. All canes or crutches must have rubber tips and these should be checked periodically; if they are worn out, a cane or a crutch on a slippery surface is more hazardous than no cane at all. For the patient with painful wrists, a platform crutch, with its trough to support the forearm, minimizes stress on the wrists and elbows by distributing weight over the whole forearm. Thickened or padded handles on all types of crutches or canes minimize the grip needed, thus reducing strain on arthritic finger joints. Details on gait training and different types of walking aids are readily available in many publications.[13]

A major problem for many patients with musculoskeletal disorders is transfer ability. A patient may be able to walk but has great difficulty arising from a bed or a chair. Basic to rehabilitation programs for those with musculoskeletal disorders is ability to turn or get out of bed, particularly if wearing heavy casts, following orthopedic surgery. In a hospital, a bed with elevating head and footrests and an overhead trapeze and siderails is essential to help such patients move about but such beds are not generally available at home. Rather than advising the patients to buy an expensive hospital bed for use at home, a rope ladder or braided bed pull attached to the foot of the bed may be all that is needed. These are commercially available or can be made from cord or thin rope with dowels placed to suit the person. Free standing trapezes for beds are also available.[3]

A common complaint of patients with arthritis in the knees and hips is inability to get up from low chairs. Chairs or other furniture can be raised by recessed wooden blocks placed under the feet. A commercially available item, Pedi-4-Legs,"* can adapt most chairs with legs safely and easily to any height required. Rather than elevating the chair, it is often simpler to provide a firm seat cushion two to four inches thick depending on height required. Some arthritic patients have found chairs with a spring or motor-driven elevating seat well worth the additional cost but these chairs may be unsafe for the very frail or partly paralyzed patient.[9]

As most accidents happen in the bathroom or bedroom where people move about to dress and bathe, these rooms for arthritic patients should have chairs with arm supports for stability and firm seats no lower than knee height.

Unfortunately, in spite of advances in joint replacement and improvement in drug therapy, not all patients with arthritis can retain their independence and ambulation. Although a wheelchair may be considered by some a sign of medical failure for the person determined to maintain independence and mobility, it may become a necessity. When a person is unable to walk, the whole contact with the environment revolves around the wheelchair. Therefore, if a wheelchair is needed permanently, it must be carefully chosen to fit all of the patient's requirements. Because of the bewildering number of models and sizes available, professional advice is usually necessary and better obtained from a rehabilitation department than from a wheelchair dealer. Hospital equipment vendors can be very helpful but may suggest needlessly expensive solutions if a wheelchair prescription is not subject to a review by a rehabilitation professional. Detailed descriptions of wheelchair configurations are beyond the scope of this chapter but are readily available from many manufacturer's catalogs or the references.[5,8]

If a permanent wheelchair is not needed, many patients with lower limb pain may even benefit from wheeled seats (caster chairs) or stools that can be used indoors while performing household or vocational tasks. Rehabilitation departments usually have some of these as well as various wheelchair models for evaluating patients.

Lately, three-wheeled battery-powered vehicles, such as the Amigo,† have become very popular with arthritic patients. They are very efficient, readily portable, and can often pass through narrow openings unfit for wheelchairs. They are not as stable as wheelchairs, however, and patients should be warned of this problem. Like all powered mobility aids, they also place less demand on the patient to exercise. Because the goals in many arthritics is to maintain physical fitness, motorized vehicles should be prescribed only if reducing stress on joints is considered more important than maintaining fitness.

Most wheelchairs should be provided with cushions; foam cushions are usually sufficient, but if the patient has limited seating tolerances or poor sensation, special cushions

---

*Pedi-4-Legs: Roloke Company, Los Angeles, CA
†AMIGO, 6693 Dixie Highway, Bridgeport, MI 48722

filled with air or special gels may be needed. Air cushions have an advantage over the gels or water-filled ones because of their light weight. Other pads may be needed in the chair, particularly in the lumbar area to improve posture. For nonambulatory patients with severe musculoskeletal deformities, some rehabilitation centers have started seating clinics. A team consisting of physician, occupational therapist, and orthotist evaluate patients and then prescribe and build custom made seats to control posture while seated in the wheelchair or other seating arrangement.[7]

All other things being equal, the availability and quality of service for a wheelchair should be a final consideration when furnished for a person with a permanent disability. Fortunately, with the increasing competition in the medical equipment market, services are available in many more communities than in the past, but the availability of repairs should be reviewed prior to any wheelchair prescription.

Depending on the mobility impairment of the patient, the home may need to be adapted to reduce musculoskeletal stress and conserve energy. This is best done through a home visit by a rehabilitation professional but a few general points follow. If the patient is confined to a wheelchair, entrances should be ramped and all outside entrances provided with hand rails, whether or not a wheelchair is needed. Doorways should be at least 30 inches wide but preferably 36 inches and door knobs and latches fitted with levers. For example, a rubber lever that fits over a door handle is shown in Figure 7-1. Floors should be kept in good repair with nonskid surfaces. Shaggy carpet and loose throw rugs are difficult surfaces not only for arthritics but even for elderly people who walk unaided. If climbing stairs is impossible, it is usually preferable for the family to modify the house so the disabled person can live on the main floor rather than install expensive wheelchair stair lifts or elevators.

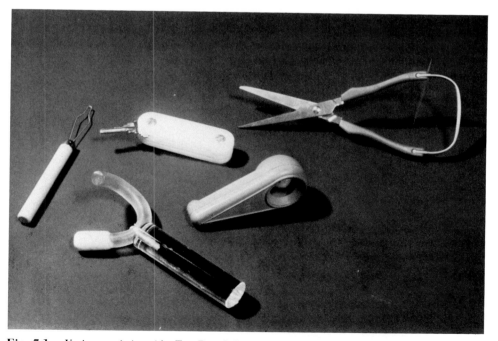

Fig. 7-1. Various assistive aids: Top Row (left to right): button hook, adapted key grip, adapted scissors Bottom Row: car door opener, rubber door opening lever that fits over a door handle.

The automobile is an essential component of mobility for almost everyone. Any disturbance of joint function may create problems for the automobile driver. It is now possible to provide many special automobile adaptations to facilitate access and provide driving control to most handicapped persons. For example, an automobile door latch opener is shown in Figure 7-1. Special programs are widely available to assess the driver's capability and adaptability to automobile modifications in most rehabilitation centers. Parking in public places has always been a problem for those in wheelchairs. A space at least 12 feet in width is needed to permit patients with wheelchairs, braces, and crutches to get in and out of cars on a level surface. Fortunately, with the new legislation favoring the handicapped, many more handicapped spaces are available to the public than in the past. This, along with curb cuts and special entrances, have made life somewhat simpler for disabled patients, but much remains to be done, particularly in the area of public transportation.

Eating Aids

Medical supply houses now have available many attractive and durable eating aids for those with poor grasp and disorders affecting the shoulder and elbow. Special utensils may not be necessary as objects and utensil handles may be enlarged with foam padding, bicycle grip handles, or even foam from a hair roller. One should avoid adding too much weight for badly weakened hands. A universal cuff that slips around the hand is widely used to hold utensils in a special pouch (Fig. 7-2). If the forearm is fixed in pronation, swivel and bent angled utensils may be necessary. For loss of range of motion in the elbow and shoulder, extended handles can compensate. A wingnut on the extension handle will allow the angle of the utensil to vary and permit it to be removed conveniently. Patients

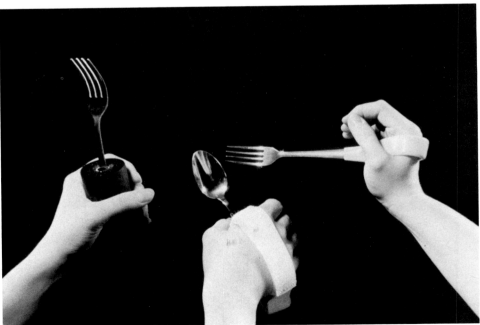

Fig. 7-2.   Eating aids (left to right): foam-enlarged handle, universal cuff, Quad-Quip fork holder.

may also be helped by plate guards, scoop dishes, or suction cups. Dycem mats will hold the plate firmly on the eating surface. Light weight plastic mugs or glasses are preferable to more conventional ones for patients with hand and wrist involvement and drinking straws are very helpful.

When it comes to preparing meals, most occupational therapy departments are equipped to provide advice to families about meal preparation, specialized adaptive equipment, and advice concerning the convenient locations of cabinets, use of roll-around carts to avoid heavy lifting, and other work simplification suggestions. An example of only one of many handy kitchen appliances is the jar opener in Figure 7-3. An excellent description of mealtime aids and food preparation as well as general advice on housekeeping for disabled persons is found in the book by Hale[3] and a "Mealtime Manual" covers a large variety of equipment techniques and resources as well as some recipes and gives prices and sources of all equipment and supplies covered in the book.[4]

Dressing Aids

Independent dressing for the physically disabled person is only partly solved by aids. Types of clothing must be considered. Garments should be adjustable and expandable, easily put on and taken off, and reinforced against wear by braces and crutches. Because self-esteem for the disabled person is most important, attractive and carefully selected clothes will greatly enhance physical appearance and concealed defects or appliances. Today's fashions emphasizing comfort and informality encourage individual expression— a welcome notion to those who have disabilities.

Clothing should be chosen with openings and sleeves, easily loosened and fastened. Garments with front openings are the easiest to don and doff, for example, fastening a

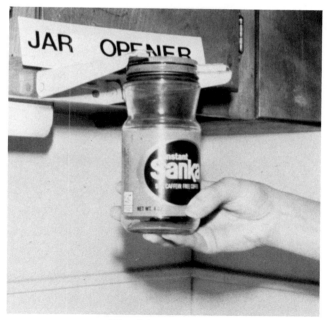

Fig. 7-3.   Jar opener.

brassiere in front is much easier than fastening it in back. Velcro closures are great substitutes for buttons and, if carefully applied, can be used without changing the appearance of common garments such as shirts and slacks. If buttons are used, they should be as large as feasible but button hooks can be very helpful. Zippers are easier to use than buttons and can be easily opened and closed with adaptive aids (Fig. 7-4).

A dressing stick, a dowel with a coat hook on one end and a cup hook on the other, is of great assistance to many arthritics for picking up and pulling on clothes and slipping shirts over stiffened shoulders (Fig. 7-5). It also allows older arthritic patients to remain seated while dressing and thus decreases risks of falling.

Patients with limited reach and stiff lower limbs have the greatest difficulty in dressing with shoes, socks, and trousers. A long-handled shoe horn and boot jack may help put on and remove slipon shoes or tie shoes modified with elastic laces. A stiff plastic stocking gutter with pull tabs makes it possible to put on stockings without bending. Researchers also can help obtain articles otherwise out of range while dressing or performing other tasks and several styles are available.

All occupational therapy departments will have suggestions or resources for aids for dressing and adaptive clothing and most textbooks on rehabilitation can also be consulted for ideas.[6,10] In addition, there are several companies that are specializing in designing clothing for the disabled and elderly (See list at end of chapter).

Hygiene Aids

Aids to personal hygiene such as toothbrushes, razors, brushes, and combs, can have either enlarged or extended handles, such as those described for feeding devices. Washing

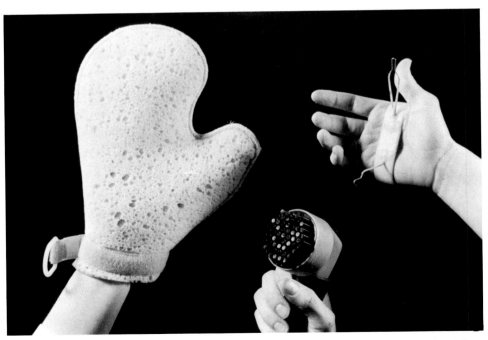

Fig. 7-4. Miscellaneous aids (left to right): wash mitt, multi-purpose turning handle, Quad-Quip buttonhook, and zipper pull.

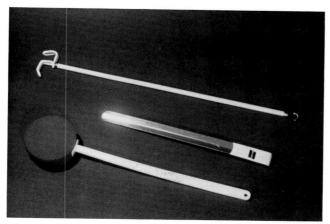

Fig. 7-5. Dressing and bathing aids (from top down): dressing stick, long-handled shoe horn, long-handled bath brush.

aids include wash mitts, soap on a rope, brushes with suction cup, and long-handled sponges (Figs. 7-4, 7-5).

As the bathroom with its narrow space and slippery floor is probably the most dangerous place in the house for anyone with a disability, grab bars should be placed where needed around tubs, showers, and toilets. In the tub and shower, nonskid strips or mats should be placed on lower surfaces. For those with weakness or stiffness in the lower limbs, raised toilet seats are readily available in most medical supply stores, and seats for bathtub or shower along with bath lifters are common. If a person cannot sit down in the bottom of the tub, a bathtub seat placed over the tub and a hand-held shower that plugs into the faucet will often solve the problem of bathing. When a person cannot walk into the bathroom—bathroom entrances are usually hopelessly small for wheelchair entry—a bed-side commode may need to be substituted for the toilet in the bathroom. The commode should be provided with sidearms and arranged to permit the feet to touch the floor. Toilet activities for a person with unilateral limitation of hip and knee flexion may be accomplished with a raised commode seat, having one sloping side. A special toilet adaptation is even available to cleanse the anal area for persons with limited reach who cannot do this for themselves.

Communication Aids

Reading, writing, and the use of the telephone as well as radio and television are essential for disabled persons to keep in touch with others and not be deprived of normal sources of intellectual and emotional stimulation.

For reading, large print books, special magnifiers, even special magnified television screen systems are available for those with poor vision. For patients with musculoskeletal disorders, the main problem is usually to hold reading matter in a comfortable position. A variety of aids can provide help including angled book stands that can be placed on tables, over beds, or even on the floor like a music stand. Difficulty turning pages can be overcome using rubber thimbles or rubber pencils to grip the pages.

For writing, there are a number of alternatives such as implements held on fingers with metal rings (Fig. 7-6). Handles on writing implements can be enlarged by rubber

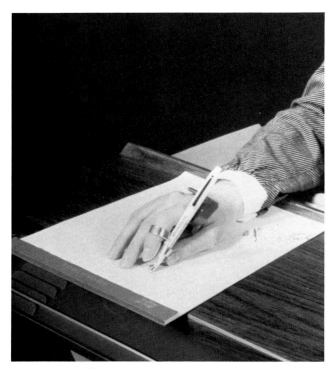

Fig. 7-6. Wanchik writing aid.

bands or foam rubber or even by sticking a pen through a plastic golf ball. Clipboards are often helpful in writing to stabilize paper if it is awkward to hold the page steadily.[3]

Electric typewriters have been a great benefit to persons who lack strength or have pain in their joints on using the controls on a manual typewriter. Electric typewriters have now been succeeded by computers with printers that most patients with musculoskeletal disorders have little difficulty operating because of the very light touch required.

For telephone communication, advances in design of telephones have made it much easier for disabled to send or receive calls. A telephone should obviously be placed for most efficient and comfortable use, especially if reach is limited. Probably it is easier to use a touch type telephone than dials for most patients with arthritis and giant push button telephone adapters are currently available to make this even easier. The need to dial can be completely eliminated by a call maker that will call up automatically at the press of a button or insertion of a card into a slot. If it is painful to hold the telephone for any length of time, a person can have the telephone mounted on a gooseneck arm or use a headset or even place a conventional telephone entirely by dial microphone and speaker set in a special boxed unit. All telephone companies can easily help handicapped persons with the advice as to the options available.

Radios and telephone and television sets, of course, can be adapted by special handles on the sets or remote controls and so do not usually present too much of a problem for handicapped persons. A new device, recently introduced, has a series of plastic or metal rods that depress to conform to a surface that needs tight pinch such as a television dial. This is a very versatile device and relatively inexpensive (Fig. 7-4). One practical solution for persons who have difficulty getting in and out of chairs yet who wish to have a variety of communication resources close at hand is a rolling utility cart. With three shelves, it is possible to keep a telephone, TV control dials, stationery items, books, magazines, and other items all within handy reach.

Patients with special problems in communication that may exist along with a musculoskeletal disability should be advised to seek a speech and hearing therapist. Most rehabilitation centers can provide this service but local chapters of American Speech and Hearing Association can usually suggest how to obtain these services.

Recreation Aids

Only by participation in recreational activities can many disabled persons resume life in the community again and make new friends or escape from an institutional setting. Therefore, physicians should encourage those with permanent musculoskeletal disability to participate not only in group exercises or outdoor sports but in any recreational activity of interest. There are many sports that have been adapted for disabled persons; for example, bowling can be done with a long-handled ball pusher or even a special bowling ball ramp is available for those confined to a wheelchair who have limited upper limb function. Boards and playing pieces for table games such as checkers, cribbage, backgammon, and chess can be enlarged and made from light plastic for those with problems with grasp or poor coordination. Special tools for gardening and shop work have been developed for specific handicaps. Hales's book is an excellent guide to recreational activities and also lists various organizations promoting leisure activity for the handicapped.[3]

CONCLUSION

The aim of this chapter has been to provide a limited guide to assistive devices that are available for persons with musculoskeletal impairments, as it is impossible to provide great detail in any area. We have listed in the reference section a number of sources that could be consulted for further information. Rehabilitation centers or rehabilitation medicine departments in hospitals are always available as sources of information along with local hospital supply houses.

Because such a profusion of equipment for the disabled exists, a national program is now available to assist handicapped people and others in obtaining information about commercially available rehabilitation equipment. It is called the ABLEdata system, and is funded by the National Institute of Handicapped Research. The National Rehabilitation Information Center, 4407 Eighth Street, Washington, D.C., operates this system. The ABLEdata system is a computerized list of all commercially available rehabilitation products including manufacturers, distributors, and national distributors with mail order product catalogs. Access to the computerized system can be provided by a local information broker. Names of information brokers may be obtained from the State Vocational and Rehabilitation Division, usually in the state capital or by contacting the National Rehabilitation Information Center.

Another commercial computerized data base on products for the disabled is Accent on Information. Data entry is organized by categories of equipment and by specific functional loss. Included are ideas about how to make or adapt equipment, organizations of interest to disabled persons, and a list of approximately a thousand companies, developers, and organizations. Each data entry lists product name, cost, and brief description. There is also an Accent Buyer's Guide that developed from this information system; it lists manufacturers, distributors, and organizations classified by product and type of function. For further information, contact Accent on Information, P.O. Box 700, Bloomington, IL 61701.

REFERENCES

1. Cordery J: The Conservation of Physical Resources as Applied to Activities of Patients with Arthritis and the Connective Tissue Diseases. Study Course III, 3rd International Congress, World Federation of Occupational Therapy, William C. Brown Co., Dubuque, IA 1962, p. 22
2. Fahland V, Grendahl VC: Wheelchair Selection: More Than Choosing A Chair With Wheels. Rehabilitation Publication #713, Sister Kenny Institute, Minneapolis, MN, 1976
3. Hale RG: The Sourcebook for the Disabled, Philadelphia, W.B. Saunders, 1979
4. Institute of Rehabilitation Medicine, New York University Medical Center, Klinger, JL (ed): Mealtime Manual (ed. 2). Camden, NJ, Campbell Soup Co., 1978
5. Kamenetz HL: Wheelchairs and Other Indoor Vehicles, in Redford JB (ed): Orthotics Etcetera, (ed. 2). Baltimore, Williams and Wilkins, 1980, pp. 443–493
6. Leslie LR: Training for Functional Independence and Training in Homemaking Activities, in Kottke FJ, Stillwell GH, Lehmann JF (ed): Krusen's Handbook of Physical Medicine and Rehabilitation (ed. 3). Philadelphia, W.B. Saunders, 1981, pp. 501–517
7. Motloch WM: Seating for the Physically Impaired. Orthotics Prosthetics 32:11–21, 1977
8. Peizer E: Wheelchairs in American Academy of Orthopedic Surgeons (ed): Atlas of Orthotics. St. Louis, C.V. Mosby, 1975, pp. 431–453
9. Redford JB, Broky WS, Zilber S: Electrical Power-Assisted Seat Lift: Is It Helpful? An Appraisal of Its Function. Orthotics Prosthetics 33:25–31, 1979
10. Rusk HA: Rehabilitation Medicine (ed. 4). St. Louis, C.V. Mosby Co., 1977, pp. 143–151
11. Swezey RL: Arthritis: Rational Therapy and Rehabilitation. Philadelphia, W.B. Saunders Co., 1978, pp. 97–102
12. U.S. Veterans Administration, Directory of Living Aids for the Disabled Person, Superintendent of Documents, U.S. Government Printing Office, Washington, DC, 1983
13. Varghese G: Crutches, Canes, and Walkers, in Redford JB (ed): Orthotics Etcetera (ed. 2). Baltimore, Williams and Wilkens, 1980, pp. 432–442

SOURCES OF SELF HELP CLOTHING

1. Caddell, K, Textile Research Center, Box 4150, Lubbock, TX 79409
2. FashionABLE, Rocky Hill, NJ 08553
3. Geri Fashions, Newberg, OR 97132
4. Leinenweber, Inc., 60 W. Washington St., Chicago, IL 60602
5. PTL Designs, Inc., Box 364, Stillwater, OK 74074
6. Sears Company Home Health Catalog, Chicago, IL 60602
7. Smith Co., 7674 Park Avenue, Lowville, NY 13367

GENERAL REFERENCES

1. Enders A (ed): Technology for Independent Living Source Book, Rehabil. Engineering Society of North America, 4405 East-West Highway, Bethesda, MD, 1984
2. Goldsmith S: Designing for the Disabled: A Manual of Technical Information, Institute of British Architecture, London, England, 1963
3. Hamilton L: Why Didn't Somebody Tell Me About These Things? Intercollegiate Press, Shawnee Mission, KS, 1984

4. Klinger JL: Self Help Manual for Arthritis Patients, Arthritis Foundation, Atlanta, GA, 1980

5. Kreisler M, Kreisler J: Catalog of Aids for the Disabled, McGraw-Hill Book Co., New York, NY 16020

6. Laurie G: Housing and Home Services for the Disabled: Guidelines and Experiences in Independent Living, Harper and Row, Hagerstown, MD, 1977

7. Lowman EW, Klinger JL: Aids to Independent Living: Self Help Aids for the Handicapped, McGraw-Hill Book Co., New York, NY, 1969

8. May EE, Waggoner NR, Hotte EB; Independent Living for the Handicapped and Elderly, Houghton Mifflin Co., Boston, MA, 1974

9. Melvin JL: Rheumatic Disease: Occupational Therapy and Rehabilitation (2nd Edition) F.A. Davis Co., Philadelphia, PA, 1982

10. National Handicapped Housing Institute Inc., Product Inventory of Home Hardware Equipment and Appliances for Barrier-Free Housing Design, Minneapolis, MN

11. Robinault IP (ed): Functional Aids for Multiply Handicapped, Harper and Row, Hagerstown, MD, 1973

PART 2

Specific Problems

Steven F. Brena
Stanley L. Chapman

8

Chronic Pain:
Physiology, Diagnosis, Management

The word *pain** is an abstraction, a relative concept useful to rationalize whatever choices are made out of its multiple meanings. To the philosopher, pain is a challenge to test human fortitude; to the sociologist and the psychologist, pain may be a way to study behaviors of people; to the physiologist, pain is a perceptual phenomenon based on physical sensations; while to the physician it is a signal to be decoded and interpreted for the diagnosis of diseases. A common abstraction, which oftens clouds a clear understanding of the phenomenon of pain, is the question of real pain vs. psychogenic pain. Every painful experience must be assumed to be real to the individual sufferer in the presence, as well as in the absence, of organic pathology. As in all sensory perceptions, pain involves an interplay between physical sensations and their emotional and cognitive interpretations. In every painful experience there are always psychogenic components and neurophysiological components. These components constantly mutually interact, making a determination of organic versus psychological pain inoperative.

It may be safely assumed that every painful experience in humans is 100 percent psychological and 100 percent physiological at the same time. Two other sources of semantic confusion are the terms *acute pain* and *chronic pain.* Usually acute pain indicates a high intensity painful experience of recent onset; while chronic pain merely implies a time factor (Greek: chronos = time) added to an ongoing painful perception. Thus, the two words are not defined along the same dimensions: *acute* refers not only to time but also implies an affective dimension of severity; *chronic* only refers to a temporal dimension.

Probably the most effective way to study the experience of pain in humans is to consider it a multi-level phenomenon which is shown in Figure 8-1:

*The English word "pain" is derived from the Sanskrit root "pu," meaning sacrifice, and from the Latin word "poena," meaning "punishment." These two roots clearly indicate religious undertones in the human experience of pain, both in Western and Eastern cultures.

PRINCIPLES OF PHYSICAL MEDICINE AND REHABILITATION
IN THE MUSCULOSKELETAL DISEASES

NOCICEPTIVE* DETERMINANTS

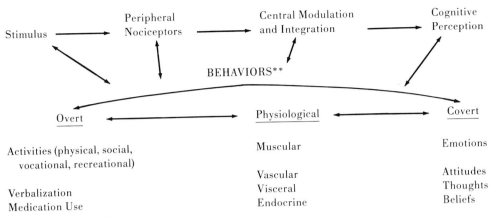

*Latin: Nocere—to damage.
**Established through processes of operant and classical conditioning and social modeling.

Figure 8-1. Nociceptive determinants.
(From Brena SF, Chapman SL: Acute vs. Chronic Pain States: "The Learned Pain Syndrome" In Clinics in Anaesthesiology, Chronic Pain: Management Principles, Saunders Publishing Company, London, 1985. (In Press).

NOCICEPTIVE DETERMINANTS

In this chapter a brief mention will be made of the pathophysiology of nociception (Latin: Nocere = to damage) and the processes of conditioning. Clinical classes of chronic pain states will be described as part of the diagnostic process of chronic pain patients. Treatment modalities will be discussed within the framework of Pain Control Programs.

The Pathophysiology of Nociception

The processing of nociceptive information includes a sequence of events, many of them still poorly understood: (1) a transduction of energy changes from an area of tissue damage into sequential nerve impulses, generated peripherally and passed centripetally; (2) a nociceptive afferent system over the sensory, cranial, and spinal nerves; (3) a modulation and integration of the nociceptive information within the central nervous system (CNS) until it becomes a cognitive awareness, which is the painful experience. Modulation and integrative processes can be understood in terms of molecular biology or, more traditionally, by resorting to psychological terminology.

Transduction

The skin, the subcutaneous tissues, and the deep somatic tissues contain a variety of transducer-like structures, mostly bare nerve endings of high threshold, which are fired only by energy changes of such magnitude as to threaten tissue homeostasis. These structures, which respond only to nociceptve stimulation, are called *nociceptors*. Some nociceptors are responsible mainly to mechanical injury, while others are activated by noxious thermal and chemical stimuli (polymodal nociceptors). It is now well established that nociceptors are mostly activated by local accumulation of many algesic substances, such as potassium chloride, hydrogen ions, histamine, bradykinins, and various prosta-glandins. Algesic accumulation usually occurs following cellular damage by injury or through acute inflammatory processes. Certain physiological conditions may also enhance nociceptor excitability. For instance, the nociceptors of the tendons and muscles are activated—or at least primed—by the excessive tone of the skeletal muscles as occurs in poor habits of body mechanics and in various muscle-contraction syndromes.[19,64] Visceral nociceptors have been little investigated when compared with somatic nociceptors; how-ever, research has shown that specific visceral nociceptors do exist.[20] Distension or pro-longed isometric muscle contraction of the hollow viscus seems to be an adequate nociceptive stimulus.

Nociceptive Afferent Pathways

Recordings from single nerve fibers have demonstrated that nociceptive information in primates is conveyed to the spinal cord from somatic structures mainly by two types of primary afferent fibers: myelinated A-delta fibers and the unmyelinated C-fibers. Around 25 percent of A-delta fibers and 50 percent of C-fibers are nociceptive afferents. Visceral impulses travel mainly through C-fiber afferents. The relationship between perception of pain and afferent nociceptive stimulation has recently been reviewed.[23]

Ascending Fiber Networks: CNS Modulation and Integration

The fibers conveying nociceptive information terminate in the upper dorsal horn, mostly in laminae 1 and 2 (the substantia gelatinosa). Immunohistochemical methods have located a number of peptides in the dorsal root ganglion cells, which may play the role of neurotransmitters: somatostatin, neurotensin, Substance—P, etc.[38] The relative specificity of the peripheral nociceptive system has little counterpart in the CNS. There is no *central pain center* as a receiving station comparable to the cortical projections of other sensory systems. Neurophysiologic investigation in animals has helped to throw some light in the way that the CNS processes peripheral nociception. It is now well accepted that central neurons do not simply reflect discharges of nociceptors, but that peripheral nociceptive information is profoundly modified in the CNS via complex phenomena of modulation and central integration that occur postsynaptically at multiple levels of the CNS. Table 8-1 summarizes the nociceptive system in its peripheral and central-integratory mechanisms.

THE NOCICEPTIVE SYSTEM

Stimulation of several brain areas inhibits the excitation of many dorsal horn neurons to nociceptive stimulation. Such areas include the periaqueductal gray of the midbrain, the raphe magnum of the medulla, and the lateral reticular areas of the caudal medulla.[30] Transmitters involved in such antinociceptive phenomena include the following: (1) the opioid peptides: the opio-melanocortin group, the pro-enkephalin group, the dynorphin group; (2) 5-hydroxytryptamine (serotonin); (3) noradrenalin; and (4) glycine and gamma-aminobutyric acid. The complex neurophysiology of the opioid peptides in antinociceptive inhibition has been reviewed by Duggan.[28] Documented high concentrations of opioid peptides in the caudate nuclei, in the globus pallidus and in the limbic system link together pain suppressing mechanisms with motor systems, stress responses, and the sympathetic system via the limbic loop to the hypothalamus.[3]

Table 8-1
The Nociceptive System

Anatomy	Physiology	Clinical Equivalent
Peripheral Nociceptors	Chemosensitive to algesic agents, Mechanosensitive, Polymodal	Threshold for Pain Perception is higher than Nociceptors' Threshold
A-Delta Fiber Network C-Fiber Network	Peripheral afferents. Neurotransmitter: Somatostatin, Neurotensin, Substance P, Others	
Spinal Dorsal Horn (Mostly Laminae I, II, V, VI)	First synaptic relay. Links to motor and sympathetic segmental reflexes	Segmental motor and sympathetic activation
Ascending Pathways (Mostly via spinothalamic and spinoreticular tracts)	Transmission of nociceptive information	
Brain Stem: Reticular formation; periaqueductal grey; Raphe nuclei	Anti-nociceptive modulation, via descending inhibitory tracts to spinal neurons (Dorsolateral funiculus?)	Some are activated by direct electrical stimulation; blocked by naloxone
Diencephalon: Nonspecific thalamic nuclei	Anti-nociceptive integration; nonspecific suprasegmental activation of autonomic and motor systems (?)	Nonspecific, aversive responses to nociception (?)
Hypothalamus: several nuclei (Caudateglobus pallidus)		
Cerebrum: Limbic system	Motivational—affective dimension of pain (?)	Suffering (?) Learned pain Behaviors (?)
Neo-cortex	Cognitive perception of pain (?)	Learned coping skills (?)

From Brena SF: Nerve Blocks and Chronic Pain States: An Update. Part 1: Post-Grad. Med., 1984 (In press). With permission.

Acute vs. Chronic Pain: Nociceptive Determinants

Physiological Phenomena

The bulk of evidence from research in nociception—antinociception seems to demonstrate that such phenomena are primarily organized to subserve the experience of pain associated with trauma and inflammation. The release of opioid peptides both modulates nociceptive stimulation and reduces the firing of motor neurons in response to multiple peripheral inputs. It seems that antinociception and muscle activity are linked together as likely protective mechanisms in the face of a bodily threat. Together they induce a generalized pattern of bodily inactivity that may be deemed necessary for healing to occur. Moreover, release of endogenous peptides in response to tissue injury results in a generalized emotional hyporesponsiveness to environmental stimuli that, in turn, enhances a general sluggishness in bodily movements.

From the data presently available from research in anti-nociception, the relationship depicted in Figure 8-2 characterizes acute pain states.

Acute Pain

Likewise, in Figure 8-3 it is shown that if this relationship is reversed, a pattern of events may follow which seems to characterize, at least clinically, many chronic pain states.

Chronic Pain

Voluntary muscle activity is a learned behavior with little, if any, genetic inheritance. Feedback is one of the most important concepts in learning control of movements and behaviors in a healthy person. Feedback impulses from the central nervous system usually evoke patterns of normal, painless functional activity. A state of wellness requires a proper balance of physical activity and rest. When this balnace is upset in either direction, serious malfunctions are likely to occur. Feedback impulses are modified by the lack of function, and, in turn, evoke patterns of decreased and even more painful muscular work in a progressively deteriorating cycle. Inactivity is one of the most prevalent features in many chronic pain patients.[53] Several factors are likely to be associated with patterns of progressive inactivity: (1) the process of aging with the concomitant constellation of physical and emotional changes; (2) serious emotional maladjustment, including states of depression

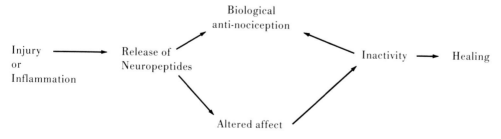

Figure 8-2. (Acute pain. From Brena SF, Chapman SL: Acute vs. Chronic Pain States: "The Learned Pain Syndrome" In Clinics in Anaesthesiology, Chronic Pain: Management Principles, Saunders Publishing Company, London, 1985, (in press). With permission.)

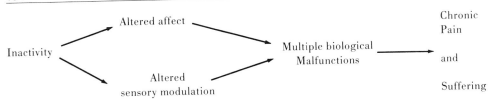

Figure 8-3. Chronic pain. From Brena SF, Chapman SL: Acute vs. Chronic Pain States: "The Learned Pain Syndrome" In Clinics in Anaesthesiology, Chronic Pain: Management Principles, Saunders Publishing Company, London, 1985, (in press). With permission.

and "learned helplessness"[59]; (3) failure to modify a habit of inactivity, biologically unjustified, long past natural healing from an injury or a disease process; (4) An on-going, progressive, pathological condition; and (5) mistaken fears that physical harm or unbearable pain will accompany activity.

The literature on the physiology of inactivity has received an impetus from research concerning bodily responses to states of weightlessness experienced by astronauts during space flights.[51,52] From this and related research, an inactivity syndrome and its likely dysfunctional mechanisms can be described as summarized in Table 8-2.

The Inactivity Syndrome

Overt Behaviors

The classical Pavlovian conditioning process can be summarized as follows:

U S (Unconditioned Stimulus) ⟶ U R (Unconditioned Response)
    (Food)   (Salivation)

C S (Conditioned Stimulus) ⟶ C S (Conditioned Response)
    (Bell)   (Salivation)

The same sort of process occurs in the experience of pain:

U S (Unconditioned Stimulus) ⟶ U R (Unconditioned Pain Response)
    (Injury, disease)

C S (Conditioned Stimulus) ⟶ C R (Conditioned Pain Response)
    (People, places, feelings,
    thoughts)

According to this process, mental stimuli such as being with certain people or in certain places or situations can continue to evoke pain responses merely through association with an original injury. Classically conditioned acute pain has been demonstrated with humans in the laboratory using a laser beam applied to the hand as the unconditioned stimulus to produce pain and a sound as the conditioned stimulus.[27] Classically conditioned pain behaviors are likely to decrease over time in normal circumstances when the unconditioned stimulus of injury or disease is no longer present. This process can be accelerated by teaching the patient alternative responses to make in the presence of a conditioned stimulus. Removing the patient from the environment where he or she has experienced pain may also serve to decrease the intensity of classically conditioned pain

Table 8-2
The Inactivity Syndrome

Musculoskeletal System	Activation of patient's latent T.P.'s*—Loss of muscle mass. Loss of coordination. Osteoporosis. Fibrosis and stiffness of joints.
Cardiovascular System	Activation of the sympathetic system. Adrenergic preponderance. Increased basal rate. Decreased cardiac reserve. Dysfunctional anginal pain following efforts in physical activity.
Respiratory System	Decreased strength of respiratory muscles may cause restrictive respiratory impairment.
Digestive System	Decreased gastrointestinal motility and digestive secretion. Altered eating habits. Constipation. Possible malnutrition. Obesity.
Urinary System	Hypercalcemia. Urinary retention. Urinary tract infection.
Central Nervous System	Decreased sensory inputs result in altered sensation. Autonomic imbalance may cause poor adaptation to changes in exercise levels. Depression. Cognitive stagnation and confusion. Disordered sleep problems.
Immune System	Decreased secondary immune-activity from stress and malnutrition (?).

Modified from Vallbona C: Bodily Responses to Immobilization, in Kottke FJ, Stillwell GK, Lehman JF (eds): Krusen's Handbook of Physical Medicine and Rehabilitation. Saunders, London. 1982. With permission.
*T.P.=Trigger Point

responses. Pain responses that initially are classically conditioned, however, often become strengthened with time through other learning processes, such as operant conditioning.[31] This conditioning process refers mainly to the strengthening of behavior followed by a positively reinforcing consequence and the weakening of behavior followed by negative or no reinforcement. Unlike classical conditioning, operant conditioning depends upon the consequences of response rather than on what preceded the response. Potential rewards contingent upon pain behavior include the following:

Financial gain.   Present legislation for compensation after injury and the Social Security Disability Program are particularly apt to reinforce pain behavior as the benefits can be competitive with those available through work.

Relief from responsibility or stress.   Our social values often stigmatize psychological difficulties while not holding an individual responsible for physical problems and thereby create the opportunity for socially acceptable avoidance of stresses or responsibilities.

Social reinforcement.   Sympathy and attention contingent upon pain behaviors can come from any person in the patient's close environment. One aspect of social reinforcement that is often neglected is the role of the care-giver who perceives great satisfaction from being the strong one in a relationship and resists strongly any attempt to change such a relationship.

Drugs.   Many drugs given for pain create pleasant feelings of tranquility, leading to conditioned increase in drug intake. In addition, the temporary acute discomfort from drug withdrawal can maintain drug-taking behavior. Once physical or psychological dependence has developed, pain behaviors and drug-taking behaviors mutually reinforce each other.

Pain behaviors can also be learned through observation of the behavior of others in a process known as social modeling. The importance of social modeling in acute and chronic pain states has been repeatedly suggested by findings from numerous studies.[4,36,67]

Covert Behaviors

Studies performed on acute pain have revealed that variables related to cognition and emotion can infuence pain responses markedly. Most of these studies have involved exposing volunteers to a controlled stimulus and measuring such variables as subjective pain intensity and pain tolerance. Results have indicated that the pain experience is exacerbated if subjects expect that the stimulus will be intense if they have no perceived control over it, if they are anxious, and/or if they focus attention on the stimulus. These factors can influence chronic pain behaviors to an even greater extent. Many chronic pain patients have learned to expect pain to such a degree that it is assumed to be their lifelong companion, and they see themselves as having no control over the pain. Their behavior often resembles the learned helplessness syndrome found in animals who have been exposed repeatedly to stimuli over which they have no control.[59] This syndrome is characterized by psychomotor depression and impaired ability to learn in new situations.

Pinsky[55] has emphasized demoralization as the characteristic personality dimension in intractable chronic pain patients. Others have identified chronic pain to be a *masked depression* implying that pain complaints are a means of expressing depressed feelings.[58] Feelings of fatigue, hopelessness, uselessness, and discouragement are common clinical findings in chronic pain patients. Tension and anxiety also play prominent roles. Many patients have become conditioned to focus their attention and center their lifestyle and identity on pain and in the process have programmed themselves to experience it more acutely. Pain and anxiety often exist in a kind of vicious cycle in which each increases the other until one is relieved. The beneficial effects of relaxation training procedures in chronic pain sufferers gives clear testimony to the contribution of anxiety and muscular tightness in the experience of chronic pain.

The Learned Pain Syndrome

Brena and Chapman[11] have described a particular syndrome of chronic pain, which they called the *Learned Pain Syndrome* to emphasize the prominent role of conditioning factors. The syndrome is characterized by the following sets of symptoms: *Dramatization of complaints* with choices of words with high effective content; *Disuse*, which refers to the consequences of inactivity upon bodily systems; *Disability*, that is, a perceived, conditioned inability to work; Drug misuse[†]; and Dependency. (The "Five D's" Syndrome.)

The Diagnostic Process

The Unidimensional Approach

Clinical information generated by competent pain control centers in the United States has well documented the existence of a cluster of sensory impairments, which have been called *The Chronic Pain Syndrome*.[46] Though chronic pain can represent many different syndromes, its existence as an illness entity is no longer in dispute. The problem has now shifted to how to diagnose chronic pain in relationship to its pathological, emotional, and social components and how to classify its multiple clinical manifestations. The classical medical approach in the diagnosis of diseases, based on the analysis of biological malfunctions that are categorized into diagnostic judgments, seems to be quite inadequate when applied to many cases of chronic pain patients. On the other hand, the Third Edition of the *Diagnostic and Statistical Manual of Mental Disorders* (DSM-III) has a group of diagnoses—the Somatoform Disorders—that describe some patients with chronic pain in whom psychological malfunctions are predominant.[56]

However, the DSM III is a psychiatric diagnostic handbook, which necessarily fails to consider other categories of chronic pain patients with less prominent psychiatric features. The same point can be made for the six taxonomic groups described by Pilowsky and Spence.[54] Their classification of chronic pain patients is based on a one-dimensional hierarchical strategy: The Illness Behavior Questionnaire (IBQ). The IBQ has been designed to measure different aspects of abnormal illness behavior. Unfortunately, it fails to correlate behaviorial data with traditional medical findings of biological disorders and physical dysfunctions.

Agnew, Crue, and Pinsky[1] have proposed a "temporal classification of pain complaints," which tries to correlate within a time frame both pathological factors in various stages of nociceptive activity and psychosocial factors expressed in clinical judgments of competent and incompetent coping. The authors have described the various pain states as follows:

[†]Drug misuse can be defined as: (1) use of a drug that is inappropriate to the condition,such as use of a sedative in a functional patient; (2) overdosage; (3) incorrect time schedule for drug administration.

1. Acute Pain: Pain of a few days, of varying intensity from a presumed nociceptive input from an inferred or documented pathological condition.
2. Sub-Acute Pain: Pain of a few days to a few months; similar to acute pain in its nociceptive mechanisms.
3. Recurrent Acute Pain: From a recurrent or continued nociceptive input triggered by an underlying chronic pathological condition.
4. On-going Acute Pain: From a continued nociceptive input due to an uncontrolled, progressive neoplastic process.
5. Chronic Benign Pain: Nonneoplastic, usually over six months with no identifiable nociceptive peripheral input; likely central defect in pain modulation; adequate coping by the patient.
6. Chronic Intractable Benign Pain Syndrome (CIBPS):   Chronic benign pain with incompetent coping by the patient, who becomes obsessed by the continuing painful experience.

The taxonomy of pain proposed by Agnew, Crue, and Pinsky[1] adequately describes all possible types of pain patients. Unfortunately it relies on the use of nonquantified clinical judgment and of rather vague time references.

The Multidimensional Approach

Probably a more meaningful classification of chronic pain states can be obtained by a cross-matched evaluation of pathological, dysfunctional, emotional, and social factors. Several models for quantification of chronic pain states have been proposed.

Black and Chapman[7] have designed a three-factor index for assessment of pain states, using estimates of Somatic inputs, Anxiety, and Depression, the so called "SAD Index." The patient's total painful experience is represented by the vector sum of these three factors. The SAD model fails to incorporate relevant social and environmental factors and, therefore, is of limited diagnostic value, as the authors themselves have recognized. Duncan et al.[29] have designed a computerized "pain profile" for classification of each patient with pain. The model is based on mathematical comparison of three indices representing various pain dimensions: pathological, psychosocial, and behavioral aspects. The Duncan model is an excellent tool for teaching and research but it is time-consuming and, therefore, of limited clinical value. Moreover, it has never been tested as to its practical reliability and validity.

In 1975 Brena and Koch[14] presented a model for quantification and classification of chronic pain states that has stood the test of time and has been found to be reliable and valid (Fig. 8-4).[12,13,15,37]

THE EMORY PAIN ESTIMATE MODEL (EPEM)

The EPEM is an operational definition of a pain patient obtained through analysis of data pertaining to biological nociception from observable pathological and dysfunctional abnormalities—as assessed through medical examination; assessment of pain behaviors and correlation between medical and behavioral data. Table 8-3 shows the scoring criteria for the EPEM. The medical scores are depicted on a horizontal line and the behavioral scores are depicted on a vertical line, which intersect each other at midpoint as shown in

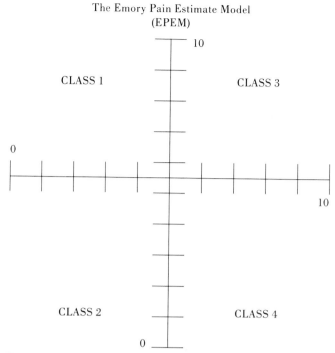

Figure 8-4. The Emory Pain Estimate Model (EPEM).

Figure 8-4. This arrangement yields four different classes of chronic pain patients, each of which is likely to require different therapeutic management. Table 8-4 summarizes traits of patients belonging to these four classes of the EPEM.

CLASSES OF CHRONIC PAIN STATES

Class I describes patients with a primary learned pain syndrome, characterized by inactivity, misuse of several drugs for pain and prominent ecological stressors. Consciously or unconsciously, Class I pain patients play various sick roles, which have been described by Pilowsky.[54] Anecdotal labels in the literature that try to describe Class I patients include: *psychogenic pain disorder, doloric patients,*[61] and *CIBPS*. These patients are intractable by conventional medical treatments, which may actually reinforce their sick roles. On the contrary, they are good candidates for referral to competent pain control facilities for appropriate psychophysiologic reactivation. Class II describes patients with often highly dramatized pain complaints within ill-defined anatomical patterns who generally show close-to-normal ADL and minimal misuse of drugs. Primary care of Class II patients should be designed to keep them functional despite their complaints through directive counseling and relaxation training. Unwise use of medication, suggestions of inactivity, unnecessary hospitalization for extensive diagnostic workups, and/or surgery for pain is likely to iatrogenically displace Class II patients into Class I. Class III describes patients with secondary learned pain syndrome associated with a documented pathologic

Table 8-3

Emory Pain Estimate Model

Medical Ratings:		Points
1) Physical Examination: (0–5 points)		
Joint Mobility	(Restricted)	
Cervical Spine	Above mid-range of motion:	0.5
Lumbar Spine		
Each of Four Extremities	Below mid-ROM:	1
Muscle Strength:		
	Movement against some resistance:	0.5
For each group of muscles	Movement against gravity only:	1
	Loss of movement:	2
Trigger Points and/or Splinting: (for each anatomic location)		0.5
Enlarged Organ or Abnormal Mass: (depending on size)		0.5–1
Systemic Functions: Abnormality in each parameter (depending on severity)		0.5–1
Loss of Reflexes: (for each reflex)		0.5
Sensory Abnormality:		
Segmental:		1
Non-segmental:		0.5
Loss of Vibration:		1
Motor Abnormality:		
(muscle atrophy, dystrophy, spasticity depending on severity, for each)		0.5–1
Loss of Coordination:		1
Other Abnormality: (depending on severity)		0.5–1
2) Diagnostic Procedures:		
Radiological studies: (for each abnormality)		
Severity:		0.5–2
Diffusion:		0.5–2

Other Studies: (for each abnormality)

    Severity: 0.5–2

    Diffusion: 0.5–2

Behavior Ratings: (0–10 Points)

1) Activity Profile

Uptime
(Feet on the floor while sitting or walking)
(Normal value: above 14 hours daily*)

10–14 hours:	0.5
8–10 hours:	1
6–8 hours:	1.5
4–6 hours:	2
Below 4 hours:	2.5

2) Pain Verbalization:

Pain Density: (intensity $\times$ frequency $\times$ duration†)

10–29	0.5
30–49	1.0
50–69	1.5
70–89	2.0
90–100	2.5

3) Drug Profile:

    Drug Dependence: 2.5

    Drug Dosage: (for each drug) within suggested doses   0.5

    Above clinically suggested doses   2.5

4) Personality Profile: (MMPI)

    For each clinical scale with a T-score between 70 and 84:   0.5

    For each clinical scale with a T-score of 85 or above   1.0

---

*Uptime measures may be obtained through use of a daily diary.

†Density is defined as mean subjective pain intensity at any moment in time. It can be calculated by multiplying the proportion of the time the person reports pain by the mean pain intensity rating when pain is present. Example: Pain present half the time with a mean intensity = 60, Density = 1/2 of 60 = 30.

Table 8-4
Classes of Chronic Pain States

	Clinical scores	Nociception	Psychology	Management
Class I	Behavior High: B > 5 Medical Findings Low: M < 5 Dysfunctional	Mostly from inactivity and poor body mechanics. Side effects from high drug usage.	Highly conditioned pain behaviors. Multiple emotional and environmental factors contribute to pain experience.	Multimodal structured psycho-physiological reactivation.
Class II	Behavior Low: B < 5 Medical Findings Low: M < 5 Functional	Mostly from stress-related muscle-contraction syndromes.	Conditioning factors include: Poor self-pacing skills, effects of stress and chronic anxiety.	Training in relaxation and stress management. Other brief targeted therapies.
Class III	Behavior High: B > 5 Medical Findings High: M > 5	Both from a documented pathological condition and from inactivity. Side effects from high drug usage.	Incompetent coping with the disease process and stress.	Stabilization of the pathological condition. Multimodal, structured pain rehabilitation programs.
Class IV	Behavior Low: B < 5 Medical Findings High: M > 5	From a documented pathological condition.	Competent coping with the disease process and stress.	Therapeutic restraint to avoid upsetting competent coping. Education, relaxation, self-hypnosis, and other brief targeted therapies.

condition. Competent coping with the pathologic disorder has been lost. These patients demonstrate high intensity illness behavior, characterized usually by inactivity, inadequate or misused medications for pain, and emotional maladjustments. Ecological stressors and socioeconomic rewards are often present. Proper treatment strategy for Class III patients should include both primary correction or stabilization of the pathologic condition and secondary referral to a pain control center. Class IV describes patients who are able to contain illness behavior and conserve competent coping in the presence of documented organic disease. An anecdotal label in the literature describes some of these patients as *stoics.*[61] Primary care of Class IV patients should show restraint in aggressive medical interventions to avoid impairing their functional levels and transferring them to Class III. Management of these patients should include careful education about the nature of their condition, correct and adequate by-the-clock medication, directed counseling for proper ADL, and relaxation training.

Brena and Chapman's[12] analysis of 250 patients (207 with back pain and 45 with headaches) treated at the Emory Pain Control Center showed that 50 percent of sufferers with chronic low back pain fell in Class I and that 66.7 percent of these Class I patients had a pending disability claim. On the contrary, 83 percent of patients with chronic headache were found to be Class II patients. Brena et al[13] have studied the relationship between impairment, disability, and classes of chronic pain patients in 101 consecutive referrals for vocational evaluation at the Emory Pain Control Center. Results have indicated that Class III patients show significantly higher ratings of impairment and disability than did Class I patients, who in turn show significantly higher ratings of impairment and disability than Class II patients. The difference between Class I and Class II patients in impairment and disability ratings can most likely be attributed to conditioned rather than to medical factors, as both of these groups by definition show low levels of medical findings.

Pain Control Programs

Definition

The Commission on Accreditation of Rehabilitation Facilities (CARF) has defined chronic pain control programs as follows:

> A program organized to reduce pain, improve quality of life and decrease dependence on the health care system; for persons with chronic pain which interferes with physical, psychosocial and vocational functions; through the provision of coordinated, goal oriented, interdisciplinary team services in an inpatient or outpatient setting.

> In a broader sense a pain control program could be defined as a strategy of treatment designed to reverse patients' illness behaviors into health behaviors.‡

The Pain Team

The CARF Standards Manual for Facilities Serving People with Disabilities has recommended that the following services should be available on a regular and continuing basis: physician services, psychologist or psychiatrist, and physical therapy. For inpatient

---

‡The World Health Organization (WHO) has defined health in the following terms: "A state of complete physical, emotional and social well-being." (Constitution of the World Health Organization, Geneva, Switzerland, 1964).

programs it also has recommended specialized nursing care for pain patients, pharmacy, dietetics, and social services. Other services, such as occupational therapy, vocational services, chaplaincy, recreation therapy, etc., should be made available through affiliation arrangements dependent upon the need of patients served and specific goals of the program. All services should be available around the clock. All members of the pain team play different and equally important roles that should be clearly understood and respected by all members of the team. The crucial role played by the pain team for successful outcome of treatment has been emphasized by all reputable pain control centers.[53] In traditional biologically-oriented medicine, the physician is viewed as the "knower" and the "provider" for a "cure" of the disease; the patient usually casts himself into a totally passive role of the recipient of external interventions, sometimes with no perceived need for a personal commitment return to a state of health. The role of paramedical personnel is largely viewed as secondary. On the contrary, in rehabilitation and behavioral medicine, the physician is an educator and is supported in this role by all members of the pain team. The patient is taught to become involved in the rehabilitation process and given counseling for self-maintenance of health. The goal is not cure but adjustment, a change from a perceived state of illness to a perceived state of wellness.

Patient Population

Patients with various sensory impairments perceived as chronic pain may be candidates for pain control programs. The painful sense of impairment may be independent from any documented pathologic condition (primary *learned pain syndrome*—Class I patient according to EPEM) or associated with a documented pathological abnormality (secondary *learned pain syndrome*—Class III patient according to the EPEM). This second group of patients includes nonterminal cancer patients. Studies have demonstrated that a large percent of patients with cancer at all sites demonstrate emotional and physical problems, such as altered ADL, generalized weakness, ambulation difficulties, anxiety, and depression, which are amenable to therapeutic intervention and improvement through rehabilitation.[40] Functional patients, with or without a well-identified pathological condition (Class II and Class IV pain patients, respectively) may also benefit from a pain control program, limited to fewer treatment modalities, mostly centered around stress management.

Leading pain control centers in the United States and Canada report a remarkable uniformity of data concerning patients characteristics, program structures, and treatment outcome.[5,53] Most chronic pain patients have reached middle age with no significant difference between males and females and no specific work pattern. About 60 percent (range 52–77 percent) are injured workers on Workers' Compensation Benefits. About 70 percent (range 50–90 percent) of all chronic sufferers treated showed the back as the primary pain location.[§] A large number of the chronic pain patients with no terminal illness misuse one drug or another. Seventy percent have evidence of iatrogenic complications that may include the following: medication, unnecessary surgery, wrong counseling for inactivity, dependence, and disability. The single most common reinforcer for illness behavior seems to be the excused escape from everyday responsibility. The most difficult

---

[§]Characteristically, most of the pain control centers from industrialized countries in Western Europe, New Zealand and Australia report also that back pain patients are predominant among chronic sufferers. (People-to-People Pain Delegation to New Zealand and Australia: Brena, S.F. [Ed.] 1984 Report).

patients seem to be those who show severe personality trait disturbances; that is, chronic, manipulative patients with long histories of incompetent coping in situations of daily living.

Treatment Programs

Because the common characteristic of pain-disabled patients (Class I, Class III) is inactivity, with its clusters of secondary impairments, the main thrust of a pain control program is psychophysiological reactivation through rehabilitation.

Within this broad approach strategy, several-tactical goals may be identified: (1) detoxify patients in cases of drug misuse and physical dependence; (2) desensitize patients to particular sensory inputs which they have learned to perceive as unpleasant (hyperstimulation analgesia and nerve blocks); (3) teach patients new skills for competent coping in situations of distress (relaxation training, biofeedback, psychological and occupational therapy); (4) train inactive patients to increase body mobility and activity levels, and teach them specific exercises of physical therapy; (5) coach patients away from excessive attention to body cues; (6) educate family members to reinforce health behaviors rather than of illness behaviors; and (7) assess impairment and disability in patients with pending disability claims and provide vocational assistance to help them in returning to productivity.

Because rehabilitation for pain control requires the capability of insight and motivation for self-change, patients who lack these qualities are poor treatment candidates. The following disabilities usually disqualify patients from pain rehabilitation: major cognitive deficits from cerebral vascular accident or dementing illness; patients with severe hearing deficits, not improved by hearing aids; patients with severe cardiopulmonary impairment; patients with significant language barriers concerning the primary language used at the pain control facility.

Therapeutic goals of a pain control program can be achieved both by inpatient and outpatient management. Each offers its own advantages.

Inpatient management. Structured therapeutic communities can be developed; continual accurate observation of patients behavior is facilitated; environmental cues for pain behavior are eliminated; more intensive interaction between patients is possible.

Outpatient management. Reduced cost; the opportunity to observe problems and progress in the patient's home environment; the opportunity for patients to continue working or participating in other productive activities of daily living while receiving treatment; easier programming of maintenance of behavior changes; patients do not see themselves as being sick because they are in the hospital. The majority of inpatients at the Emory Pain Control Center fall in Classes I and III, while Class II and Class IV patients are mostly candidates for outpatient management.

Treatment Modalities

Hyperstimulation analgesia. The term *hyperstimulation analgesia* has been proposed by Melzack[45] to indicate changes in subjective pain intensity following a variety of techniques of intense sensory stimulation. Three major properties of hyperstimulation analgesia can be identified: a moderate, intense sensory input is applied to the body; the sensory input is sometimes applied at a site distant from the painful region; and the sensory input of brief duration (from a few minutes to 30 minutes) may result in changes in pain intensity that may last for days, weeks and even longer. Neurophysiologically, these properties of hyperstimulation analgesia are explained by postulating that intense and repeated sensory stimulation at distant sites may activate powerful brain stem descending inhibitory mechanisms that may result in blocking nociceptive inputs at the posterior spinal horn. Melzack[44,45] conceptualized these antinociceptive effects as a "central biasing mechanism" that would act as an inhibitory feedback system. Melzack[45] and Melzack and Wall[50] have reviewed clinical and research evidence that painful inputs sometimes produce persisting memory traces in the spinal cord or in the brain, which may evoke the perception of pain long after the initiating nociceptive event has healed or has been removed. Intense and repeated sensory stimulation could block these sensory memories by direct spinal inhibition or by activation of the structures that comprise the central biasing mechanism. If the decreased pain intensity is matched by increased physical activity, the added sensory inputs would tend to prevent the recurrence of the abnormal neural activity and the resulting painful perception.

Analgesia through sensory stimulation has been known for a long time and recorded in almost all world cultures; historically these procedures were labeled as *counter-irritation* and included the following: cupping, cauterization, applying a vesicant to the skin, and moxibustion (a Chinese technique of stimulation, which consists of allowing a cone made from the leaves of the Mugwort plant to burn slowly at a bodily site until it approaches or reaches the skin).[18]

More modern and sophisticated forms of hyperstimulation analgesia include the following: dry needling, electro-acupuncture, and transcutaneous electrical nerve stimulation (TENS).

Dry needling.   During the 1950s several investigators independently discovered that the insertion of a needle into a trigger zone in patients suffering from myofascial syndromes dramatically relieved their discomfort for long periods of time.[60,64] In reviewing the literature on dry needling, Lewit[41] called this phenomenon the *needle effect.* This effect is maximal when the needle is inserted at the point of maximum discomfort; in Lewit's observations, the brief shot of pain produced by the needle resulted in decreased pain intensity in 86.8 percent of cases of myofascial pain for months and even longer in about 50 percent of these cases. These very positive results need to be replicated in controlled studies.

Acupuncture.   Traditional acupuncture is a form of Chinese folk medicine, which is based on metaphysical theories and still widely practiced by the so-called "barefoot" doctors in rural China. Over the last 15 years, scientific investigation in Western countries and in China has focused sharply on the physiology underlying this ancient therapeutic modality. Several well-studied observations have emerged: (1) acupuncture has a significantly greater effect on the perception of pain than does placebo intervention[22,62]; (2) partial analgesia can be produced in animals such as monkeys and mice,[57] further demonstrating that acupuncture analgesia is not simply a placebo effect; (3) the distribution of acupuncture points is similar to that of trigger points[65]; every trigger point reported in the western literature has a corresponding acupuncture point, with a close correspondence (71 percent) between the pain syndromes associated with the two kinds of points[18]; (4) intense stimulation in patients with chronic low back pain at acu-points and trigger points results in decreased pain intensity, with neither procedure statistically more effective than the other[33,42]; (5) acupuncture changes the transmission of nociceptive impulses at several levels of the central nervous system.[39] In current Western technology, both in Western and oriental countries, traditional acupuncture is now supplemented by electrical stimulation; when electrical stimulation is carried at acu-points the technique is known as electro-acupuncture; when it is targeted at trigger points, it is known as percutaneous electrical nerve stimulation (PENS).

Transcutaneous Electrical Nerve Stimulation (TENS). Following the publication by Melzack and Wall[49] of their famous paper on the "the Gate Theory," stimulation of the posterior tracts of the spinal cord via implanted electrical devices became popular in the late 1960s. With the popularization of spinal cord stimulation, it soon became clear that similar analgesic effects could be produced by skin stimulators; Medtronics, the manufacturer of the first spinal cord stimulators, soon introduced a well-designed, well-engineered generator for transcutaneous electrical nerve stimulation. Since the early 1970s TENS has gained an enormous popularity and its technological devices have multiplied in geometrical proportion, each manufacturer claiming that its stimulator is the best. Present models are quite sophisticated devices, allowing choices of high or low frequency stimulation, two or four electrodes, built-in programs that vary the pulse duration to prevent adaptation of the sensory nerves, adjustable intensity, pulse frequency, and pulse duration for each of the channels. TENS has triggered controversy among physicians as to its actual value in significantly changing subjective pain intensity, both in acute and chronic pain syndromes. As so often occurs in topics dealing with painful perceptions, the confusion has arisen because of poorly designed studies, poor definition of classes of chronic pain patients, and poor monitoring of results. At the present the following points seem to be well documented: (1) TENS is another form of hyperstimulation analgesia, which has the advantage over acupuncture and dry needling of being noninvasive; (2) this advantage, however, is likely counterbalanced by the potential for over-use and exploitation of TENS by therapists; and (3) TENS pain-relieving effects are comparable to those obtained with ice massage in a patient suffering both from acute dental pain[16] and in patients with chronic low back pain[47] (About 65 percent of patients reported decreased pain intensity greater than 33 percent with each method. In some patients ice massage appears even more effective than TENS); and (4) according to present medical information, TENS is dramatically effective in peripheral neuropathies; it is very useful in acute myofascial pain problems and less valuable in many chronic myofascial pain syndromes; it is ineffective in disease affecting the central nervous system, such as pain from spinal cord injuries and in the thalamic syndrome; it is totally ineffective as the sole treatment for patients who are judged to have primarily psychosocial problems (Class I EPEM patients).[43] Fried et al[34] have reported significant long-term success with the use of TENS in the treatment of chronic posttraumatic pain, mostly chronic back pain. However, this report is substantially contaminated by the fact that in addition to TENS, all patients received full range of therapy appropriate to their disability, such as conventional modalities of physical therapy (ultrasound, heat, cold, massage), occupational therapy, physical fitness exercises, and psychological and vocational counseling, when indicated.

Neural blockade. Since the first book on pain, published in 1894,[25a] in which Corning described clinical applications of local anesthetics for the relief of pain, nerve blocks have been a time-honored modality for pain relief in surgery, obstetrics, and in the management of the chronic pain patient.[8,26] Depending on the site affected by the neural blockade, nerve blocks may be classified as subarachnoid blocks, epidural blocks, somatic nerve blocks, sympathetic nerve blocks, peripheral nerve blocks, and local blocks (mostly infiltration of trigger points). The pharmacologic duration of a nerve block is related to the injected chemical and may last for a few hours, if a local anesthetic agent has been used, to weeks and months after using a neurolytic agent (alcohol or phenol). The value of nerve blocks in chronic pain states is presently under review, as knowledge about the physiology of nociception, the impact of inactivity, the interplay between pathological conditions and learned illness behaviors and the placebo phenomenon accumulates.[10] At present, few nerve block techniques are standing the criticism of time and clinical experience:

Epidural blocks. Patients with recent onset of low back pain and radicular spinal pain should be given an early trial of this technique with a local anesthetic agent, alone or in combination with a steroid drug. If successful, the epidural block, which has few iatrogenic risks in experienced hands, may return the patient to function in a relatively short time and possibly prevent onset of a chronic pain syndrome through prolonged inactivity. More controversial, and still unproven, is the use of epidural blocks in patients with chronic low back pain.

Sympathetic blocks. Blocks of the sympathetic ganglia are useful in changing pain perception, not only through their peripheral vasomotor effects, but also through their blockade of deep somatic and visceral nociceptive afferents as they traverse the sympathetic ganglia, inbound toward the posterior spinal roots. The blocks of the splanchic segments (celiac plexus block) with a neurolytic agent stands virtually alone as one of the few neurolytic blocks proven reliable in controlling pain from terminal malignancy of the upper abdominal organs. The classical and best documented indications for sympathetic blockade remains causalgia and other forms of reflex sympathetic dystrophy of recent onset; more controversial is its effectiveness in peripheral vascular diseases, in vasospastic syndromes, in the early stages of herpes zoster infection,[24] and in chronic back pain.[16,17]

Local blocks (blocks of TPs). The most common finding, if properly looked for, in patients with chronic pain is evidence of soft-tissue abnormality, clinically manifested through small circumscribed and hypersensitive areas in muscles and the connective tissues that are visualized through thermographic studies as "hot spots".[66] Typically, pressure upon these tender spots triggers pain in distant bodily areas. The presence of trigger points has created a large number of waste-basket diagnoses, such as "muscular rheumatism," "myalgia," myogelosis," "fibrositis," "myofascitis," etc. In the absence of a well-documented pathologic condition, soft tissue abnormalities could be viewed as signs of a nonspecific, nonmetameric disuse syndrome, commonly associated with inactivity, postural defects, stress, and their mutual interactions.[19] Among the numerous TP syndromes, four are particularly worth mentioning since their misdiagnosis usually leads to expensive, repetitive and often stress-producing medical investigations. Table 8-5 summarizes their clinical features.

Repeated infiltrations of TPs with a local anesthetic agent, eventually supplemented by hyperstimulation techniques for analgesia and appropriate stretch exercises, will result in long-term disappearance of the TPs.

There is evidence in the literature that a needle effect may be involved in the pain-relieving mechanisms of neural blockade. Frost et al,[35] in a double-blind comparison of mepivacaine and saline injected into trigger points of patients with myofascial syndrome,

Table 8-5

Clinical Features of Trigger Point Syndrome

Syndrome	TPS	TZ	Associated Symptoms	Mistaken Diagnosis
Anterior chest wall Syndrome (Tietze's syndrome)	Great and small pectoralis muscles (contracted fibers of the pectoralis minor may entrap the auxillary artery)	Anterior chest; ulnar side of upper limbs	"Tightness" of the chest. Aspecific cardiac arrhythmias	Ischemic heart disease when symptoms on the left side Thoracic outlet syndrome
Thoraco-lumbar paraspinal syndrome (Lumbago)	Superficial and deep paraspinals	Around the chest wall; up to the shoulders; down to buttocks and posterior aspect of the thighs	Restricted spine ROM Restricted total body mobility	Intercoastal neuralgia. Degenerative disc disease. Sciatica.
Abdominal wall Syndrome	Mostly Rectus Abdominis. Less frequently: the oblique transverse and pyramidalis muscles	All abdominal quadrants; anterior chest wall; dorsal back region	Nausea, vomiting, diarrhea, and multiple other visceral symptoms	Multiple visceral disease, according to associated symptoms.
Pelvic Floor Syndrome. (Tension myalgia; Pyriformis syndrome, coccygodynia.)	Levator ani and Pyriformis muscles. Less frequently: ligaments and fascia of the pelvic diaphragm.	Low back region. Lower limbs; Coccyx.	Disorders in bowel movements, Dyspareunia. "Tightness" of the perineal region.	Sciatica, urinary and rectal diseases. Sexual abnormality.

From Brena SF: Nerve Blocks and Chronic Pain States—An Up-Date. Post-Graduate Medicine, 1984, (in press).

209

documented that saline injections resulted in a significantly greater relief of pain (80 percent) than mepivacaine injections (52 percent). Similarly, Brena et al[17] in a double-blind, cross-over design study have shown significant mean reduction in subjective pain intensity lasting up to 3 months after treatment in 20 patients with low back pain of long duration from documented degenerative spine changes. Each subject received 12 lumbar sympathetic blocks, 6 with normal saline and 6 with 0.25 percent bupivacaine. No significant difference was found between the results of the analgesic and saline blocks. Results were discussed in terms of massive placebo effects and the analgesia obtained through deep stimulation of various tissue structures.

Techniques of Behavior Medicine

Biofeedback therapy.   EMG biofeedback is an established procedure that is often useful for relief of muscle tension and as an adjunct to operant conditioning and relaxation training. It has been used in combination with education with results of very significant long-term improvement in muscle contraction and migraine headaches, though its utility in back pain is unproven. EMG biofeedback may have a useful effect in increasing the awareness of the role of stress in pain problems, in motivating patients to practice relaxation, in leading some patients toward psychotherapy, and in helping patients gain a sense of self-efficiency and self-control. It is now realized that pain problems rarely can be addressed solely through a mechanistic provision of biofeedback, but that biofeedback provided in the context of a comprehensive program of pain management can be a powerful therapeutic tool.

Relaxation.   There are various techniques for relaxation, through muscle exercises, breathing techniques, imagery, and self-hypnosis. Relaxation often can be fostered through practice with audio-training tapes. Individual psychological counseling must be added when indicated.

Behavior modification.   Behavior modification refers to a systematic structuring of the environment in such a way as to exercise the frequency of desired health behaviors and reduce the frequency of pain-related behaviors. Pain programs generally address not only observable or overt behaviors such as verbal complaints, activity levels, and drug intake, but also to covert behaviors such as thoughts, attitudes, and self-statements regarding the pain experience. Techniques of behavior modification are based on principles of learning and are the core of most advanced multimodal pain programs.[32]

In general, single modality treatments may be useful in managing patients with recent onset pathogenic pain or functional patients with chronic pain (Class II and IV EPEM). All professionals in competent pain control centers in the United States unanimously agree, however, that interdisciplinary programs are necessary when applied to dysfunctional chronic pain patients (Class I and III EPEM). All treatment modalities for these patients should be structured in contingency management; a "P.R.N." treatment approach to these chronic pain patients is rarely useful and should be discouraged.

Table 8-6 shows rating of the various treatment modalities as reported by patients at the Emory Pain Control Center.[21]

Table 8-6

Patient Ratings of Helpfulness of Treatment Modalities

Modality	Number of Patients Treated	Rating			
		Very Helpful	Somewhat Helpful	Not Helpful	Harmful
Activity increase	215	48%	43%	7%	2%
Drug withdrawal	114	53	33	14	0
Group counseling	234	53	43	4	0
Life Skills Program (OT)	137	38	52	10	0
Sympathetic nerve blocks	222	22	45	31	3
Physical therapy	221	60	35	5	0
Relaxation Training	237	60	35	5	0
Biofeedback therapy	30	63	27	10	0
TENS	16	25	50	25	0

From Brena SF, Chapman SL: Management of Patients with Chronic Pain, Spectrum Publications, Inc, New York, 1984, p. 157. With permission.

Treatment Results

Twenty long-term follow up studies from competent pain control centers in the United States and Canada have been recently reviewed.[5] Most of these studies were completed through mailed questionnaires and telephone interviews with patients and relatives. The following information was generally requested: changes in ADL, changes in PI (Pain Intensity), changes in drug habits, changes in usage of the health care system, and changes in the working status. While the results from these 20 studies differed in detail, a general trend is common in all of them. Up to five years after treatment is completed, a majority of patients interviewed reported increased ADL, decreased PI, decreased perception of need for drugs, and decreased usage of the health care system. Four studies have revealed no differences in treatment outcome in patients with or without pending disability claims; percentages of patients returning to work at follow-up from 11 months to 2 years post-treatment generally ranged from 30 percent to 50 percent. The usefulness of structured pain control programs versus traditional sequential medical interventions for cost containment also has been investigated. Stieg and Williams[63] have computed the cost effectiveness of a pain rehabilitation program to the workers' compensation insurance carriers. Fifty-three histories of chronic pain patients who had completed a pain rehabilitation program were reviewed. Financial data were provided by the insurance carriers based on studies of at least one year before and one year after the pain treatment. Information included the following: the annual cost of medical treatment prior to admission to the pain control center (mean value dollar $9,311), the annual cost of medical treatment after the treatment program (mean value dollar $5,190), the annual cost of disability payments before treatment (mean value dollar $6,766), the annual cost of disability payments after treatment (mean value dollar $3,000) and the total cost of the treatment program ($1,860). A simple formula to estimate the total benefit in dollars over a patients lifetime after proper pain control management, assuming maintenance of successful changes, was developed. It was concluded that the net saving over a patient's lifetime from the group of 53 patients tabulated in the study was an astounding quarter of a million dollars for each patient. Though a control group of equivalent patients who did not receive treatment at a pain control facility would have helped to clarify these results, the authors concluded that treatment at the pain control center had resulted in a large financial savings.

PAIN CONTROL FACILITIES

Historically, pain clinics have evolved within the biomedical model as multidisciplinary groups of physicians who will act in a consultant capacity in difficult pain problems.[8,9] Most early pain clinics were actually equated with "nerve block clinics" when nerve blocks represented the only nonsurgical treatment modality besides drugs for pain control. In 1979 the American Society of Anesthesiologists[2] published an International Directory for Pain Centers—Clinics. In the directory, the committee on pain therapy of the ASA proposed several definitions.

Major comprehensive pain center. To be qualified as such the following prerequisites are necessary: Space and beds assigned solely to the pain center; full-time professional staff of more than one discipline; full-time support staff; organized process for screening and selecting of patients; records review and maintenance; participation of consultants of multiple disciplines; routine psychological assessments; ongoing research activities; organized training programs; availability of therapy appropriate to the needs of patients served; periodic evaluation of treatment results.

Comprehensive pain centers. To be identified as such, at least two-thirds of the criteria listed under major comprehensive pain centers should be met.

Syndrome-oriented pain centers. A facility organized to provide in-depth management of all aspects of a particular pain syndrome. Examples of syndrome-oriented pain centers would be: low back pain centers, headache pain centers, cancer pain centers, etc.

Modality-oriented pain centers. A facility that offers the chronic pain patient the appropriate therapy as defined by the specialty of the center. Examples of such a center would include nerve block clinics, TENS clinics, acupuncture clinics, etc. Table 8-7 shows the distribution of various clinical models and of various medical specialties with primary responsibility[2] among pain control facilities.

From the experience of pain control facilities in the United States a new breed of physicians has emerged: the Algologist, the medical expert in diagnosis and treatment of pain (Greek: Algos=pain; Logos=study). The concept of the science of Algology is slowly gaining acceptance in the United States as witnessed by the foundation in 1983 of the American Association of Algology (A.A.A.) to support the growth of the new specialty and to obtain recognition of an American Board of Algology. Membership in the A.A.A. is limited to physicians who have demonstrated outstanding contribution in pain management by their excellence in the field from past clinical work and/or past research. Some state agencies have officially recognized the algologist as a physician particularly qualified to render clinical opinions in cases of pain-disabled patients. For instance, the Georgia Department of Human Resources has added Algology as a specialty to be represented on the Vocational Rehabilitation panel.

Over the last several years pain control facilities have proliferated in geometric

Table 8-7

Distribution of Pain Control Facilities

	Asia	Australia New Zealand	Canada	Europe	Latin America	United States
Major Comprehensive Pain Centers	1	1	1	6	0	41
Comprehensive Pain Centers	10	7	9	17	1	78
Modality-Oriented Pain Clinics	13	2	13	40	1	97
Syndrome-Oriented Pain Clinics	6	1	4	16	1	62
Department With Primary Responsibility						
Anesthesiology	14	7	11	35	3	96
Neurosurgery	2	1	1	6	0	31
Orthopedic Surgery	0	0	0	1	0	8
Psychiatry	0	1	2	0	0	9
Psychology	1	0	2	0	0	7
Oral Surgery	1	1	3	0	0	13
Rehabilitation Medicine	2	0	2	3	0	35
Others	1	1	4	13	0	18

From Brena SF, Chapman SL (Eds.): Pain Clinics, Clinics in Anesthesiology. Saunders Publishing Company, London, 1984, (in press). With permission.

progression. A report published in the Medical World News in 1976 listed only 17 pain clinics in the whole United States; the ASA Directory (1979) lists over 225 pain control facilities; the American Pain Society estimates that there are at least 800 pain control facilities currently operating in the United States. Such growth is most gratifying to the pioneers of the field but it is also a source of serious concern.

Some of these facilities are being staffed by physicians and other health professionals who have little or no training or experience in managing patients with chronic pain. Some of these are well intentioned clinicians who have been attracted to the science of Algology because currently it is fashionable to "treat pain." Of even greater concern is the fact that some so-called pain clinics are being run by unscrupulous physicians and therapists to exploit patients, as occurred in some acupuncture clinics during the early 1970s. Many such clinics are actually selling under a new label several old treatment modalities, such as drugs and surgery, which reflect the skills of the clinic director or participants. Eventually the combination of a Board of Algology and the standards set by CARF for Certification of Pain Control Programs should eliminate non-professional operations and guarantee quality care for chronic pain patients.

CLOSING REMARKS

More research on pain has been done over the last ten years than in any previous decade in the history of medicine. Research findings have completely changed the scientific perspective of pain, defining it from a mere symptom of disease to an extraordinarily complex sensory experience. Some of these findings have been successfully applied in the clinical management of patients with pain, mostly in its chronic syndromes. Because of the complexity of pain, no one single scientist or clinician can master in depth the full range of knowledge available today in the field. The only available alternative is the scientific multidisciplinary approach and the concept of the clinical algology-pain team as the best managing unit for chronic sufferers. The bulk of experience from competent pain control centers around the world has also demonstrated that no single physician, because of the skills gained through any current medical specialty, can be competent enough to serve as a medical director of an algology team. This gap, which is growing ever more evident as experience accumulates, can likely be filled by the algologist, a physician especially trained in basic neurophysiology, psychology, and pharmacology science dealing with pain phenomena, and also competent in biological and behavioral medicine. To a certain extent the same considerations can be made for other members of the pain team: psychologists, nurses, and therapists all need to gain special knowledge and training in pain, which is not easily available in their respective training and practices. All present indicators demonstrate that a successful approach to chronic pain can be best achieved with the establishment and recognition of the science and practice of algology, for research, training, and clinical services to patients.

REFERENCES

1. Agnew D, Crue BL, Pinsky J: A Taxonomy Form for Diagnosis and Information Storage for Patients with Chronic Pain. Bull Los Angeles Neurol Surg 44:84–86, 1979

2. American Society of Anesthesiologists. Dictionary of Pain Clinics-Centers, 1979

3. Anderson KV: Endogenous Opioid Peptides and the Control of Pain, in Brena SF, Chapman SL

(eds): Management of Patients with Chronic
Pain, New York, Spectrum Publications, 1983, pp
33–46

4. Apley G: The Child with Abdominal Pains,
Oxford, Blackwell Press, 1975

5. Aronoff GM, Evans WO, Sanders PL: A Review
of Follow-up Studies of Multidisciplinary Pain
Units. Pain 6:1–11, 1983

6. Black R: The Chronic Pain Syndrome. Surg Clin
No Amer 55:999–1011, 1975

7. Black RG, Chapman CR: The SAD Index for
Clinical Assessment of Pain, in Bonica JJ, Albe-
Fessard D (eds): Advances in Pain Research and
Therapy. New York, Raven Press, 1975, pp 301–
305

8. Bonica JJ: Clinical Application of Diagnostic and
Therapeutic Nerve Blocks. Springfield, Charles
C Thomas, 1959

9. Bonica JJ: The Management of Pain. Philadelphia, Lea and Febiger, 1953

10. Brena SF: Nerve Blocks and Chronic Pain States:
An Up-Date. Postgrad Med 1985 (in press)

11. Brena SF, Chapman SL: The "Learned Pain Syndrome." Postgrad Med 69:53–62, 1981

12. Brena SF, Chapman SL: The Validity of the
Emory Pain Estimate Model Anesthesiol Rev
9:45, 1982

13. Brena SF, Chapman SL, Stegall PG, et al:
Chronic Pain States: Their Relationship to Impairment and Disability. Arch Phys Med Rehab
660:378–389, 1979

14. Brena SF, Koch DL: The "Pain Estimate" for
Quantification and Classification of Chronic
Pain States. Anesthesiol Rev 2:8–13, 1975

15. Brena SF, Koch DL, Moss RM: The Reliability of
the Pain Estimate Model. Anesthesiol Rev 3:28–
29, 1976

16. Brena SF, Unikel IP: Nerve Blocks and Contin-
gency Management in Chronic Pain States, in
Bonica JJ, Albe-Fessard D (eds): Advances in
Pain Research and Therapy. New York, Raven
Press, 1975, pp 707–710

17. Brena SF, Wolf SL, Chapman SL, et al: Chronic
Back Pain: Electromyography, Motion and Beha-
viorial Assessments Following Sympathetic
Nerve Blocks and Placebos. Pain 8:1–10, 1980

18. Brockbank W: Ancient Therapeutic Arts. London, Heinemann, 1954

19. Cailliet R: Disuse Syndrome: Fibrositic and
Degenerative Changes, in Brena SF, Chapman
SL (eds): Management of Patients with Chronic
Pain. New York, Spectrum Publications, 1983, pp
63–71

20. Cervero F: Deep and Visceral Pain, in Kosterlitz
HW, Terenius LY (eds): Pain and Society.
Weinheim, Verlag Chemie, 1980, pp 263–282

21. Chapman SL: Behavior Modification, in Brena
SF, Chapman SL (eds): Management of Patients

with Chronic Pain. New York, Spectrum Publications, 1983, pp 145–159

22. Chapman CR, Wilson ME, Gehrig JD: Compara-
tive Effects of Acupuncture and Transcutaneous
Stimulation on the Perception of Painful Dental
Stimuli. Pain 2:265–283, 1976

23. Chery-Croze S: Painful Sensation Induced by a
Thermal Cutaneous Stimulation. Pain 17:109–
138, 1983

24. Colding A: The Effect of Regional Sympathetic
Blocks in Treatment of Herpes Zoster. Acta Anesthesiol Scand 13:133–141, 1969

25. Commission on Accreditation of Rehabilitation
Facilities (CARF). Standards Manual for Facilities Serving People with Disabilities. Chronic
Pain Management Programs. Tucson, CARF,
1983, pp 23–27

25a. Corning LL: Pain: Its Neuropathologic, Diagnostic and Neurotherapeutic Relations. Philadelphia, J. B. Lippincott, 1894

26. Cousins MG, Bridenbaugh PO (eds): Neural
Blockade in Clinical Anesthesia and Management of Pain. New York, JB Lippincott, 1980

27. Crue BL: Taxonomy of Pain: Is Pain a Sensation?
Presentation at the Fourth Annual Emory University Conference on Pain, Snowmass, Colo-
rado, 1980

28. Duggan AW: Electrophysiology of Opioid Peptides and Sensory Systems. Brit Med Bull 39:65–
70, 1983

29. Duncan GH, Gregg GM, Ghia JN: The Pain Profile: A Computerized System for Assessment of
Chronic Pain. Pain 5:275–284, 1978

30. Fields HL, Basbaum AI: Brainstem Control of
Spinal Pain—Transmission Neurons. Ann Rev
Physiol 40:193–221, 1978

31. Fordyce WE: Behavioral Methods for Chronic
Pain and Illness. St. Louis, Mosby, 1976

32. Fordyce WE: A Behavioral Prospective on
Chronic Pain. Br J Clin Psychol 21:313–320,
1982

33. Fox EJ, Melzack R: Transcutaneous Electrical
Stimulation and Acupuncture: Comparison of
Treatment for Low Back Pain. Pain 2:141–148,
1976

34. Fried T, Johnson R, McCracken W: Transcutaneous Electrical Nerve Stimulation: Its Role in
the Control of Chronic Pain. Arch Phys Med
Rehab 65:228–231, 1984

35. Frost FA, Jessen B, Siggaard-Andersen J: A Con-
trolled Double-Blind Comparison of Mepivacaine
Injection vs. Saline Injection for Myofascial
Pain. Lancet 1:499–501, 1980

36. Gentry WD, Shows WD, Thomas M: Chronic
Low back Pain: A Psychological Profile. Psychosomatics 15:174–177, 1974

37. Hammonds W, Brena SF: Pain Classification and
Vocational Evaluation in Chronic Pain States, in

Melzack R (ed): Pain Measurement and Assessment. New York, Raven Press, 1983, pp 197–203

38. Hokfelt T, Skirboll L, Dalsgaard CJ, et al: Peptide Neurons in the Spinal Cord with Special Reference to Descending Systems, in Sjolund Bjoiklund J (ed): Brain Stem Control of Spinal Mechanisms. Amsterdam: Elsevier Bio-Medical Press, 1982, pp 89–118

39. Kerr FWL, Wilson PR, Nijensohn DE: Acupuncture Reduces the Trigeminal Evoked Responses in Decerebrate Cats. Exper Neurol 61:84–95, 1978

40. Lehmann JF, DeLisa JA, Warren, CG, et al: Cancer Rehabilitation: Assessment of Need, Development, and Evaluation of a Model of Care. Arch Phys Med Rehab 59:410–419, 1978

41. Lewit K: The Needle Effect in the Relief of Myofascial Pain. Pain 6:83–90, 1979

42. Liatinen J: Acupuncture and Transcutaneous Electrical Stimulation in the Treatment of Chronic Sacrolumbalgia and Ischialgia. Amer J Chinese Med 4:169–175, 1976

43. Long DM: A Peripheralist View of Chronic Pain: Observations in Transcutaneous Electrical Stimulation. Seminars in Neurol 3:341–346, 1983

44. Melzack R: Phantom Limb Pain: Implications for Treatment of Pathological Pain. Anesthesiology 35:409–419, 1971

45. Melzack R: The Puzzle of Pain. New York, Basic Books, 1973

46. Melzack R, Guite S, Gonshor A: Relief of Dental Pain by Ice Massage of the Hand. Canad Med Assoc J 122:189–191, 1980

47. Melzack R, Jeans ME, Stratford JC, et al: Ice Massage and Transcutaneous Electrical Stimulation: Comparison of Treatment for Low Back. Pain 9:209–217, 1980

48. Melzack R, Stillwell DM, Fox EG: Trigger Points and Acupuncture Points for Pain: Correlations and Implications. Pain 3:3–23, 1977

49. Melzack R, Wall PD: Pain Mechanisms: A New Theory. Science 150:972–979, 1965

50. Melzack R, Wall PD: The Challenge of Pain. Harmondsworth, Penguin Books, 1982

51. NASA Biomedical Results in Apollo. 368, 1975

52. NASA Biomedical Results in Skylab. 377, 1977.

53. Ng LKY (ed): NIDA Research Monograph 36 New Approaches to Treatment of Chronic Pain: A Review of Multi-disciplinary Pain Clinics and Pain Centers. U.S. Dept. of Health, Education and Welfare, Washington, DC, 1981

54. Pilowsky I, Spence ND: Illness Behavior Syndromes Associated with Intractable Pain. Pain 2:61–71, 1976

55. Pinsky JJ: Psychodynamics and Psychotherapy in the Treatment of Patients with Chronic Intractable Pain, in Crue BL (ed): Pain: Research and Treatment. New York, Academic Press, 1975, p 34

56. Reich J, Rosenblatt RM, Touping J: DSM-III: A New Nomenclature for Classifying Patients with Chronic Pain. Pain 16:201–206, 1983

57. Sandrew BB, Yang RCC, Wang SC: Electro-Acupuncture Analgesia in Monkeys: A Behavioral and Neurophysiological Assessment. Archives Internationales de Pharmacodynamie et de Therapie 231:274–284, 1978

58. Schaffer CB, Dowland PT, Britter RM: Chronic Pain and Depression: A Clinical and Family History Survey. Amer J Psychiat 133:1151–1154, 1976

59. Seligman MEP: Helplessness. San Francisco, W. H. Freeman Press, 1975

60. Sola AE, Williams RL: Myofascial Pain Syndromes. Neurology 6:91–95, 1956

61. Steger HG, Fox CD, Feinberg SD: Behaviorial Evaluation in Management of Chronic Pain, in Bishop DS (ed): Behavior and the Disabled: Assessment and Management. Baltimore, Williams and Wilkins, pp 272–320, 1980

62. Stewart T, Thompson J, Oswald D: Acupuncture Analgesia; an Experimental Investigation. Brit Med J 1:67–70, 1977

63. Stieg RL, Williams RC: Chronic Pain as a Bio-Social Cultural Phenomenon: Implications for Treatment, in Crue BL (ed): Seminars in Neurology—Pain, 3:370–376, 1983

64. Travell G, Rinzler SH: The Myofascial Genesis of Pain. Postgrad Med 11:425–434, 1952

65. Travell JG, Simons DG: Myofascial Pain and Dysfunction: The Trigger Point Manual. Baltimore, Williams and Wilkins, 1983

66. Wexler CE: Lumbar, Thoracic and Cervical Thermography. J Neurol Orthoped Surg 1:37–41, 1979

67. Woodrow KM, Freedman GD, Siegelaub AB, et al: Pain Tolerance According to Age, Sex and Race. Psychosom Med 34:548–556, 1972

Arlene Feinblatt
Frances Sommer Anderson
Wayne Gordon

9

Psychosocial and Vocational Considerations

Musculoskeletal disorders are associated with various degrees of functional limitations and pain. For this reason rehabilitation efforts are of prime importance. Psychological and social factors influence the degree to which functional rehabilitation will be achieved. This chapter will delineate the impact of these factors on the patient's rehabilitation progress. The critical role of the physician in facilitating optimal adjustment to an impairment will be explored. Lastly, specific issues that arise in dealing with chronic pain problems will be explored.

THE IMPACT OF DISABILITY

Significant variables affecting the impact of disease and disability have been discussed by a variety of rehabilitation experts.[42,50] Critical demographic variables include level of education, socio-economic status, and marital status. Also important are the nature of the onset and age of onset of disability, prognosis, and degree of visibility of the disability. Further, the individual's view of illness or disability will affect their receptivity to rehabilitation. Attitudinal as well as architectural barriers must be removed to assure the patient's optimum vocational adjustment following a change in physical functioning.

Educational Level

Educational level and occupation must be considered when dealing with the patient. For example, a college graduate who is professionally employed may be able to utilize considerable intellectual resources and consider a wide variety of alternative responses to their situation. They may be able to utilize their professional skills in a new way, such as moving from a practice model of employment to a teaching model. These patients, however, are more likely to question and, at times, even reject treatment due to their own curiosity and sophistication. An unskilled and less educated patient may have a totally different response to becoming disabled and to his or her relationship with the physician. If their ability to switch occupational roles is impaired, their status as breadwinner may be more seriously threatened. This patient may behave in a more compliant fashion toward

PRINCIPLES OF PHYSICAL MEDICINE AND REHABILITATION
IN THE MUSCULOSKELETAL DISEASES

the physician, perhaps even becoming dependent upon them. In other cases, the patient may be fearful of the technological and scientific milieu and reject the aid of the physician.

Socio-economic Level

The loss of income that usually accompanies severe disability can place a strain on the family. Not only are there fewer resources available, but spouses might need to take on the caretaking role if funds are not available for attendant care. Furthermore, without sufficient financial resources, modifications in family living cannot be made that will enable the disabled person to function more independently. For example, ramps may be needed to replace stairs, elevators installed, and doorways widened. From the rehabilitation management standpoint, the physician would benefit from an assessment of the economic resources of the patient in making a treatment plan. A variety of social service agencies may have to be relied upon to help meet the financial needs of the less economically advantaged.

Marital Status

The marital status of the individual can have great bearing on the patient's adjustment, as can the interpersonal attachments made by the disabled person prior to the trauma. At the onset of trauma, the person who is "ill" becomes a rallying point for friends and/or family. As time passes it becomes clear, as the day-to-day requirements of disability become routinized, that the patient is no longer in danger. Soon, fewer individuals come to visit and to assist the person. In addition, frequently the patient's focus narrows to cope with physical needs. Thus, for any number of reasons, the individual is less involved in social activities. Social deprivation can lead to a withdrawn, depressed, and isolated patient[2,3] who has no motivation for compliance with a medical treatment regimen or for further rehabilitation. This narrowing of focus is lessened when a large family or supportive spouse is present and continues to include the disabled person in outside activities.

Family members may react to the disabled person in a variety of ways. Some may find the financial and physical demands burdensome. They may become resentful and hostile. Some members may attempt to overprotect and shelter the disabled person, creating an atmosphere in which the patient is encouraged to assume the "invalid" role. Indeed, recent data indicates that upon return to home after completing their medical rehabilitation, quadriplegics become more dependent in their activities of daily living. This is explained in part by family members being more willing to do for that patient what he/she "can do" for himself/herself.[8a] These various patterns of familial reaction obviously have implications for the patient's adjustment to disability.

Age at Onset

The difficulties in acceptance of illness or disability vary from patient to patient, of course, but the age of onset is one variable that deserves scrutiny. "Taking age of onset into account is important for understanding the particular life circumstances, tasks, and problems with which the individual with disability must cope..."[50] (p. 236). There are a variety of resources available, as well as pressures, at various life stages. The immobilization and long term hospitalization of a child may have profound impact on the young person's future adjustment, may even be the root of social isolation and fears of abandonment. Young adults, middle-aged persons, and older individuals have their own unique responses to the same situation. While the younger person probably has greater physical stamina and immediate family upon which to draw for help, the older individual may possess greater maturity and experience less peer pressure to be more physically active. Thus, the variables brought to bear by the patient's age deserve attention. Unfortunately, the relationship of such factors as age of disablement and the nature of the impairment, ie, congenital or traumatic, and adjustment have not been systematically studied.

Nature of Onset

Those traumas that occur suddenly as the result of an accident will probably affect an individual differently than those whose progress is insidious, slow, and progressive. In the former, the individual has no warning but learns of his impairments at once and must adjust to the full impact of the trauma. Athelstan and Crewe[5] found that manner of onset of injury was related to adjustment in a sample of spinal cord injured men that they studied. Those who were rated as active victims, ie, driving the car, were rated as better adjusted than those who were rated as innocent victims, ie, hit by the car. Thus, the more responsibility the person was judged as having for their accident, the better was their outcome. A degenerative prognosis, on the other hand, requires continued reassessment and readjustment to prevailing conditions.[2,3] Clear-cut limitations, such as those brought on by total paralysis may make functional limitations very clear while generalized or diffuse weakness may cause doubt and uncertainty. Anxiety arises when ambiguity of disease is continuous.

Cognitive-Affective Processes

Physical rehabilitation experts have emphasized the importance of cognitive-affective processes affecting the impact of disability.[42,50] Wright[50] minimizes the relationship between physical disability and adjustment, as illustrated in the following:

> . . . There is no substantial evidence to indicate that persons with impaired physique differ as a group in overall adjustment from their able bodied counterparts . . . (p. 240)
> . . . There is also no clear evidence of an association between type of physical disability and particular personality characteristics . . . (p. 240)

A variety of studies have investigated the existence of specific personality patterns associated with particular musculoskeletal disorders. Spergel, Ehrlich, and Glass,[43] in a study of individuals with rheumatoid arthritis, did not find a homogeneous personality pattern in their patient population. Rather, their data "reinforce the traditional theory of individual differences frequently stressed psychologists . . ."[43] They caution against using a personality stereotype of patients with rheumatoid arthritis.

For many individuals with musculoskeletal disorders, the disability is invisible. That is, the casual observer is unaware from appearance that the disabled person is functionally limited. Pain and stiffness are not always detectable. For the individual with a disability that is not highly visible, eg, a person with back, neck, or shoulder pain, people's interpretations of the individual's behavior may be inaccurate. For example, if the individual has difficulty performing a specific activity, the disability may not even be considered a cause. There are few role models for the individual to identify with when the disability is visible. Denial on the part of the patient, as well as those around the patient, is easier; and it may be more difficult for the professional to diagnose or to recognize the disability, particularly if vague symptoms are present. Diagnosis may even be delayed, leading to further difficulties. From the outsider's perspective, there is a less tangible loss for the person with an invisible disability, and futhermore, less social support for their grief.

Unless the individual has a clear self-concept that can incorporate their invisible problem, they, as well as their families, friends, and peers, are more likely to defend against the impact of the impairment. This might hamper rehabilitation efforts.[12] The better the individual is able to integrate the disabled part of their body into their self-concept, the greater will be the acceptance of their limitations. The greater the self-acceptance, the more satisfied the patient will be with rehabilitation efforts. Studies have shown that, "a poorly integrated deformity seemed to favor dissatisfaction with the operative result, whereas a clear concept of the body image seemed rather to predispose to postoperative satisfaction."[5] (p. 232).

Although the self-esteem of most individuals will be shaken by disability, its effects can vary. Studies have found that events involving the face and torso have been more closely connected with self-concept than events associated with the appendages.[50] Traumas that occur to a basic aspect of the individual's identity, such as events that affect gender identification or occupational status have a crucial impact on the individual's self-concept.[50]

There are many aspects of the individual's personality that, however, may have positive effects upon the individual whose self-esteem has been assaulted by the emotional, financial, and social effects of disability. Perseverance, independence, intelligence, internal control, creativity, aggressiveness, and moral stamina have been found conducive to adjustment.[50]

Perceiving a larger scope of values, subordinating physical attributes relative to other values, containing the effects of disability and transforming comparative status values into asset values enhance the opportunities for acceptance and decrease the view of disability as devaluating.[50]

Opportunities for employment in today's society increase for the disabled by the use of technological improvements that decrease functional limitations, eliminate architectural and legal barriers, and increase job variety. Attitudes have improved with the use of educational programs for the public, advertising, and the greater visibility of the disabled community in general.

Vocational potential can be enhanced by the elimination of a variety of barriers. Interpersonal barriers can be reduced by overcoming devaluating social attitudes. Educational barriers can be lowered by providing facilities for the disabled and by eliminating architectural barriers. The assets of the individual must be considered rather than centering attention on loss and handicap.[50]

PHYSICIAN-PATIENT ISSUES

The attitude of the patient toward the physician and other helping professionals, as well as toward the disability, will have great impact upon treatment and rehabilitation. Many patients are able to adjust successfully to the use of professional staff including physicians, physical therapists, occupational therapists, social workers, and psychologists, to name a few, to help in rehabilitation efforts. Others will have a need to deny loss or disability and may, therefore, postpone contact with their physician. Still others may find secondary gain in disability and take comfort in the role of being ill or physically impaired.

There are few areas as important as the history-taking portion of the clinical workup. The patient's attitudes become apparent, particularly with regard to issues of compliance and resistance. In addition, observations regarding interfamilial behavior, work history, attitudes of shame and fear, become apparent during this initial phase and will have profound effect upon the course and success of treatment. Has the patient come alone? Does the patient require assistance? In what manner is such assistance given, by whom, and how is it received? Who answers the physician's questions? How are the questions answered? What is the mood of the patient? If the patient is depressed, can their mood be lightened in any way? In the case of profoundly depressed individuals it is important to keep in mind the professional staff available to the physician for referral.

The manner in which the physician presents his findings, prognosis, treatment options, and recommendations may result in compliance or resistance on the part of the patient. For this reason, it is important to encourage the patient's cooperation and confidence. In a study of mothers' visits to an emergency clinic, "friendliness on the part of the doctor was positively related to the mothers' satisfaction and compliance with the recommendations. Amount of time spent with the doctor was not related to client satisfaction."[25](p. 74). Wright[50] has suggested that the physician and patient act as comanagers in treatment: "Inner strength and self respect grow in a relationship when the person has a significant role in planning his or her life, when the person's suggestions and feelings are regarded as important."[50](p. 418). Wright further emphasizes the fact that motivation increases when patients share in planning.

Kubler-Ross,[26] in her work with the terminally ill, also stresses the significance of shared information and decision-making with patients. The patient's readiness for information as well as their right to have such facts are major issues discussed in her work. Many individuals wish to be informed of the true nature of their illnesses. In a study of 300 patients with multiple sclerosis, 90 percent believed that they would be told its nature.[18] For these patients, there were many motives involved. Freedom to plan their lives, freedom from the strain of uncertainty, a wiser use of financial resources, better arrangements for their physical care, and removal of the fear that they might be neurotic were cited as reasons for wanting knowledge about disability.

Thus, for the physician, a basic respect for the patient, a friendly and caring attitude, as well as a consideration in the give and take of information, provide the healthiest climate in which to obtain the greatest opportunities for successful medical treatment. Avoidance of technical jargon, care with terms, use of understandable language in a manner designed to inform and educate, and the use of techniques that strengthen the functional roles of the patient and family all encourage cooperation and enhance the chances for satisfactory rehabilitation.

In recent years, bills of rights for patients and the use of patient advocates have become more widespread. Patients no longer see themselves as passive recipients of decisions made by authorities. Group counseling, peer counseling, self-help groups, specialized personnel, and agencies who deal with the disabled person's needs may provide invaluable assistance to patient and physician in the rehabilitation process.

TREATMENT OF CHRONIC PAIN

Definitions and Mechanisms

Patients with musculoskeletal disorders frequently present with pain symptomotology. Determination of the etiology of the pain can be difficult because of the complexity of the pain phenomenon. Attempts at defining pain have been varied. Melzack and Wall,[32] opposing the simple stimulus-response notion of pain, proposed the gate-control model that views pain as "involving sensory, affective, and cognitive components. Current definitions deal with both the sensation of pain as well as emotional-motivational aspects of the pain experience.[10,31] Sternbach[44] has defined pain as "a personal, private sensation of hurt; a harmful stimulus which signals current or impending tissue damage; a pattern of responses which operate to protect the organism from harm."[44] (p. 12). He has stated[46] that pain "is as likely to reflect psychological as it is physical pathology." His research has demonstrated that the experience of pain is influenced by social and cultural learning history.[47,48]

A number of investigators[14,20-22,46] have distinguished between acute and chronic pain, stressing that chronic pain is a *pattern of behaviors* that are learned over time. Acute pain is pain for which there is a known and possibly observable physiologic mechanism. Acute pain activates the autonomic nervous system and is usually accompanied by anxiety.[13,46]. The preceding investigators vary in their interpretations of the mechanism responsible for chronic pain. For example, Sternbach's[46] view is that the autonomic nervous responses habituate over a period of a few weeks or months, even if the pain persists. During that time, the patient experiences "vegetative changes" such as sleep and appetite disturbance, decreased libido, and increased irritability and social withdrawal. These changes lead to feelings of hopelessness and helplessness characteristic of depression. In his view, the physician should treat the anxiety that accompanies acute pain using explanations of the condition and reassurance and possibly anxiolytic agents. For the chronic pain patient, treatment of the depression is recommended through attempts to increase activity levels and vocational involvement. Antidepressant medications may be needed to accelerate the process.

Another view of the development of chronic pain has been presented by Keefe and Brown.[21] They have identified "acute," "pre-chronic," and "chronic" stages in their longitudinal studies of changes in patients' behavior[19] and attempt to separate cognitive, overt behavioral, and physiologic responses of chronic pain patients.[20,22] These investigators suggest that decreases in activity and the use of medication immediately following an injury are adaptive behaviors. They also view muscle spasms during this stage as a protective reaction of the musculoskeletal system to immobilize joints and protect from further injury. The anxiety that accompanies an injury can be a motivator to seek treatment and to comply with it. Two to six months postinjury, as healing takes place, the typical patient will attempt to return to preinjury activity patterns. Those individuals who gradually resume activity without experiencing flare-ups of pain are more likely to become pain-free. Patients who are either unable (because of job or financial pressures, for example) or unwilling (because of personality style, eg, superachievers and workacholics) to gradually resume preinjury activity patterns are more likely to experience exacerbation of pain and to resort to rest and the use of medication. With each attempt to resume activity that fails, the patient becomes more and more cautious and fearful of activity, which leads to shortening of muscles, increased muscle spasm, and fatigue. The patient's self-evaluation becomes negative and depression ensues. This stage is referred to as "pre-chronic." These investigators view the role of social consequences of pain behaviors as critical at this and the later chronic stage. After six months postinjury, there is usually little or no evidence that tissue damage is responsible for the pain. An alternative is that the positive attention received from spouse, family, and friends, the opportunity to avoid work and/or other responsibilities, and possible financial compensation become very powerful positive reinforcers of the pain behaviors.

The view of chronic pain as a pattern of behaviors that are learned over time has not been accepted by all investigators. Mersky and Spears,[33] for example, identified hysterical personalities in an outpatient female population. Blumer and Heilbronn[7] have focused on underlying depression as the mechanism responsible for the chronic pain syndrome. There is some evidence that homogeneous subgroups of chronic pain patients can be identified, which strongly suggests that there is not one underlying mechanism responsible for chronic pain. Bradley, Prokop, Margolis, and Gentry,[8] using multi-variate statistical techniques, identified three homogeneous MMPI subgroups of low-back-pain patients: (1) essentially normal profile, (2) elevations on scales Hs, D, and Hy, and (3) a "psychopathologic" profile with elevations on the majority of clinical scales. Sternbach[45] identified four subgroups of MMPI profiles in chronic pain patients: (1) Hypochrondriasis—extremely elevated Hs, generally poor treatment outcome, (2) Reactive depression—elevated D (T-score above 70), favorable response to antidepressant medication and positive treatment outcome, (3) Somatization reaction—"conversion V" (elevated Hs and Hy compared with low D), moderately successful treatment outcome, and (4) Manipulative reaction—Pd scale elevation nearly as high as neurotic scales, poor treatment outcome.

Sarno[37-39] has proposed that there are two major types of back pain that are related to psychological mechanisms. The first, psychogenic regional pain, is essentially a conversion reaction in which the pain does not conform to any anatomic or physiologic configuration and there are negative laboratory or clinical findings. The other type of back pain is a result of tension myositis.[40] Tension myositis, or TMS, is a physiologic manifestation of tension. Sources of tension are external/environmental, eg, life situations, working conditions, etc., and internal/intrapsychic, eg, personality characteristics such as compulsivity, perfectionistic tendencies, etc., and emotional responses such as fear and anxiety which can create further tension. In Sarno's view, excess tension and emotional responses that are unacceptable to the individual are channeled into the body through the *psychophysiologic mechanism* of tension myositis, ie, "physical changes caused by some emotional phenomenon"[40] (p. 57). He cites other psychophysiologic disorders such as heartburn, gastritis, ulcer and hiatus hernia, colitis, spastic colon, tension and migrane headaches, hives eczema, hay fever, and asthma.[40]

Sarno[40] defines tension myositis syndrome, TMS, as a "change of state of muscle (*myo*). The change is circulatory; tension constricts the blood vessels feeding the involved muscles, and the resultant blood deprivation leads to painful muscle spasm and nerve pain."[40] (p. 15) The mechanism is the autonomic nervous system's response to stress. In addition to heat, cold, hunger, and fatigue, emotions are potent activators of the autonomic nervous system. The autonomic nervous system controls the body's circulation of blood and TMS is seen as "the result of tension-induced alterations in local circulation resulting in blood deprivation, called *ischemia*. Tension causes the arterioles to close partly (vasoconstriction), and this slows the circulation of blood in a given area, thereby depriving the tissues of their normal blood supply."[40] (pp.63–64). Spasms are caused by oxygen deprivation to the muscles due to the reduced circulation. Further, the reduced circulation to the nerves means a reduced oxygen supply and this results in nerve pain and possibly numbness.

Clearly, more research is needed to determine what relationships exist among affective responses, overt motor behaviors, and physiologic responses in the chronic pain population to help identify the most effective treatment interventions. Meanwhile, the physician who is confronted with a patient with pain symptomology can benefit from knowledge of the categories into which the individual with pain may be classified, using the Third Edition of the *Diagnostic and Statistical Manual of Mental Disorders* (1980). The two major relevant categories are the Somatoform disorders and Psychological Factors Affecting Physical Condition. A detailed description of these categories follows.

Somatoform Disorders[1]

In this group of disorders, the patient presents with physical symptoms that suggest physical disorder but for which no demonstrable organic evidence can be found and for which there is no known physiologic mechanism (Table 9-1). Instead, there is either positive evidence or strong suggestion that the symptoms are associated with psychological factors or conflicts. These disorders are not under voluntary control.

Somatization disorder. The patient presents multiple, recurrent somatic complaints that are chronic and occur in a fluctuating course. The complaints usually begin before the age of 30 years. Although the patient's concerns are presented in a dramatic, vague, or exaggerated manner, it is necessary to rule out physical diseases that may have vague, multiple, or confusing symptoms, eg, multiple sclerosis or systemic lupus erythematosus. The patient has often received treatment from a number of physicians. Criteria for inclusion in this category include having at least 12–14 symptoms, from a list of 37, for which the patient has seen a physician, taken medication, or changed their life pattern. Some examples of the symptoms that are commonly reported are difficulty swallowing, loss of voice, abdominal pain, shortness of breath, or chest pain. Patients in this category present the appearance of being depressed and anxious.

As is apparent by the number, duration, and vagueness of the symptoms presented by patients suffering from this disorder, the patient will require firm reassurance. Due to their dependence upon physicians, as well as the numerous medical examinations they have undergone, such patients are often willing to submit to unnecessary surgery. They are also likely to become addicted to medications. When firm reassurance and clearly given support fail to provide relief to the patient, psychotherapy should be considered as the patient is likely to be experiencing occupational, interpersonal, and/or marital problems. Certainly, such problems could arise the longer the symptoms persist.

Conversion disorder. The loss of or alteration in physical functioning as an expression of a psychological conflict or need characterizes the conversion disorder. The patient achieves primary gain by keeping an internal conflict or need out of awareness, and, in some cases, achieves secondary gain by avoiding an activity or getting emotional and/or financial support as a result. A conversion disorder usually develops suddenly under stress. Upon examination, the patient's attitude will belie a deep concern about their symptom. "La belle indifference" has been used to characterize the patient with conversion symptoms. Such attitudes, however, may be found in seriously ill patients who need to defend against illness and differential diagnosis must be made with care. Conversion disorders are found in all age groups. They are usually of short duration and have an abrupt onset and resolution. Marked impairment may produce serious complications such as contractures and/or atrophy. Common conversion symptoms are hysterical paralysis, seizures, and blindness.

Etiology is of prime significance in this group of patients. In cases where an internal conflict is being repressed from awareness, psychotherapy is essential because of the danger that removal of the symptom can precipitate a psychosis. Generally, long-term supportive counseling with gradual uncovering of the repressed material is advised. This approach may result in total resolution of the symptom. When issues of secondary gain are involved, behavioral methods of treatment may provide the only method of relief. In such cases, helping family members to become aware of their patterns of behavior that reinforce the sick role is essential. Behavioral treatment can help the patient learn more adaptive behaviors to use in a situation that is producing conflict. Psychiatric assessment and psychological testing may be necessary in order to identify the appropriate treatment approach.

Psychogenic pain disorder. In this category, the predominant symptom is pain. Evidence that psychological factors mediate the pain symptom is necessary. Often, the location of the pain is inconsistent with the anatomical distribution of the nervous system. The patient makes frequent visits to doctors and may make excessive use of analgesics without obtaining relief. The concern about the pain is less intense than would be expected given the reported severity of the pain. The mood of the patient is often dysphoric. Although psychogenic pain occurs at any time, it is most frequent among adolescents and young adults. The duration of symptoms varies but the pain often appears suddenly and increases in severity. Sources of stress can usually be identified by the interviewer. The degree of impairment varies with the degree of pain. Examples of psychogenic pain disorder are paraesthesias and muscle spasms.

In those cases of psychogenic pain where stress and tension have clearly produced the symptoms, rest and long-term efforts to create a less pressured life style can prove helpful. Stress management clinics, meditation, and yoga exercises can be beneficial for some individuals. Moderate exercise that helps reduce stress will also aid patients with tension-induced muscle spasms. Hypnosis can be helpful with some patients. Psychological counseling may be necessary in cases of severe stress reactions. In cases where secondary gain can be identified as a predominant factor, behavioral methods may be indicated.

Hypochondriasis. Hypochondriacal patients present unrealistic interpretations of physical signs or sensations. They are preoccupied with the possibility of developing a serious disease. Despite persistent medical reassurance their symptoms often cause functional limitations in social as well as occupational situations. The patient often presents the medical history in great detail and at great length. They may appear anxious and depressed and are often angry and frustrated. Hypochondriasis occurs most commonly in adolescence but it may appear at any age. Symptoms are chronic but there is a fluctuation of complaints. Complications can include risks from undergoing repeated diagnostic procedures. True pathology can be missed if the patient is labeled hypochondriacal and the symptoms are not taken seriously. Firm, reassuring support following adequate medical testing remains the best approach to treatment of these patients. In cases where hypochondriacal tendencies have interfered with occupational and interpersonal situations, psychotherapy seems indicated to help the patient discover the need for such preoccupation. Underlying affect such as guilt, grief, and repressed anger may result in hypochondriacal tendencies.

Atypical somatoform disorder. This category is used for patients whose symptoms do not fit clearly in any of the preceding categories. An example would be that of a patient who is preoccupied with some imagined defect in their physical appearance that is out of proportion to any physical abnormality that might exist. Treatment would consist of firm reassurance and support. If this is ineffective, psychotherapy should be considered to help the patient gain understanding as to the reasons for the exaggerated focus on a relatively minor problem.

Table 9-1

Somatoform Disorders

Disorder	Age of Disorder	Course	Impairment	Presentation	Mood	Duration
Somatization disorder	Begins before 30	Recurrent	Multiple, fluctuating	Complaints presented in dramatic, vague or exaggerated way.	Anxious and depressed	Chronic
Conversion disorder	Any age	Sudden onset, often under stress. Sudden resolution	Mild to marked	Lack of concern	"la bell indifference"	Usually short
Psychogenic disorder	Any age, most frequently adolescence or early adult	Sudden, under stress	Varies with pain	Concern regarding pain less intense than severity.	dysphoric	Varied
Hypochondriasis	Any age, most common in adolescence	Waxing and waning	Socially and occupationally functionally impaired	Presents history at length in great detail; often angry and frustrated	Anxious and depressed	Chronic

Atypical Somatoform Disorder is a residual category

Psychological Factors Affecting a Physical Condition

The diagnosis is made on the evidence of a temporal relationship between an environmental stimulus (eg, argument) and the exacerbation of a physical condition. This category is used when the patient has demonstrable organic pathology that is clearly affected by psychological factors. Examples are neurodermatitis and asthma.

Treatment of Chronic Pain

Chronic pain is the most common and most difficult problem that the physician must treat.[13,19,40] The cost of chronic pain in terms of hospitalizations and other medical treatments, loss of income, disability payments, and cost of litigation is enormous. A recent estimate of a cost of $60 billion annually made by the National Institute of Neurological and Communicative Disorders and Stroke, was cited by Fey and Fordyce.[13] The rehabilitation programs that have received most attention within the last 10 years and that have been subjected to the most rigorous evaluation are based on the multimodal behavioral model developed by Fordyce and his colleagues.[14,15] An alternative model based on Sarno's[37-40] theory of TMS was described by Kirshbaum, Mihovich, and Feinblatt[24] and is used at the Institute of Rehabilitative Medicine—New York University Medical Center, New York City. These two treatment approaches will be described below.

Behavioral Rehabilitation

The behavioral approach to rehabilitation of the chronic pain patient defines pain as "behavior" and requires visible or audible expressions as evidence that the person is experiencing pain.[14,16,44] Further, pain behavior that is sensitive to its consequences, either positive or negative, can become independent of nociceptive stimuli, ie, can be exhibited because of its consequences. Thus, chronic pain behavior can be a result of a combination of early medical management strategies, social contingencies, and previous psychological problems that make being ill reinforcing. Fey and Fordyce[13] have identified direct positive reinforcers for pain behavior: (1) The family's responding positively *only* to pain behaviors, not to other behaviors; (2) The interest and caretaking provided by the health care system to the pain patient, as well as the prescription of medications; (3) Monetary compensation in the form of disability payments that become contingent on pain behaviors, leading to a disincentive for non-pain behaviors (c.f. Peck, Fordyce, and Black, 1978[34]); (4) Rest and inactivity leads to a reduction in pain levels and thus becomes a positive reinforcer for pain behaviors. The cite equally powerful indirect reinforcers of pain behaviors: (1) Pain removes the person from a difficult situation; (2) Compensatory body positions and ambulation aids indirectly reinforce pain behaviors because the patient is conditioned to avoid pain by using them; (3) Pain behaviors are learned from family members through modeling and imitation.

Treatment programs using the behavioral approach developed by Fordyce[14] and Fordyce, Fowler, and de Lateur[15] have been instituted at the University of Minnesota, Department of Rehabilitation Medicine, Minneapolis,[4,35] Rancho Los Amigos Hospital, Downey, California,[9] Portland Pain Center, Portland, Oregon[41] and Emory University, Atlanta, Georgia.[11] As identified by Fey and Fordyce,[13] the aim of these programs is the elimination of pain behaviors by reducing the social reinforcement from staff and family while reinforcing well behaviors. Changing the treatment and home environments to develop and to sustain responses that are incompatible with sick behaviors is fundamental to this approach. These programs address a variety of behaviors: Physical disability and inactivity, verbal and nonverbal pain behaviors, narcotic addiction, depression, sexual dysfunction, and vocational problems. Fordyce[14] and Fordyce and Steger[17] have delineated the evaluation, treatment, and follow-up stages of these treatment programs.

The evaluation phase of the treatment program[13] is necessary to determine the nature and extent of the pain behaviors and disability as a basis for defining specific treatment goals and as a means of evaluating the effectiveness of the interventions. Generally, the patient's medical history is reviewed to rule out conditions that could be treated medically. A preadmission record of activity, medications, and pain ratings is required of each patient. Behavioral evaluations by a psychologist of the patient, spouse, and other family members are carried out to determine the relationship among pain behaviors, physical activity, and environmental consequences. The patient's pain patterns and sleep patterns are also examined. The "class" of pain behaviors, eg, sounds, grimaces, postures, is identified, circumstances that activate and diminish the pain behaviors are determined, and the relationship of pain behaviors to stress, tension, anxiety, and changes in the couple's activities together is examined. A comparison of the patient's reported use of medication prior to admission to actual use during the initial inpatient admission is made. A baseline of physical therapy and occupational therapy activity levels is obtained on admission. An assessment of vocational needs and current legal status is made before treatment interventions begin.

The treatment phase of the behavioral model has been described in detail by Fordyce[14] and summarized recently by Fey and Fordyce.[13] Generally, the goals of a 4–6 week inpatient admission are as follows: (1) medication detoxification—changing from a pain-contingent to time-contingent regimen; (2) physical reactivation—setting physical and occupational therapy activity level quotas below baseline level to reduce the reinforcement value of rest, to build physical strength gradually, and to teach pacing of activity; (3) increase well behaviors; (4) reduce attention and social reinforcement for pain behaviors; (5) vocational counseling—using practice jobs prior to a return to the work situation; (6) stress-reduction—using muscle relaxation techniques and biofeedback, hypnosis, and cognitive-behavioral techniques.

Recent reviews of the behavioral approach to treatment of chronic pain generally conclude that the results are promising.[13,19,27] A decrease in reports of pain is often found, along with an increase in activity level, return to employment, and a decrease in the use of medication. The reviewers consistently identify the lack of control groups, vague criteria for determining treatment outcome, a lack of or imprecise follow-up, and lack of evaluation of the effectiveness of each component in a multi-model treatment program as obstacles to evaluating the effectiveness of the treatment.

Psychodynamically Oriented Treatment

The Psychophysiological Pain Program (PPP) at the Institute of Rehabilitation Medicine—New York University Medical Center, New York City, treats patients with the psychogenic regional pain and TMS described by Sarno[37-40] and referred to earlier in this chapter. The PPP utilizes a holistic approach to treatment, recognizing that the patient's pain has both physiological and psychological determinants that interact. The principles of psychodynamic psychotherapy are used, along with cognitive-behavioral techniques.[23,30] The evaluation and treatment components of the program are described below.

Sarno[40] describes the patients in the Psychophysiological Pain Program as individuals who are "conscientious, responsible, hard-working and often compulsive."[40] He states further that they have "a need to accomplish, or live up to some ideal role."[40] Many factors are involved in the development of chronic psychophysiological back pain. Frequently, life experiences such as loss, minor injury, or a change in social or economic status can pose a serious threat to the individual's rigidly defined self-image. This emotional stress triggers the psychophysiologic mechanism underlying TMS. Many of the patients have family situations in which they have appeared to be the "rock"; they have been the one upon whom others have depended. They often state that they have always felt that if something had to be done correctly, they were the only one who could do it. They highly value their ability to take charge, to be independent, to be in control. These abilities are strongly integrated into their self-concept. This personality style often conceals a wish for and fear of dependence, and a strong fear of helplessness and vulnerability.

The need to be competent and in control proves to be a heavy burden for the individual and places great stress on the autonomic nervous system, which prepares the body to take action.[40] The constant internal pressure to perform "perfectly" results in feelings of exhaustion and frustration. The compulsive caring for others results in a neglect of the individual's own needs—needs that may not become apparent until the chronic pain and disability manifests itself. Paradoxically, being disabled by pain provides a measure of relief from the environmental demands, yet, at the same time, results in the surfacing of feelings of incompetence and dependence—the very feelings that the patient has repressed through their "competent" orientation. Further, the patient begins to feel tremendous resentment and anger at the insensitivity of people around them, because those people can rarely be as sensitive and competent at caretaking as the patient was with them. The awareness of their own dependency needs is very painful.

Candidates for the intensive inpatient program are examined by the medical director and are required to undergo a psychological evaluation consisting of a clinical interview and a standard psychological test battery. Not all individuals are amenable to psychodynamically-oriented treatment, nor are all patients capable of benefitting from such an approach. In the selection process, particular attention is paid to the patient's strengths and to those factors that have been found to contribute to success in dynamic psychotherapy.[28] Specifically, the quality of interpersonal relationships of the patient, their capacity for insight, intellectual potential, and the array of their coping mechanisms are assessed.

Patients exhibiting subnormal intelligence, organic brain syndrome, florid psychosis, or overt suicide potential are not accepted into the program, due to the stress encountered in the uncovering psychotherapeutic approach, as well as the anxiety engendered by the rehabilitation setting. Further, these patients may not have the capacity for intellectual challenge or may lack the psychic energy required for such an uncovering approach. In some cases, decompensation might occur as a result of the confrontational aspects of psychodynamic treatment. For some individuals, a psychiatric milieu may be required. Those patients who are not accepted into the program are referred elsewhere for appropriate treatment.

Certain prognosticators of successful treatment have been identified during the evaluation process. Patients who persevere throughout the lengthy evaluation procedure and who continue to apply themselves to the task at hand during psychological testing, despite apparent discomfort or even severe pain, have proven to be more successful in treatment. In addition, those patients who are aware of their deficits and who attempt to utilize alternative methods of coping have also been found to do better in treatment. These patients are likely to be highly motivated to lose their pain and eager to resume their premorbid lifestyle. Patients who experience their pain as overwhelming, who cannot attend to tasks at hand, and who are unable to discuss other aspects of their life without referring to their pain, have generally been found to be poor candidates.

Patients who appear to receive secondary gain from their pain, whether it be familial attention or financial compensation, are sometimes poor candidates for the PPP. Their behavior is often characterized by a constant referral to their pain and an inability to relate to other situations or people not directly involved with their pain. In addition, they exhibit a great deal of reluctance to perform the tasks required of them. This behavior, coupled with a paucity of defensive styles, indicates that, for these patients, pain may serve a vital function because few alternative compensatory coping mechanisms are available. Such patients have proven to be poor risks. Requesting help from the examiner to a moderate or extreme degree, requiring frequent rest periods, refusing to perform tasks, and denying and evading the examiner's questions are behaviors indicative of someone with a dependent personality who may be quite resistant to the uncovering psychodynamic approach. These patients frequently have longer treatment histories.

The goals of the PPP are (1) to educate the patient regarding the role of psychological factors in somatic symptom formation, (2) to reduce stress, (3) to prepare the patient for continued psychotherapy, (4) to identify and explore specific tension-related patterns of experience and behavior, and (5) to provide the opportunity for experimentation with new roles and styles of relating. In this regard, hospitalization provides a microcosm of the real world in which such goals may be achieved. In some cases, stress reduction is accomplished by removing the patients from the home environment. In addition, the hospital is viewed as a protective setting in which the patient is free to relate more openly and without fear of punitive social consequences, thus further reducing stress. Hospitalization, as well as the group experience, affords patients the opportunity to share with others like themselves the emotional concerns of individuals with chronic, often debilitating pain. Sharing the process with others also reduces the stigma of psychotherapeutic treatment. Trying out new coping styles with other patients in a safe milieu provides opportunity for rehearsal with alternative behavior patterns.

When treatment begins, the Medical Director gives each patient an explanation of the psychophysiologic process underlying their symptomatology. These didactic explanations, as well as lectures, are presented throughout the patient's inpatient treatment program. Their goal is to provide the patient with the correct framework in which to view their treatment process. Emphasis upon the underlying psychological conflict is maintained, creating a more motivated psychotherapy patient. Corrections in medical misinformation are also provided in this manner so that patients do not focus on the physical aspects of their disorder.

Preparation for continued psychotherapy is considered an essential goal of treatment. Although the intense therapeutic experience may prove beneficial, many patients experience deep-seated, longstanding emotional problems that may require longer treatment than that of the brief hospitalization period. Continued outpatient individual and/or group psychotherapy is available to facilitate consolidation of gains made during inpatient treatment and to stimulate further improvement.

Resistance to psychological etiology of somatic symptoms is well documented.[6,36,49] For back pain patients in particular, resistance may be even greater, especially if the patient has been through the medical "mill" and has been seen by a variety of specialists. Their addiction to explanations of their pain as due to poor alignment, herniated discs, pinched nerves, sciatica, and scoliosis is profound. Fear of being helpless and being told they may become totally wheelchair bound or may never take part in sports or any other athletic activity, create individuals hesitant to utilize muscles and limbs that can become atrophied by disuse. Resistance, then, to a psychogenic etiology may be overwhelming. Further entrenching resistance is the face-saving quality of a physical condition. In addition, cognitive dissonance often requires that patients maintain their view of their disorder as purely physical. When a patient has undergone surgery(ies), painful manipulative procedures such as traction, and even addiction to narcotic medications in order to ease their discomfort, it is difficult to get them to reformulate their understanding of their pain. Frustration, resentment, fear, and guilt become readily apparent. Patients frequently and mistakenly assume that their physician is implying that they "wanted" their pain, that they "brought it on themselves," or that "it is all in their head." The ongoing educational aspects of the program provided by the physician in the PPP provide a much needed forum for dispelling such myths.

In addition, due to the anticipated intimacy of psychotherapeutic treatment with its analysis and exploration of possibly unknown feelings, desires, and needs, patients often experience anxiety. Dependency needs that lie at the core of some of these patient's problems can be exacerbated by the hospitalization experience and the closeness of the psychotherapeutic relationship. The patient often views the procedure as one of being taken care of and their dependency needs are manifested to an extreme degree in their relationships with the nurses, physical therapists, occupational therapists, psychologists, and other hospital personnel.

The conflicts, fantasies, attitudes, and behaviors from the patients' everyday lives are brought to the hospital experience.[24] Significant relationships from the past are recreated in the intense atmosphere of hospital life. Rivalries, jealousies, and angers are often aroused and become available for exploration in psychotherapy. For example, the Medical Director, physical therapists, and cotherapists, who are often seen as authority figures, serve as suitable targets for the displacement of various attitudes developed in relation to authority figures in the patient's past, eg, parents and other significant adults. Other hospitalized patients, suffering from organic disabilities, who are in proximity to the pain patient may arouse intense feelings related to dependency needs. All of these experiences are available for psychotherapeutic exploration. Previous maladaptive behavioral patterns as well as new, more constructive, methods of coping are accessible once the patient becomes actively involved in making the connection between psychological experiences and pain symptomatology.

In order to develop more constructive methods of dealing with loss, injury, change in status, dependency fears, and poor self-esteem (which result in the addiction to achievement), the Psychophysiological Pain Program attempts to make patients aware of these feelings. Support and confrontation are the main techniques utilized in the short-term inpatient treatment approach. Support is evident in the hospital atmosphere, in the self-help aspects of group psychotherapy, as well as in the didactic medical lectures given to patients. Rapport with therapists and other patients is easily established in such a milieu. Once a positive commitment to the goals of the program is established, a more confrontational approach can be implemented. Thus, repressed feelings are encouraged to surface when the anxiety they engender can be tolerated. The somatization that aided in the repression of affect is then no longer necessary. Patients frequently verbalize increased feelings of anxiety at the time that their physical symptomatology decreases or abates altogether.

This therapeutic program requires constant communication between all therapists involved. Confrontations undertaken with patients before they are prepared to handle them may precipitate panic reactions. Patients may not be ready to accept interpretations and in some cases might even leave treatment due to the threatening nature of the interaction. Constant communication between staff members also allows for the free exchange of ideas and aids therapists in understanding the stages through which the patient is going in their treatment.

In summary, the psychodynamic treatment of the Psychophysiological Pain Program at the Institute of Rehabilitation Medicine attempts to educate the patient about the etiology of their symptomatology, to reduce stress, to prepare the patient for continued psychotherapy, and to identify and explore behavioral patterns that have led to anxiety and somatic manifestations. In addition, the program attempts to aid the patient in developing new constructive coping strategies. This may result in more conscious anxiety, but will not require the repression of affect resulting in somatization. After inpatient treatment, outpatient individual and group psychotherapy may be recommended to help the patient consolidate gains made during the intensive inpatient phase.

There have been no adequate follow-up studies of the effectiveness of this treatment approach. Further, no control groups are used and the criteria for determining treatment outcome are not defined. The effectiveness of the various components of the program, eg, education, physical and occupational therapy, individual and group psychotherapy, has not been evaluated. Clearly, a systematic procedure to assess the effectiveness of this program is greatly needed. The only follow-up reported to date is that described by Sarno,[40] who conducted a telephone survey in 1982 of 177 TMS patients. All were patients who had been diagnosed by Sarno as having TMS and who had been instructed by him regarding the nature of TMS. Some had had a course of physical therapy. It was not reported whether or not these patients had received inpatient treatment and/or outpatient treatment that included psychotherapy. Included in the survey were only those patients whose treatment had concluded at least one year prior to the survey. The results of the survey indicated that 76 percent were "relieved of significant pain," 62 percent were "totally relieved," and 14 percent had "minor recurrences of no importance."[40] (p. 102). Sixteen percent were treatment failures.

REFERENCES

1. American Psychiatric Association. Diagnostic and Statistical Manual of Mental Disorders, Third Edition. Washington, D.C.: American Psychiatric Association, 1980

2. Anderson F, Bardach JL: Sexuality and neuromuscular disease: A pilot study. Int Rehabil Med 5:21–26, 1983

3. Anderson F, Bardach JL, Goodgold J: Sexuality and neuromuscular disease. Rehabilitation Monograph #56. New York: The Institute of Rehabilitation Medicine and The Muscular Dystrophy Association, 1979

4. Anderson T, Cole T, Gullickson G, et al: Behavior modification of chronic pain: A treatment program by a multidisciplinary team. Clin Orthop Related Research 129:96–100, 1977

5. Athelstan G, Crewe NM: Psychological adjustment to spinal cord injury as related to manner of onset of disability. Rehabil Counseling Bull 22:311–319, 1979

6. Bastiaans J: Psychoanalytic psychotherapy, in Wittkower ED, Warner H (eds): Psychosomatic medicine: Its clinical application. New York: Harper and Row, 1977, pp 86–93

7. Blumer D, Heilbronn M: Chronic pain as a variant of depressive disease. J Ner Ment Dis 170(7):381–406, 1982

8. Bradley LA, Prokop CK, Margolis R, et al: Multivariate analysis of the MMPI profiles of low back pain patients. J Behav Med 1:253–272, 1978

8a. Brown M, Gordon WA, Diller L: Functional assessment and outcome measurement: an integrative review, in Pan E, Backer T, Vash C (eds) Annual Review of Rehabilitation, 3:93–120, New York, Springer, 1983

9. Cairns D, Thomas L, Moonery V, et al: A comprehensive treatment pain approach to chronic low back pain. Behav Ther 8:621–630, 1977

10. Casey KL: Physiological mechanisms of pain perception, in Weisenberg M (ed): The control of pain. New York: Psychological Dimensions, 1977, pp 227–259

11. Chapman S, Brena S, Bradford A: Treatment outcome in a chronic pain rehabilitation program. Paper presented at the 56th Annual Session of the American Congress of Rehabilitation Medicine, Honolulu, 1979

12. Falno DR, Allen H, Maki DR: Psychosocial aspects of invisible disability. Rehabilitation Literature 43(1-2):2–6, 1982

13. Fey SG, Fordyce WE: Behavioral rehabilitation of the chronic pain patient, in Pan EL, Backer TE, Vash CL (eds): Annual review of rehabilitation—Vol. 3. New York: Springer Publishing Company, 1983, pp 32–63

14. Fordyce WE: Behavioral methods for the control of chronic pain and illness. St. Louis, Missouri: C.V. Mosby, 1976

15. Fordyce WE, Fowler RS, de Lateur B: An application of behavior modification technique to a problem of chronic pain. Behav Res Ther 6:105–107, 1968

16. Fordyce WE, Fowler R, Lehmann J, et al: Some implications of learning in problems of chronic pain. Journal of Chronic Diseases. 21:179–190, 1968

17. Fordyce WE, Steger JC: Behavioral management of chronic pain, in J Brady, O Pomerleau (eds): Behavioral medicine: Theory and practice. Baltimore, Williams and Wilkins, 1978

18. Harrower HR, Herrmann R: Psychological factors in the care of patients with multiple sclerosis for use of physicians. New York: National Multiple Sclerosis Society, 1953

19. Keefe FJ: Behavioral assessment and treatment of chronic pain: Current status and future directions. Consult Clin Psychol 50(6):896–911, 1982

20. Keefe FJ, Block AR: Behavioral treatment of pain, in Surwit RS, Williams RB, Steptoe A, Biersner R (eds): NATO symposium on behavioral medicine: Behavioral treatment of disease. New York, Plenum Press, pp 371–388, 1982

21. Keefe FJ, Brown C: Behavioral treatment of chronic pain, in Boudewyns P, Keefe FJ (eds): Behavioral medicine in general medical practice. Menlo Park, California, Addison-Wesley, pp 19–41, 1982

22. Keefe FJ, Brown C, Scott DS, et al: Behavioral assessment of chronic pain, in Keefe FJ, Blumen-

thal JA (eds): Assessment strategies in behavioral medicine. New York, Grune & Stratton, pp 321–350, 1982

23. Khatami M, Rush AJ: A pilot study of the treatment of outpatients with chronic pain: Symptom control, stimulus control and social system intervention. Pain 5:163–172, 1978

24. Kirshbaum K, Mihovich EG, Feinblatt A: The Assessment and treatment of chronic psychogenic back pain: A holistic psychodynamic approach. Paper presented at American Psychological Association Annual Convention, New York City, 1979

25. Korsch BM, Negrete VF: Doctor-patient communication. Scientific American 227(2):66–74, 1972

26. Kubler-Ross E: On death and dying. New York: MacMillian, 1969

27. Latimer PR: External contingency management for chronic pain: Critical review of the evidence. Am J Psych 139(10):1308–1312, 1982

28. Luborsky L, Spence DP: Quantitative research on psychoanalytic therapy, in Bergin AE, Garfield S (eds): Handbook of psychotherapy and behavior change. New York: Wiley, 1971, pp 408–438

29. Macgregor FC, Abel TM, Byrt A, et al: Facial deformities and plastic surgery. Springfield, Illinois: Charles C Thomas, 1953

30. Meichenbaum D, Turk D: The cognitive-behavioral management of anxiety, anger, and pain, in Davidson PO (ed): The behavioral management of anxiety, depression, and pain. New York, Brunner/Mazel, 1976, pp 1–34

31. Melzack R: The puzzle of pain. New York: Basic Books, 1973

32. Melzack R, Wall PD: Pain mechanisms: A new theory. Science 150:971–979, 1965

33. Mersky H, Spears FG: Pain: Psychosocial and psychiatric aspects. Baltimore, Williams and Wilkins, 1967

34. Peck CJ, Fordyce WE, Black RG: The effect of the pendency of claims for compensation upon behavior indicative of pain. Washington Law Review 53:251–278, 1978

35. Roberts AH, Reinhardt L: The behavioral management of chronic pain: Long-term follow-up with comparison groups. Pain 8:151–162, 1980

36. Ross WD: Musculoskeletal disorders, in Wittkower ED, Warner H (eds): Psychosomatic medicine: Its clinical applications. New York, Harper and Row, 1977, pp 296–306

37. Sarno JE: Psychogenic backache: The missing dimension. J Fam Pract 1(8):8–12, 1974

38. Sarno JE: Chronic back pain and psychic conflict. Scandinavian J Rehab Med 8:143–153, 1976

39. Sarno JE: Psychosomatic backache. J Fam Pract 5(3):353–357, 1977

40. Sarno JE: Mind over back pain. New York, William Morrow, 1984

41. Seres J, Newman RI, Yospe LP, et al: Multidisciplinary treatment of chronic pain: A long-term follow-up of low back pain patients. Pain 4:283–292, 1978

42. Shontz FC: Physical disability and personality theory and recent research. Psychol Aspects Disabil 17:51–69, 1970

43. Spergel P, Ehrlich GE, Glass D: The rheumatoid arthritic personality: A psychodiagnostic myth. Psychosomatics 19(2):79–86, 1978

44. Sternbach RA: Pain: A psychophysiological analysis. New York, Academic Press, 1968

45. Sternbach RA: Pain patients: Traits and treatment. New York, Academic Press, 1974

46. Sternbach RA: Psychological aspects of chronic pain. Clin Orthop Relat Research 129:150–155, 1977

47. Sternbach RA, Tursky B: Ethnic differences among housewives in psychophysiological and skin potential responses to electric shock. Psychophysiology 1:241–246, 1965

48. Tursky B, Sternbach RA: Further physiological correlates of ethnic differences in response to shock. Psychophysiology 4:67–74, 1967

49. Wolfe HH: The psychodynamic approach to psychosomatic disorders: Contributions and limitations of psychoanalysis. Br J Med Psychol 41:343–348, 1968

50. Wright BA: Physical disability: A psychosocial approach. Second Edition. New York, Harper and Row, 1983

John H. Bland

10

Preventive Management and Rehabilitation in Rheumatoid Arthritis of the Cervical Spine

Rheumatoid arthritis (RA) has emerged as an immunologic-infectious disease with strong genetic implications. It is difficult to determine both the population incidence and prevalence as well as the natural course of the disease. Its very definition remains imprecise. Recognition and diagnosis of rheumatoid arthritis in its earliest stages is sometimes impossible because it may have a variable nonspecific pattern for months or years before emerging as "characteristic." Using the American Rheumatism Association criteria of 1957 for rheumatoid arthritis, 3.2 percent of the adult noninstitutionalized population have the disease[25] (Table 10-1). Extrapolated to 1976 this is 5,000,000 persons with rheumatoid arthritis in the United States.[19] By the same criteria a prevalence of 0.3 percent was found in adults under age 35, this figure increasing exponentially in subsequent decades exceeding 10 percent in persons 65 years and older. The overall sex ratio is about 3 females to 1 male. Males have an abrupt increase in prevalence at 60 years and over, while females predominate in a ratio of 5 to 1 under age 60. At age 60 the sex ratio is approximately 1.4 to 1. Clinical studies suggest an equal sex ratio in new cases of rheumatoid arthritis in the elderly.[5]

The principle lesions of RA are in the diarthrodial joints and to a lesser degree in tendons, tendon sheaths, bursae, and the periarticular subcutaneous tissue (Fig. 10-1). The inflammatory lesions of joints involve the synovium primarily with a proliferation of granulation tissue capable of secretion of enzymes destructive to connective tissues (Fig. 10-2). The subchondral bone is secondarily affected as is the articular cartilage, ultimately being destroyed. (Fig. 10-3). About 20 percent of patients with peripheral rheumatoid arthritis develop the characteristic subcutaneous nodules (Fig. 10-4). Tendons and ligaments may be involved in varying magnitude, from clinical tenderness to anatomic rupture. Striated muscles, peripheral nerves, arteries, small blood vessels, particularly the post-capillary venules, are all involved. Immune complexes play a major role in initiating the inflammatory process. Cardiac involvement in RA is frequent but not commonly symptomatic. Pericarditis and pleuritis are common. Spleen, lymphoid tissues, and bone marrow may be involved as are lungs, eyes, and the exocrine gland system.

PRINCIPLES OF PHYSICAL MEDICINE AND REHABILITATION IN THE MUSCULOSKELETAL DISEASES

Table 10-1
Criteria for Diagnosis of Rheumatoid Arthritis American Rheumatism Association
(with modification)

1. Morning stiffness
2. Arthritis in at least one joint (active synovitis)
3. Swelling of at least one joint (tissue and synovial fluid)
4. Swelling of at least one other joint
5. Symmetrical, simultaneous swelling of two or more joints
6. Typical subcutaneous nodules
7. Characteristic radiologic changes
8. Positive agglutination test (Latex, sheep cell agglutination test, Bentonite flocculation test—anti-immunoglobulin identification)
9. Poor mucin clot test; pathologic increase in polymorphonuclear leucocyte in synovial fluid: total protein concentration greater than 3.5 gm %.
10. Typical histologic characteristics of synovial biopsy
11. Typical histologic characteristics of subcutaneous nodule

Ratings:
1. Classical: 7 criteria present (1 to 5 must be present for at least 8 weeks)
2. Definite: 5 criteria present (1 to 5 must be present for at least 8 weeks)
3. Probable: 3 criteria present (1 to 5 must be present for 5 weeks)
4. Possible: At least two of the criteria below:
   a. morning stiffness
   b. history of observation of joint swelling
   c. recurrent arthritis (synovitis) for at least 8 weeks
   d. subcutaneous nodules
   e. increased erythrocyte sedimentation rate
   f. iritis

So nonspecific is rheumatoid arthritis that a series of exclusions has been developed. If these diagnoses or characteristics are present rheumatoid arthritis may be excluded (unless there is coexistent diseases). Each entity listed below can precisely mimic clinical rheumatoid arthritis.

Exclusions to the Diagnostic Criteria for Rheumatoid Arthritis (appended)

Exclusions to the Diagnostic Criteria for Rheumatoid Arthritis

1. Typical rash of dissiminated lupus erythematosus
2. High concentration of lupus erythematosus cells
3. Histologic evidence of polyarteritis nodosa
4. Weakness of neck, trunk and pharyngeal muscle or persistent muscle swelling of dermatomyositis
5. Definite scleroderma
6. Clinical picture characteristics of rheumatic fever
7. Clinical picture characteristic of gouty arthritis
8. Tophi
9. Clinical picture characteristic of acute infectious arthritis
10. Tubercle bacilli in the joints or histologic evidence of joint tuberculosis
11. Clinical picture characteristic of Reiter's syndrome
12. Clinical picture characteristic of shoulder-hand syndrome
13. Clinical picture characteristic of hypertrophic pulmonary osteoarthropathy
14. Clinical picture characteristic of neuroarthropathy
15. Hypothyroidism and myxedema

Table 10-1
Criteria for Diagnosis of Rheumatoid Arthritis American Rheumatism Association
(with modification) *Continued*

16. Hyperparathyroidism
17. Acromegaly
18. Erosive osteoarthritis
19. Calcium pyrophosphate dihydrate crystal deposition disease
20. Homogentisic acid in the urine detectable grossly with alkalinization
21. Histologic evidence of sarcoidosis or positive Kveim test
22. Multiple myeloma
23. Characteristic skin lesions of erythema nodosum
24. Leukemia or lymphoma
25. Agammaglobulinemia

For more specific and extensive description see Textbook of Rheumatology, Eds. Kelley, Harris, Ruddy and Sledge. W.B. Saunders Co., Philadelphia, 1981, p. 928–931

For the purpose of this chapter dealing with management, prevention, and rehabilitation of RA of the cervical spine, only cases with well established clinical, radiologic, and immunologic diagnoses are considered.

PREVALENCE OF CERVICAL SPINE INVOLVEMENT IN RHEUMATOID ARTHRITIS

In 1890 Garrod who first identified RA as a clinical entity noted that 178 of 500 patients with rheumatoid arthritis had cervical spine disease (28 percent).[8] Sharp et al found the cervical spine clinically involved in 40 percent of 44 patients.[26] Bland et al found radiologic evidence of RA of the cervical spine in 86 percent of 100 patients with classic or definite disease.[3] Conlon et al[7] also noted 88 percent of 333 patients with RA had symptoms referrable to the neck and 167 (50 percent) showed radiologic changes of RA. Bland et al[4] developed radiologic criteria for the diagnosis of RA of the cervical spine and compared the X-ray films of the cervical spine in 100 patients with definite to classic RA with 113 patients with no evidence of RA. The criteria proved very dependable and were used in the study.[4] Table 10-2 Radiologic Criteria of RA of the cervical spine.

The cervical spine is the second most common set of joints involved in RA with metatarsal phalangeal joints being the most common, the cervical spine second, and the metacarpophalangeal joints following.[1,2,26] Most patients with RA have cervical spine involvement and constitute a group of great interest to rheumatologists, physiatrists, orthopedists, and rehabilitation experts.

ETIOLOGY AND PATHOGENESIS OF RHEUMATOID ARTHRITIS OF THE CERVICAL SPINE

The mechanisms by which tissue damage occur in the cervical spine are the same as in diarthrodial joints elsewhere. Figure 10-5 is a schematic representation of etiology and pathogenesis of RA. It is presumed that antigen X initiates an immune response, either autoimmune or an environmental antigen or both, and a self perpetuating immunological series of events follows with chronic, proliferative synovitis, loss of normal structure and

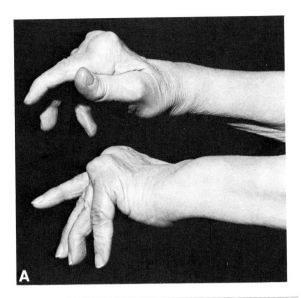

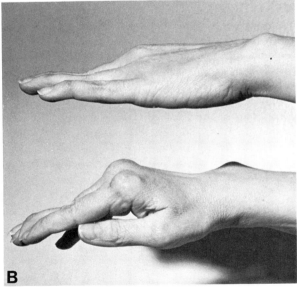

Fig. 10-1. (A) Hands of a patient with rheumatoid arthritis illustrating involvement of joints, tendons, ligaments, bursae, and periarticular connective tissue; note gross subluxation MCP and wrist joints, swollen tendon sheaths, and synovial cyst formation volar surface right hand. (B) Involvement multiple tissues in and around MCP and PIP joints. Note swan-neck deformity.

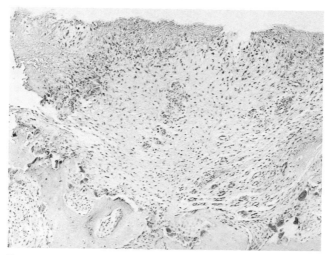

Fig. 10-2. Proliferating pannus of rheumatoid arthritis destroying bone in section taken from a Luschka joint in the cervical spine. Lower portion of section is bone with extreme proliferation of multiple cell types in the pannus.

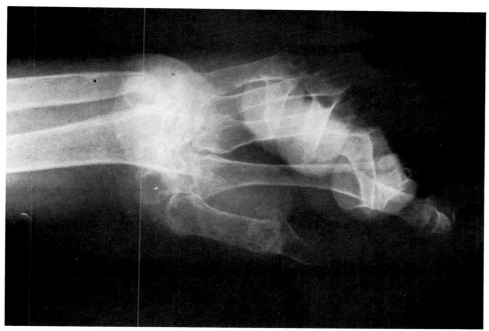

Fig. 10-3. Gross destruction of bones and joints of the wrists and MCP joints by extremely destructive pannus in rheumatoid arthritis. Subchondral bone completely destroyed followed destruction of the bony structures themselves.

239

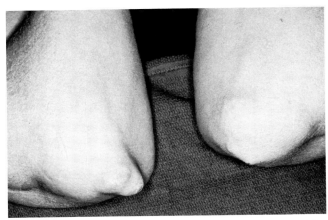

Fig. 10-4. Characteristic rheumatoid subcutaneous nodules over the olecranon processes.

function of the components of the joints, weakening and disruption of the joint capsules, ligaments and tendons, erosion of cartilage and bone, sometimes rupture of tendons and fall in the viscosity and multiple other changes in the synovial fluid. The earliest lesion in rheumatoid arthritis is a proliferation of the lining layer of the synovium in the presence of many inflammatory cells. A broad spectrum of different types of cells occupy the synovium, mainly T-lymphocytes. Polymorphonuclear leukocytes are in the joint fluid itself. A pannus forms and spreads over the surface of the articular cartilage, or on to the subchondral bone. The pannus includes both types of synovial cells, secretory and phagocytic, lymphocytes T and B, plasma cells, monocytes, other macrophages, fibroblasts and the proliferating endothelial cells of blood vessel walls, (Fig. 10-6). Both collagen and proteoglycans are degraded by lysosomal enzymes released from the many millions of polymorphonuclear cells dying each day.

In the cervical spine there are five areas that become involved in varying magnitude. These are: (1) The connective tissue structures, joints including capsules, synovium, hya-

Table 10-2
Radiologic Criteria for Diagnosis of Rheumatoid Arthritis of the Cervical Spine

1. Atlanto-axial subluxation of 2.5 mm or more
2. Multiple subluxations of C2-3, C3-4, C4-5, C5-6
3. Narrow disc spaces with little or no osteophytosis
   a. Pathognomonic at C2-3 and C3-4
   b. Probable at C4-5 and C5-6
4. Erosions of vertebrae, especially vertebral plates
5. Odontoid, small, pointed, eroded, loss of cortex
6. Basilar impression ("Platybasia")
7. Apophyseal joint erosion; blurred facets
8. Osteoporosis, generalized, cervical spine
9. Wide space (5 mm or more) between posterior arch of atlas and the spinous process of the axis (Flexion to extension)
10. Osteosclerosis, secondary, atlanto-axial-occipital complex

If five criteria or more are present, the diagnosis of rheumatoid arthritis is assured.

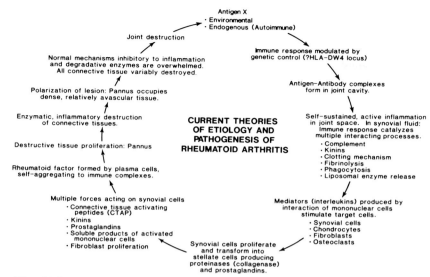

Fig. 10-5. Current Theories of Etiology and Pathogenesis of Rheumatoid Arthritis.

line cartilage, subchondral bone, ligaments, tendons and muscles—though the primary lesion begins in and dominates the synovium. (Fig. 10-7). (2) Nerve roots both within the spinal canal and as they enter the intervertebral foramina and exit to become the anterior and posterior rami. (Fig. 10-8 A and B). (3) The spinal cord, with the myelopathy of rheumatoid arthritis (Fig. 10-9). (4) The vertebral artery with the many syndromes consequent to its compression or superimposed artherosclerotic lesions complicating the rheumatoid arthritis (Fig. 10-10). (5) The esophagus—with upper cervical spine subluxation impinging on the superior pharyngeal muscles and occasionally lower down, subluxations compromise esophageal function mechanically. (Fig. 10-11).

CLINICAL CHARACTERISTICS OF CERVICAL SPINE RHEUMATOID ARTHRITIS

The clinical manifestations of RA of the cervical spine varies from no symptoms or signs to severe head, neck, occipital, temporal or retro-orbital pain, arm and leg pain, paresthesias, weakness of both upper and lower extremities, loss of or exaggeration of deep tendon reflexes, hemiparesis or quadriparesis, atrophy of peripheral muscles—Brown-Sequard syndrome, cardiac or respiratory arrest, loss of proprioception and vibratory sense as well as pain and temperature, drop attacks, and death itself. [1,3,6,10,21,26]

Pain is the most frequent symptom occurring in 52 to 63 percent of patients with radiologic evidence of RA of the cervical spine. It has a deep aching and persistent quality, perceived in the upper cervical, occipital, temporal and retroorbital regions if the pain sensitive structures are in the upper cervical spine and down the sides of the neck and over the clavicles if the pain sensitive structure is at C3–4. The scapular and deltoid region is the site of pain if the rheumatoid involvement is at C5–6, also down the arm. Cervical muscle spasm contributes to the pain. A full range of painless neck movement may be possible in association with seemingly severe radiologic and pathologic rheumatoid

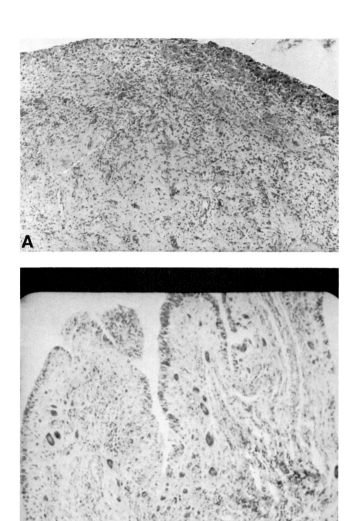

Fig. 10-6. (A) Biopsy of synovium of severe case of proliferative synovitis, note intense surface proliferation of synovial cells and plasma, macrophage and mononuclear cell infiltration of the deeper layers. (B) Close-up of synovial villus with multiple cell types infiltrating and plasma cells, mononuclear and giant cells infiltrating with production of large amounts of destructive enzymes.

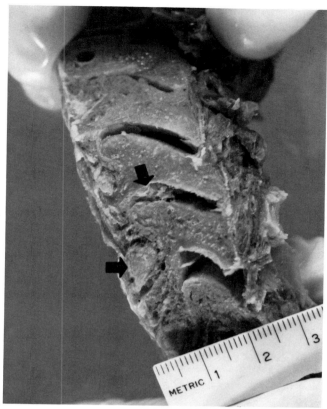

Fig. 10-7. Saggital section through whole human cervical spine. Upper arrow points to pannus spread over the hyaline cartilage surface. All joints were involved. Note the lower arrow points to the spinal nerve root in the intervertebral foramen.

changes. Tenderness of the musculature as well as weakness is common. With neck flexion a bony prominence can sometimes be seen in the suboccipital region in the midline as the atlas and the skull subluxate anteriorly as a unit. (Fig. 10-12). The prominence is the spinous process of the axis and may be reduced by pressure posteriorly on the forehead while pressing with the thumb on the spinous process of the axis. A posterior sliding motion of the head and atlas en bloc occurs in relation to the axis. With grossly abnormal and sudden cervical movement, severe lancinating pain, unresponsive to analgesics or corticosteroids may be precipitated. The head may be rotated and tilted sideways, sometimes permanently because of asymmetric slipping of the eroded atlanto-occipital or atlanto-axial facets and bony destruction of the lateral masses of the atlas and the axis. Normal occipito cervical lordosis may be lost with the head carried in a peculiar forward position.

Crepitus or a "clunking" on flexion or lateral flexion is common with gross subluxations of the atlas with stretching and traction on it and on the axis. The greater occipital nerve, C2, may give rise to severe occipital neuralgia. Weakness of the neck muscles and "heaviness" of the head occur with inability to hold the head up or raise the chin from the chest, arm and leg weakness with atrophy of the intrinsic muscles of the hand, pyramidal

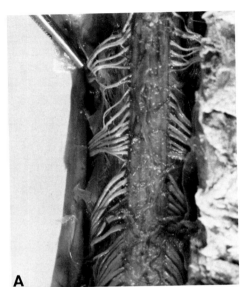
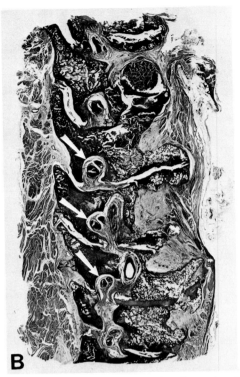

Fig. 10-8.   (A) Posterior view cervical spinal cord showing posterior rootlets entering the cord and going forward to join the anterior motor rootlets and roots to enter the dural root sleeves and the intervertebral foramina. Here they are in close relationship to the zygapophyseal and Luschka joints and may be involved in the inflammatory process with consequent clincal signs of a radiculopathy. (B) A saggital histologic section of 5 levels in the cervical spine showing (white arrows) intervertebral foramina containing the anterior and posterior roots. Note the close apposition to the zygapophyseal and Luschka joints.

signs usually appear late. Vertigo, nystagmus, loss of consciousness, quadriplegia, and transient blindness (intermittent compression and obstruction of the vertebral arteries), anterior spinal arteries may be stretched, compressed, or thrombosed with anterior horn cell damage and upper motor neuron syndromes. Drop attacks without loss of consciousness occur if proprioceptive pathways from the limbs to the cerebellum are compressed resulting in abrupt loss of skeletal muscle tone. Severe subluxation of atlas on axis may compress the respiratory center in the medulla or result in other symptoms of medullary compression, quadriplegia, and Brown-Sequard syndrome.

The time of onset in the course of RA of atlas-axis subluxation is difficult to determine but has been reported as early as 2 weeks to as late as 13 years after the onset. [15,22]

Chronic myelopathy, due to intermittent or chronic spinal cord compression causes, first, hyper-reflexia and ultimately loss of deep tendon reflexes and extensive or localized muscle atrophy, frequently attributed to the primary disease. Common presenting features include paresthesias and other sensory disturbances, diminished or absent vibration sense, flexor spasms, urinary retention or other bladder disturbances, absent superficial abdominal and cremasteric reflexes, and difficulty with walking due to spastic weakness of the legs. Such may appear only during neck flexion—or extension or perhaps during a sneeze

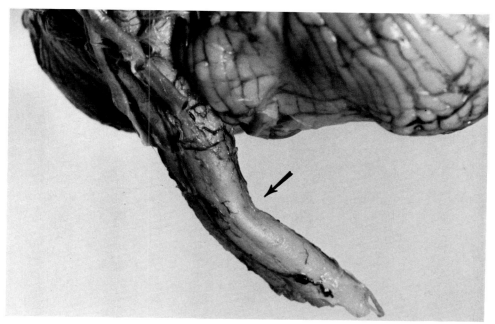

Fig. 10-9.   Brain and upper spinal cord with rheumatoid arthritis, atlanto-axial subluxation with chronic cord compression. Note the notch in the spinal cord.

or cough. Paresthesias first felt in the distal portions of the limbs localized to one hand or one whole extremity may later be felt over the trunk. Positive Babinski sign and ankle clonus are common.

Neurologic manifestations begin insidiously and may regress and reappear over months. In many patients their significance is undetected and unsuspected until a rapidly changing neurologic picture occurs—or death comes abruptly due to medullary compres-

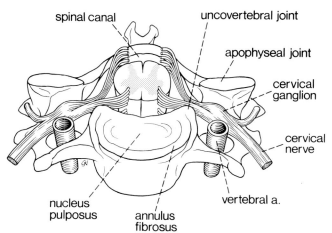

Fig. 10-10.   Drawing showing close anatomical relationship between the vertebral artery, the Luschka (uncovertebral) and zygapophyseal joints and the intervertebral foramen. Rheumatoid pannus can involve the anterior and posterior roots, the ganglion or the vertebral artery.

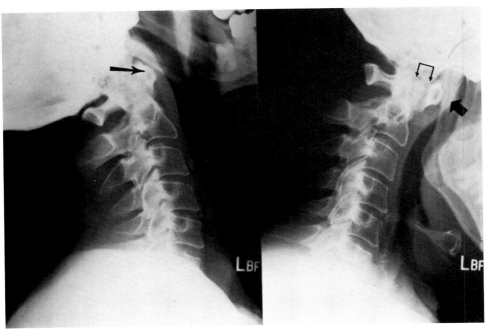

Fig. 10-11. Left: Radiograph of the cervical spine in extension in a patient with rheumatoid arthritis. The arrow points to the anterior arch of the atlas, only a few mm from the pharynx and upper esophagus. Right: The spine in flexion with an 11 mm atlas axis subluxation and a gross bulge into the pharynx. Note the change from extension to flexion with compression and bulging of the pharynx. The large arrow points to the bulging pharynx; the small arrow points to the space between the odontoid and the anterior arch of the atlas. Note the shadow of the pharynx above, the esophagus below. Subluxation may cause dysphagia.

sion. Neurologic changes are often reversible with early diagnosis and appropriate treatment. It is thus important that these expressions of cervical spine disease be sought.

Vertical subluxation (pseudobasilar impression) may occur into the foramen magnum following extensive erosive changes in the odontoid, the bone of the foramen magnum, or severe osteoporosis. Bone absorption in the basilar processes of the skull and occipital condyles can occur. Odontoid erosion, absorption or fracture with separation of the body of the axis is occasionally seen (Fig.10-13).

THE CERVICAL SPINE COMPONENT OF THE OVERALL REHABILITATIVE MANAGEMENT OF RHEUMATOID ARTHRITIS

Primarily it is of the utmost importance to carry out a total program of management of RA, systematically assessing the magnitude and duration of disease, systemic manifestations (weakness, fatigue, depression, insomnia) and general attitude toward themselves, family, and their medical attendants. It is necessary to assess personality structure and the patient's ability and willingness to participate in an overall program (including the cervical spine), attention to each joint involved and a clinical judgement of the possibility of arresting, reversing, or increasing functional capability. The American Rheumatism Asso-

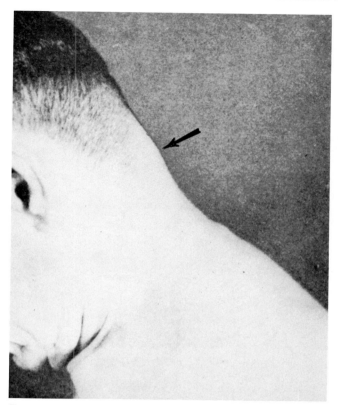

Fig. 10-12. Note the prominence on the posterior neck (arrow). It is the underlying spinous process of the axis, brought out by the atlas and skull subluxation forward as a unit. (Reproduced by kind permission of Dr. Harold S. Robinson, Vancouver.)

ciation functional criteria are useful in these initial assessments. You should review activities of daily living, capability of eating, dressing, overall hand activities, personal hygiene, brushing teeth, combing hair, shaving, toileting. The degree of mobility should be reviewed; getting off and on a toilet, getting in and out of a chair, driving a car, walking inside and outside the home, and climbing stairs. A consideration of various household activities such as gardening, cooking, cleaning, laundry, shopping—also the ability to continue working at their occupation—assess how tired the patient is after so many hours or a full days activity. All of these should be given some quantitative assessment. Table 10-3 lists the functional criteria of the American Rheumatism Association.[28] There are a number of indicators of a poor prognosis that aid in overall current assessment and predictive planning (Table 10-4).

A review of the past history of what management has been, ie, physician, duration of relationship with the physician, occupational and physical therapists, physiatrists, orthopedic and neurologic consultation, any use of splints, canes, crutches, collars, braces, wheelchairs, and walkers. The management and rehabilitation of the cervical spine should never be initiated to the exclusion of overall management of the disease, rheumatoid arthritis.

The sophisticated use of rest and exercise, much more of the former in active and

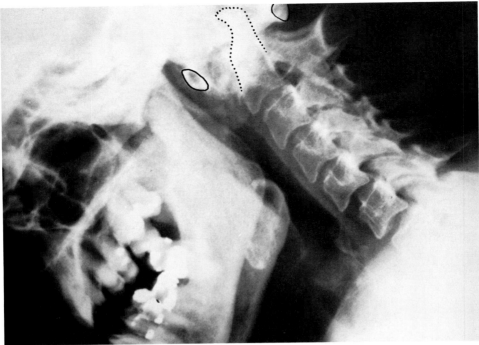

Fig. 10-13. Lateral view cervical spine with severe anterior and vertical subluxation of atlas-axis odontoid complex (superior migration of the odontoid) and the odontoid process is in the foramen magnum resulting in spinal cord compression and myelopathy. The dotted line outlines the severely eroded and partially destroyed odontoid process. The solid lines outline the anterior and posterior arches of the atas. Note the anterior space is much larger than the posterior space, leaving little room for the spinal cord at its junction with the medulla oblongata.

acute inflammation, and more of the latter as the disease process tends to diminish. Drugs are aimed at controlling the inflammatory process or suppressing the exuberant and ultimately damaging immunologic storm.

There is general medical misconception that all neck pain occurs from neural compression. Any pain-causing disease or condition affecting peripheral joints and the musculoskeletal system generally may and often does involve the cervical spine resulting in pain. Pain in the neck, chest, shoulder, arm, and hand may be caused by direct compression of

Table 10-3
Functional Criteria of the American Rheumatism Association

Class I	Complete Able to carry on all usual duties without handicaps
Class II	Adequate for normal activities, despite handicap of discomfort or limited motion of one or more joints
Class III	Limited Can perform little or none of duties of usual occupation or self care
Class IV	Largely or wholly incapacitated Bedridden or confined to a wheelchair; little or no self care

Table 10-4

Indicators of a Poor Prognosis in Rheumatoid Arthritis

1. Being female
2. Insidious onset
3. Symmetrical disease
4. Initial marked rheumatoid activity that persists
5. Early multiple joint effusions
6. Early constitutional symptoms.
7. Early appearance of subcutaneous nodules
8. Extraarticular manifestations, especially vasculitis
9. Early appearance of x-ray erosions in joints
10. Early high titer rheumatoid factor
11. Prolonged interval between onset of disease and final medical evaluations

cervical nerve roots or their peripheral nerves, spinal cord compression, central spinal cord disease (syringomyelia), osteoarthritis, intervertebral disc disease, primary or secondary bone, muscle, ligament, tendon or joint capsule lesions and instability, or abnormal and excessive cervical spine mobility. The radiation of pain involves dermatome, myotome, and sclerotome distribution, a clinical point often unappreciated. In general, pain arising from deep somatic nerve endings in bone, joint, ligament, or capsule results in inner scapular pain, aching in arm and forearm and associated with generalized paresthesias of the hand.

An early sign of neural compression is pain (before paresthesia), regarded as ischemic in etiology as intrinsic blood supply to nerve roots and cord is blocked before axoplasmic flow and physiologic nerve function ceases. Patients are often very tender to pressure over the cervical vertebral spinous process of the segment or segments causing the pain. Nonoperative management serves in most uncomplicated cases, ie, soft or rigid collar, intermittent immobilization, specific exercises, cervical pillows, nonsteroidal antiinflammatory drugs, muscle relaxants, and analgesics selectively and judiciously used.

A good general formulation is as follows: (1) No clinical problems: patient able to perform all usual activities without handicaps—should be managed with overall management of RA. (2) Mild without disability: a program in prevention of cervical spine disease in as far as this can be accomplished. (3) Moderate RA with disability: prevention and active rehabilitative methods and techniques applied maximally. (4) Severe with major disability: including nerve root involvement, muscle weakness, myelopathy, atlanto-axial subluxation, and subaxial subluxations. See below.

SYSTEMATIC APPROACH TO MANAGEMENT OF RHEUMATOID ARTHRITIS OF THE CERVICAL SPINE

Rehabilitation treatment programs are in sharp contrast to standard medical care in which the physician concentrates on curing the patient's anatomic and pathologic changes and assumes function will spontaneously return. The patient is left alone to cope with residual changes. The basic difference in curative and rehabilitative medicine is in the direction of effort. Rehabilitation medicine utilizes a broad spectrum of treatment and management designed to minimize the consequence of permanent or protracted disability. The ideal is to have both approaches going forward in tandem in so far as is reasonable and possible, integrating curative with rehabilitative methods, simultaneous attention to the pathology and to function. There is a continuum of gradually shifting emphasis on control of pathology to restoration of function. The overall management rehabilitative job is to maintain and restore function, prevent contractures, increase muscle strength, stimulate latent control, train the patient to use residual function to a maximum, learn proper use of assistive devices and guide and educate both the patient and the family.

Rest

Localized rest, immobilization of joints, as well as overall global rest can and will reduce the magnitude of the inflammatory process in rheumatoid arthritis.[14,20] Immobilization of rheumatoid joints for as much as four weeks will reduce inflammation without loss of joint mobility, taking great care to take them out of casts or splints twice daily for range of motion exercises, active if possible, passive at least. Strength is compromised, however.[9,11,18,20] Delay of strengthening exercises are necessary until the inflammatory process is suppressed and controlled, an achievable goal in the hands of a physician informed in etiology and pathogenesis of the disease. A specific problem in the cervical spine is that true immobilization of the upper cervical spine (C1-2-3), where it is most needed, is very difficult to achieve.

Mechanical stress damages joints that are inflamed and have ligamentous laxity. Rest position in bed should include use of specific cervical pillows to allow the cervical spine, ie, Wal-Pil-O or Cervi-Pillo, a tubular shaped contour pillow. These pillows aid greatly in promoting sleep and maintaining optimum posture during rest by supporting the neck in a supine position and the head in the side-lying position.

Education of the patient in relaxation techniques is of great importance to the patient with rheumatoid arthritis. Stretching exercises cannot be optimally carried out unless the patient can attain muscular relaxation. One to 3 20-minute periods daily of muscular relaxation practice are recommended, not only to relieve the pain of continuous and sustained muscle spasm but because relaxation allows metabolic and biochemical recovery of physiologic muscle function.

Exercise

Exercise can be categorized as active, passive, against resistance, assisted active exercise, strengthening exercises, isometric, isotonic, and isokinetic exercises. In rehabilitation, exercise management is prescribed to achieve specific treatment goals, eg, maintain or increase joint mobility or increase strength—always attempting to improve function. The rationale for all therapeutic exercise is to restore as much as possible the physiologic characteristics of the tissues involved, minimizing the constraints of the disease and avoiding complications of immobilization. Total immobilization is virtually never indicated.

Stretching exercises are to prevent contracture or augment range of motion after contracture has occurred. Exercise will not reverse weakened and lax ligaments. One uses exercises in this instance to maintain a poor status quo.

Contractures occur in any immobilized tissue, particularly about the joints. Joint capsules and ligaments as well as synovium develop fibrotic reactions and over produce collagen. Each joint capsule is different than all others in the physiologic lightness or looseness and the specific weave of the collagen fibers, ie, molecular randomness, linear array, varying degrees of structural characteristics. This is as true in the neck as it is elsewhere. Capsules, muscles, tendons, and ligaments undergo adaptive shortening with immobilization even with active inflammation in process. Connective tissue degradation goes on and remodeling is accelerated during active inflammation. One must avoid excessive stretching during active inflammation. Collagen is more susceptible to collagenase enzyme action when stretched or over-heated.

Stretching exercises should be within the constraints of pain, should not be performed if they produce pain that lasts more than two hours, should be sufficient to maintain joint mobility for that day, and are best performed when the stiffness is least, ie, not in the early morning.

Strengthening Exercises

The histologic characteristics of muscle, mitochondrial size and number, rate of contractile protein synthesis, enzyme production, strength, and endurance are clearly induced by conditioning stresses, ie, customary daily activity or prescribed exercise. It has been shown in normal humans that one daily brief maximal isometric contraction for 10 seconds will stimulate an increase in static muscle strength.[18] The advantage of this brief nonfatiguing exercise for a patient who has chronic areas of inflammation all over their body is that their muscles are not weakened by the inflammatory process and can maintain or even gain in static strength. Thus, such activities of daily living as combing the hair, dressing, eating, light housekeeping and walking are exercise. Fatigue occurs much more promptly in repetitive tasks requiring more than 20 percent of the available static strength. The movements of the cervical spine in activities of daily living should be carried out with a "business as usual" point of view.

Active Gravity Assisted Exercises for the Neck (Fig. 10-14)

A useful cervical spine stretching technique is to ask the patient to let his neck flex passively on the chest so that the chin approaches the chest, then roll one ear to a shoulder, and then the occiput rolls backward and the chin rolls to the opposite shoulder and back again to the chest. This exercise is done with the whole neck and torso as relaxed as it can be. The patient who has subluxation of atlas and axis should do this only with caution—such a patient should be standing and warned that it may cause vertigo.

A passive exercise done by the therapist is to support both sides of the patient's head while the patient contracts muscles on the painful side by attempting to push the head against the therapist's hand as forcefully as possible, ie, isometric contraction held for 5–10 seconds—then relaxed. During the relaxation the head is rotated or further flexed as permitted by muscle relaxation. Such can be repeated daily or twice daily and the patient may be taught to use this technique independently similar to manually resisted cervical isometric exercises. The patient may carry out this exercise using his or her own hand as illustrated in Figure 10-15.

Cervical isometric exercises should always be used if patients are wearing a brace or collar, systematically done, and regarded as having great importance. Weakness due to immobilization is inevitable if the patient must wear a collar much or most of the time. Manual resistance with palm pressure for 10 seconds against the forehead, the occiput and each temporal area is a simple twice daily exercise regimen.[12] Figure 10-16A and B illustrate respectively extension and rotation of the neck against resistance.

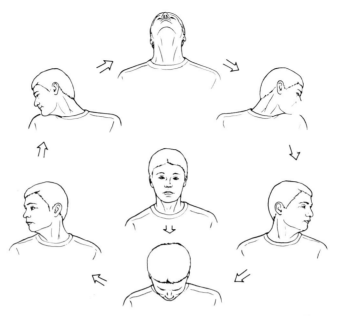

Fig. 10-14. Active gravity assisted exercises for the neck (Please see text).

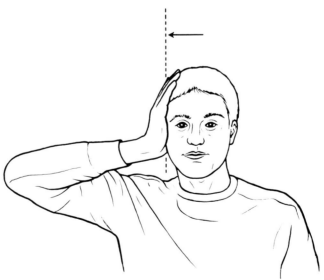

Fig. 10-15. Patient laterally flexing the neck against resistance that she exerts.

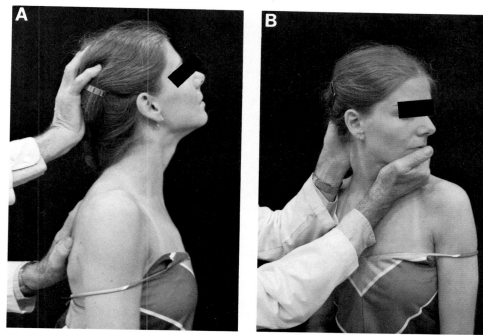

Fig. 10-16. (A) Isometric extension of cervical spine against resistance. (B) Isometric rotation of cervical spine against resistance.

Drug Therapy

By and large drug therapy is regarded as constituting only 10–20 percent of the total management program for rheumatoid arthritis. Nevertheless, well selected anti-inflammatory medication is important in rheumatoid arthritis, an immunologic, probably infectious, inflammatory disease. The spectrum of nonsteroidal anti-inflammatory agents grows apace. My position is that aspirin remains the drug of choice administered in full dosage and is the most effective single drug for relief and control of inflammation, pain, and stiffness. There are no perfect drugs and each patient requires clinical survey regarding past experience with aspirin, allergic diathesis, personal belief in the drug, and the well known contraindication to its use.

Aspirin being the drug of choice in my view, I prescribe it using a special method. A printed flier is supplied to educate the patient in pharmacologic mechanism of action, desirable and undesirable effects and how to avoid the latter, recognition of overdose by noting tinnitus and deafness, and the technique of getting and maintaining maximum anti-inflammatory effect on a continuing basis. This is done by giving the aspirin, in a sense, as food. Take 3–4 tablets in the middle of a meal; that is, eat half the breakfast, take the aspirin, and then finish breakfast. The same method is repeated with the other meals providing an average ingestion total of 10–14 tablets per day. The patient is asked to crush or chew the aspirin in order to accelerate absorption and is taught to take the drug until tinnitus occurs. Then, he or she stops the drug completely and allows 3–4 days to pass, making certain the tinnitus disappears, thus assuring that the tinnitus was caused by the aspirin. Then aspirin therapy with a dose, one tablet lower than the previous dose, is restarted. Aspirin therapy need not be continued forever. If the patient becomes asymptomatic and functional, it is recommended that he or she continue to take aspirin for 3–4 months after a satisfactory clinical state has been reached, and then stop. From that time on, the patient must maintain the program of rest, exercise, activity, and intermittent use of drugs if need be.

There is always a place for other anti-inflammatory drugs at the discretion and clinical judgement of the clinician. Gold, penicillamine, methotrexate, and the cytotoxic immunosuppressive agents all have their indications and their advocates. Corticosteroids continue to have a place in drug therapy but require very sophisticated, knowledgeable judgement in their use. There is no role for intra-articular corticosteroids in cervical spine rheumatoid arthritis.

Posture and Gait

Maintenance of normal posture and body biomechanics are essential in the prevention of damage in cervical spine rheumatoid arthritis. The patient should be taught proper postures, standing, walking, sitting, and the spread of work postures specific for him. The maintenance of skeletal alignment minimizes joint, muscle, and ligamentous stresses, preserving maximum mobility and function. Optimum posture and body alignment is achieved when the center of gravity is in the center of the body axis. Simply said, a plumb line from the level of the external auditory meatus level (centering on the skull) should transect the lateral tip of the acromion, the greater trochanter of the femur and the midpoint of the lateral aspect of the knee reaching the lateral malleolus or just in front of it. Normal posture implies cervical lordosis, thoracic kyphosis, lumbar lordosis, and sacral kyphosis. The pelvis tips posteriorly enough to minimize the lumbar lordotic curve. Normally one should be able to stand with heels 3–4 inches from the wall and rotate the pelvis (pelvic tilt) so that the occiput, dorsal, and lumbar spine and buttocks are all touching the wall. With the head centered and shoulders level, there should be no gross knock knee or bow leg of the knees (or varus or valgus of the foot) the patient should ideally be able to approximate the medial femoral condyles of the knees and the medial malleolae when standing. With the center of gravity in the midline the least stress and hence minimal muscular effort is demanded to maintain a standing posture.

Optimum sitting posture is a function of what the person is doing seated. The central consideration is that during all seated activities, alignment of the spine is such as to minimize musculoskeletal stress, ie, a straight back chair may be too straight, and not allow room posteriorly for buttock protrusion, secretarial chairs may have the lumbar pad too high or too low accentuating lumbar lordosis, or a soft chair or stuffed soft piece of furniture may necessitate extension of the legs creating abnormal posterior tilting of the pelvis and strain from hamstring muscle tension.

Other considerations are neck position, shoulder and elbow angles to perform work, the lighting, the desk height, and the degree of muscle stress on the neck and back necessary to maintain visual work. The posture lying down is equally important. Avoid a soft yielding mattress, use special therapeutic pillows, do not sit semi-propped in bed with the dorsal spine rounded and the neck hyperflexed with flexed hip and knee. Remember in the rheumatoid arthritis patient with multiple active synovitis in many joints a loss of mobility in one joint results in increased stress in other joints necessary to compensate for the lost motion, clearly true in the cervical spine.

Attention to gait is an important part of rehabilitation. Normal gait is efficient, heel to toe, energy conserving, and maintains strength and power. Postural deformities, weakness, joint disease, ligamentous laxity, and subluxation result in awkward, inefficient gait patterns, causing increased strains on connective tissue structures in and about joints. Proper gait training, ie, as near normal gait as possible, the use of properly fitted canes, crutches, walkers, and braces to minimize the stress may allow the patient to continue to maintain his cervical spine in a normal posture. A necessity to efficient gait is normal joint motion and absence of contractures. Maintenance of normal motion in the cervical spine prevents pathologic alterations of gait with joint and ligamentous stress with consequent compensation by articular and periarticular structures. Attention to shoes, correction of leg length discrepancies, bracing and splinting, and general gait training are important applications.

Collars and Braces for the Neck

The most severe and compromising characteristic of rheumatoid arthritis of the cervical spine is the progressive ligamentous laxity, subluxations at the atlas-axis level, subaxial subluxations, and vertical subluxations into the foramen magnum. A subluxation of more than 5–6mm at the atlas axis junction is regarded as pathologic instability; more than 8mm is potentially dangerous. Between C2 and C7 a subluxation anteriorly of more than 3.5mm of one or more vertebrae on another is defined as unstable. Any similar translatory displacement of vertebral bodies or angulation between vertebrae of more than 11 degrees (compared to adjacent disc interspaces) is, by definition, unstable. Soft collars though they are quite comfortable, can be used night and day but play no role in immobilizing the cervical spine. Immobilization of the upper cervical spine may be necessary to avoid neural damage to both nerve roots and the spinal cord. It is likely that the ordinary hard, plastic submandibular collar is effective in regulating the degree of movement, at least early in upper cervical spine RA. The plastic collar restricts motion by 50 percent. The plastic collar/brace, occipito-mental-sternal (Philadelphia collar) is comfortable and it does restrict motion by 75 percent but is often irritating to the skin. A four poster brace is quite good in immobilization, particularly in the lower cervical spine while the long two poster cervical brace is better for the upper cervical spine. The only brace that restricts motion almost completely is the halo, resulting in only 5 percent or less of residual motion when it is in place. Figure 10-17 illustrates the spectrum of available collar types. Real immobilization of the occiput-atlas axis complex is only achieved with the plastic collar brace (Philadelphia collar), one of the poster type, the Halo, or the Minerva.

In one study of 130 patients with rheumatoid arthritis of the cervical spine and subluxation, no measureable effect occurred in arresting the progress of subluxation from the wearing of cervical collars.[27] Sound scientific evidence that cervical collars and bracing favorably influences the natural course of C1–C2 subluxations in RA is lacking. Many patients with RA have a reduction in pain, by wearing the hard plastic collar or semirigid Philadelphia collar, particularly during any exacerbation of the disease. The latter provides some soft tissue support. Collars may provide real protection against potentially severe damage to the spinal cord, or even death on flexion-extension injury or fall. During travel, whether driving or being driven, the collar should be worn at all times. Therapeutic pillows also provide a measure of cervical support and support the neck in the supine position and the head in the side lying position minimizing flexion or extension of the neck in supine or prone position.

The following recommendations are made for collar prescription: (1) In the absence of any neurologic signs or symptoms, past or present, for management of cervical, occipital, head, shoulder and arm pain, both night and day as needed, the soft collar, plastic

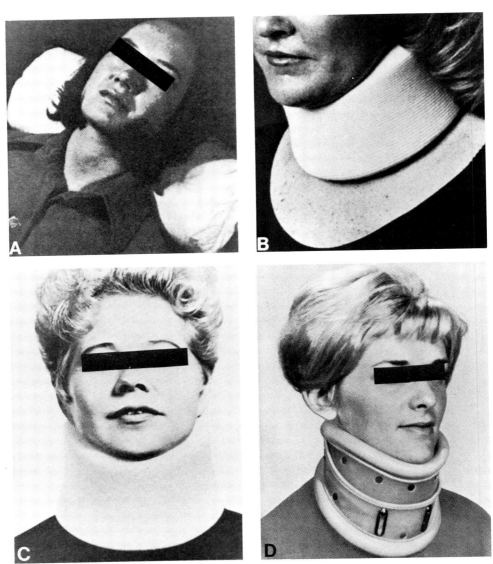

Fig. 10-17. The spectrum of available collars and braces for the cervical spine in rheumatoid arthritis. (A) Cervical pillow, (B) Low cut soft collar, (C) High cut soft collar, (D) Firm hard plastic, sumandibular collar, completely adjustable, (E) Philadelphia collar-plastizote, (F) Rigid four poster brace (Tangential view) (Reproduced with permission of Pel Supply Company, Cleveland, Ohio and LO-CAL, CAMP AOA, Spencer Medical and Bell-Horn manufacturers of prosthetic, orthotic and medical supplies.), (G) Rigid four poster brace (side view) (Reproduced with permission of Pel Supply Company, Cleveland, Ohio and LO-CAL, CAMP AOA, Spencer Medical and Bell-Horn manufacturers of prosthetic, orthotic and medical supplies.), (H) Rigid four poster brace (back view) (Reproduced with permission of Pel Supply Company, Cleveland, Ohio and LO-CAL, CAMP AOA, Spencer Medical and Bell-Horn manufacturers of prosthetic, orthotic and medical supplies).

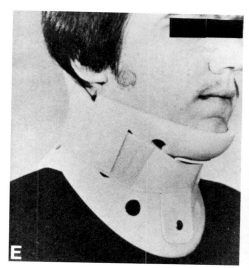

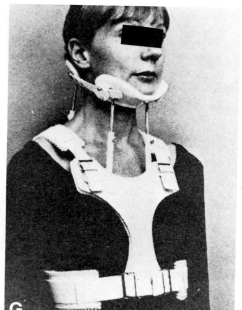

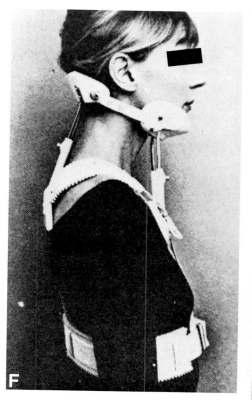

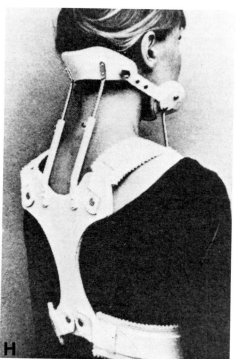

submandibular collar or the plastic Philadelphia collar brace. (2) For atlanto axial and subaxial clinical and radiologic instability (atlanto axial subluxation greater then 5mm) and neurological symptoms and/or signs, the long two poster, plastic Philadelphia collar, brace or the four poster brace. (3) For atlanto axial, subaxial instability and vertical subluxation into the foramen magnum, with greater than 8mm atlanto axial subluxation (threat of catastrophic neurologic event) use halo fixation or long two poster. (4) For mid cervical (subaxial) instability with severe pain and non-life threatening neurologic symptoms and/or signs, (shoulder and arm and hand symptoms and signs) use long two poster, plastic Philadelphia collar brace or the four poster. (5) For low cervical spine severe pain and instability with moderate neurological signs (shoulder, scapula, arm and hand) use four poster, long two poster, or plastic Philadelphia collar brace.

Surgical Intervention

The rheumatoid lesions of the cervical spine tend to stabilize under conditions of optimum management.[27] The real natural history of RA of the cervical spine is not yet completely defined. One must observe untreated patients in order to ever learn the true natural history. Rheumatoid arthritis may become arrested for reasons we do not understand; it is not necessarily a progressive disease. X-ray evidence progresses to a greater degree than does neural involvement, which is the usual reason for surgical intervention. Eighty one percent of 106 patients had radiographic deterioration but only 36 percent had progressive neural abnormality.[21] Pellicci et al[21] recommend the following indications for operation: (1) intractable pain associated with progressive neural deterioration, (2) Progression of neural dysfunction in the presence of known subaxial subluxation or superior migration of pre-existing atlanto-axial subluxation, (3) Rapid progression of neural dysfunction over weeks to months. At the most only 10 percent of patients with radiographic evidence of disease progression reach a point at which surgery must be considered. A cautionary point—10 percent of patients who have a posterior surgical arthrodesis of the cervical spine—still deteriorate neurologically.[24]

Meijers et al[17] recommends surgical intervention at the appearance of "alarm signals" that appear and rapidly worsen. These are: (1) severe neck pain, often radiating to the occiput, (2) disturbed bladder function, varying from incontinence to urinary retention, (3) diminished motor power in arms and legs, (4) jumping legs, as a consequence of spinal automatism, (5) tingling and paresthesias of fingers and feet or just numbness (dysesthesia), and (6) "marble sensation" (heaviness in the limbs and trunk), a sense of disturbance of deep sensibility. In general most patients do not manifest these symptoms until the neurological lesion is rapidly progressing requiring prompt surgical management.

There is no relationship between the degree of subluxation and the neurological signs. We stress the importance of distinguishing between subluxations that remain fixed on flexion-extension views, rarely leading to neurological deficits and the more common, quite mobile subluxations that are more likely to do so.[16,23]

My experience leads me to justify a policy of conservatism in management. A very difficult problem is that of severe, vertebral instability by X-ray with little or no associated pain and no neurological abnormalities. In such cases I urge and provide an adequate stiff collar with advice to wear it constantly—and within the constraints of the collar to move and conduct ones life in a "business as usual" way—this seems to stabilize and even encourage ankylosis of unstable segments and the risks are few if the collar is continually worn, exercises are done daily, and the patient is well educated in the nature of the lesion and its rehabilitation. It is difficult to get compliance in wearing a cumbersome and awkward collar continuously for a long period. Among those who have, I have observed stabilization of initially mobile displacements, but never under a period of six months.

I regard this plan as the best in the mobile atlanto-axial subluxations in which the odontoid process is projecting above the foramen magnum with the object of protecting from sudden medullary death. In any patient with RA it is extremely important to know the status of the cervical spine, since apart from any specific treatment for the cervical arthritis it has an important bearing on the patients general management.

Elective or routine surgical stabilization with arthrodesis (prophylactic) even with radiographic or neural evidence of disease is not indicated. The person with radiographic subluxation and no neural dysfunction should understand the potential seriousness of the problem. Occasionally patients themselves in full discussion may elect to proceed with the surgery rather than risk neural deterioration. A firm cervical plastic collar or Philadelphia collar is needed—depending again clinically on the magnitude of pain and the degree of compliance. Such people should be examined about each 2–3 months with established criteria for assessment of stability or advance of the disease process. Conservatism is the best basic approach to the problem but should not be substituted by complacency. Constant consideration of the potential problems must be maintained with vigilance in follow-up observation.

Traction

Traction is seldom effective in RA. Because the disease is characterized by so much ligamentous laxity it would be indicated only under very unusual circumstance. If there is progressive neurologic dysfunction gentle traction may be used to determine whether favorable neurologic changes will follow. This use has merit and is recommended. Optimum traction, on the other hand, in cervical osteoarthritis is usually effective.

Heat

Superficial heating supplies symptomatic relief. Moist heat is a most effective way of relieving continuous and sustained muscle spasm. Such means as infrared lamps, ordinary light bulbs, heating pads, hot packs, hot water, and electric blankets are all symptomatically useful. The threshold for pain is surely raised in man and other animals by the use of superficial or deep heating. Hot tub baths or showers are symptomatically useful.

Cold

Instinctively patients with rheumatoid arthritis avoid cold applications. Nevertheless very acute inflammation is effectively managed by cold compresses, ice packs, or ice massage. It has relatively little application in the cervical spine since the structures involved are too deep below the surface to be influenced by cold.

Diathermy (Heating Through)

Diathermy occurs by short-wave, microwave, or ultrasound. It has been shown to affect the viscoelastic properties of collagen and alter the creep (plastic stretch) of ligamentous structures placed under tension.[13] Though microwave and ultrasound bring heat to structures well below the surface, I know of no real evidence of its efficacy in the management of rheumatoid arthritis of the cervical spine.

Massage and Manipulation

Massage induces muscle relaxation of skeletal muscles when they are in continuous and sustained spasm. It may have a place in cervical spine RA. I know of no evidence for effectiveness of manipulation of the cervical spine in RA. Much more damage than good is likely to be done. Chiropractic teaching is that all illnesses of man are a consequence of spinal subluxations, cured by spinal adjustments, all unsubstantiated by scientific evidence. In very skilled hands manipulation may be useful in cervical osteoarthritis; I see no place for it in RA.

Transcutaneous Nerve Stimulation Operant Conditioning, Biofeedback, Electrical Stimulation, Acupuncture, and Vapo-coolant Sprays

Intractable pain in the cervical spine may be improved by these techniques. I have had occasional good experiences in clinical problem solving using operant conditioning, biofeedback techniques, acupuncture, electrical stimulation or vapo-coolant sprays but predictability is lacking. Fluori-methane is a vapo-coolant now preferred over the flammable ethyl chloride. This has been effective in pain relief in the cervical spine—again without predictability.

Local Anesthetic Injections for Focal Muscle Pain

Local anesthetic injection is only occasionally useful, particularly about the sternocleidomastoid muscle and the trapezius in cervical spine rheumatoid arthritis.

SUMMARY

Though the majority of patients with established and secure diagnosis of RA have cervical spine involvement many remain asymptomatic, requiring only the optimum management of the overall disease process. Because atlanto-axial subluxation may be present and produce no symptoms, all patients who have active and definite RA should have cervical spine X-ray films. Collar immobilization in varying degree may have a favorable effect on the increasing degree of subluxation, and an estimated 8–10 percent may require decision making regarding surgical intervention. The program in management and rehabilitation of cervical spine RA include extensive patient education, active and passive exercises, strengthening isometric exercises, and exercises against resistance as well as stretching exercises. Prescribed rest, hydrotherapy, collar immobilization with a stiff plastic collar, special pillows, postural and gait training, and application of the physical therapeutic modalities, heat, sometimes cold, massage, and sometimes biofeedback, electrical stimulation, TENS, and education in relaxation.

REFERENCES

1. Bland JH: Rheumatoid arthritis of the cervical spine. J Rheum 1:391–342, 1974
2. Bland JH, Brown EW: Seronegative and seropositive rheumatoid arthritis, clinical, radiologic and biochemical differences. Ann Intern Med 60:88–94, 1964
3. Bland JH, Davis PH, London MG, et al: Rheumatoid arthritis of the cervical spine. Arch Intern Med 112:892–898, 1963
4. Bland JH, VanBuskirk FW, Tampas JP, et al: A study of roentgenologic criteria for rheumatoid arthritis of the cervical spine. Am J Roentgenol Radium Ther Nucl Med 95:949–954, 1965
5. Brown JW, Sones DA: The onset of RA in the Aged. J Am Ger Soc 15:873–881, 1967
6. Christophides N, Huskisson EC: Misleading symptoms and signs of cervical spine subluxation in rheumatoid arthritis. Brit Med J 185:364–365, 1982
7. Conlon PW, Isdale IC, Rose BS, et al: Rheumatoid arthritis of the cervical spine. Ann Rheum Dis 25:120–126, 1966
8. Garrod AE: A treatise on rheumatism and rheumatoid arthritis. London, C. Griffin and Company, 1980
9. Gault SJ, Spyker JM: Beneficial effect of immobilization of joints in rheumatoid and related arthritides: A splint study using sequentia analysis. Arth Rheum 12:34–44, 1969
10. Halla JT, Fallaki S, Hardin JG: Nonreducible rotational head tilt and lateral mass collapse. Arth Rheum 15:1316–1324, 1982
11. Harris R, Capp EP: Immobilization of the knee joint in RA. Ann Rheum Dis 21:353–359, 1962
12. Kendall PH: Exercise for Arthritis, in Licht S (ed): Therapeutic exercise. 2nd edition. New Haven, E. Lichts, 1965, pp. 707
13. Leahmann JF, Warren CG, Sham SM: Therapeutic heat and cold. Clinical Orthopedics and Related Research 99:207–245, 1974
14. Lee P, Kennedy A, Anderson J, et al: Benefits of Hospitalization in RA. Quart J Med 43:205–214, 1974
15. Margulies ME, Katz I, Rosenberg M: Spontaneous dislocation of the atlanto-axial joint in rheumatoid spondylitis; recovery from quadriplegia following cervical decompression. Neurol (Minn) 5:290–294, 1955
16. Marks JS, Sharp J: Rheumatoid cervical myelopathy. Quart J Med 199:307–319, 1981
17. Meijers KAE, Van Beusekom GTH, Luyendijk W, et al. Dislocation of the cervical spine with cord compression in rheumatoid arthritis. J Bone Joint Surg 56B:668–680, 1974
18. Muller EA: Influence of training and of inactivity on muscle strength. Arch Phys Med 51:449–462, 1970
19. National Commission on Arthritis and Related Musculoskeletal Diseases. In Arthritis. Out of the Maze. 2. Work Group Reports. DHEW Publication #76-1151
20. Partridge REH, Duffy JJR: Controlled trial of the effect of complete immobilization of the joints in RA. Ann Rheum Dis 22:91–99, 1963
21. Pellicci PM, Ranawat CS, Isairis P, et al: A prospective study of the progression of rheumatoid arthritis of the cervical spine. J Bone Joint Surg 63A:342–350, 1981
22. Pratt TL: Spontaneous dislocation of the atlanto-axial articulation occurring in ankylosing spondylosis and rheumatoid arthritis. J Faculty Radiol (London) 10:40–43, 1959
23. Rana NA, Hancock DO, Taylor AR, et al: Atlanto axial subluxation in rheumatoid arthritis. J Bone Joint Surg 55B:458–470, 1973
24. Ranawat CS, O'Leary P, Pellicci, et al: Cervical spine fusion in rheumatoid arthritis. J Bone Joint Surg 61A:1003–1010, 1979
25. Roper, Bennett, Cobb et al: 1958 Revision of diagnostic criteria for rheumatoid arthritis. Bull Rheum Dis 9:175–179, 1958
26. Sharp J, Purser DW, Lawrence JS: Rheumatoid arthritis of the cervical spine in the adult. Ann Rheum Dis 17:303–313, 1958
27. Smith PH, Sharp J, Kellgren JA: Natural history of rheumatoid cervical subluxations. Ann Rheum Dis 31:222–223, 1972
28. Steinbrocker O, Traeger CH, Batterman RC: Functional criteria for rheumatoid arthritis. 140:659–663, 1949

James S. Lieberman

11

Cervical Soft Tissue Injuries and Cervical Disc Disease

Conditions causing neck pain and referred pain into adjacent body areas are among the most frequent musculoskeletal disorders seen by both primary care physicians and specialists. Neck pain may be caused by many diseases in all categories including trauma, tumors, infections, inflammatory disease, degenerative diseases, and congenital anomalies. An encyclopedic discussion of all causes of neck pain is beyond the scope of this chapter. Rather, the chapter will concentrate on cervical soft tissue injuries and cervical disc disease including spondylosis. The cervical spine manifestations of rheumatoid arthritis (RA) are covered in Chapter 10.

PATIENT EVALUATION

Obviously, the evaluation of a patient presenting with a complaint of neck and related pain requires an appropriate and thorough history and physical examination. The history and examination, however, can often be augmented by observation of the patient and the patient's behavior during the interview and examination.

While the patient is under observation, close attention should be paid to the patient's posture, gait, head and neck position, use of the upper extremities, motion of the head and neck, facial expressions indicating pain, and the emotional content of the description of pain symptoms. In addition, it is important to assess the patient relative to consistency of behavior in different situations, ie, during sitting, standing, lying down, walking, and while the patient is not aware of being under observation.

The History

The assessment of the patient with neck pain depends upon a comprehensive and detailed history that elicits that information needed for a diagnostic impression. A convenient format is shown in Table 11-1.

PRINCIPLES OF PHYSICAL MEDICINE AND REHABILITATION IN THE MUSCULOSKELETAL DISEASES

Table 11-1

Assessssment Format for Neck Pain Patients

1. Age, occupation and handedness of the patient.
2. Description of the pain complaint.
    a. Date of onset, date of injury and whether sudden onset or gradual onset as well as whether acute or chronic.
    b. Relationship to other events—ie, trauma, febrile illness, systemic disease, systemic symptoms, etc.
    c. Pain distribution including neck, head, upper limb, chest, and breast.
    d. Character of pain.
        (1) Sharp/dull/burning/lancinating
        (2) Constant/intermittent
        (3) Daytime/nighttime/anytime
    e. Relationship to position of head and neck.
    f. Activities that worsen or lessen pain.
3. Neurologic symptoms.
    a. Motor system.
    b. Sensory system.
    c. Coordination.
    d. Sphincter function, sexual function.
    e. Special senses, cranial nerves.
        (1) Visual—blurring, eye pain
        (2) Aural/labyrinthine—tinnitus, dizziness, vertigo
        (3) Pharyngeal—dysphagia, hoarse voice
    f. Loss of consciousness, seizures
4. Course.
5. Treatment and effects of treatment including medications.
6. Work history relative to pain complaint.
7. Past history relative to neck complaints or injuries.
8. Past history and system review for systemic processes relevant to neck pain.
9. Litigation or other secondary gain factors.

It has been estimated that as many as 90% of cervical spine disorders are related to injury. When a history of trauma has been obtained, specific detailed information about the event(s) should be elicited:

Detailed Injury Assessment by Type of Injury

1. Auto accident.
    a. Impact—head-on, rear end, side impact, speed of impact.
    b. Driver versus passenger in front seat, rear seat.
    c. Use of restraints; what restraints.
    d. Position of patient in vehicle.
        (1) Facing forward, rotated, facing backward.
    e. Injuries to other occupants.
    f. Associated head injury, trunk or extremity injuries.
    g. Road conditions, car stationary or moving, brakes on or off.
2. Falls.
    a. How patient fell.
    b. Where patient fell, on what surface.
    c. Position on impact.
    d. Height of fall.
    e. Associated head, trunk or extremity injuries.

Table 11-1

Continued

---

3. Blows.
   a. Location—head, neck, face, back.
   b. Object causing blow.
   c. Height/weight of falling object.
   d. Associated head, trunk, extremity injuries.
4. Sports injuries.
   a. What sport, where played, what position.
   b. Protective equipment.
   c. Condition of field.
   d. Exact description of event.
   e. Associated head, trunk, extremity injuries.

Examination of the Patient

Physical examination of the patient with neck pain should actually have begun with the observational assessment noted above. Patients with significant neck pain tend to splint the neck and reduce head and neck motion. The patient who exhibits significant spontaneous head and neck motion probably has little or no neck pain.

The specific examination of the neck requires that the patient and examiner be correctly positioned. Ideally, the patient should be seated on a chair or stool with the examiner standing behind the patient for most of the evaluation.

Range of motion of the neck, both passive and active, should be tested. The movements tested are flexion, extension, lateral bending, and rotation. The average range of motion for flexion and extension is 45° in each direction.[1] For assessment without a goniometer, the average person should be able to flex so that the chin touches the sternum. For every finger breadth of missing flexion approximately 10° of flexion is lost.[33] Similarly, the average person can extend the neck so that the occiput touches the first thoracic vertebra spinous process. As in flexion, each finger breadth of missing extension suggests a loss of 10° of extension.[33] Careful observation of the patient and neck palpation during motion is helpful in checking that motion is occurring smoothly throughout the cervical spine. Lateral bending should reach 40°[33] to 45°[1] of motion to either side from neutral position, while rotation should be from 80°[1] to 90°[33] to either side from the neutral position. Complaints of pain during motion testing should be recorded. Care should also be taken to record patient resistance to passive motion and jerky motions of the neck as they may indicate voluntary attempts to reduce motion.

Following range of motion testing, palpation of both soft tissue and bony structures of the neck should be performed. Soft tissue palpation should include an assessment of both tenderness and muscle spasm. Soft tissues to be examined include the lymph node chains, thyroid gland, parotid gland, carotid artery, superior nuchal ligament, supraclavicular fossa, and greater occipital nerves as well as the musculature. The following muscles should be palpated: Sternocleidomastoid, trapezius, lateral and anterior neck muscles, suboccipital muscles, rhomboids and suprascapular musculature. Deep cervical paraspinal muscles are difficult to palpate because of overlying muscles. However, it is sometimes possible to palpate deeper structures by pushing up the upper trapezius over the cervical spine in relaxed cooperative, suitably built patients. It is frequently helpful to palpate muscles for spasm while the patient is performing range of motion as it may be apparent only during motion of the neck. Soft tissue palpation can be accomplished with the patient seated.

Bony palpation is best accomplished with the patient supine as neck muscle relaxation occurs and bony structures are more easily felt.[30] Structures to be palpated include the hyoid bone, thyroid cartilage, first cricoid ring, and carotid tubercles, anteriorally. Posteriorally, the occiput, inion, superior nuchal line, mastoids, spinous processes, and facet joints should be palpated. With the patient seated, spinous processes can also be percussed to assess tenderness. The reader is referred to Hoppenfeld's textbook[30] for details of bony palpation.

Although there is no direct counterpart of the straight leg raising test for assessing cervical root symptomatology, various head and neck compression maneuvers provide useful information. Direct vertical compression of the head on the neck in the neutral position may increase or cause pain. Pain radiating into the upper extremities suggests radicular pathology while neck pain suggests a cervical joint or soft tissue problem. Variants of vertical compression in the neutral position include performing compression with the head flexed, extended, or tilted. When compression is done with the neck extended and laterally rotated it is called Spurling's sign. This maneuver may produce radicular symptoms on either side depending on whether symptoms occur secondary to root stretch or foraminal compression. Finally, a shoulder depression test may be useful.[33] The patient's head is tilted to one side and downward force is applied to the opposite shoulder. This may produce root pain.

In addition to the tests mentioned above, evaluation of neck pain patients should include testing Tinel's sign over median, radial, and ulnar nerves at wrist and elbow as well as performance of all three thoracic outlet syndrome tests.[40] These include: Adson's maneuver, in which the radial pulse is palpated with the arm dependent, with the patient holding his breath, extending his neck, and rotating his head side to side; the exaggerated military posture (costoclavicular) maneuver in which the radial pulse is palpated with the arm dependent after shoulders are drawn backward and downward; and the hyperabduction maneuver in which the radial pulse is palpated with arm abducted from the dependent to hyperabducted position. Finally, shoulder motion and function should be thoroughly assessed to rule out primary shoulder disorders with secondary or referred neck pain.

The last step in the clinical evaluation of the neck pain patient is a complete neurologic examination including testing of mental status, cranial nerve function, motor and sensory performance, coordination, gait and reflex function including the presence of pathological reflexes. To assess atrophy above and below elbow circumferences should be measured using a specific reference point so that subsequent measurements are done at the same place on the limb. Sphincter function should be assessed by a rectal examination.

Radiologic Evaluation

An adequate radiographic examination should be obtained in all patients with neck pain. The minimum acceptable study should include anteroposterior, lateral, oblique, and odontoid views. Flexion and extension views are the most common additional studies. In addition, other "routine" views are recommended by some clinicians. These include a caudal-angled view and pillar views.[33,61] Particular care must be taken to be sure that the entire cervical spine is visualized. The C_7–T_1 area is the one most often seen poorly. The lateral view may have to be done with the patient holding sandbags in each hand to drop the shoulders.

In addition to routine radiographs, a number of special radiologic procedures are available for use in certain circumstances.[33,34] These include: (1) Cineradiographs to study spine motion, (2) tomography, (3) xeroradiography, a technique which shows bony and soft tissue detail on a single film, (4) stereoradiography, (5) magnification radiography, and (6) computerized axial tomography (CAT) with or without contrast material. In addition, myelography with or without CAT and discography are available where indicated. Myelography should be reserved for patients suspected of having spinal cord symptoms or signs, or for patients with radiculopathy who are being considered for surgery. Discography is a controversial technique and many specialists feel it is unnecessary. However, it is still used in some centers.[33,34] Vertebral angiography may be considered when the cervical spine disorder is suspected of causing pathology to these blood vessels. Finally, nuclear magnetic resonance (NMR) of the spine is becoming available in many centers. A very preliminary study suggests, however, that CAT and myelography may be more sensitive than NMR in cervical disc disease.[49]

Electrodiagnostic Testing[39]

Electromyography (EMG) and nerve conduction velocity (NCV) studies provide objective evidence of pathology to neural structures that may be involved in a patient with a cervical spine disorder. In addition, an experienced electromyographer can assist in deciding whether a patient's apparent weakness is organic or functional. The studies should be scheduled at least three weeks after symptom onset because that is the time course for the appearance of typical electrical changes after neural injury.

Within the context of cervical spine disorders, the tests are particularly valuable in the evaluation of suspected radicular or peripheral nerve pathology. In some centers these studies are ordered routinely while they are rarely ordered in other centers. While routine electrical studies are not "necessary" for the evaluation of clinically obvious radicular syndromes, the information obtained from routine studies provides a valuable baseline when the clinician must evaluate a patient with persistent or recurrent symptoms. The ability of the electromyographer to date lesions approximately and assess acuity of changes is particularly helpful in this setting. This task is made more difficult, however, when baseline studies are not obtained. In addition, combinations of radiculopathy and entrapment neuropathy can be detected prior to treatment. For these reasons the author recommends routine electrodiagnostic testing in suspected radicular symptoms.

CLINICAL DISORDERS

Cervical Soft Tissue Injuries

Cervical soft tissue injuries typically occur during a traumatic event that impacts a sudden acceleration, deceleration, or lateral force causing sudden uncontrolled head and neck motion. The most common event is an acceleration injury producing acute hyperextension of the neck and head. Sudden deceleration forces produce acute neck and head flexion. While serious spinal column pathology occurs in deceleration injuries, soft tissue injuries in this situation are less common and frequently less severe. Lateral impacts produce acute side to side head and neck motions. Lateral impact trauma may cause either spinal column or soft tissue injury. However, lateral impact injuries are the least frequent. This section will focus upon the acceleration-hyperextension cervical soft tissue injury.

Historical Background

As early as the mid-nineteenth century, railway passengers began to complain of neck injuries when a stationary train suddenly accelerated. This condition was termed "railway spine" and was a medico-legal problem even at that time.[34] Recent interest in acceleration-hyperextension injuries began with neck disorders seen in pilots who underwent catapult-assisted take-offs from aircraft carriers.[43] However, this type of injury assumed its current prominence after the end of World War II, when the increased use of automobiles lead to large numbers of cervical injuries.[13] In recent times, the term "whiplash" has been applied to those injuries.

The introduction of the term whiplash has been attributed to Crowe in 1928.[43] Other experts, however, credit Davis with introducing the term in 1944 or 1945.[33] The term was popularized by subsequent articles including those by Gay and Abbott,[21] Gotten,[23] and Zatskin and Kreton.[67] Unfortunately, the term whiplash is often used as a diagnosis when, in fact, it was initially only used to describe the motions occurring during injury. As a diagnostic term, whiplash should be discarded and replaced by terminology appropriate to the situation, eg, cervical acceleration-hyperextension injury or cervical soft tissue injury.

Mechanism of Injury[13,43,44,46]

A vehicle struck from the rear is suddenly accelerated forward. At the time of acceleration, the seat back is pushed into the occupant and the person's body is accelerated forward. If there is no head rest, or if the head rest is not properly adjusted, there is no similar acceleration force applied to the head and neck. Therefore, the body is accelerated forward but the head and neck are not. This produces extension motion of the head and neck. When the limit of normal soft tissue stretch is exceeded, an extension strain is placed upon the neck. The neck extension and backward rotation of the head stretches the anterior cervical musculature. When their tone is overcome, only the anterior longitudinal ligament and anterior annulus fibers are available to resist the extension of the head and neck. If there is a sufficient extension force, head and neck extension may not stop until the head strikes the thoracic spine. If the neck and head are rotated, the normal extension range of motion is less than when the head and neck are straight. Thus, hyperextension injuries occur with a lesser degree of extension when the head and neck are rotated at the time of impact. In addition to neck hyperextension, the maxilla and mandible undergo relative separation as the head rotates and temporomandibular joint injury may occur.

When the vehicle's acceleration ceases, the head and neck will move forward into flexion, partly as a result of deceleration and partly as a result of an induced flexor stretch reflex. When forward flexion occurs, it is limited by the fact that the chin strikes the chest well within the normal range of motion of the neck. However, the head may strike objects ahead of it, such as sun visors, dashboard, or windshield.

In addition to acceleration and deceleration forces, there are vertical forces applied to the vehicle at impact. The vehicle is compressed and is, thus, of shorter length but taller. This vertical force may push the occupant up until the head strikes the roof of the car, or the person may be thrown into the back seat if restraints are not in use. Finally, the vertical force may cause the person's head to fall over the head rest top if it is not positioned level with the top of the occiput.

In the typical rear end acceleration type collision, the degree of injury appears to be dependent on the rate of acceleration. The acceleration is determined by the force of impact and the inertia of the object that has been struck. The force is a product of the mass and velocity of the striking object. The inertia of the struck object depends on its mass, but also upon factors that allow it to move forward easily. Examples of such factors include road conditions, whether the struck vehicle is slowly moving or stationary, and whether brakes are on or off when a stationary vehicle is struck. Such information should be obtained during history taking.

Interestingly, in collisions where the impact speed is less than 15 mph, the right front seat passenger has a greater risk for injury than the driver, since the driver can frequently brace himself with the steering wheel. Impact speeds of greater than 20 mph usually produce greater risk of injury for the driver than the front seat passenger. In this situation, the extension force on the passenger is diminished by a forward motion of the pelvis. On the driver's side, however, the steering wheel prevents the forward pelvic motion and the extension force on the driver's neck is increased. It is important to note that lap seat belts without a shoulder harness prevent this forward motion and may lead to more severe hyperextension injuries of the neck. In this regard the combination lap belt and shoulder harness is superior in injury prevention especially when a head rest is properly adjusted.

Pathology

Almost all of the information concerning the pathology of cervical soft tissue injuries comes from animal experiments since the nature of the injuries precludes pathologic examination of human victims.

A number of pathological lesions have been described by various authors.[25,31,43,44,46,62] These include:

1. Muscle injury including tearing and hemorrhage in the longus colli, longus capitis, scalenes, and sternocleidomastoid. This may vary from a small tear to complete rupture. Tears of longus colli may result in a retropharyngeal hematoma.
2. Apophyseal joints may be fractured or sprained. In addition, facet joints may be injured or fractured.
3. Anterior and posterior longitudinal ligaments undergo stretch and possible tearing. The anterior ligament is more severely involved than the posterior ligament. Disc injury and disc separation have been seen. Both ligament and disc injury have been confirmed at surgery in human victims.[25,31]
4. Esophageal damage, laryngeal hyperemia, and damage to the cervical sympathetic nerves was documented. Stretch of the larynx has been reported.[8]
5. The vertebral arteries may be stretched and injured.
6. Associated neural injuries occurred in many animals studied by Wickstrom.[62] These include brain damage in 32 percent, spinal cord damage in 5 percent and cervical root damage in 0.7 percent.

The obvious conclusion from the experimental studies and human observations is that the events occurring during cervical accelerations-hyperextension injuries lead to significant tissue pathology. The symptom complex in the human patient is much easier to understand when it is assessed in relation to the pathology described above.

CLINICAL FEATURES

Pain[13,34,46]

Patients may complain of some neck pain immediately or experience a delay of severe pain onset varying from a few minutes to 24–48 hours.[8,13] The delay may be due to the time required for the onset of the traumatic edema and hemorrhage in damaged soft tissues.[34] The pain may be localized to the neck or may radiate into one or both shoulders. In addition, there may be intrascapular pain and pain radiating into the arms. While intrascapular pain and arm pain may suggest radiculopathy, this may simply be referred pain in this type of injury. Occipital headache may be present and may radiate forward to the vertex and bitemporal region. Occasionally, neck pain will be minimal or absent and pain may be present only in the shoulders, arms, or occipital region. Persistent headaches are often seen in more severe injuries and this has been thought to be as a result of trauma to upper cervical nerves.[21] According to Macnab,[43] if the head is rotated at the time of impact, the pain symptoms are maximal on the side to which the chin was rotated.

Dysphagia, Hoarseness

Dysphagia may be experienced by the patient either early or late after the injury. Dysphagia occurring early may be as a result of pharyngeal edema or retropharyngeal hematoma,[43] although hemorrhages into the muscular layers of the esophagus are also reported.[46] The early occurrence of dysphagia suggests a serious injury.[43,46] The occurrence of late dysphagia may imply an emotional origin.[43,46]

In addition to dysphagia, hoarseness of voice is reported.[8] This may be secondary to laryngeal stretch[8] or hyperemia.[62]

Visual Symptoms

Patients may complain of intermittent blurring of vision.[38,43,46] Ocular pain may also be present.[38] These symptoms are thought to be due to cervical sympathetic chain or vertebral artery injury.[43] A Horner's syndrome may occur.[43]

Dizziness

A feeling of dizziness or vertigo may be a complaint. Patients may also complain of veering on ambulation. Vertigo may be due to vertebral artery damage or spasm or an inner ear problem.[46] The veering may be secondary to an impaired neck-righting reflex as a result of neck muscle spasm.[43,46] Vertigo may also be secondary to over activity of beta-receptors in injured neck muscles.[26]

Tinnitus

Buzzing in the ears, or other tinnitus-like complaints may be present.[6,43] This symptom may be due to vertebral artery or inner ear injury. Tinnitus does not appear to have prognostic value.[43] Additional otic complaints including decreased hearing and loudness recruitment are reported.[22]

The symptom complex of headache, tinnitus, vertigo, visual disturbance, ocular and otic pain is sometimes referred to as Barre's syndrome.[26]

Temporomandibular Joint Symptoms

As noted above, temporomandibular joint injury can occur. This may be strain or even dislocation.[46] When this occurs, patients may complain of pain on mastication and limited, painful opening of the mouth.[46] These symptoms may be increased by a traction halter during treatment.

Thoracic Outlet Syndrome (TOS)

Symptoms that are thought to be typical of TOS are reported in cervical soft tissue injuries.[5] These include pain, heaviness, and fatiguability of the arms, and numbness and tingling in ulnar innervated fingers. Unfortunately, these symptoms are not specific for TOS and heaviness and fatiguability of the arms is a common complaint in cervical soft tissue injury.

Physical Findings

Within the first two hours after injury, findings on examination are usually minimal. In fact, a completely normal examination may occur.[29] After several hours, limitation of neck motion, tightness, muscle spasm, and tenderness of both *anterior and posterior* neck structures is present.[29,46] Swelling of anterior musculature may be present.[34] Patients who have suffered an acceleration-hyperextension injury should have both anterior and posterior neck findings. Those who exhibit only posterior tenderness should be viewed with some skepticism.[46]

Neurologic examination in these patients should be normal. If there is evidence of neural dysfunction, further investigation must be carried out to localize the findings to cord, root, plexus, or peripheral nerve levels. Findings that suggest a possible concomitant head injury should also be fully investigated.

It is wise to remember that physical findings in cervical soft tissue injury are usually less spectacular than severity of symptoms would predict. In addition, physical findings usually disappear before symptoms subside.

Radiologic Findings

Most early X-ray studies are normal[13] or reveal evidence of pre-existing degenerative changes. On occasion, initial X-rays reveal evidence of bony injury such as posterior joint crush fractures or minimal subluxation.[43] However, the most common "pathologic" X-ray finding in the acute phase is straightening of the normal cervical lordotic curve.[28] Care must be taken in interpreting this finding as being of clinical significance since this may be seen with only a small degree of voluntary neck flexion at the time of X-ray.[33,61] Soft tissue swelling or anterior displacement of prevertebral structures may be visualized. Occasionally, a widened disc space may be noted. This suggests a severe extension injury with damage to the anterior longitudinal ligament and anterior disc.[7,8] In sharply localized lesions, segmental motion changes may be seen in flexion-extension views.[34] Follow-up X-rays are indicated in cases with persistent symptoms.[28,29] These may show late cervical disc space changes[28,29] that provide objective evidence of more serious injury than was suspected initially. This may modify treatment.

Management

Appropriate management begins during the initial contact with the patient. A thorough history, physical examination, radiologic evaluation, and reassuring discussion with the patient are mandatory. Patients should have the injury and its consequences, as well as expected symptom duration, explained to them clearly. Statements such as "there is nothing wrong" when it is obvious to the patient that there is a problem, should be avoided.[34] It is unfortunate that physicians frequently undertreat cervical soft tissue injuries, or do not treat them correctly. This failure of adequate treatment may be responsible for some of the poor treatment results seen.[43]

Rest and splinting of the neck are necessary in most cases of cervical soft tissue injury. Rest of the neck may be accomplished solely by activity restriction in very mild cases, while moderate cases require a neck collar and a short course of bed rest.[38,43] Severe cases require a collar and more prolonged bed rest, which in some cases may require hospitalization.[38,43]

The neck orthosis suitable for most cases is the soft cervical collar.[4,13,22,29,33,38,43,46] This should be fit in slight flexion and must fit the patient. Ideally, the collar should be fabricated for each individual.[4] A soft cervical collar splints but does not immobilize the neck. The device is comfortable, well accepted by patients, and serves as a reminder to the patient to restrict activity.[64] The neck collar or a collar made from a towel should be worn at night early in the treatment program if pain is awakening the patient or there is a problem sleeping.

The duration of collar use in cervical soft tissue injury is somewhat controversial. Cailliet[4] recommends no longer than two weeks in the usual acute injury, while Jackson[33] suggests three to eight weeks. Prolonged collar use leads to (1) disuse atrophy of neck muscles, (2) soft tissue contracture, (3) shortening of muscles in sustained contraction, (4) thickening of facet capsular tissues, and (5) increased dependency and enhancement of functional overlay.[4] This author usually recommends no more than two weeks of continuous collar use in typical injuries, with longer use in very severe cases. It is critical that collar use not be stopped abruptly.[4,33] A program of collar weaning should be employed, with periods of time in and out of the collar in a progressive manner, eg, one hour out, three hours in for three to four days, then two hours out, two hours in for three to four days, and then three hours out, one hour in for three to four days. The weaning program should be accomplished in conjunction with a neck exercise program (vide infra).

Failure to use a collar weaning/exercise program may perpetuate pain complaints and collar use. In this scenario, the patient is told to abruptly cease collar use but has an increase in pain secondary to soft tissue changes induced by collar use and no exercise. The patient is then placed back in a collar for a further period and it is again discontinued abruptly. The patient is now in more pain because of further loss of adequate soft tissue function. The patient is then placed back in the collar. This continues until chronic collar use and chronic pain are present. At that time, the patient is considered to be neurotic or a malingerer when, in fact, the problem may be, to a considerable degree, iatrogenic.

Bed rest is useful for most patients although hospitalization is rarely necessary unless other injuries have occurred. Macnab[43] suggests an initial trial of 12–24 hours. If the patient is relatively symptom free at that time bed rest is discontinued. A cervical pillow may be of long term benefit to the patient,[4,33] both acutely and chronically. If symptoms are still present at 24 hours, bed rest is continued for 1 week. Macnab[43,46] feels that most patients should be able to return to work at the end of one week. Heavy manual labor jobs are an exception. However, the patients need instruction on avoiding extension strains to the neck. Furthermore, patients should be counseled that their resumption of activity may lead to some increase in pain during some activities. They should also be counseled that the symptom increase does not mean that they are causing an increase in neck damage by that activity. In fact, patients should be firmly encouraged to resume activities. Macnab[16] has developed a neck sparing routine that provides specific suggestions in the areas of sleeping, sitting, tension, driving, reaching, lifting, and sports. That routine is as follows:

Neck Sparing Routine*

Sleeping. If you have discomfort at night the following changes may be helpful. Sleep on your back with the back and neck supported by five pillows, so that you are in the reclining or semisitting position. It is important when doing this to try to keep the neck and the rest of the spine in a straight line. If you still have discomfort, or if you are unable to sleep on your back, it will be necessary for you to wear a soft, supporting collar. This can be provided for you. Go to bed early. Even if you do not sleep the whole time, it is advisable to try to get ten hours rest at night during the acute phase of your trouble.

Sitting. Avoid adopting any position in which your head is tilted backwards, for example, resting your chin on your hand. Try to sit with your neck and spine in a straight line—your shoulders braced back and your chin tucked in—the sort of posture you expect your children to adopt when you tell them to "sit up straight."

Tension. Any form of emotional tension will aggravate the pain. It does so because in states of tension we adopt the "fight position," with the chin thrust forward. When such situations arise, make a deliberate effort to relax the muscles. Be more conscious than ever of the need to keep your chin tucked in and the neck and spine in a straight line.

Driving. Prolonged driving commonly aggravates pain in the neck. This is caused by a combination of tension and bad sitting posture. Avoid the tendency to thrust your chin over the top of the steering wheel. If you are short, sit on a firm cushion so that you do not have to crane your neck to see out the window. Bring the seat as close as possible to the steering wheel so that you can sit with your back supported by the back of the car seat, with your spine held straight.

Reaching. Avoid reaching or looking up at high objects—both activities demand that you tilt your neck backwards. If this is repeated or prolonged it will hurt your neck.

Lifting. Avoid carrying any object over ten pounds. When your neck is painful do not wear heavy overcoats. Do not pull, or attempt to move, heavy objects of furniture.

Sports. When your symptoms are severe, all sports should be avoided. Golf, bowling, and gardening put severe strains on the neck. Swimming—except for swimming on the back—will aggravate the pain. Diving should be avoided until you are completely free from all symptoms.

Local heat is a commonly used modality. However, heat applied in the first 72 hours after injury may increase tissue reaction and pain. During the initial 72 hour period, the application of ice may be tried for periods of 15–20 minutes.[4] If the patient cannot tolerate

---

*(Reprinted from Macnab I: Acceleration Extension Injuries of the Cervical Spine, in Rothman RH, Simeone FA (eds): The Spine, 2nd edition. Philadelphia, W.B. Saunders, 1982, pp 657-658. With permission)

icing, it may be better to use nothing rather than heat during this first 72 hour period. Heat can then be used after the acute period after injury. Heat makes the patient feel better but does not speed up tissue healing. The heat can be applied by a heating pad, hot shower, or hot moist towels. Heat treatments such as ultrasound or diathermy, given in a physical therapy unit are usually unnecessary and may be ill advised, particularly if they prevent the patient from resuming usual activities because of the appointments.

Traction has been advocated by some authors.[28,33,34,43,46] However, it may aggravate symptoms in some patients,[4] and has even been considered to add to the trauma of the injury.[60] There is little agreement as to traction method, weight, treatment duration, or frequency and only the neck position and direction of traction force are agreed upon.[4] The neck should be slightly flexed and the direction of pull should cause the patient to feel it at the mastoids. Traction may be prescribed for home use or in the physical therapy unit. Home traction is difficult to use without proper instruction and probably should be avoided in most cases.[4] Traction in the therapy unit can be administered in the supine or sitting position and pull can be intermittent or continuous during each session. The choice of method varies with physician, therapist, and patient tolerance. Very forceful traction should be avoided early after acute injury,[4,34] and traction should be discontinued if it aggravates symptoms. Traction may be more useful for patients with cervical radiculopathy[59] than those with soft tissue injury. This author uses home traction only for very reliable patients and avoids traction in the therapy unit in most patients because it prevents patients from normal activities because of time spent in therapy. If traction is used, its continuation must be justified by symptom reduction and reduced use of analgesics. In addition, its duration should be limited.[3]

Injections of local anesthetic into neck muscles as well as stellate ganglion and occipital nerve blocks have been advocated by some authors.[3,8,57] However, they are not used by most clinicians.

Various pharmaceutical agents have been recommended in cervical soft tissue injury. These include analgesics, anti-inflammatory drugs, proteolytic enzymes, muscle relaxants, sedatives, and tranquilizers. As a general rule, minimal medication use is recommended and controlled substances should be used with caution. Mild analgesics or combined analgesic/anti-inflammatory agents such as the various nonsteroidal anti-inflammatory drugs may be useful. Occasionally, narcotics are needed but should not be given longer than one week.[3] Muscle relaxants may be of limited value although this author has not been impressed with their efficacy. Sedatives and minor tranquilizers may be valuable during the very early phase, especially if bed rest is needed. However, the abuse potential of these agents limits their usefulness.

Exercise programs are also of value in cervical soft tissue injury. Cervical isometric exercise may be begun in the collar after the acute phase subsides. They are particularly useful as an adjunct to collar weaning. They strengthen neck muscles and improve posture.[24,28] They are easy to perform in any location and easy to teach to the patient.

Cervical isometric exercises are performed in four positions: Flexion, extension, and lateral motion to each side. A simple technique is illustrated in Figure 11-1. These can also be done by having the patient perform contraction against the resistance of their hands pushing against the movement. Initially, the exercises should be done twice a day, with five repetitions in each of the four positions. Each contraction should be held for ten seconds. Over a two week period repetitions should be increased to ten in each position. The frequency of isometric exercise can be increased to four times a day or more as tolerated. When frequency is increased, however, repetitions should be reduced to five and built up again. They should be continued after collar use is discontinued. Cailliet[4] advocates

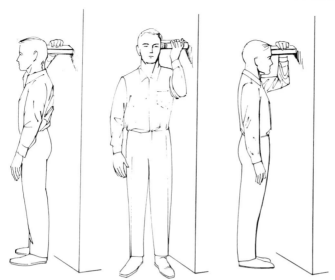

Fig. 11-1. Drawing illustrates the correct position for the performance of cervical isometric exercises. A padded book or block of wood is used for support. Note that the cervical spine is maintained in a neutral position during the performance of these exercises. (Reprinted from DePalma AF, Rothman RH: The Intervertebral Disc, Philadelphia, W.B. Saunders Company, with permission of the publishers.)

rhythmic stabilization exercises, a form of active-assisted-resistive exercise, after the acute phase. In this form of exercise the patient resists neck movement imposed by the therapist. The disadvantage of this type of exercise is that a therapist is involved while isometrics can be done by the patient alone. Further, Cailliet[4] advocates neck range of motion exercise in the convalescent phase after injury. The value of this type of exercise is disputed, however.[33]

Surgical treatment in cervical soft tissue injury is rarely needed. Occasionally, however, it may be of value in patients with symptoms lasting more than two years[46] if strict criteria are met. Surgery should only be contemplated when symptoms can be clearly determined to be arising from one or, at most, two vertebral levels. These patients require extensive investigation including repeat plain X-rays, myelography, and even discography.[28,46] Anterior cervical discectomy and fusion is the usual surgical procedure.[28,46] There is not complete agreement as to the efficacy of surgery. Some authors[28,46] favor it and some advocate surgery only if radicular symptoms are present.[13] In carefully selected cases, however, results may be gratifying.

Prognosis

An accurate prognosis is difficult in cervical soft tissue injury and this topic has been the subject of a number of reports.[18,23,24,28,34,46,51] Macnab[46] states that if a patient's symptoms are severe enough to warrant a week of bed rest, daily discomfort will be present for six weeks. If at the end of 6 weeks the patient still has some discomfort all day long they may have intermittent symptoms for an additional 6–12 months.[46] In another study,[18] median duration of symptoms was 66 days (range 3–158) for minor injuries, 99 days (range

8–954) for moderate injury and 101 days (range 8–266) for severe injury. Median work days lost were 0 for minor injuries, 5 for moderate injury, and 15 for severe injury, a statistically significant figure. The difficulty in accurate prognosis is clearly shown by the range of work days lost in that study: 0–332 days for minor injuries, 0–141 days for moderate injury and 0–120 days for severe injury. Note that the patient with most work days lost had a minor injury.

Factors that have been felt to lead to a poor prognosis include (1) arm numbness and pain,[24,28,34,51] (2) pre-existing cervical degenerative disease,[34,51] (3) shoulder and cranial pain,[34] (4) persistent pain,[28,34] (5) radiographic evidence of restricted motion at one level,[28] or pre-existing degenerative disease, (6) severe initial symptoms or history of unconsciousness,[34] (7) emotional factors,[18,20] and (8) the necessity for prolonged treatment[18,29] and litigation.[18,34]

The role of litigation is particularly controversial. In Gotten's 1956 report[23] of 100 cases, 88 recovered after litigation or claims were settled, regardless of the verdict; 12, however, did not. Macnab,[42,43,46] however, emphasizes that 12 percent of Gotten's cases still had significant disability after settlement. Gotten concluded that patients used their injury as a lever for personal gain.[23] In his own study, Macnab[42,43,46] reports a series in which only 55 percent of 266 litigation cases recovered after settlement. However, he qualifies his report by stating that these were selected, not average cases. Macnab[42,43,46] does make an important observation: Patients' associated injuries, such as extremity fractures or sprains, recovered quickly as did those patients with flexion or lateral impact injuries. It was difficult for Macnab to accept litigation neurosis restricted to cervical extension injury complaints only.[42,43,46]

In other reports[18,27,34] litigation is felt to adversely affect prognosis. However, other authors[5,10,51,55] do not support this conclusion. There is some evidence to support the concept that symptom duration is prolonged in litigation cases[18,27] whether or not settlement of litigation leads to recovery.

Flexion and Lateral Impact Injuries[34]

Flexion injuries and lateral impact injuries tend to produce less significant soft tissue injury although, as noted above, significant spinal injury can occur in these circumstances. Flexion and lateral bending are limited by the chest and shoulders, respectively. The motion induced by impact is thought to be well within the physiological normal range of motion that is thought to be why less soft tissue damage occurs in these injuries. Lateral impact injuries can produce brachial plexus lesions, however. In general, evaluation and management of these injuries is similar to that of extension injury.

Cervical Disc Disease

Cervical disc disease may be acute or chronic. Acute cervical disc herniation is similar to typical lumbosacral disc herniation in that it is secondary to acute extrusion of nucleus pulposus through the annulus fibrosus with compression of neural structures. It differs from lumbosacral disc herniation in that the spinal cord may be compressed as well as nerve roots. Chronic cervical disc degeneration produces bony changes in the spinal column and these osteophytes may also compress the spinal cord, nerve roots, or both. In addition, the vertebral arteries may be compressed. Chronic cervical disc degeneration is known by several synonyms including cervical spondylosis.

Acute Cervical Disc Herniation

Pathogenesis

In acute cervical disc herniation, nuclear material extrudes through the annulus fibrosus. At the time of extrusion it may be contained by the posterior longitudinal ligament, or the ligament may be broached resulting in a free fragment within the epidural space. The events that allow this to happen have been extensively studied in reports examining the pathophysiology of disc disease and the effects of aging on the intervertebral disc.[2,19,52] In brief, a series of biochemical and biophysical changes occur in both the nucleus pulposus and annulus fibrosus. These include a decrease in water content of the nucleus as well as alterations in the collagen and acid amino glycans. The nucleus loses its normal gel function and ceases to transmit forces equally in all directions to the annulus. High forces are thus transmitted to selected areas of the annulus. At the same time, changes occur in the annulus, which cause it to lose structured integrity. Small cracks appear in the annulus and nuclear material extrudes into the annulus. The process continues until frank extrusion of nuclear material through the annulus occurs. In addition to the biochemical and biophysical alterations, there is evidence that genetic and auto-immune phenomena play a role as well.[56] Herniation of the disc may be central producing cord compression. Centro-lateral producing cord and root compression, or lateral producing root compression only.

Clinical Findings

Acute cervical disc herniation may be sudden and acute or may be delayed 24–48 hours after the causative insult.[53] Symptoms may or may not be related to trauma. In those patients with a nontraumatic onset, pain is frequently first noted on awakening in the morning.[48,53] In a recent epidemiological study of acute disc herniation[36] several factors were found to be strongly associated with the clinical condition. These included: Frequent heavy lifting, diving from a diving board, and cigarette smoking (probably secondary to chronic cough). Other statistically significant activities included operating or driving vibrating equipment and a large amount of time spent in a motor vehicle. The most common occurrence was in the fourth decade and the male:female ratio was 1.4:1. The most commonly affected levels were C_{6-7} (C_7 root) and C_{5-6} (C_6 root). Similar results as to level have been described in other studies.[37,47,50,65] These vertebral levels of greatest incidence correspond to regions of maximum flexion and extension[41,63] of the neck.

The patient may complain of neck pain or neck pain may be minimal.[48] Radicular pain and symptomatology should be present and may predominate. This consists of pain in the shoulder, intrascapular region, arm, hand, fingers, and even the anterior chest wall or breast. The pain may be increased by neck motions that stretch the involved root or by Valsalva maneuver producing activities such as cough, sneeze, or straining.[53] Headache may also be present.[33] When acute cervical myelopathy is present, the pain is frequently poorly localized and it often does not radiate. It may be referred to the thighs, buttocks or subcostal area.[53] With myelopathy leg weakness and symptoms of sphincter dysfunction may be present.

Physical findings may be nonspecific or localizing. Nonspecific findings include decreased range of motion of the neck and paravertebral muscle spasm. Palpation of neck muscles may cause discomfort and percussion of vertebral spinous processes may produce pain that may be helpful in localization. The various neck compression maneuvers described in the evaluation section of this chapter may reproduce the patient's neck and radicular pain.

A detailed neurological examination will usually reveal the level of the involved nerve root(s). The neurological findings for the various root levels are shown in Table 11-2. In addition, the examiner should carefully check for upper motor neuron findings including a sensory level, hyperactive reflexes, pathological reflexes, and signs of sphincter dysfunction.

Radiologic Evaluation and Electrodiagnosis

Plain cervical spine films may be normal or reveal straightening of the lordotic curve. Degenerative changes may be seen, however, they must be carefully correlated with the patient's clinical findings. Myelography and CAT with contrast material should be performed prior to surgery. Plain CAT studies in the cervical region may fail to show a herniated disc.[11] Discography has been used but it is controversial, as noted above.

The advantages of electrodiagnostic testing have been described above. In recent years, combined root and nerve lesions have been described (the double crunch).[58] Electrodiagnostic testing is invaluable for evaluating this situation.

Conservative Treatment

The conservative management of acute cervical disc herniation is similar in many respects to the management of acute cervical soft tissue injuries. A majority of patients with acute cervical disc herniation respond to a program of conservative management.

Rest and splinting of the neck are important modalities. A short period of bed rest may be of value as in soft tissue injury. The patient should be fitted with a soft cervical collar in slight flexion. Collar use may be more prolonged than that for soft tissue injury. Full time use may be for two to three weeks with another two to three week period of weaning.[53] Patients should be told that at least six weeks may be needed for recovery.[53]

The use of traction is also controversial in acute cervical disc herniation injury. Some authors advocate traction[14,35] either at home or in a therapy unit. Traction several times a day is usually used.[14,35] Other authors do not advocate traction except in rare instances.[53,54] This author utilizes traction in acute cervical disc herniation because its best results appear to be in radiculopathy.[59] However, home traction is used only for very reliable patients. The time and expense of therapy unit traction are thought to be justified in an attempt to avoid surgery. As a final resort before surgery, continuous traction with the patient reclining in bed may be attempted. The reader is cautioned to start with very low weights (six pounds) even though outpatient traction has been unsuccessful at much higher weights.

Local heat using superficial heat modalities such as hot packs, a heating pad, or infrared lamp may be of benefit. Icing may be beneficial in the first few days of symptoms. Deep heat modalities such as ultrasound and diathermy are unnecessary and may be harmful by increasing nerve root edema.[35]

Cervical isometric exercises are also recommended after the acute phase has subsided[53,54] usually two to three weeks after onset. The exercise program should be begun while the patient is still in the collar.

Finally, infiltration of local tender areas (trigger points) with local anesthetics may be

Table 11-2
Clinical Findings in Cervical Radiculopathy

Disc space	Involved roots	Pain distribution	Sensory dysfunction	Motor dysfunction	Reflex change
C_4–C_5	C_5	Neck, tip of shoulder and anterior arm	Deltoid area	Spinati, deltoid, biceps and other elbow flexors	Decreased biceps reflex
C_5–C_6	C_6	Neck, shoulder, medial scapular border, lateral arm, dorsum of forearm, thumb and index finger	Thumb, index finger, radial forearm	Biceps, other elbow flexors, extensor carpi radialis	Decreased biceps reflex and brachioradialis reflex
C_6–C_7	C_7	Neck, shoulder, medial scapular border, lateral arm, index and middle fingers	Middle finger, midportion of forearm	Triceps, extensor carpi ulnaris, pectoralis major	Decreased triceps reflex and pectoralis reflex
C_7–T_1	C_8	Neck, medial scapular border, ulnar side of arm and forearm, ring and little fingers	Ring and little fingers	Intrinsic hand muscles, flexor carpi ulnaris, sometimes triceps	None or decreased finger flexors

beneficial. Injections may be repeated at intervals as close as every three days, if needed.[53,54]

Drug therapy for acute cervical disc herniation is similar to that for soft tissue injury. Analgesics, anti-inflammatory agents, and muscle relaxants are recommended.[14,35,53,54] Large doses of narcotics are usually unnecessary, but narcotic medication may be useful for the first week. The use of a short course of high dose oral steroids has also been recommended.[35] This consists of an initial dose of 80 mg of Prednisone or its equivalent. The dosage can be decreased 10 mg/day for a course of eight days or 20 mg/day for a course of four days. The use of oral steroids will possibly increase the recovery rate in a patient who is recovering very slowly. This author has not seen a dramatic recovery in an otherwise stable or worsening patient simply by adding steroids.

Manipulation of the cervical spine should be avoided in cases of cervical disc disease as many untoward results have occurred.[54] General measures such as use of a cervical pillow, reducing automobile travel, and avoiding excessive neck flexion, extension and rotation should be employed.[54]

Using conservative management, DePalma and Rothman[9] reported 29 percent complete recovery, 49 percent partial recovery and 22 percent no recovery in a series of 225 patients treated for 3 months.

Surgical Treatment

The indications for surgical treatment of acute cervical disc herniation are cord compression, persistent or worsening neurologic deficit, and persistent or recurrent pain.

Cord compression. Signs of cord compression are an indication for immediate surgical decompression.

Persistent or worsening neurologic deficit. Motor deficits are particularly worrisome. Prolonged delay in surgical therapy may lead to residual motor dysfunction. C_8 root compromise should be treated more promptly than any other motor syndrome because of the severe disability with residual deficit. Motor deficits in other cervical root distributions can be tried longer on conservative therapy unless the motor deficit would hamper particular vocational activities. With significant motor deficit at any level, conservative management for more than one week without improvement is probably contra-indicated.[14] Sensory deficits can be treated conservatively longer.

Persistent or recurrent pain. When pain is incapacitating after several weeks of conservative therapy, or when symptoms recur after successful conservative therapy is terminated, surgery is probably indicated. This indication is more controversial than the two above.

Surgical approaches vary from surgeon to surgeon. The approaches include anterior surgery with or without fusion, a lateral approach, and a posterior approach. The choice of surgical approach frequently depends upon which procedure the surgeon is most comfortable with. However, the anterior approach is recommended for midline soft cervical disc herniation, while either the anterior or posterior approach is suitable for lateral acute disc protrusion.[56] With the anterior approach the postoperative course may be less painful with earlier ambulation and mobility.[56] However, in the individual patient the specific advantages and disadvantages of the various approaches must be considered by the surgeon. High rates of success are reported for all approaches,[14,56] with success rates approaching 90–95 percent.

Chronic Cervical Disc Degeneration— Spondylosis

Pathogenesis

The series of biochemical and biophysical alterations in the disc, which were described above for acute disc herniation, are also significant in the pathogenesis of cervical spondylosis. These changes may be regarded as the first stage in degeneration of the disc. If there is no acute disc herniation, degeneration of the disc continues in a predictable and progressive fashion. At first the vertebral segment becomes mechanically unstable secondary to the degenerated disc.[45] The unstable segment is then quite susceptible to trauma, which increases degeneration. Eventually, narrowing of the disc space occurs and finally, osteophyte formation occurs at several locations. As osteophytes increase in size they may encroach upon nerve roots in the nerve root exit canal or narrow the spinal canal leading to cord compression.

Bony changes are only part of the picture of cervical spondylosis. The neurologic features of the disorder, cord compression, root compression, or a combination, are not necessarily due to osteophyte formation alone. In fact, there are four interrelated areas of pathology that interact to produce the neurologic picture of cervical spondylosis.

The four areas[15] are pathologic encroachment from osteophytes, a developmentally shallow spinal canal, biomechanical effects of altered cervical motion, and circulatory factors. Rarely is a single factor, or even a combination of two or three factors, responsible for the neurologic manifestation of cervical spondylosis.[15] In the majority of cases, all four factors are participating in the production of neurologic manifestations.

Clinical Findings

Chronic cervical disc degeneration produces a clinical picture that falls into one or a combination of five areas:[12] (1) Radiculopathy, (2) neck and shoulder pain, (3) headache, (4) myelopathy, and (5) vertebral-basilar insufficiency. Generally speaking, patients with symptomatic chronic cervical disc degeneration are older (sixth decade onset) than patients with acute cervical disc herniation. The male:female ratio is about 1:1.

The patient's complaints are similar to those in acute cervical disc herniation. Neck pain may be minimal and shoulder and radicular pain may be more severe.[45] Generally, symptoms begin insidiously although an acute onset or acute exacerbation grafted onto chronic complaints may occur. Myelopathic clinical features span the range of cord syndromes. Transverse lesions, motor syndromes, central cord syndrome, Brown-Sequard syndrome, and combined root and cord syndromes are all reported.[12] Myelopathy usually develops insidiously.

Lateral osteophytes may compress the vertebral arteries. The clinical manifestation of cervical spondylosis induced vertebral-basilar symptoms run the gamut from transient ischemic symptoms such as vertigo, drop attacks, and diplopia, to a completed Wallenberg's lateral medullary syndrome secondary to infarction in the territory of the posterior inferior cerebellar artery.

Physical findings in patients with symptomatic chronic cervical disc degeneration will be similar to those seen in the acute disorders. Typical radicular or cord signs will be present depending upon the site of neural pathology.

Radiologic Findings

The typical radiologic findings in cervical spondylosis are[34]:

1. Intervertebral disc space narrowing.
2. Anterior and posterior osteophyte formation at this vertebral body margin.
3. Sclerosis of the bone beneath the vertebral end plate.
4. Osteophyte formation adjacent to the neurocentral lip.
5. Osteoarthritic changes in apophyseal joints with osteophyte formation.
6. Narrowing of the sagittal diameter of the spinal canal.

Clinicians should be aware that the normal sagittal diameter of the canal from C_3 to C_7 is 13–18 mm. A sagittal diameter of 12 or 13 mm suggests possible cord compression, while values of 11 mm or below are very significant for a correlation with cord compression.[14,16] Measurement of this sagittal diameter is shown in Figure 11-2.

Myelopathy and CAT are suggested in the preoperative evaluation of spondylosis patients with root or cord syndromes.

A major caveat must be mentioned. As many as 80 percent of people over 55 have typical radiologic changes of cervical spondylosis.[66] Many of these patients have no symptoms at all. Furthermore, symptoms may be coming from an area of minimal, rather than maximal, X-ray changes. The clinician must do careful clinical/radiological correlation, especially when surgery is being considered, lest the surgeon operate on an abnormal area that is not producing symptoms.

Management

Patients with radiculopathy secondary to chronic cervical disc degeneration may be managed in a similar fashion to the acute syndromes. Similar physical measures are employed. However, chronic radiculopathy patients should receive little in the way of controlled substances. Frequently, similar measures such as a neck collar, heat, and traction may also relieve the spondylosis induced headaches. Use of a neck collar may also reduce neck motion enough to prevent flexion-extension induced vertebral-basilar insufficiency symptoms. Patients with myelopathy do not respond well to conservative measures and surgical decompression is recommended in most cases.

The indications for surgical intervention in chronic cervical disc degeneration are[12,15-17,32,66]:

1. Acute or progressive signs of cord pathology.
2. Radicular deficit which does not resolve with conservative management.
3. Intractable pain—a controversial area.
4. Significant vertebral artery compression.

Again, the surgical approach may be anterior or posterior.[56] A definite indication for the anterior approach is cervical instability secondary to degenerative disease or trauma.[56]

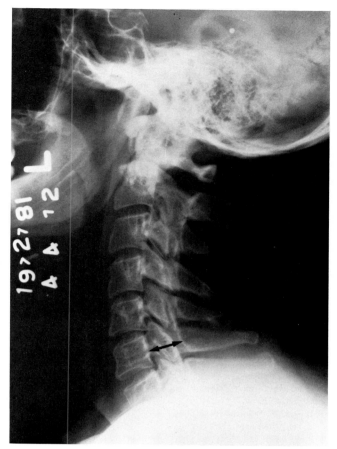

Fig. 11-2. Lateral cervical spine x-ray indicating anatomic points for measuring the sagittal diameter of the spinal canal.

Definite indications for the posterior approach include degenerative cervical disc disease with myelopathy and multiple areas of compression and compression of the cord above C_{2-3} or below $C-T_1$.[56] These areas cannot be accessed by an anterior approach. Either approach may be appropriate for a laterally placed hypertrophic chronic disc herniation or a single midline hypertrophic spur causing cord compression.[56]

Results of surgery are variable. In radicular syndromes, more acute cases probably do better than more chronic ones.[32] In cases with myelopathy, results may depend upon how much irreversible damage has occurred within the cord,[14,32] ie, patients operated earlier in the course of their myelopathy do better. The multi-level cord compression patients treated by posterior surgery appear to have the poorest results.[56]

The term "failed neck syndrome" has been coined for those patients who fail to do well after neck surgery. Causes of the failed neck syndrome are said to be[17]:

1. Selecting the incorrect patient for surgery. This is usually surgery done for pain only without neural deficit. This is also said to occur with poor judgment in operating on certain litigation cases.

2. Performing an incorrect operation—eg, an operation at the wrong level, failure to decompress the root or cord properly, unwarranted surgery at additional levels, or unusual surgical trauma.

3. A misleading or confusing diagnosis—eg, radiographic and clinical findings not correlated.

4. Hazardous situations—eg, intubation of the myelopathy patients worsening them, postoperative quadriplegia with history suggesting this might occur.

The diagnosis and treatment of patients with neck pain and pain in related body areas secondary to cervical soft tissue injury is challenging. Hopefully the material in this chapter will provide the basic guidelines for meeting the challenge.

REFERENCES

1. American Medical Association, Guides to the Evaluation of Permanent Impairment, 2nd edition. Chicago, American Medical Association, 1984

2. Brown MD: The Pathophysiology of Disc Disease. Orthop Clin North Am 2:359–370, 1971

3. Burney RG, Moore PA, Duncan GH: Management of Head and Neck Pain. Int Anesthesiol Clin 21:79–96, 1983

4. Cailliet R: Neck and Arm Pain, 2nd edition. Philadelphia, FA Davis, 1981

5. Capistrant TD: Thoracic Outlet Syndrome in Whiplash Injury. Ann Surg 185:175–178, 1977

6. Chrisman OD, Gervais RF: Otologic Manifestations of the Cervical Syndrome. Clin Orthop 24:34–39, 1962

7. Cintron E, Gilula LA, Murphy WA, et al: The Widened Disk Space: A Sign of Cervical Hyperextension Injury. Radiology 141:639–644, 1981

8. Cloward RB: Acute Cervical Spine Injuries. Clin Symp 32:2–32, 1980

9. DePalma AF, Rothman RH: The Intervertebral Disc, Philadelphia, W.B. Saunders, 1970

10. DePalma AF, Subin DK: Study of the Cervical Syndrome. Clin Orthop 38:135–142, 1965

11. Dublin AB, McGahan JP, Reid MH: The Value of Computed Tomographic Metrizamide Myelography in the Neuroradiological Evaluation of the Spine. Radiology 146:79–86, 1983

12. Dunsker SB: Cervical Spondylotic Myelopathy: Pathogenesis and Pathophysiology, in Dunsker SB (ed): Cervical Spondylosis. New York, Raven, 1981, pp 119–134

13. Dunsker SB: Hyperextension and Hyperflexion Injuries of the Cervical Spine, in Youmans JR (ed): Neurological Surgery, 2nd edition. Philadelphia, W.B. Saunders, 1982, pp 2338–2343

14. Ehni G: Extradural Spinal Cord and Nerve Root Compression from Benign Lesions of the Cervical Area, in Youmans JR (ed): Neurological Surgery, 2nd edition. Philadelphia, W.B. Saunders, 1982, pp 2562–2573

15. Ehni G: Cervical Arthrosis, Chicago, Year Book, 1984

16. Epstein BS, Epstein JA, Jones MD: Anatomicoradiological Correlation in Cervical Spine Discal Disease and Stenosis. Clin Neurosurg 25:148–173, 1978

17. Fager CA: Failed Neck Syndrome: An Ounce of Prevention. Clin Neurosurg 27:450–465, 1980

18. Farbman AA: Neck Sprain, Associated Factors. JAMA 223:1010–1015, 1973

19. Fenlin JM Jr: Pathology of Degenerative Disease of the Cervical Spine. Orthop Clin North Am 2:371–387, 1971

20. Fleming JFR: The Neurosurgeon's Responsibility in "Whiplash Injuries." Clin Neurosurg 20:242–252, 1973

21. Gay JR, Abbott KH: Common Whiplash Injuries of the Neck. JAMA 152:1698–1704, 1953

22. Gibson JW: Cervical Syndromes: Use of a Comfortable Cervical Collar as an Adjunct in Their Management. South Med J 67:205–208, 1974

23. Gotten N: Survey of 100 Cases of Whiplash Injury after Settlement of Litigation. JAMA 162:865–867, 1956

24. Greenfield J, Ilfeld FW: Acute Cervical Strain. Evaluation and Short Term Prognostic Factors. Clin Orthop 122:196–200, 1977

25. Harris WH, Hamblen DL, Ojemann RG: Traumatic Disruption of Cervical Intervertebral Disk from Hyperextension Injury. Clin Orthop 60:163–167, 1968

26. Hinoki M, Niki H: Neurological Studies on the Role of the Sympathetic Nervous System in the Formation of Traumatic Vertigo of Cervical Origin. Acta Otolaryngol Suppl 330:185–196, 1975

27. Hirschfeld AH, Behan RC: The Accident Process. JAMA 186:193–199, 300–306, 1963

28. Hohl M: Soft Tissue Injuries of the Neck in Automobile Accidents: Factors Influencing Prognosis. J Bone Joint Surg 56A:1675–1682, 1974

29. Hohl M: Soft Tissue Injuries of the Neck. Clin Orthop 109:42–49, 1975

30. Hoppenfeld S: Physical Examination of the Spine and Extremities. New York, Appleton-Century-Crofts, 1976

31. Howcroft AJ, Jenkins DHR: Potentially Fatal Asphyxia Following a Minor Injury of the Cervical Spine. J Bone Joint Surg 59B:93–94, 1977

32. Hunt WE: Cervical Spondylosis: Natural History and Rare Indications for Surgical Decompression. Clin Neurosurg 27:466–480, 1980

33. Jackson R: The Cervical Syndrome, 4th edition. Springfield, Charles C Thomas, 1978

34. Jeffreys E: Disorders of the Cervical Spine. London, Butterworths, 1980

35. Johnson EW: Conservative Management of Cervical Disc Disease, in Dunsker SB (ed): Cervical Spondylosis. New York, Raven, 1981, pp 145–153

36. Kelsey JL, Githens PB, Walter SD, et al: An Epidemiological Study of Acute Prolapsed Cervical Intervertebral Disc. J Bone Joint Surg 66A:907–914, 1984

37. Kondo K, Molgaard CA, Kurland LT, et al: Protruded Intervertebral Cervical Disk: Incidence and Affected Cervical Level in Rochester, Minnesota, 1950 through 1974. Minnesota Med 64:751–753, 1981

38. LaRocca H: Acceleration Injuries of the Neck. Clin Neurosurg 25:209–217, 1978

39. Lieberman JS: Neuromuscular Electrodiagnosis, in Youmans JR (ed): Neurological Surgery, 2nd edition. Philadelphia, W.B. Saunders, 1982, pp 617–635

40. Lord JW Jr, Rosati LM: Thoracic Outlet Syndromes. Clin Symp 23:3–32, 1971

41. Lysell E: Motion in the Cervical Spine. An Experimental Study on Autopsy Specimens. Acta Orthop Scand Suppl 123, 1969

42. Macnab I: Acceleration Injuries of the Cervical Spine. J Bone Joint Surg 46A:1797–1799, 1964

43. Macnab I: The "Whiplash Syndrome." Orthop Clin North Am 2:389–403, 1971

44. Macnab I: The Whiplash Syndrome. Clin Neurosurg 20:232–241, 1973

45. Macnab I: Cervical Spondylosis. Clin Orthop 109:69–77, 1975

46. Macnab I: Acceleration Extension Injuries of the Cervical Spine, in Rothman RH, Simeone FA (eds): The Spine, 2nd edition. Philadelphia, W.B. Saunders, 1982, pp 647–660

47. Martin GM, Corbin KB: An Evaluation of Conservative Treatment for Patients with a Cervical Disk Syndrome. Arch Phys Med Rehabil 35:87–91, 1954

48. Marvel JP Jr: The Clinical Syndrome of Cervical Disc Disease. Orthop Clin North Am 2:419–433, 1971

49. Modic MT, Weinstein MA, Pavlicek W, et al: Magnetic Resonance Imaging of the Cervical Spine: Technical and Clinical Observations. AJR 141:1129–1136, 1983

50. Murphey F, Simmons JCH, Brunson B: Ruptured Cervical Discs. 1939 to 1972. Clin Neurosurg 20:9–17, 1973

51. Norris SH, Watt F: The Prognosis of Neck Injuries Resulting From Rear-End Vehicle Collisions. J Bone Joint Surg 65B:608–611, 1983

52. Rothman RH: The Pathophysiology of Disc Degeneration. Clin Neurosurg 20:174–182, 1973

53. Rothman RH, Marvel JP Jr: The Acute Cervical Disk. Clin Orthop 109:59–68, 1975

54. Rothman RH, Marvel JP Jr, Baker R: The Conservative Treatment of Cervical Disc Disease. Orthop Clin North Am 2:435–441, 1971

55. Schutt CH, Dohan FC: Neck Injuries to Women in Auto Accidents. A Metropolitan Plague. JAMA 206:2689–2692, 1968

56. Simeone FA, Rothman RH: Cervical Disc Disease, in Rothman RH, Simeone FA (eds): The Spine, 2nd edition. Philadelphia, W.B. Saunders, 1982, pp 440–499

57. Tenicela R, Cook DR: Treatment of Whiplash Injuries by Nerve Block. South Med J 65:572–574, 1972

58. Upton ARM, McComas AJ: The Double Crush in Nerve Entrapment Syndromes. Lancet 2:359–362, 1973

59. Valtowen EJ, Kiuro E: Cervical Traction as a Therapeutic Tool. Scand J Rehabil Med 2:29–36, 1970

60. Weinberger LM: Trauma or Treatment? The Role of Intermittent Traction in the Treatment of Cervical Soft Tissue Injuries. J Trauma 16:377–382, 1976

61. Weir DC: Roentgenographic Signs of Cervical Injury. Clin Orthop 109:9–17, 1975

62. Wickstrom JK, Martinez LJ, Rodriguez R Jr, et al: Hyperextension and Hyperflexion Injuries to the Head and Neck of Primates, in Gurdjian ES, Thomas LM (eds): Neckache and Backache. Springfield, Charles C Thomas, 1970, pp 108–117

63. White AA III, Panjabi MM: The Basic Kinematics of the Human Spine. Spine 3:12–20, 1978

64. Wolf JW Jr, Johnson RM: Cervical Orthoses, in The Cervical Spine Research Society (eds): The Cervical Spine. Philadelphia, J.B. Lippincott, 1983, pp 54–61

65. Yoss RE, Corbin KB, MacCarty CS, et al: Signifi-

cance of Symptoms and Signs in Localization of Involved Root in Cervical Disk Protrusion. Neurology 7:673–683, 1957

66. Young AC: Radiology and Cervical Spondylosis, in Brain R, Wilkinson M (eds): Cervical Spondy-

losis and Other Disorders of the Cervical Spine. Philadelphia, W.B. Saunders, 1967, pp 133–196

67. Zatskin HR, Kreton F: Evaluation of the Cervical Spine in Whiplash Injuries. Radiology 75:577–583, 1960

Andrei Calin

12

The Spine in Ankylosing Spondylitis and Related Conditions

The following chapter will focus on low back pain, lumbrosacral strain, and the different mechanical problems affecting the spine. We now turn to inflammatory spinal disease. It is self-evident that back pain is a vast problem that affects inummerable patients and costs society billions of dollars. The first problem for the physician is to determine whether a patient who presents with back pain has an inflammatory or mechanical problem. The differences in the history and physical findings are summarised in tables 12-1 and 12-2.

Until the last ten years most interest in rheumatology focused on rheumatoid arthritis and systemic lupus erythematosus. Recently there has been an enormous growth in the clinical importance of ankylosing spondylitis and the spondylarthropathies. In part this is because of their close association with HLA, and in part because of the recognition that a substantial number of patients suffer from different forms of these disorders. Professionals in many branches of medicine have been fascinated by developments in this area. It is probable that no other field offers the same chance of unravelling the intricacies of the relationship between genetics and the environment in the pathogenesis of disease. For example, a specific infective agent (eg, Shigella) has been found to precipitate a clearly-defined clinical disorder (Reiter's syndrome) in a genetically-susceptible individual (HLA B27). Over the years, immunogeneticists, geneticists, epidemiologists, bacteriologists, membrane biologists, clinicians (both adult and paediatric), and other investigators have joined in the attempt to clarify our understanding of ankylosing spondylitis, Reiter's disease, psoriatic arthropathy, and other interrelated conditions.

Within the last 20 years ankylosing spondylitis has been clearly demarcated from rheumatoid arthritis. The major forces leading to this separation have included careful clinical observation, painstaking epidemiologic work, attention to pathology, closer radiologic observation, and the development of immunogenetics. These different steps have been summarized in the monograph of Wright and Moll[25] and more recently in a multinational text.[4]

Ankylosing spondylitis itself is an inflammatory arthritis of the spine that always affects the sacroiliac joints and less commonly the peripheral joints. The term derives from

PRINCIPLES OF PHYSICAL MEDICINE AND REHABILITATION IN THE MUSCULOSKELETAL DISEASES

Table 12-1

Differential History in Back Symptoms of Mechanical
and Inflammatory Type

	Mechanical	Inflammatory
Past history	Variable, episodic	Persistent
Family history	Negative	Positive
Onset	Acute	Insidious
Age at onset	15–90	<40
Sleep disturbance	Minor	Often marked
Morning stiffness	Minimal	Marked
Involvement of other systems	Negative	Positive
Effect of exercise	Worse	Better
Effect of rest	Better	Worse
Radiation of pain	Anatomical (S1, L5)	Diffuse (Thoracic, buttock)
Sensory symptoms	Positive	Negative
Motor symptoms	Positive	Negative

ankylos, Greek for *bent or crooked* and *spondylos,* the Greek for vertebra. The term has many eponyms, reflecting both national pride and aetiological conjecture. In the past terms have included *spondylitis ankylopoetica, spondylitis deformans, atrophic spondylitis, Marie-Strumpell's disease, rheumatoid spondylitis* and several other names.

The seronegative spondylarthritides as a group are characterized by involvement of the sacroiliac joints, by peripheral inflammatory arthropathy, and by the absence of rheumatoid factor. The term refers to an inflammatory disease of both the spine and peripheral joints. Additional features include:

1. Pathologic changes concentrated around the enthesis (ie, the site of ligamentous insertion into bone) rather than the synovium. Nonenthesopathic changes may also develop in the eye, the aortic valve, lung parenchyma, and skin.
2. Clinical evidence of overlap occurs between the various seronegative spondylarthritides. Thus, a patient with psoriatic arthropathy may well develop uveitis or sacroiliitis; a patient with inflammatory bowel disease may develop ankylosing spondylitis or mouth ulcers.

Table 12-2

Differential Findings on Examination between Back
Pain of Mechanical and Inflammatory Type

	Mechanical	Inflammatory
Scoliosis	Frequent	Absent
Range of movement decreased	Asymmetrically	Symmetrically
Local tenderness	Local	Diffuse
Muscle spasm	Local	Diffuse
Straight leg raising	Decreased	Normal
Sciatic nerve stretch	Positive	Absent
Hip involvement	Absent	Frequent
Neurodeficit	Positive	Negative
Other systems	Negative	Positive

3. A tendency toward familial aggregation, with the suggestion that these entities breed true within families.

INFLAMMATORY VERSUS MECHANICAL BACK PAIN

Until recently there was little interest in ankylosing spondylitis and perhaps the majority of patients with this condition were wrongly diagnosed and therefore inappropriately treated. The physician must have a low threshold for diagnosing ankylosing spondylitis. Unless every patient who presents with back pain is questioned regarding the nature of the symptoms, the possibility of diagnosing ankylosing spondylitis will be forgotten. We have previously shown that certain features are characteristic of inflammatory rather than mechanical back pain. Specifically, one should consider the possibility of ankylosing spondylitis if three or more of the following aspects are present:

1. Age of onset below 40 years of age,
2. Insidious onset over weeks rather than hours,
3. Duration greater than three months when the patient first presents,
4. Association with morning stiffness,
5. Improvement with exercise.

These features became apparent during a controlled study of different forms of back pain.[9]

Other differential features have been summarized in tables 12-1 and 12-2. It should also be appreciated that patients may present with a pleuritic-like chest pain. This pain is worse on inspiration and is due to insertional tendinitis of the many costosternal and costovertebral muscle insertions.

CLINICAL SUBSETS

The interrelated group of conditions making up the spondylarthopathies (Table 12-3) have a variety of signs and symptoms that emanate from most of the body systems. Even in the reactive arthropathies where the specific infective trigger is recognized, the pathogenesis of these conditions is poorly understood. One can assume that numerous genes interact to define the specific phenotypic expression. Nevertheless, there is overlap and we have to remember that it is never certain whether apparently different disorders are indeed distinct diseases or simply different parts of the same clinical spectrum. [4,12]

The spondylarthropathies include ankylosing spondylitis, Reiter's syndrome (both the postvenereal, or endemic, and the postinfective, or epidemic, forms), the reactive arthritides (due to infections by Yersinia and Salmonella), certain subsets of juvenile arthropathy (juvenile ankylosing spondylitis and the seronegative enthesopathic arthropathy syndrome), enteropathic sacroiliitis (ulcerative colitis and Crohn's disease), psoriatic arthropathy, and perhaps a group of rarer disorders (Behcet's syndrome, Whipple's disease, and pustulotic arthro-osteitis).

These disorders can be categorized according to the specific periarticular or articular involvement. The various spondylarthropathies can be distinguished from one another according to the particular peripheral joints involved, the associated clinical features (ie, urethritis, conjunctivitis, skin involvement), and the manner in which the disease progresses (ie, remission or relapse).[5]

Table 12-3
Individual Conditions that Overlap to
form the Spondylarthropathies

Psoriatic arthropathy
Reiter's Syndrome/Reactive arthropathy[1]
Enteropathic spondylitis (Crohn's Disease & Ulcerative colitis)
Uveitis
Ankylosing spondylitis
JAS[2]
SEA[3]
Pustulotic arthro-osteitis[4]
Behcet's Disease
Whipple's Disease
Undifferentiated spondylitis[5]

1. Campylobacter, Yersinia, Shigella, Salmonella
2. Juvenile ankylosing spondylitis
3. Seronegative enthesopathic arthropathy syndrome
4. Considered by Japanese to be part of spondylarthropathy spectrum (rare in USA and Europe).
5. Undifferentiated spondylitis (ie subset of patients who have spondylo-arthropathic features but who fail to meet criteria for ankylosing spondylitis, Reiter's syndrome or other condition eg dactylitis, uveitis plus unilateral sacroiliitis).

GENETIC BACKGROUND

In contrast to the situation with the various mechanical forms of back pain, hereditary factors are well recognized and play an important role in the development of the spondylarthropathies. Approximately 10–20 percent of HLA B27-positive individuals develop ankylosing spondylitis following an unknown environmental event or develop Reiter's syndrome after exposure to Shigella or other environmental agents.[6,7] The offspring of an individual with HLA B27 have a 50 percent chance of carrying the same antigen and thus, an overall 10 percent chance of developing ankylosing spondylitis or Reiter's syndrome if exposed to a specific arthritogenic trigger. The risk for the B27-postive individual, however, is not as straightforward as suggested above. We now know that randomly selected individuals with HLA B27 may have only a 2–10 percent chance of developing disease,[20] whereas the risk for B27-positive relatives of B27-positive patients with ankylosing spondylitis ranges from 25 to 50 percent.[8,24]

The explanation for the link between HLA B27 and the spondylarthopathies remains unknown. Hypotheses include: (1) B27 acts as a receptor site for an infective agent; (2) B27 is a marker for an immune response gene that determines susceptibility to an environmental trigger; or (3) B27 may induce tolerance to foreign antigens with which it cross-reacts.

The genetics of the HLA system is becoming both better defined and more complicated. For example, it is now recognized that over 30 genes code for the heavy chains of Class I antigens (HLA A, B, and C molecules). The HLA region is now known to include the Class I molecules, Class II molecules (HLA D/DR, the DP antigens, and DQ antigens), and the Class III molecules (the complement allotypes C2, Bf, C4a, and C4b). The recent progress can be summarized by saying that: (1) There are many more allelic series than the well-known HLA A, B, C, D/DR; (2) A single Class I or II molecule carries many different epitopes; and (3) Class I and II molecules in part resemble immunoglobulins. This last point is of particular interest and data now suggest that Class I molecules can interact with not only a large number of foreign exogenous molecules but also with, perhaps, hormones and other autologus molecules.[21]

ANKYLOSING SPONDYLITIS

Criteria for Diagnosis

The criteria for diagnosing ankylosing spondylitis have been evolving in recent years. The New York criteria (Table 12-4) have limitations.[1] For example, precisely what constitutes reduced spinal mobility has not been adequately defined. Also, the criterion based on limitation of chest expansion is somewhat imprecise: it is difficult to measure chest expansion accurately, and the reduction below 2.5 cm occurs late in the course of the disease. A simpler approach defines ankylosing spondylitis as the presence of symptomatic sacroiliitis. A patient with back discomfort and radiologic evidence of sacroiliitis would be diagnosed as having ankylosing spondylitis. Symptomatic sacroiliitis is usually associated with a decreased range of spinal mobility.

Prevalence

Once considered a rare disease, the illness is now known to have a prevalence comparable to that of rheumatoid arthritis. Twenty percent of HLA B27-positive blood donors have symptomatic sacroiliitis. The figure for an open population ranges from 2–20 percent. Because the B27 antigen occurs in 6–14 percent of white individuals, approximately 0.4–1.6 percent of whites have ankylosing spondylitis. For many the disease is unrecognized. The distribution follows the population frequency of HLA B27, being more common in whites than blacks.

Ankylosing spondylitis has often gone undiagnosed; inappropriate diagnostic proce-

Table 12-4
New York Criteria for Diagnosis and Grading of Ankylosing Spondylitis (1966)

A. Diagnosis
  1. Limitation of motion of the lumbar spine in all three planes—anterior flexion, lateral flexion, and extension
  2. History or the presence of pain at the dorsolumbar junction or in the lumbar spine
  3. Limitation of chest expansion to 1 inch (2.5 cm) or less, measured at the level of the fourth intercostal space
B. Grading
  Definite as:
  1. Grade III–IV bilateral sacroiliitis with at least one clinical criterion
  2. Grade III–IV unilateral or Grade II bilateral sacroiliitis with clinical criterion 1 (limitation of back movement in all three planes) or with both clinical criteria 2 and 3 (back pain and limitation of chest expansion)
  Probable as:
  Grade III–IV bilateral sacroiliitis with no clinical criteria

dures lead to erroneous diagnoses (ie, mechanical back disease). Such patients often receive incorrect therapy.

Although ankylosing spondylitis was formerly considered a predominantly male disease, several studies now suggest that there may be a more uniform sex distribution.[6,20] Female patients are less frequently diagnosed, perhaps because physicians and radiologists may be reluctant to diagnose a disease that they consider to be rare in females. The disease may be milder in females and present with a greater number of peripheral joint manifestations.[15] In the past, many women with ankylosing spondylitis were inappropriately diagnosed as having seronegative rheumatoid arthritis.

Clinical Presentation

If several of the screening questions summarized above are positive, radiologic evidence will be needed to confirm the diagnosis of ankylosing spondylitis. In essence, sacroiliitis is sufficient. There may or may not be ascending spinal disease. It remains unknown why some patients develop severe sacroiliac involvement with no additional signs of ankylosing spondylitis while others may have minimal sacroiliitis with lumbar, thoracic, and cervical spine disease. Many radiologists have been unfamiliar with rheumatologic joint disease and have diagnosed ankylosing spondylitis only when there was evidence of major ankylosis of the sacroiliac joints and spine. Ankylosing spondylitis can be diagnosed, however, in the presence of only minimal sacroiliitis. The severity of sacroiliitis is graded from 0 to IV based on the amount of radiographically observed joint distortion. In many patients, the disease does not progress beyond Grade II or III.

Early change in the lumbar spine is manifested as squaring of the superior and inferior margins of the vertebral body. This phenomenon is due to inflammatory disease at the site of insertion of the outer fibres of the anulus fibrosus (ie, enthesopathy). Later changes result in the classic, though rare, bamboo spine. Comparable spinal changes are seen in primary ankylosing spondylitis and in the spondylitis associated with the inflammatory bowel disease. In spondylitis associated with Reiter's syndrome and psoriatic arthropathy, however, the changes tend to be asymmetric and random.

Radionuclide scans, computed tomography, and other advanced radiologic techniques have been suggested to evaluate the condition of the sacroiliac joints, but a simple anteroposterior radiograph usually suffices.

Physical Examination

Examination of the spine may reveal muscle spasm and loss of the normal lordosis. In contradistinction to mechanical spinal disease, mobility is usually decreased symmetrically in both anterior and lateral planes. The degree of restriction of forward flexion can be documented by measuring the distraction, on flexion, of two points—the lower point at the level of the lumbosacral junction and the upper point 10 cm above this level. Evidence of a neurodeficit or other signs of nerve entrapment will not be found in patients with inflammatory disease.

Peripheral joint involvement, especially in the lower limb, occurs at some stage in approximately 20–30 percent of cases; the frequency increases with the severity of the disease. Inflammatory disease of the hip and shoulder may produce progressive disability. Enthesopathic features include plantar fasciitis, costochondritis, and Achilles tendinitis.

Laboratory Findings

HLA B27 testing should not be used as a routine screening procedure; it is expensive and usually unnecessary.[3] A diagnosis of ankylosing spondylitis does require radiologic evidence of disease. B27 is present in over 95 percent of white patients.

Other laboratory changes are less striking. Elevation of the erythrocyte sedimentation rate occurs in most patients but may be normal despite severe disease. Elevation of serum IgA[19] and the presence of immune complexes suggest aberrant immunity.[16] Serum creatine phosphokinase and alkaline phosphatase may be raised. Lymphocytes predominate in the synovial fluid, and synovial histologic findings are nonspecific.

Pathology[2]

The synovial lesions of ankylosing spondylitis and rheumatoid arthritis share identical histopathologic characteristics: intimal cell hyperplasia; a diffuse lymphocyte and plasma cell infiltrate; formation of lymphoid follicles; and plasma cells containing IgG, IgA, and IgM. IgM is found less frequently in ankylosing spondylitis than in rheumatoid disease. Synovitis per se, however, does not explain the propensity toward ligamentous ossification and widespread new bone formation observed in ankylosing spondylitis. Inflammation at the enthesis accounts for the unique pathology, or enthesopathy, of ankylosing spondylitis; new bone formation appears to be a specific reparative process occurring at the enthesopathic site. Complications of severe spinal disease include fractures and spondylodiskitis after minimal trauma.

Extra-Skeletal Involvement

Extra-articular features include fatigue, weight loss, and low-grade fever. Cord compression due to spinal fractures or the cauda equina syndrome may cause neurologic symptoms. The effects of systemic involvement and of radiotherapy on the decreased survival of patients with ankylosing spondylitis are well recognized.

Eye Involvement

Uveitis develops in up to 25 percent of patients during their illness. It occurs most often in HLA B27-positive patients with peripheral joint disease but shows no correlation with the severity of the spondylitis. The visual episodes are usually self-limiting but may require local steroid therapy. Progressive visual impairment is more common in Reiter's syndrome than in ankylosing spondylitis.

Pulmonary Disease

Patients with severe disease may exhibit chronic infiltrative and fibrotic changes in the upper lung fields that mimic tuberculosis. Pulmonary ventilation is usually well maintained by the diaphragm, despite the chest wall rigidity. The pulmonary fibrosis is occasionally clinically silent, but most affected patients present with cough, sputum, and dyspnoea. Cyst formation and subsequent Aspergillus invasion may cause haemoptysis.

Cardiovascular Disease

Aortic incompetence, cardiomegaly, and persistent conduction defects occur in 3.5–10 percent with severe spondylitic disease. Cardiac involvement may be clinically silent, or it may dominate the picture. Thickened aortic valve cusps and scar tissue in the root of the aorta represent the major histologic changes.

Amyloidosis

Amyloid deposition is an occasional complication of ankylosing spondylitis, particularly in Europe. It may be present in up to 10 percent of patients, although it appears to be of little clinical significance in most cases.

The Kidney

In contrast to patients with rheumatoid arthritis who may show renal impairment as an expression of disease, renal glomerular function is usually unimpaired in ankylosing spondylitis, despite recognized pathologic changes. An IgA neghropathy, however, has been described in patients with seronegative spondylarthropathy.

Prognosis

Ankylosing spondylitis is a gratifying condition to recognize and treat early: much can be accomplished toward ameliorating symptoms and, perhaps, preventing spinal deformity. The primary objectives are to relieve pain, decrease inflammation, begin remedial strengthening exercises, and maintain good posture and function.

For the individual patient the natural history of disease remains poorly defined. Some patients are destined to have minimal symptoms with pelvic involvement and little or no spinal or extra-spinal disease. For other patients a progressive, widespread disease results in poor functional outcome and even death. Why some patients do well and others do poorly remains unknown. Presumably, additional genes determine the phenotypic expression.[10]

REITER'S SYNDROME

The most common cause of an inflammatory oligoarthropathy in a young male is Reiter's syndrome. This classical triad of urethritis, conjunctivitis, and arthritis represents the one chronic rheumatic disorder related to both a specific genetic background (HLA B27) and a specific infection. Reiter's syndrome is often not self limiting. Progressive disease may result in major disability. The disease may be defined as an episode of arthropathy within one month of urethritis or cervicitis.[23]

Whether a dysentric (epidemic) or a venereal (endemic) infection is the most common precipitating event remains a matter of controversy. In young children, however, the former is the rule. In many cases, the distinction between urethritis as a precipitating factor and urethritis as an integral manifestation of the syndrome remains unclear; the association with veneral disease, however, creates a sense of guilt for the patient. In postvenereal Reiter's syndrome both Chlamydia and Mycoplasma have been implicated. In a patient with a specific predisposing genetic background, a variety of different organisms may be responsible.

Prevalence

The prevalence of Reiter's syndrome remains unknown. The disorder develops in at least 1 percent of patients with nonspecific urethritis. Shigella dysentery is followed by Reiter's syndrome in 1–2 percent of cases (ie, 20 percent of B27-positive patients).

The sex distribution of Reiter's syndrome is difficult to define because the syndrome is diagnosed only with difficulty in females, in whom urethritis is often clinically inapparent. Formes frustes of the syndrome are now being recognized. A woman presenting with uveitis and an inflammatory arthropathy of the knee in association with the HLA B27 antigen may have Reiter's syndrome. Similarly, the disorder is difficult to recognize in children; a diagnosis will usually be made only if an epidemic of dysentery is present and Reiter's syndrome has been recognized in other family members. Postdysenteric Reiter's syndrome almost certainly has an equal sex distribution.

Clinical Picture

Reiter's syndrome should be considered a symptom complex rather than the association of three specific features. The syndrome may present as a tetrad (ie, with the addition of buccal ulceration or balanitis to the classic triad); alternatively, only two of the three cardinal features may be present. Several of the classic features may appear insignificant and be overlooked. For example, the urethritis may be mild, perhaps forgotten; the discharge may be minimal and remembered by the patient only after direct questioning. Balanitis may not be evident unless the prepuce is retracted and the glans penis closely inspected. Buccal ulceration is usually painless and apparent only on close inspection. A red eye may be forgotten or considered irrelevant, and the various skin lesions typified by keratoderma blennorrhagicum may be misdiagnosed.

Rheumatologic features include arthralgias, tenosynovitic episodes, plantar faciitis, and other enthesopathies, as well as frank arthritis. The typical sausage-shaped digit is a frequent occurence related to the disorder's enthesopathic nature.

Some 20 percent of patients with Reiter's syndrome develop sacroiliitis and ascending spinal disease. Whether spondylitis should be considered a complication of the Reiter's syndrome or a manifestation of B27 disease remains unclear. Other radiologic evidence of Reiter's syndrome includes plantar spurs and periosteal new bone formation. Cardiac complications similar to those in ankylosing spondylitis occur late in Reiter's syndrome.

The hyperkeratotic skin lesions seen in Reiter's syndrome cannot be distinguished from those in psoriasis.

Formerly considered a self-limited process, Reiter's syndrome is now known to be a more persistent disease in many patients. About 80 percent of patients have evidence of disease activity when they are re-examined after a five year period.[13]

Laboratory Evaluation

It is unclear whether the presence of HLA B27 correlates with increased severity of Reiter's syndrome. A patient with severe Reiter's syndrome may have an erythrocyte sedimentation rate in the normal range or one as high as 100 mm/hour or more. Synovial fluid analysis is rarely diagnostic, apart from the fact that it reveals a relatively high complement level (reflecting a nonspecific inflammatory reaction), rather than the low level seen in rheumatoid arthritis (reflecting immune complex disease).

Occasionally, the diagnoses of ankylosing spondylitis and Reiter's syndrome may prove difficult to disentangle. Some patients who are diagnosed as having ankylosing spondylitis may have presented originally with Reiter's syndrome, but the episodes of urethritis have subsequently been forgotten by the physician and patient. Similarly, patients diagnosed as having Reiter's syndrome may actually have ankylosing spondylitis with peripheral joint disease and a chance occurrence of urethritis.

THE REACTIVE ARTHROPATHIES[14]

Reactive arthropathy refers to an inflammatory arthritis that follows an infection, in which there is no microbial invasion of the synovial space. The B27-linked arthropathies following Shigella, Salmonella, Yersinia, and Campylobacter jejuni infection are in this group. Why some patients develop only an arthropathy whereas others have the full spectrum of Reiter's disease after exposure to one of these agents in unknown.

Yersinia Infection

Yersinia enterocolitica infection may present with fever, mild gastrointestal illness, and, following a latent period, polyarthropathy and erythema nodosum, especially in B27-positive individuals. The symptom complex may mimic acute rheumatic fever. The arthropathy may last for weeks or months, and in HLA B27-positive individuals, sacroiliitis may occur.

Salmonellosis

An arthropathy associated with Salmonella infection mimics that caused by Yersinia.

JUVENILE CHRONIC ARTHROPATHY[17]

Chronic arthritis in a child or teenager often persists into adulthood; therefore an awareness of juvenile arthropathy is relevant when attending adult patients. Until recently, the term juvenile rheumatoid arthritis was used, inappropriately, to describe all forms of childhood arthritis. As in adults, arthritis in children may be associated with psoriasis, inflammatory bowel disease, and other conditions. The acute systemic form, Still's disease, presents with fever, rash, and toxicity in young children who are negative for B27 and rheumatoid factor (IgM-anti-IgG). Still's disease is also recognized in adults.

Another subset (in the spondylarthropathy group) consists largely of adolescent males who predominantly exhibit oligoarthropathy affecting the large joints of the lower limbs: such individuals are frequently positive of HLA B27. This group may develop sacroiliitis or ankylosing spondylitis; the presence of B27 is associated with spinal disease involvement.

It remains unclear why children with ankylosing spondylitis present first with peripheral joint disease, unlike the adult. It may be that the developing sacroiliac joints and spine are not susceptible to the pathologic process or that the two entities are in fact different in spite of a shared genetic background.

Another group includes B27-negative individuals (usually females less than five years of age) presenting with an oligoarthropathy characterized by a positive fluorescent antinuclear antibody (FANA) test. These subjects are at risk for developing asymptomatic chronic iridocyclitis, in contrast to FANA-negative and B27-positive patients, who develop clinically obvious acute uveitis. A few older children (preponderantly females) develop a seropositive, nodular, and erosive disease that resembles adult rheumatoid arthritis. A B27-related syndrome known as seronegative enthesopathy and arthropathy (SEA syndrome) is now also recognized in children.

THE ENTEROPATHIC ARTHROPATHIES[18]

Two major clinical patterns of arthropathy associated with inflammatory bowel disease (ulcerative colitis and Crohn's disease) are peripheral arthropathy and spondylarthropathy.

Peripheral Arthropathy

Approximately 20 percent of individuals with severe Crohn's disease or ulcerative colitis develop an acute migratory inflammatory polyarthritis, often of abrupt onset and involving the larger joints of the lower extremities. The arthritis resolves in weeks or months. Arthritis flare-ups usually parallel exacerbations of the underlying disorder. The pathogenesis of the joint complication is unknown. B27 antigen is not present. Treatment is directed at the primary disorder and is more effective in ulcerative colitis than in Crohn's disease.

Spondylarthritis

About one patient in five with inflammatory bowel disease develops sacroiliitis and, occasionally, severe ankylosing spondylitis. The spinal disease may precede the bowel disease or follow it. There is no correlation between the severity of the bowel disorder and the spondylitis, which mimics primary ankylosing spondylitis rather than the spondylitis associated with psoriasis or Reiter's syndrome. Therapy is as for classic ankylosing spondylitis (see below). Despite the bowel disease, the nonsteroidal anti-inflammatory drugs are usually well tolerated.

About 50 percent of individuals with both inflammatory bowel disease and ankylosing spondylitis are B27-positive, a percentage lower than that found in patients with primary ankylosing spondylitis.

A postintestinal bypass syndome consisting of arthropathy and occasionally dermatitis is well recognized. Immune alterations have been described in these patients, and B27 is occasionally associated with this syndrome.

PSORIATIC ARTHROPATHY[22]

Different subsets of psoriatic arthropathy are recognized, several forms of which appear to be enthesopathic rather than purely synovitic. Uveitis, sacroiliitis, and ascending spinal disease occur in up to 20 percent of cases. Patients are seronegative for rheumatoid factor and exhibit sausage digits and characteristic radiologic changes. The disease may be markedly destructive.

Psoriasis itself is a genetically determined disease, associated with HLA B13, HLA

Bw17, and HLA Cw6. Moreover, HLA B27 is present in approximately 20 percent of individuals with psoriatic arthropathy even in the absence of sacroiliitis. HLA Bw38, HLA DR4, and HLA DR7 appear to be genetic markers for patients with peripheral arthropathy. About 50 percent of psoriatic spondylitis patients are B27-negative; thus, as with inflammatory bowel disease, other genetic or environmental factors are relevant.

Psoriatic arthropathy is a common disease, occurring in about 20 percent of individuals with psoriasis, particularly in those patients with psoriatic nail disease. Women are affected slightly more commonly than men, in contrast to the more marked sex distribution in rheumatoid disease. Several forms of psoriatic arthropathy, separated by indistinct boundaries, have been described.

1. Asymmetric oligoarthropathy. In general, there is little relationship between joint and skin activity. Patients with this common form of psoriatic arthropathy remain seronegative for rheumatoid factor. Asymmetric involvement of both large and small joints is seen; the sausage-shaped digit is common. A disparity is often observed between the clinical appearance and subjective symptoms. Any patient presenting with this form of arthropathy should be carefully examined for signs of psoriasis (scalp, umbilicus, gluteal region, and nails). In the past, many such individuals were considered to have seronegative rheumatoid arthritis.
2. Symmetric polyarthropathy resembling rheumatoid arthritis. Rarely, the pattern of arthritis may be indistinguishable from that seen in rheumatoid disease. This form may represent coincidental rheumatoid arthritis in a patient with psoriasis.
3. Arthritis mutilans. A resorptive arthropathy, arthritis mutilans is the severest form of destructive arthritis. The telescoping digits appear as the so-called opera-glass hand.
4. Psoriatic spondylitis. Approximately 20 percent of subjects with psoriatic arthropathy have radiologic sacroiliitis (ankylosing spondylitis). This is frequently silent. Indeed, quite dramatic spinal changes may be seen radiologically without any symptoms.
5. Psoriatic nail disease and distal interphalangeal joint involvement. Nail pitting, transverse depressions, and subungual hyperkeratosis often occur in association with distal interphalangeal joint disease. The relationship between the psoriasis and the arthritis remains unclear.

Laboratory Features

An elevated erythrocyte sedimentation rate, anaemia, and rarely, hyperuricaemia may occur. The frequency of positive tests for rheumatoid factor is the same as that found in the general population. The synovial tissue and fluid changes are nonspecific.

Radiologic Findings

Characteristic changes in this sometimes highly destructive disease include whittling of the distal ends of the phalanges, giving the joints a "pencil-and-cup" appearance; extensive bone resorption can result in an opera-glass hand. Erosions, ankylosis, periostitis, sacroiliitis, and ankylosing spondylitis are other typical radiologic findings. The radiological spinal changes seen in ankylosing spondylitis tend to be more symmetrical and less patchy than those seen in psoriatic spondylitis. With the latter there may be skip areas of involvement with more changes distal to the disc space itself.

MISCELLANEOUS ARTHROPATHIES

Behcet's Syndrome[11]

Behcet's syndrome is a multisystem disorder that can mimic many other diseases. Painful oral ulceration occurs in well over 90 percent of patients; genital ulceration, ocular disease, and erythema nodosum appear in 80 percent; and arthritis in 30–60 percent. Thrombophlebitis and neurologic and intestinal involvement are observed in up to one third of patients.

Most cases of Behcet's syndrome occur in the Middle East and Japan, but some are recognized in the United States and Great Britain. Men are affected twice as often as are women; the predominant age range is 15 to 40 years. Genital ulceration and erythema nodosum occur more commonly in female patients. Eye lesions include conjunctivitis, scleritis, retinal vasculitis, and optic neuritis. Because of the multi-system manifestations of Behcet's syndrome, the patient may first be examined by an ophthalmologist, dermatologist, venereologist, rheumatologist, or general internist.

Arthritis associated with Behcet's syndrome is chronic, seronegative, and usually nondestructive. Neurologic involvement may be manifested as minor episodes of brainstem dysfunction, meningoencephalitis, and cranial nerve palsies. There may be intestinal disease including recurrent colitis or occult inflammation. Vasculitis and circulating immune complexes have been noted. Certain patients, especially those in Japan, demonstrate the HLA B5 antigen. HLA B27 is present in some patients with arthritis, and HLA B12 is found in a few patients with mucocutaneous involvement.

Corticosteroid therapy usually results in improvement of symptoms, but recrudescence is common. Relapses have been managed with combined corticosteroid and azathioprine therapy. Chlorambucil has reportedly produced improvement in a few patients. Anectodal evidence suggests that colchicine in a dosage of 0.6 mg twice daily may control the cutaneous manifestations.

Whipple's Disease

Whipple's disease may be considered a very rare form of seronegative spondylarthropathy. It affects males predominantly, the ratio of male to female patients being 9:1. Manifestations include weight loss, malabsorption, fever, hyperpigmentation, and lymphadenopathy. Peripheral joint involvement mimics that seen in inflammatory bowel disease. Sacroiliitis may occur. Diagnosis requires the demonstration of PAS-positive inclusion bodies in macrophages on intestinal biopsy. Prolonged antibiotic therapy has a favorable response.

MANAGEMENT SUMMARY

There is no cure for ankylosing spondylitis. Problems in the managment of this condition are summarized in Table 12-5. The major aims are listed in Table 12-6.

The delay in reaching a diagnosis is the major problem in the management of ankylosing spondylitis. Once the condition is recognized therapy is directed towards education of both patient and family. Following an understanding of the nature of the

Table 12-5
Problems in Management of
Ankylosing Spondylitis

Failure to reach diagnosis
Few or no controlled studies
No cure
Wide spectrum of severity
Uncertain prognosis, varied course
Skeletal and extra-skeletal disease
No known disease modifying agents
NSAIDs all associated with toxicity
Inappropriate expectations of patients

Table 12-6
Major Aims in
Management of
Ankylosing Spondylitis

Patient education
Family education
Genetic counseling
Drug therapy—NSAIDs
Cessation of smoking
Day and night posture
Extension exercises
Swimming
Sex counselling
A multidisciplinary approach:
    Surgery
    Physiotherapy
    Occupational therapy
    Ophthalmology
Patient groups and self-help

disease, the patient is prescribed nonsteroidal anti-inflammatory drugs to decrease the symptoms and increase the well-being. At the same time an aggressive exercise programme is introduced and advice must be given regarding posture, rest, and pleasure activities and type of bedding. For those with severe disease a multidisciplinary approach is of paramount importance.

Indomethacin may be considered the drug of choice and a flow chart suggesting appropriate use is provided in Figure 12-1.

Occasionally emergency conditions develop requiring immediate management and these are summarized in Table 12-7.

Therapy in Reiter's syndrome is more complicated since the course is particularly varied. The major errors in management of this condition are summarized in Table 12-8. The difficulties in management are listed in Table 12-9. The major goals in the treatment are summarized in Table 12-10. A flow chart focusing on drug therapy is given in Figure 12-2.

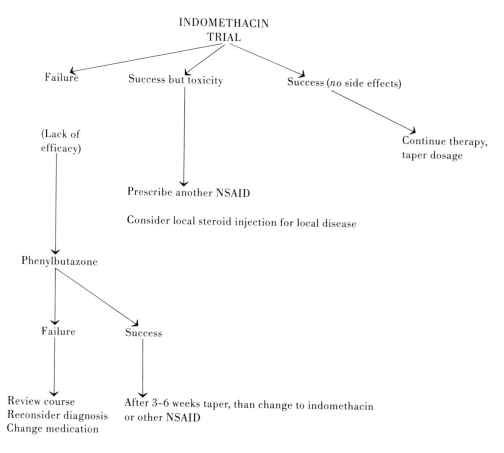

Fig. 12-1. Flow chart of drug therapy in ankylosing spondylitis.

Table 12-7
Emergency Conditions and Appropriate Management in
Ankylosing Spondylitis

Event	Management
Acute knee synovitis and popliteal rupture	Aspirate and intra-articular injection
Spondylodiskitis	Rest
Spinal fracture	Neurosurgical evaluation
Severe uveitis	Ophthalmological evaluation
Cardiac conduction defects	Consider pacing
Drug reaction (various)	Variable

Table 12-8
Major Errors in Management of Reiter's Syndrome

Failure to reach diagnosis
Inability to provide patient with insight
Danger of thrusting feelings of guilt on patient
Recourse to corticosteriod therapy
Too many NSAIDs without appropriate plan
Failure to try phenylbutazone
Loss of contact with patient because of patient's loss of confidence

Table 12-9
Major Difficulties in Management
of Reiter's Syndrome

Inability to define prognosis
Multisystem disease with 'unusual' problems
Tendency towards 'doctor-shopping'
Lack of 'expected' response to therapy
Toxicity of available drugs
Frustrated patients, frustrated doctors

Table 12-10
Major Goals in Management of
Reiter's Disease

Explanation, insight
Family counseling
Indomethacin—Phenylbutazone
Exercise programme as able; swimming is best
Attention to spine, if involved
Occasional use of local steroid injection
Early eye care for inflammatory eye disease
Avoidance of fragmented care
Azathioprine, methotrexate
Physical modalities as needed (foot care, and so on)
Selected referrals for complications, for example:
    Ophthalmology
    Cardiovascular

Principles of Treatment

The patient should be aware that attention to general health is important. Particularly, smoking must be abandoned and an adequate exercise program followed. The avoidance of excess weight should also be considered of paramount importance.

The patient must know that exercises are designed to maintain mobility and posture. Thought must be given to posture while working, playing, and while asleep at night. The purpose of anti-inflammatory drug therapy is to decrease pain and stiffness in order to allow an aggressive exercise program to be followed. Once pain is controlled, a regular exercise program will be feasible and patients will soon appreciate that pain itself is lessened by active exercise. Drugs therefore become less necessary and in general the patient will have a happier disposition regarding the underlying inflammatory disease.

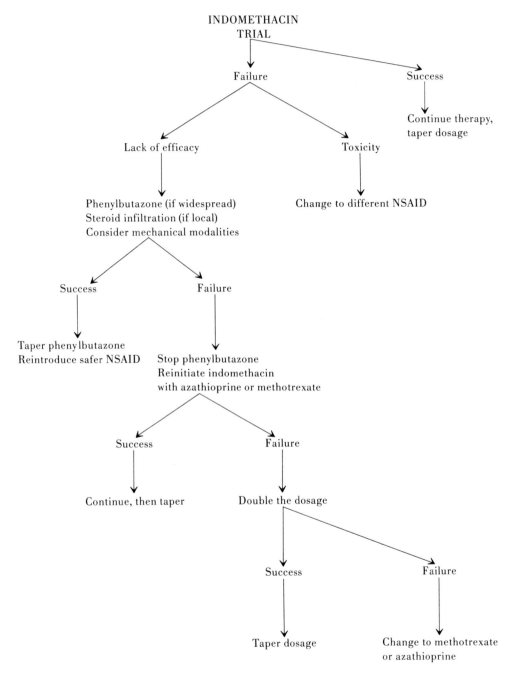

Fig. 12-2. Flow chart detailing drug therapy in Reiter's Syndrome.

Rest

Although rest itself is an anathema for most patients with ankylosing spondylitis, there may be periods when the systemic nature of the disease is such that fatigue becomes an increasing problem. When lying in bed it is important that the back is flat and that no more than a single pillow is used. Lying flat on the abdomen is also useful and provides an appropriate position while resting.

The bed should be firm and if the mattress is not providing sufficient support, a board should be placed between the mattress and the bed frame. A sheet of plywood or chipboard 70 × 150 × 1 cm is ideal. While traveling, many patients find it helpful to put the mattress directly on the floor.

Seating

High chairs with a firm seat and upright, firm back are better for posture of the spine than the more conventional "comfortable" chair. The seat of the chair should not be too long from front to back because the sufferer finds difficulty in placing the lower spine into the base of the back of the chair. Low, soft chairs are to be avoided. After a period of sitting, patients usually find that going for a short walk or at least standing for a few moments is helpful for the back.

Heat

Heat in its various forms often helps with the pain and stiffness. A hot bath or shower is a useful practice before carrying out a specific exercise program.

Back Supports

Corsets and braces are of no value and indeed frequently make ankylosing spondylitis worse. It is important to develop the patient's muscles in order to retain a good posture by natural means. Any support—if it works—allows the muscles to become wasted and weakened, complicating the poor posture. While at work, positions that require stooping are to be avoided. Usually it is simply a question of altering the height of the seat or the desk. The ideal job is one that gives a variety of sitting, standing and walking positions.

Driving

Long journeys by car can be a problem for the patient. Stopping for five minutes every one or two hours is a useful approach. A short, brisk walk will often relieve symptoms. Special mirrors can be fitted to help driving, and particularly reversing. Head rests are advisable to avoid sudden deceleration injuries to the neck.

Exercise

Regarding sporting activities, most body contact sports should be avoided. By contrast, regular swimming is an excellent activity and enhances good posture, muscle strength, and general well-being. Cycling is also beneficial, provided a long-term stooped posture is not maintained.

The author's approach is to discuss with the patient a series of exercises that should be carried out at least twice daily. If one has the good fortune to have available good physiotherapists (ie, physiotherapsts who have an interest in rheumatology and a specific understanding of ankylosing spondylitis) then their help is of great value. One or two good sessions with a physiotherapist will often suffice. Thereafter the patient can be reviewed at six-monthly intervals to make sure that the appropriate exercises are being followed.

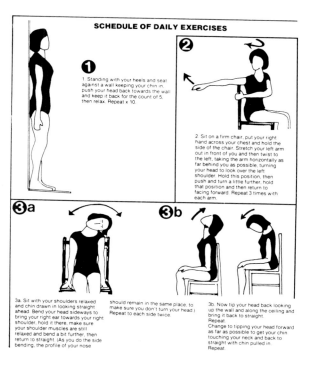

SCHEDULE OF DAILY EXERCISES

1 1. Standing with your heels and seat against a wall keeping your chin in, push your head back towards the wall and keep it back for the count of 5, then relax. Repeat x 10.

2 2. Sit on a firm chair, put your right hand across your chest and hold the side of the chair. Stretch your left arm out in front of you and then twist to the left, taking the arm horizontally as far behind you as possible, turning your head to look over the left shoulder. Hold this position, then push and turn a little further, hold that position and then return to facing forward. Repeat 3 times with each arm.

3a 3a. Sit with your shoulders relaxed and chin drawn in looking straight ahead. Bend your head sideways to bring your right ear towards your right shoulder, hold it there, make sure your shoulder muscles are still relaxed and bend a bit further, then return to straight. (As you do the side bending, the profile of your nose should remain in the same place, to make sure you don't turn your head.) Repeat to each side twice.

3b 3b. Now tip your head back looking up the wall and along the ceiling and bring it back to straight. Repeat. Change to tipping your head forward as far as possible to get your chin touching your neck and back to straight with chin pulled in. Repeat.

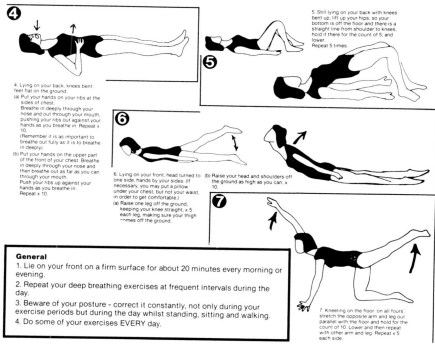

4 4. Lying on your back, knees bent, feet flat on the ground.
(a) Put your hands on your ribs at the sides of chest. Breathe in deeply through your nose and out through your mouth, pushing your ribs out against your hands as you breathe in. Repeat x 10. (Remember it is as important to breathe out fully as it is to breathe in deeply).
(b) Put your hands on the upper part of the front of your chest. Breathe in deeply through your nose and then breathe out as far as you can through your mouth. Push your ribs up against your hands as you breathe in. Repeat x 10.

5 5. Still lying on your back with knees bent up, lift up your hips, so your bottom is off the floor and there is a straight line from shoulder to knees, hold it there for the count of 5, and lower. Repeat 5 times.

6 6. Lying on your front, head turned to one side, hands by your sides. (If necessary, you may put a pillow under your chest, but not your waist, in order to get comfortable.)
(a) Raise one leg off the ground, keeping your knee straight, x 5 each leg, making sure your thigh comes off the ground.
(b) Raise your head and shoulders off the ground as high as you can, x 10.

7 7. Kneeling on the floor (on all fours), stretch the opposite arm and leg out parallel with the floor and hold for the count of 10. Lower and then repeat with other arm and leg. Repeat x 5 each side.

General
1. Lie on your front on a firm surface for about 20 minutes every morning or evening.
2. Repeat your deep breathing exercises at frequent intervals during the day.
3. Beware of your posture - correct it constantly, not only during your exercise periods but during the day whilst standing, sitting and walking.
4. Do some of your exercises EVERY day.

Fig. 12-3. Daily exercise regimen for Ankylosing Spondylitis

The purpose of the exercises is to make the patient conscious of the posture and to enhance mobility. My approach is to tell the patient that if they are 5 feet 6 inches today, they should be 5 feet 7 inches by Christmas. By the end of next year they should reach 5 feet 8 inches. If the patient can understand that the purpose of the exercise is stretching upwards, extending all joints, then they will achieve the correct approach to the exercise program. A specific schedule of daily exercises is summarized in Figure 12-3. This schedule has been devised in conjunction with the National Ankylosing Spondylitis Society—for an annual subscription of about $10 a year patients can become a member of this Society, benefiting from an excellent newsletter and a wealth of information (National Ankylosing Spondylitis Society, 6 Grosvenor Crescent, London SW1X 7ER, England. Director: Fergus Rogers [or contact Dr. A. Calin, NASS Medical Adviser, Royal National Hospital for Rheumatic Diseases, Upper Borough Walls, Bath BA1 1RL, England]).

Surgery

Surgery has only a minimal place in the management of ankylosing spondylitis. Arthroplasty may be appropriate for markedly damaged joints and rarely spinal osteotomy for ridding the patient of an undue degree of spinal flexion.

REFERENCES

1. Bennett PHJ, Burch TA: New York symposium on population studies in the rheumatic diseases. Bull Rheum Dis 17:453, 1967

2. Bywaters EGL: Pathology of the spondylarthropathies, in Calin A (ed): Spondylarthropathies. Orlando, Grune & Stratton, 1984, pp. 43–68

3. Calin A: HLA-B27 in 1982: reappraisal of a clinical test (editorial). Ann Intern Med 96:114, 1982

4. Calin A (ed): Spondylarthropathies. Orlando, Grune & Stratton, 1984, pp. 1–427

5. Calin A: Spondylarthropathies: an overview, in Calin A (ed): Spondylarthropathies. Orlando, Grune & Stratton, 1984, pp. 1–8

6. Calin A, Fries JF: Striking prevalence of ankylosing spondylitis in healthy W27 positive males and females: A controlled study. N Engl J Med 293:835, 1975

7. Calin A, Fries JF: An experimental epidemic of Reiter's syndrome revisited: Follow-up evidence on genetic and environmental factors. Ann Intern Med 84:564, 1976

8. Calin A, Marder A, Becks E, et al: Genetic differences between B27 positive patients with ankylosing spondylitis and B27 positive healthy controls. Arthritis Rheum 26:1460, 1983

9. Calin A, Porta J, Fries JF, et al: Clinical history as a screening test for ankylosing spondylitis. JAMA 237:2613, 1977

10. Carette S, Graham D, Little H, et al: The natural disease course of ankylosing spondylitis. Arthritis Rheum 26:186, 1983

11. Ehrlich GE: Behcet's syndrome, in Calin A (ed): Spondylarthropathies. Orlando, Grune & Stratton, 1984, pp. 241–252

12. Engleman E, Bombardier C, Hochberg MC: Conference on epidemiology of rheumatic diseases: specific needs of developing and developed countries, Santa Ynes, California, November 1–5, 1982. J Rheumatol 10(suppl 10):1, 1983

13. Fox, R, Calin A, Gerber J, et al: The chronicity of symptoms and disability in Reiter's syndrome: an analysis of 131 consecutive patients. Ann Intern Med 91:190, 1979

14. Leirisalo M, Repo H: Reactive arthritis, in Calin A (ed): Spondylarthropathies. Orlando, Grune & Stratton, 1984, pp. 403–412

15. Marks SH, Barnett M, Calin A: Ankylosing spondylitis in women and men: a case-controlled study. J Rheumatol 4:624, 1983

16. Rosenbaum JT, Theofilopoulos AN, McDevitt HO, et al: Presence of circulating immune complexes in Reiter's syndrome and ankylosing spondylitis. Clin Immunol Immunopathol 18:291, 1981

17. Schaller JG: Chronic childhood arthritis and the spondylarthropathies, in Calin A (ed): Spondylarthropathies. Orlando, Grune & Stratton, 1984, pp. 187–208

18. Schumacher HR: Enteropathic arthropathies, in Calin A (ed): Spondylarthropathies. Orlando, Grune & Stratton, 1984, pp. 209–240

19. Trull AK, Panayi GS: Serum and secretory IgA

immune response to Klebsiella pneumoniae in ankylosing spondylitis. Clin Rheumatol 2:331, 1983

20. van der Linden SM, Valkenburg HA, De Jongh BM, et al: The risk of developing ankylosing spondylitis in HLA-B27 positive individuals. A comparison of relatives of spondylitis patients with the general population. Arthritis Rheum 27: 241–249, 1984

21. van Rood: HLA as regulator. Ann Rheum Dis 43:665–672, 1984

22. Vasey FB, Espinoza LR: Psoriatic arthropathy, in Calin A (ed): Spondylarthropathies. Orlando, Grune & Stratton, 1984, pp. 151–186

23. Willkens RF: Criteria, in Calin A (ed): Spondylarthropathies. Orlando, Grune & Stratton, 1984, pp. 9–20

24. Woodrow JC, Nichol FE, Whitehouse GH: Genetic studies in ankylosing spondylitis. Brit J Rheumatol (suppl 2) 22: 12–17, 1983

25. Wright V, Moll JMH: Seronegative Polyarthritis. Amsterdam, North Holland, 1976.

Myron M. LaBan

13

Low Back Pain, Lumbosacral Strain, and Lumbar Disc Disease

Lumbosacral pain, like the common cold, has until only recently remained a diagnostic enigma, often refractory to treatment. A quality of life impaired by the marked physical, psychological, social, and economic consequences of chronic low back pain has been historically neglected by medical research. Helping to dispel some of the frustration previously associated with the diagnosis and treatment of this syndrome are recent advances in understanding the pathophysiology and mechanical function of the lumbar spine. These newer diagnostic techniques, which include water soluble contrast medium for myelography, computerized body tomography, magnetic resonance imaging, discograms, and electroneuromyography, are helping to redirect clinical treatment. Increasing diagnostic sophistication has been paralleled by long overdue recognition that the vast majority of back pain complaints are not surgical problems and are amendable to appropriate medical treatment. As a corollary, it is equally important to emphasize the imperatives of identifying a surgical problem early, as to minimize postoperative disability as a consequence of permanent neurologic impairment. As with medical therapy, a rational and informed opinion, with respect to surgical treatment, must be predicated on an accurate diagnosis, a failure of appropriate, conservative therapy, and a recognition of surgical indications.[23]

PREVALENCE OF LOW BACK PAIN

Lumbosacral pain affects 70–80 percent of the population of most industrialized countries, 10–15 percent of which are affected annually.[43] Hult, in a study of Swedish industrial and forest workers, reported an 80 percent frequency of low back pain and a 60 percent incidence in light and heavy industry workers between ages 25 and 59 years of age.[10,11] The majority of cases having incapacitating lumbosacral pain experienced their initial symptoms before the age of 30.

In the United States back and spinal disability are the most frequent chronic condi-

PRINCIPLES OF PHYSICAL MEDICINE AND REHABILITATION
IN THE MUSCULOSKELETAL DISEASES

©1986 Grune & Stratton, Inc.
ISBN 0-8089-1773-0 All rights reserved.

tions limiting vocational activity in patients younger than 45 years of age.[15] Between the ages of 45 and 65, back pain ranks third after heart disease and arthritis as a major cause of chronic disability. With respect to days of restricted activity, bed confinement and loss of work time, injuries ranked second only to respiratory disease. Of this number 33 percent or 24.5 million injuries consisted of sprains, strains, dislocations, and/or fractures. Extrapolating statistics for 1980 from the State of California, Bonica estimates that of this number there were approximately 11 million low back injuries producing 120 million days of restricted activity, 30 million days of bed confinement, and a loss of 25 million working days.[4]

In an epidemiologic survey of the psychological and social factors associated with lumbosacral pain, Nagi,[36] in a random sample, interviewed 1135 respondents of whom 18 percent reported frequent episodes of low back pain. The incidence of low back discomfort was greater among females, equal between blacks and whites, increased directly with age, and varied inversely with education. As might be expected, the less well educated were more likely to perform heavier labor.

As an immediate and growing medical and economic problem the number of patients with disabling back pain in the United States appears to be epidemic. An estimated 2 percent of all employees annually experience either their initial or recurrent episodes of compensable back injury. Both the frequency of occurrence and, to a greater extent, related costs are accelerating at rates in excess of those associated with other injuries. There has been a concurrent increase in the number of surgical procedures performed for low back disorders. In nonfederal hospitals during 1975, 149,000 discectomies, 33,000 spinal fusions, 11,000 operations for spinal fractures, and 4000 laminectomies for spinal cord pathology were performed.[37]

Surgery, like more "conservative" medical therapy, has pain relief as its immediate goal. To the degree that this goal has not been obtained by antecedent treatment, surgery can still be regarded as a salvage procedure applicable to only the most intractible situations, where progressive neurological dysfunction or intransigent pain of neurogenic origin persists despite definitive medical therapy. The reported rate of success for disc excisions varies greatly with the presenting symptoms. Sciatica is the symptom most likely to be responsive to surgery. When lumbosacral pain preeminates the postoperative course is less successful. Many large series have demonstrated an acceptable 50 percent postoperative pain-free state[8] with subsequent successive surgery often counterproductive. Waddell[47] reported that after the third surgical procedure, the patients were in more pain than they had experienced preoperatively.

The antecedent discussion has suggested by cited example the wide spread prevalence of low back pain in our society. Some of the determinants involved in this ubiquitous problem have been discussed. When the patient fails to respond to acute pain management and the disability becomes chronic, iatrogenic complications, including drug dependency and the sequelae of failed surgery including the battered root syndrome, may intrude. Persistent pain can also predispose to additive psychological, social, and economic deprivation.

Psychological factors associated with chronic back pain tend to "color" the diagnosis and treatment effort. Rarely, however, are psychological issues primarily responsible for the initial episode of low back pain. They may, however, contribute to the circumstances predisposing to an industrial accident. Later in the rehabilitation process, they can become paramount and in these circumstances should be recognized early and dealt with in the course of treatment.

Lumbosacral pain remains primarily a symptom of an underlying physical disorder. Its etiology is as diverse as are the many anatomic structures of the lumbosacral spine itself and their complex interreactions. Additionally, pain of visceral, vascular, and neurogenic origin extrinsic to the lumbosacral spine, can initially present as a complaint of low back pain. Pathology of the spine itself however, or its contiguous structures, remain the primary cause of low back pain. This discomfort is usually experienced as pain confined to the low back only or can be associated with leg pain. Typically it is relieved by bed rest and aggravated by activity.

Lumbosacral pain will be discussed with reference to the structures involved, including the osseous components, the pelvic articulations and hips, the spinal cord and lumbosacral roots, the paraspinal muscles and associated soft tissues. In this regard the time honored diagnosis of "acute lumbosacral strain," although hallowed by tradition, should be forever banned as an acceptable diagnostic entity. Contemporary practice demands a more sophisticated and accurate diagnosis to which an appropriate treatment program can be tailored. Presented is a clinician's approach to the management of both acute and chronic lumbar pain, which philosophically depends on the team approach, utilizing the multivaried skills of the physiatrist, neuroradiologist, physical and occupational therapists, and, when necessary, the surgeon or psychiatrist.[23]

Pathomechanics of Lumbar Spinal Osteoarthritis

A rational approach to the diagnosis and treatment of low back pain and/or sciatica should be predicated on an understanding of the degenerative spinal process. Initially beginning with an alteration in the hydroscopic quality of the nucleus pulposus, it can progress from annular degeneration of a singular disc to multilevel involvement. Sequential disc degeneration with associated zygoapophyseal joint compromise can be associated with relatively infrequent disc prolapses. More often progressive posterior facet disease is associated with foraminal or spinal canal encroachment, producing symptoms of lateral or central spinal stenosis.

The three joint complex formed by the disc anteriorly and the paired posterior articulations are mechanically interlinked. Alteration of function due to pathology at any one of these articulations ultimately contributes to dysfunction and ensuing pathology at the others, as well as at the spinal segments above and below.

Progressive trauma to the zygoapophyseal joints leads to degenerative osteoarthritis, typical of that seen in other true diarthrodial joints. The initial synovitis is superseded by varying degrees of articular cartilage pathology. Recurrent joint effusion and cartilage thinning produces capsular laxity and predisposes to joint instability. The proliferative phase of the osteoarthritic process leads to the development of osteophytes. The diameter of the spinal canal can be reduced by the anterior protrusion of these osteophytes on the inferior articular process, narrowing of the lateral recess by anterior-medial protrusion off the superior articulating process.

Aging and trauma both contribute to the degenerative disc process involving both the annulus fibrosis and the nucleus pulposus. Initial biochemical changes within the nucleus reduce its hydrophilic affinity and thereby predisposes the annulus to altered loading. Circumferential tears in the annulus may subsequently develop with disc narrowing, a reflection of annular bulging. These circumferential tears may coalesce to form a singular radial tear, permitting nuclear material to acutely herniate as a "ruptured disc." The posterior-lateral portion of the annulus is most vulnerable to protrusions of this type.

Predisposing factors in this regard include caudal narrowing of the reinforcing posterior longitudinal ligament, facet malalignment, and variations in the cross-sectional vertebral shape from higher to lower lumbar levels. Acute midline herniations (Fig. 13-1) occur less often, but with the potential for disasterous consequences to the cauda equina, including paraparesis and loss of sphincter control.

Combined retrogressive and proliferative changes in the disc and posterior joints result in clinical symptoms and roentgenographic changes referred to (Fig. 13-2) as the combined three-joint complex degeneration. Three distinct entities have been described associated with this condition, each having specific clinical symptoms, including degenerative spondylolisthesis, lateral, and central spinal stenosis.[20]

Degenerative spondylolisthesis occurs most often at the lumbar 4–5 level with the lumbar four vertebral body subluxed forward on the lumbar five vertebra. Segmental instability at this level occurs as a consequence of disc space narrowing and posterior joint

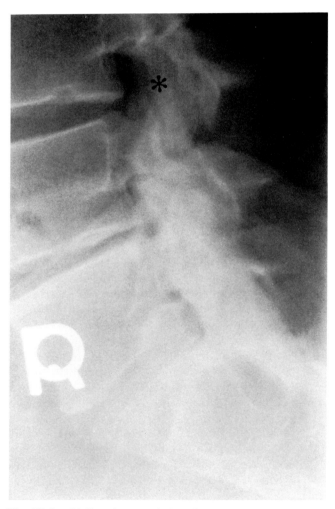

Fig. 13-1.   Midline herniated disc (*) associated with urinary retention.

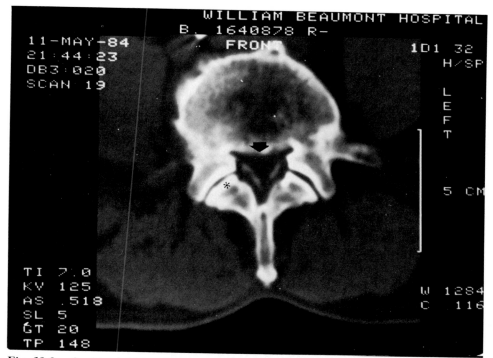

Fig. 13-2. Combined 3-jointed complex degeneration, including bulging disc anteriorly (arrow) and zygoapophyseal joints (*) posteriorly predisposing to segmental instability.

cartilage degeneration. Central, as well as lateral, spinal canal narrowing occurs with the potential for entrapment of the lumbar five root between the posterior aspect of the fifth lumbar vertebral body and the anterior displaced inferior articular process of lumbar four.

Lateral recess stenosis occurs with disc space narrowing, posterior facet degeneration, and subluxation of the superior articular process of the lower vertebrae forward and upward into the lateral spinal canal. Osteophytes and other joint proliferative changes associated with capsular thickening mechanically serve to further narrow the lateral recess, as does the position of spinal rotation and extension.

Central spinal stenosis (Fig. 13-3) with narrowing of the anterior-posterior diameter of the spinal canal is associated with the formation of osteophytes from the vertebral bodies and discal bulging. Posteriorly, redundancy of the ligamentum flava, subluxation and hypertrophy of the inferior articular processes, and thickening of the lamina can encroach on the canal. Narrowing of the lateral recesses and anterior-posterior diameter of the spinal canal produces the trefoil-shaped canal with its attendant spatial restrictions on both dural contents, including the spinal roots.

Multilevel degenerative changes may progress with successive levels of disc and joint space narrowing, predisposing adjacent levels to altered mechanical stresses. Reductions in the lumbar spinal lordosis, increased vertebral rotation, and subluxation are all direct consequences of this process. Loss of mobility at one spinal segment due to spontaneous or iatrogenic fusion also contribute to altered pathological forces at adjacent vertebral levels accelerating this process. Segmental rigidity of the spine at one level tends to shift the loss of mobility to adjoining levels in an effort to retain flexibility of movement.

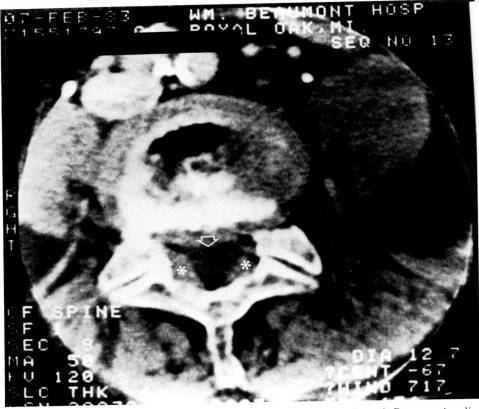

Fig. 13-3.   Central stenosis with narrowing of A-P diameter of spinal canal. Degenerative disc (arrow). Degenerative joints (*) and redundent ligamenta flavum.

Three distinct stages in the evolution of degeneration of the three-joint-complex are clinically recognized.[18] The "stage of dysfunction" is associated with complaints of pain and stiffness, often without radiographic or clinical abnormality. These patients usually respond to conservative therapy including oral analgesics, physical therapy featuring thermotherapy, exercise, and manipulative therapy.

The "stage of instability" is associated with evidence of spinal segment movement. Alteration in posture including limitation of lumbar spinal lordosis, reactive scoliosis, and limitation of both spinal flexion and extension may be associated with neurological abnormality, including reflex and strength alterations and restricted straight leg raising. Roentgenographic changes include disc space narrowing, osteophyte formation, pseudospondylolisthesis and posterior joint subluxation. Conservative treatment again in this stage is usually successful. Bed rest initially complimented with nonsteroidal anti-inflammatory agents, superficial thermotherapy, bracing, or corseting combined with progressive lumbar flexibility and strengthening exercises are appropriate for treating "mechanical" arthrogenic pain. When additionally associated with radicular signs and symptoms, intermittent pelvic traction is also beneficial.

The final "stage of stabilization" is clinically associated with a marked loss of lumbar flexibility. Stiffness as a primary complaint often supersedes pain, particularly following periods of immobility. Prolonged standing and/or walking may precipitate symptoms of either central or lateral stenosis. Localized or radicular pain with or without neuropathic signs, paresthetic complaints of numbness and tingling, and motor symptoms of "weakness" or "instability" are not uncommon. Facet, laminar, and vertebral enlargement associated with osteophyte formation progressing to vertebral fusions are characteristic X-ray features of this stage. The presence of lateral and central stenosis can be demonstrated by specialized visualization procedures, including myelography and computerized body scans.

Conservative therapy appropriate to the earlier stages of degeneration here too usually provides symptomatic relief for this group of patients. In those unresponsive to medical and physical therapy, or with progressive neurogenic deficit and/or intractible pain, surgical decompression appropriate to alleviating the inciting anatomical deficit can be recommended.[45]

Concurrent senescent changes can also occur within the paired sacroiliac joints. Early in the process there may be little to no correlation between the severity of symptoms and radiographic evidence of joint degeneration. Marked pain and disability can be associated with "normal" X-rays of the sacroiliac joints. Pain is usually experienced over the joints themselves radiating to the hips and posterior thighs in the distribution of the first and second sacral roots. The discomfort is usually worse at night, often bilateral, alternating from side to side. Acute exacerbations of pain can be precipitated by exercise or following prolonged sitting. "Weakness" is an occasional complaint, with stiffness, primarily in the morning, a predominant feature of sacroiliitis.

As in the facet joints of the spine, three stages of degeneration can be clinically identified. The *stage of dysfunction* occurs early in adult life while the sacroiliac articulations remain true diarthrodial joints, later stages develop as these joints become amphiarthrodial progressing to complete ankylosis. Degrees of mobility can be identified in these articulations varying with both age and sex of the individual. Pregnancy always increases articular mobility by the fourth month of gestation. With advancing age in both sexes this mobility is progressively reduced. In males, motion starts to diminish during the fourth decade and in females near the end of the fifth decade.[41]

During the secondary *stage of instability* pelvic X-rays with alternate leg weight bearing (Fig. 13-4) may demonstrate pubic symphysis instability in excess of three millimeters. Usually the instability is greater on the symptomatic side.[25] Any one of the "three-joint-complex" of the pelvis, the paired posterior sacroiliac joints and the anterior pubic symphysis may be painful or demonstrate concurrent X-ray evidence of progressive degenerative change.

The terminal *stage of immobilization* is associated with anatomic and functional ankylosis of these joints. Concomitant with progressive articular degeneration is the formation of osteophytes and articular fibrosis with eventual joint fusion. These changes are seen predominantly in the male, occurring as early as the third decade and progressing to complete fusion in some instances by the fifth decade. These joints normally function as shock absorbers between the pelvis and superincumbent spine, acting as a pivotal fulcrum around which a redistribution of weight occurs to both legs. During normal activity they are exposed to tremendous compressive and shear forces. Both can be increased excessively by maneuvers during lumbar extension requiring lifting and twisting, particularly when these activities occur together.

Treatment consists initially of bed rest, superficial heat, and the judicious use of oral nonsteroidal anti-inflammatory drugs. During the acute stage of sacroiliitis, injecting the symptomatic articulation with a mixture of steroid and lidocaine often produces immedi-

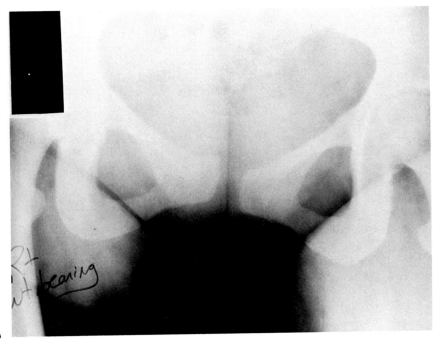

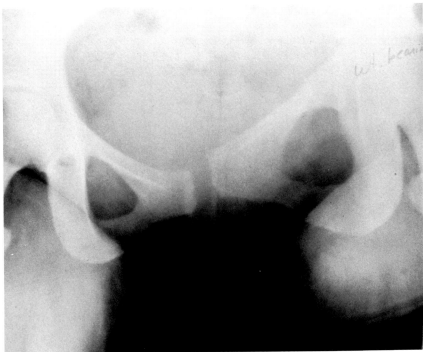

Fig. 13-4. Standing pelvic x-rays with alternate leg weight bearing demonstrating public instability as a reflection of 3-joint pelvic instability. (A) Right leg weight bearing (B) left leg weight bearing.

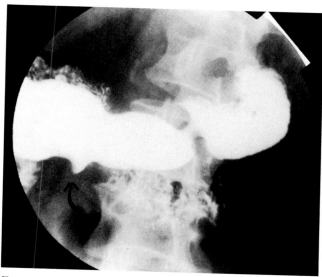

Fig. 13-5. Abdominal and lumbosacral pain associated with a malignant gastric ulcer (arrow). Patient in litigation alleging back pain residuum of a fall.

ate relief of pain. The prompt resolution of the accompanying reactive scoliosis and resumption of a comfortable erect posture can be dramatic. Later diathermy, weight reduction, lumbar flexibility, and abdominal strengthening exercises combined with corseting are together all useful treatment adjuncts.

THE CLINICAL EVALUATION

In an office setting the examiner's initial introduction to the presenting problem of lumbosacral pain is based on history. Attention to details, relative to the circumstances of the initial injury, "triggers" that cause reoccurrence, frequency of the occurrences, responses to previous treatment, the effects of postural changes, including bed rest and the limitations on ambulatory range, and, most significantly, the distribution of the pain itself are all important clues to diagnosis. Mechanical dysfunction of posture or the presence of neurologic signs, including alteration of deep tendon reflexes, weakness, atrophy, restricted straight leg raising or crossed straight leg raising signs, long tract signs, and the presence of sphincter dysfunction, are all "hard" signs of neurologic involvement. Clues to the clinical diagnosis of a musculoskeletal etiology of the presenting pain are "softer" and therefore rely to a greater extent on the details of the history, the exclusion of neurological signs, and the skill of the clinician in his or her ability to replicate as well as to reduce symptoms by appropriate anatomic maneuvers.[30] Electroneuromyography is a useful adjunct in this regard, as it can be the first objective evidence of neurogenic involvement in what might otherwise appear to be a mechanical articular problem. Likewise, X-ray examination routinely provides information that can be both diagnostic and unfortunately at times misleading relative to the etiology of the complaint. "Normal" X-rays may well be associated with a herniated disc, while roentgenographic evidence of degenerative disc disease can mask the presence of an acute sacroiliitis. In both instances clinical correlation is the sine qua non for accurate diagnosis. Confirmation of the initial problem still requires either myelogram or body CAT scan; in the later instance a therapeutic-diagnostic response to steroid lidocaine injection is usually confirmatory.[9]

In the vast majority of low back syndromes evaluated in the office the examiner is attempting to discriminate between pain of neurogenic or musculoskeletal origin. All too often in a busy practice a "mind set" occurs whereby other systems can be neglected as sources of referred back pain. The examiner must guard against system-oriented complacency (Fig. 13-6) by insisting on a thorough history, including a review of systems and a searching physical examination. In addition to neurologic testing and evaluation of the joints and soft tissue, abdominal examination, including palpation and auscultation, as well as a gait evaluation are essentials to a complete examination.

NERVE ROOT COMPROMISE

Isolated nerve root compromise as a source of lumbar pain occurs when the root is impinged by either disc or osseous distortion of the spinal or neural canals.

Disc Herniation

The description by Mixter and Barr of the ruptured lumbar disc in 1934 sparked a surgical revolution during the ensuing decades.[29] Only in recent years has experience and access to new technology freed us from the "dynasty of the disc,"[45] refocusing attention to the nerve root itself, not the disc as the site of pathology. Medical management of

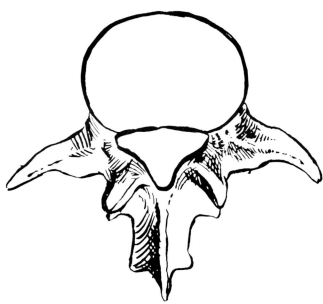

Fig. 13-6. Trefoil spinal canal predisposes to symptoms and signs of spinal stenosis.

lumbosacral pain has again regained its preeminent role in the initial management of low
back pain, even in the face of associated neurogenic involvement.[1] In this regard Nachemson[34] described impressive responses to conservative treatment of sciatica. More than 50
percent of the patients responded to medical management within a 2-4 week period.

Sciatic radiculopathy affects 2-3 percent of the population, having a prevalence of 4.8
percent in men and 2.5 percent in women older than 35 years of age. Spinal radiculopathy
has an average onset of approximately 37 years with 76 percent of the patients reporting
symptoms starting initially some 10 years earlier.[1] The initial presentation of lumbar
radicular pain clinically can be multivaried. A singular complaint of isolated lumbosacral
pain or pure sciatic pain radiation can be a harbinger of progressive radiculitis with or
without accompanying motor signs. Without aberrant motor correlate it is often difficult
to clinically quantify the degree of root compromise. In these instances of "sensory"
radiculopathy the presence of electromyographic abnormality can be diagnostic. The
identification of unilateral "H" reflex slowing is an early useful hallmark of S1 root
compromise.[3]

Although the vast majority of radiculopathies present with combined sensory and
motor symptoms and signs, the sudden onset of motor weakness alone can be a singular
manifestation of nerve root compromise. In these instances, where the acute onset of a
painless foot drop or calf weakness is associated with L5 or S1 root compromise respectively, a herniated disc must be suspected until proven otherwise. This axiom is especially
true when associated with an absent ankle jerk, restricted straight leg raising test, and/or
restricted knee extension with the hip flexed, producing "bow stringing" of the sciatic
nerve in the popliteal fossa. Counterlateral straight leg raising producing sciatic radiculopathy on the symptomatic side is highly suggestive of an impacted nerve root, particularly
in young individuals with normal lumbar spine X-rays. Paresthesias experienced in the
great toe with tenderness to palpation over the proximal sciatic notch and distal peroneal
nerve at the fibular head are corroborative evidence of L5 root compromise: S1 radiculopathy is suggested by tenderness of the tibial nerve in the popliteal fossa and within the
tarsal tunnel associated with numbness and tingling experienced over the plantar foot and
into the little toe. Anterior tibial compartment myalgias, like "shin splints," or acute calf
pain mimicking thrombophlebitis and chronically recurrent calf cramps may be manifestations of proximal nerve root compromise with distal pain radiation in the myotome
distribution of the respective L5 and S1 roots.[42]

The less frequent L4 radiculopathies may present with a combination of a reduction
in the knee jerk, anterior thigh pain, tenderness over the femoral triangle, and paresthe-
siae over the anterolateral thigh. The two most useful signs of L4 root compromise include
the presence of quadriceps weakness delineated by manual muscle testing and the dramatic resistence to hip extension testing that places the tethered L4 root on a stretch.

Although midline disc herniations can present as a singular catastrophic episode of
severe back pain with paraparesis accompanying an acute loss of bladder and bowel
function, the initial signs may be more subtle. Episodic midlumbar pain with bilateral leg
pain radiation and the perception of urinary urgency and/or precipitous incontinence may
be the only harbinger of impending paralysis.[14] Early in these special instances, reflexes
and strength may be normal. The presence of bilateral restricted straight leg raising with
postural signs of root impingement may be the only clues. These signs include "escape"
maneuvers demonstrated by the patient as they attempt to unload root tension by flexing
the knee or thrusting the ipsilateral pelvis forward, thereby reducing the lumbar lordosis.
In both instances there is an obvious unconscious effort to "lengthen" the entrapped
nerve root.

Spinal Stenosis

Congenital or acquired changes in the bony architecture of the spine can reduce the normally capacious areas of the spinal and neural canals. Functional or anatomic compression of the enclosed neurologic structures in these circumstances can precipitate the symptoms and signs of spinal stenosis.

Congenital variations of the vertebrae predisposing to spinal stenosis include foreshortened pedicles, convergent lamina, elongated and narrowed intervertebral canals, and lateral recesses.[46] In this configuration—the trefoil canal—even modest intrusions (Fig. 13-6) of either bone, disc, or ligament are not well accommodated. Although tolerated for many years without complaint, subsequent spur formation, disc degeneration, ligamentous thickening, vertebral displacement, nerve root adhesions, and increased lumbar lordosis can precipitate a wide variety of symptoms. Lumbar hyperextension often markedly increases the intensity of discomfort, particularly when the sagittal diameter of the spinal canal is reduced to less than 12 mm. Anterior spondylotic ridging and discal protrusions scissor the dural sac against the posterior enfolded ligamenta flava and hypertrophied superior articular facets. Unilateral narrowing of the lateral recess and foramina without sagittal spinal canal stenosis also can produce symptoms of claudication. In patients with spondylolysis, hyperextension also narrows the neural foramina, 10 percent in the superior-inferior diameter and up to 66 percent in the anterior-posterior diameter. Although lumbar stenosis can develop at any level, it occurs more often at L4. Spina bifida occulta at L5-S1, a transitional or sacralized fifth lumbar vertebra, and spondylolisthesis at L5 may also be seen in conjunction with spinal stenosis often predisposing to symptoms.[6]

Complaints associated with spinal stenosis are predominantly sensory and are almost always aggravated by spinal hyperextension. Neurogenic claudication secondary to spinal stenosis can mimic claudication of vascular origin in that both feature a predictable temporal pattern of exercise-pain-rest-relief. Unlike those complaints due to vascular claudication, symptoms associated with spinal stenosis are often variable with respect to distances walked and can even develop during prolonged standing or while lying down.

Classical sciatica and associated complaints of cramping calf pain are less frequent when associated with neurogenic claudication and have a distinctly paresthetic and dysesthetic quality. Sensations of coldness, burning, numbness, tingling, clumsiness, and weakness may descend from an initial saddle distribution or may conversely ascend from the feet in a sensory march. The perception of weakness always follows the onset of sensory complaints. Neurologic examination is most helpful in identifying a marked disparity between the symptom complaints and concomitant lack of motor signs. Repeated examinations, particularly at the height of the complaints, can reveal patterns of weakness, sensory alteration and reflex changes, long tract signs, and even restricted straight leg raising that may not be present after a period of rest. Bending forward or squatting characteristically alleviates these symptoms with lumbar hyperextension diagnostic in exacerbating them.

Although the pathophysiology of the symptoms associated with neurogenic claudication are as yet not well defined, neurogenic ischemia of the spinal roots has been cited as a primary precipitating cause. Claudication time has been related directly to reduced oxygen tension. In test subjects exposed to decreased ambient oxygen, exercise time to claudication is reduced. Blau and Rushworth[2] demonstrated a marked increase in the density and dilitation of blood vessels of both the spinal cord and lumbar roots in mice on the same side as an exercised limb, the hind leg having responded to prolonged, repetitive electrical stimulation. Tourniquet precipitated ischemia can exaggerate sensory complaints associated with various peripheral mononeuropathies like that of carpal tunnel, suggesting that in a similar manner even occult lesions can become symptomatic.

Nocturnal back pain associated with spinal stenosis has been related to venous congestion of Batson's paravertebral plexus distention by postural change, sudden increases in intra-abdominal and thoracic pressure, as well as in the special instance of congestive heart failure. Venous distention adjacent to presensitized nerve roots within the rigid, unyielding confines of a narrowed osseous passage "triggers" the pain, arousing the patient from sleep.[7] Elevations in central venous pressure, as occurs in a reclining position, are readily transmitted by collateral communicators to the paravertebral venous plexus, producing increased filling of the epidural plexus. Volume distention of this venous bed, a lack of valves, and multiple interlocking tributaries may divert and effectively reduce flow and oxygenation. In many patients with spinal stenosis, sheets of epidural veins come to replace the normal paired bilateral anterior-internal epidural veins contributing to reduced flow and increased venous stagnation.

Spinal roots adjacent to degenerative joints, osteophytes, or discs may become inflamed and exquisitely sensitive to even gentle manipulation. The pain experienced with nerve stimulation is variable in both intensity and degree of distal radiation, depending on the inciting magnitude of the noxious stimulus and the presence or absence of nerve inflammation. Normal nerve roots are relatively insensitive to manipulation. Chronic or recurrent nerve irritation can produce pathologic changes within the root, including intraneural fibrosis and ultimately perineural adhesions to the adjacent walls of the neural foramina. Relative ischemia can occur within the area of inflammation and subsequent fibrosis.[40]

Within the ischemic root segment, the normal balance of neural transmission can be disrupted. Spontaneous neural discharges may develop at the injury site and create the potential for ectopic foci along the distal course of the nerve. Ischemic neuritis has also been related to the development of spontaneous ephatic foci or "cross talk" between adjacent nerves with smaller, less medullated sensory fibers particularly sensitive to reduced blood flow. An absolute reduction in the normal number of functioning axons as well as the ongoing process of both dysmyelination and remyelination can interfere with the speed of segmental nerve conduction modifying the profile of afferent neurologic impulses as they enter the spinal cord. When the mix between large afferent fiber input has been altered, the phenomenon of "pathological amplification" can develop with a mild stimulus perceived as a major insult.[49]

The diagnosis of spinal stenosis rests primarily upon history as the clinical manifestations may be quite variable. Motor signs ranging from partial extremity paresis to a nonmeasurable perception of weakness, sensory phenomena varying from distal foot and toe numbness to severe pain restricting ambulatory range are not uncommon. The symptoms are invariably bilateral with multiroot involvement. Electromyographic abnormalities when present may predominate in one lower extremity with sensory complaints preeminent in the opposite extremity.

Electrodiagnostic evidence of root compromise may be confined only to the paraspinal muscle. In this regard they can be confused with the presentation of occult paraspinal muscle metatasis (Fig. 13-7) with isolated denervation of the posterior primary ramus.[24] In the latter instance the electromyographic representation of denervation is more likely to be unilateral and less widespread. In both instances the anterior rami may be spared with the neurologic examination normal, although straight leg testing is more likely to be restricted in metastatic disease. Even in the presence of severe sciatica with

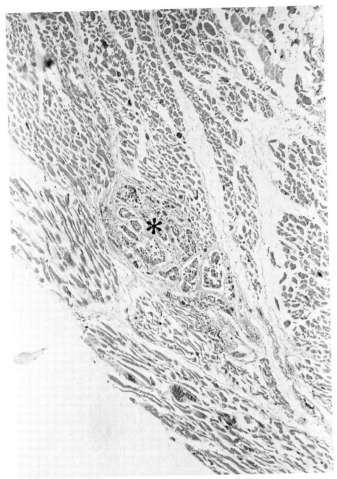

Fig. 13-7. Paraspinal muscle metastasis (*) of bronchogenic
carcinoma. Electromyographic evidence of isolated posterior primary ramus denervation in otherwise neurologic and x-ray normal
patients.

spinal stenosis, straight leg raising tolerance is often unrestricted. Compressive radiculopathies associated with herniated discs comparatively present with impacted root signs,
including limited tolerance to sciatic nerve stretch.

The recent advent of the body CAT scan and magnetic resonant imaging (MRI) has
made it possible to visualize structural abnormality of the vertebral canals beyond the
perusal of myelography. The nerve root sheaths are more efficiently outlined by the newer
water soluble contrast mediums employed in contemporary myelography. However, in
lateral entrapment syndromes of the nerve roots due to spinal stenosis or sequestration of
a lateral disc (Fig. 13-8) the myelogram can be normal. In the presence of central stenosis
"hour glassing" of the contrast column at the disc spaces (Fig. 13-9) is diagnostic with
reports of "cutting-off of the root sleeves" suggestive of lateral spinal stenosis. The CAT
body scan demonstrates skeletal spinal defects, both osseous and soft tissues, permitting

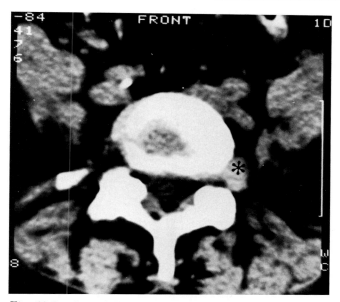

Fig. 13-8. Lateral disc fragment (*) not visualized by routine myelogram.

an accurate evaluation of dimensions of the spinal and neural canals lateral to the spinal recesses. Heretofore, electromyographers were puzzled by reports of "normal" myelograms in patients with marked signs of electrodiagnostic symptoms of root disease.[16] The CAT scan has technically superseded the epidural venograms that initially were useful in revealing the etiology of the electrodiagnostic abnormality by demonstrating incomplete filling of the pedicular venous branches adjacent to the involved nerve root.

MECHANICAL BACK PAIN

A broad variation in pathologic entities involving the musculoskeletal system can be recognized in this category. Radiologic evidence of an acute vertebral compression fracture occurring without significant trauma in an osteoporotic postmenopausal female, the presence of a sacral fracture following a fall associated with bowel incontinence, the visualization of a loss of the vertebral pedicle shadow suggesting occult metastasis, and the presence of spondylolisthesis associated with a defect in the pars interarticularis particularly in a young patient can each be diagnostic.

More often, however, the exact origin of pain related to the musculoskeletal system is not as obvious, with normal X-rays less helpful and often misleading. Joint instability at either the zygoapophyseal or sacroiliac joints cannot be recognized radiographically in its earliest clinical stages, even though associated with significant disability.[19] Vertebral segmental instability is most easily recognized and understood with reference to a model of a symptomatic spondylolisthesis with the L5 vertebrae progressively slipping forward on the sacrum, especially in adolescents or young adults. Easily visualized by lateral X-rays of the spine, the degree of instability or slip can be readily measured with spatial reference of one vertebral body to another. Here too, the measureable degree of instability often does

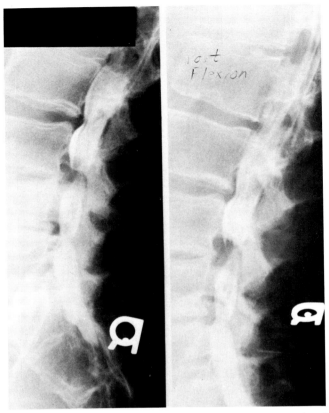

Fig. 13-9. "Hour glass" configuration of myelogram associated with multi-level disc bulging in spinal stenosis.

not correlate with the severity of clinical symptoms. This is particularly true in the older adult with recognizable spondylolisthesis and episodic lumbosacral pain and stiffness. In many instances the symptoms can be clinically attributed to cephalad vertebral articular segments or to the more caudal sacroiliac joints by their symptomatic response to appropriate treatment. The lack of radiographic evidence of structural changes at these levels can be deceptive with the spondylolisthesis inappropriately identified as the source of the discomfort. In many of these instances the spondylolisthesis may be altering mechanics at the lumbosacral junction, acting as a predisposing cause of spinal segmental instability with associated symptoms at adjacent levels.

Preservation of lumbar flexibility requires that restricted segmental mobility must be augmented at the distal and proximal vertebral articulations or supplemented by increased range of motion at the sacroiliac or hip joints. In either scenario, increased stresses are shifted to the adjacent vertebrae, predisposing them to cartalagenous and synovial damage, effusion, capsular distention, and subsequent increase in mobility. Pseudospondylolisthesis (Fig. 13-10) developing as a consequence of these progressive articular changes and concomitant disc disease is radiographically a static expression of an otherwise functional segmental spinal instability.[28] In this regard it differs from the model of true spondylolisthesis only by the presence of an intact pars interarticularis.

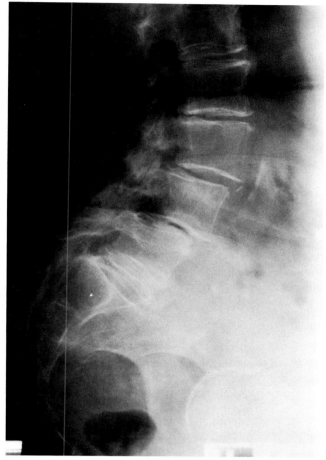

Fig. 13-10. Pseudolisthesis—vertebral instability secondary degenerative disc disease without spondylolysis.

Conversely, lumbosacral pain can be provoked by a restriction of mobility at the hips or distal extremity joints. Accommodating to a loss of hip flexibility secondary to osteoarthritis can unduly stress the pelvic and spinal joints. With pes planus, foot flexibility is reduced and forces generated by ambulation can be associated with increased sacroiliac joint arthralgias. Without the normal arches of the foot to absorb the right angle torques generated by 25 degrees of extremity rotation these forces are moved proximally to be damped at the sacroiliac joints.[27]

Eccentric loading of the zygoapophyseal joints by spinal scoliosis concomitant with unilateral trunk muscular weakness and/or asymmetrical leg length can produce spinal pain. Pain can also be produced by or increased by alteration of the gait pattern by extremity joint contracture, instability of the knee, or attempting to "walk around" a painful trochanteric bursitis or enthesitis. In these instances the converse is often also true. Postural accommodation to back pain can produce an associated trochanteric enthesitis that can mimic a radiculopathy by referring pain distally under the iliotibial band to the knee.

Pain of articular spinal origin is invariably accompanied by stiffness that varies inversely with activity. Prolonged reclining or sitting predisposes to increased stiffness with activity progressively reducing it. Articular pain is, on the other hand, increased by activity. Mechanical pressure applied to a symptomatic joint will aggravate the pain complaint, with positions likely to reduce the joint stress will alleviate the discomfort. Diagnostic maneuvers of this type help to objectify the etiology of the pain in what otherwise could be regarded as purely a subjective experience.

Pain of articular and periarticular origin have recognizable patterns of sclerotomal radiation. Complaints of diffuse flank, lower abdominal quadrant, and inguinal aching discomfort are frequent concomitant complaints associated with irritation of the sacroiliac joint. The discomfort can be severe enough to mimic the pain of intrapelvic or abdominal pathology like that of appendicitis or an acute ovarian cyst. Neurogenic symptoms accompanying acute articular inflammation is not uncommon. In many instances it is quite difficult to discriminate between pain of true radicular origin or that incurred secondary to joint involvement. Nerve roots adjacent to a degenerating facet joint; the iliolumbar component of the lumbosacral plexus carrying sensory ramifications of the L1-L4 roots lying directly anterior to the inflamed sacroiliac joints can each be secondarily involved in the inflammatory process, producing symptoms of alternating sciatica.[5] In this manner the distal lateral thigh paresthesias of the syndrome meralgia paresthetica can be a sensory expression of proximal iliolumbar trunk irritation.

The inherent sensory nerve supply of the joints can be a target of referred pain to the articulation itself, as well as a source of referred pain to other distal structures in the sclerotome distribution of joint referral. The zygoapophyseal joints are innervated by the sinuvertebral branches of the posterior primary ramus; the sacroiliac joints by branches of the S1 and S2 roots. Centrifugal spread of pain from an inflamed facet joint in an acute "facet syndrome" via the sensory nerve afferents is diffuse and follows the bilateral, multilevel ramifications of this nerve network to other facets and meninges. The symptoms of coccydynia can be a manifestation of a sacroiliitis with secondary referral via the coccygeal nerves (S1-S2) to the three-muscle sling of the pelvic floor.

When neurogenic symptoms are associated with primary articular pathology, the neurologic examination is usually normal. In most instances sensory complaints predominate. A reactive scoliosis increasing with activity is, however, a notable exception to this general impression. Although occasionally present with primary radiculopathies, this phenomena more often accompanies articular disorders, either facet syndromes or acute sacroiliitis. On occasion the scoliosis will present without pain. The patient may complain initially of lateral flank "swelling," failing to recognize its true origin as a postural manifestation of a concurrent acute, reactive scoliosis.

Gait disturbances associated with lumbar root compromise are easily recognized as a "foot slap" with L5 root dysfunction, weakness of "push off" with an S1 root and a "quadriceps plop" with an L4 radiculopathy.[38] Patients with articular disorders of the lumbosacral spine or sacroiliac joints may also have ambulatory complaints of a "leg giving out." This complaint is difficult to understand without reference to normal gait dynamics. At heel strike the knee is extended, the center of gravity resting behind the knee shifted laterally to the stance leg. Direct vector forces of pressure are transmitted proximally from the heel-ground reaction to the pelvic and lumbosacral spine. These forces are amplified by a contracted gluteus maximus muscle extending the trunk and femur on the pelvis.[27] Patients responding to an actual or anticipated increase in lumbosacral pain at heel strike fail to extend the knee. Reacting to an acute episode of lumbosacral pain, the patient accommodates by flexing the trunk on the pelvis and shifting the center of gravity posteriorly, further serving to destabilize an already unlocked, flexed knee and hip.

MEDICAL MANAGEMENT

The goals of medical management of lumbosacral disorders should include (1) relief of pain, (2) restoration of function, and (3) retardation of disease progression. Implicit in employing conservative therapy is to "do no harm" by failing to recognize the signs and symptoms of a progressive nerve root disorder more appropriately dealt with either by chemoneucleolysis or surgery—even early! Diagnostic procrastination has no role in the treatment of an acute cauda equina syndrome or in the face of progressive motor weakness, in spite of apparent appropriate medical treatment.

Acute radicular syndromes

Bed rest combined with superficial heat, preferably hydrocollator packing, is the initial treatment of choice. Bed rest as a treatment modality itself, has been demonstrated to reduce interdiscal pressure by 86 percent.[33] Positioning in lumbar flexion is advisable, either by lying prone with the abdomen over a pillow or supine with the hips and knees flexed over pillows. Reclining over a heat source in a supine position should be avoided, as this can mechanically compromise the posterior spinal elements and predispose to potential excessive heating and concomitant uncomfortable hyperemia.

Oral analgesics, the dosage and strength of the drug varying individually with the pain intensity, are utilized as required. Nonsteroidal anti-inflammatory drugs are useful over time but acutely, codeine and other narcotics, in limited amounts, may be more appropriate. Muscle relaxants that work primarily as soporifics and oral steroids are rarely effective or required in treatment.[1]

Pelvic traction can be a useful treatment tool in the management of lumbar root syndromes. As an outpatient modality, intermittent pelvic traction using a pelvic traction table, can provide significant relief for patients with ischemic radiculopathy, like that associated with spinal stenosis. Compressive neuropathies do less well, sciatica often exacerbating when associated with an impacted root secondary to a prolapsed disc. In-bed pelvic traction applied to a patient in a semiflexed hip and knee position can also be effective, in spite of scientific quantitative studies that would suggest otherwise. A traction force of 30 kg has been demonstrated to reduce interdiscal pressure by 20–30 percent,[33] often sufficient in acute root syndromes to qualitatively reduce the radicular symptoms. Pelvic traction using the body's own weight, either by suspension boots or by tilt table application, has enjoyed recent attention. Although effective in some instances, their recent popularity appears to have less to do with their lasting therapeutic efficacy than to their appeal to the faddist.

As pain subsides, progressive mobilization should be permitted over one week period. Each person's lifestyle and vocational demands vary. Therefore, no one recipe for increasing activity is applicable to every individual. However, patients should be cautioned to avoid activities that aggravate their symptoms. This includes prolonged sitting, which increases intradiscal pressure 43 percent over the standing position.[33]

Exercises designed to increase abdominal muscle strength and promote lumbar and hamstring flexibility can be initiated 2–3 weeks after pain subsides.[48] If discomfort recurs, therapy should be delayed until pain once again subsides.

Sciatic pain radiation, unresponsive to bed rest, or that recurrent with progressive mobilization, or associated with progressive motor dysfunction, deserves further diagnostic evaluation.

Electromyography is an effective tool in this regard, providing a means by which the presence and degree of motor dysfunction can be established.[3] Levels of neurogenic involvement can be determined with plexopathies differentiated from primary root syndromes that they can clinically mimic. The test is relatively innocuous, with minimal discomfort, and is cost effective in not requiring hospitalization. It provides a measure of physiologic nerve dysfunction, a baseline against which progressive or intractable radiculopathy can be compared. Three major limitations of electromyography must be recognized. Electrodiagnostic abnormality lags 10 days behind the clinical onset of symptoms, appearing earliest in the paraspinal muscles. When limited only to the paraspinal muscle the known multilevel overlap of the posterior primary ramus may mask the primary root level of involvement. Nerve root compression can be variable in its electrodiagnostic presentation, ranging from manifestations of neuropraxia, ie, segmental interruption of the nerve's ability to conduct an impulse, to frank axonal degeneration. With neuropraxia the electromyographic findings may be minimal, and yet the clinical manifestations marked. Radicular weakness or absent ankle reflex with a reduction of straight leg raising may only be associated with electromyographic evidence of a reduced number of motor units. In instances of early S1 radiculopathy, slowing or an absence of the "H reflex" relative to the uninvolved extremity may be diagnostic of a root compression syndrome that is primarily neuropraxic.[3] In these instances the prognosis for rapid postoperative recovery is relatively good.

Computerized body scans and myelography should be considered with intractable radiculopathy. CAT scanning has a decided advantage in not requiring hospitalization, while myelography provides better visualization of intradural structures. Hospitalization criteria for intractable lumbosacral pain has recently been made all the more stringent (Table 13-1) by the demands of diagnostic related groups (DRG).

Acute articular syndromes

Like radicular pain, the initial treatment of acute articular lumbosacral pain in that of bed rest. The vast majority of symptoms respond within 24 hours to a combination of superficial heat and bed rest. Oral analgesics are again useful with nonsteroidal anti-inflammatories in appropriate dosages often effective in pain control.

In less tractable cases injectable steroids combined with lidocaine can provide prompt pain relief. Facet injection under fluoroscopic control has been recommended in acute facet syndromes. Similarly, sacroiliac joint injection may not only provide relief in selected patients, but also serves to confirm the diagnosis.[23]

Using a 3 cc syringe with a 23-gauge, 2 inch needle filled with 1cc of 1 percent lidocaine and 2 cc of depo-steroid, the injection site is identified (Fig. 13-11) about halfway between the posterosuperior iliac spine and the lumbosacral spine. With the patient positioned in a flexed, prone position with a pillow placed under the abdomen, the needle is inserted at a 45 degree angle down and out (anteriorly and laterally) under the postero-superior iliac spine. With the needle positioned within the joint, 1 cc of this mixture is

Table 13-1
Admission Criteria for Low Back Pain

I. Patient Seen in Office Practice

A. Acute pain; patient requires immediate admission

Admission Criteria—Immediate
1. Paraparesis—paralysis
2. Loss of bowel-bladder function
3. L-S pain and spasticity
4. Cannot stand or sit
5. Sleeping in an upright position
6. Presence of metastatic cancer

Work Up
1. L-S spine X-rays
2. EMG/NCV/evoked potentials
3. Cystometrogram, related to bladder symptoms.
4. CBC, SMAC, protein electrophoresis, acid phosphatase, CEA, sed rate
5. Myelogram—CAT Scan-MRI

B. Acute pain; observed progression of symptoms requires admission

Admission Criteria—With Progression
1. Unilateral paresis with or without pain
2. Absent reflex
3. Atrophy
4. Intractable radicular pain unresponsive to appropriate conservative therapy (pain alone requires 2 weeks of outpatient conservative therapy)
5. Marked restriction of hip and knee extension (bow stringing)
6. Unilateral spasticity
7. Progressive EMG changes

Work Up (As Outpatient)
1. L-S spine X-ray
2. EMG/NCV/evoked potentials
3. "Therapeutic" trial of treatment, i.e., bedrest, physical therapy, corseting
4. If patient experiences the progression of the signs above and symptoms and/or is unresponsive to conservative therapy, oral or injectible medications, the patient is admitted for inpatient evaluation with myelogram/CAT Scan/MRI

Table 13-1
Admission Criteria for Low Back Pain *Continued*

C. Chronic pain after surgery:
Admission Criteria—After Surgery
1. Intractable radicular pain
2. Altered neurologic signs as progressive paresis, loss of straight leg raising, lateralizing neurological signs, atrophy
3. Progressive EMG changes and
4. Unresponsive to conservative therapy, including physical therapy, corseting, TENS, injections

Work Up
1. Myelogram
2. CAT Scan
3. EMG/NVC/evoked potentials
4. Psychometrics

D. Chronic pain with surgery
Admission Criteria—As Above in "C"
1. Progressive loss of ambulatory range—vascular vs. neurogenic "claudication"

Work Up
1. L-S spine X-rays
2. EMG/NCV/H reflex/evoked potentials
3. Myelogram—CAT Scan-MRI
4. Abdominal X-rays, ultrasound arteriogram
5. CBC, urinalysis, ZSR, protein electrophoresis, SMAC, acid phosphatase, CEA

E. Chronic pain—no surgery contemplated
Admission Criteria—As Above in "D"

Work Up
1. Psychometrics
2. Response to analgesics, mood elevators, and TENS
3. Pain clinic referral

II. Admission through the Emergency Department
Admission Criteria—Essentially the same with the addition of the following admission criteria:

Work Up
1. Second E.R. visit
2. Neuro signs
3. X-ray c̄ defects

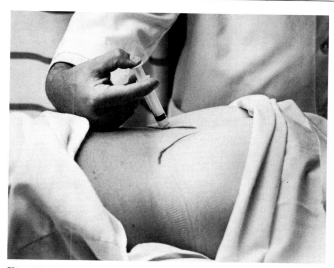

Fig. 13-11. Injection of mid-third sacroiliac joint. Subsequent adjustment of insertion angle permits injecting upper and lower joint without needle withdrawal.

injected. The needle is then withdrawn to a position just below the skin, reoriented at a 45 degree lateral angle and initially pointed downward to the inferior portion of the joint where an additional 1 cc is injected. This maneuver is then repeated, injecting the superior portion of the joint with the needle placed above the posterosuperior iliac spine.

Following injection the patient can be treated with diathermy modalities, including short wave diathermy or ultrasound, to the symptomatic joint. As pain subsides, progressive trunk flexibility and abdominal strengthening exercises can be initiated. Again, these exercises should be titrated to the patient's pain tolerance. Often with mechanical back pain trunk extension exercises may be more effective.

Bracing or corseting can be effective during recurrent, acute episodes of articular back pain. Prophylactic wearing of supports during pain free intervals, in general, cannot be recommended with the exception of pregnancy. Twenty-five percent of women experience lumbosacral pain during pregnancy. Rarely are these symptoms associated with a herniated disc.[26] Gestational corseting, appropriate exercise instruction, and occasionally the necessity of injecting a symptomatic sacroiliac joint can keep the patient functional.

These devices provide support by not only restricting trunk motion, but also by packing the abdominal viscera, thereby moving the weight bearing line forward, reducing spinal stress by 30 percent.[35] Corseting is contraindicated in patients with concurrent problems of hemorrhoids, varicosities, or hiatus hernia where increases of intraabdominal pressure can aggravate these problems. All patients recovering from acute lumbosacral pain should be encouraged to increase their activity to tolerance. Aerobic fitness programs involving activities like brisk walking, swimming, and bicycling can be recommended to increase endurance. Jogging, however, can predictably aggravate chronic recurrent back pain.

Instruction in appropriate back hygiene as a prophylactic measure should be encouraged. Compensating methods of lifting and bending, as well as information pertinent to causative factors relative to low back pain from the curriculum of the "low back school."[50]

Chronic Lumbosacral Pain

When pain of radicular or articular origin proves to be intractable to thorough diagnostic and standard medical and surgical treatment approaches, referral to a "pain program" and/or a "work disability evaluation program" is appropriate. Initially established as diagnostic and treatment centers for intractable lumbosacral pain, these pain programs with few exceptions have focused less on the management of the physical aspects of pain than on cognitive restraining to handle the personal and psychosocial ramifications of chronic, intractable discomfort. These programs also feature modification of drug regimens, as well as the use of transcutaneous electrical nerve stimulation (TENS) as a salvage procedure for pain control in patients unresponsive to other treatment modalities.[39]

Work disability evaluation programs are primarily prevocational in nature, focusing on the patient's residual work capacities, tolerances, skills, and aptitudes for substitute work categories.[32] Fortunately, relatively few patients require either of these two programs, as the vast majority of acute lumbosacral pain syndromes are either self limiting or responsive to interventional medical therapy.

REFERENCES

1. Bell GR, Rothman RH: The conservative treatment of sciatica. Spine 9:54–56, 1984
2. Blau JN, Rushworth G: Observations on the blood vessels of the spinal cord and their responses to motor activity. Brain 81:354–363, 1958
3. Braddom RL, Johnson EW: H-Reflex: Review and classification with suggested clinical uses. Arch Phys Med Rehabil 55:161–166, 1974
4. Bonica JJ: The Nature of the Problem, in Carron H, McLaughlin RE (eds): Management of Low Back Pain, Boston, John Wright—PSG Inc, 1982, pp 1–15
5. DePalma AF, Rothman RH: The Intervertebral Disc. Philadelphia, WB Saunders, 1970, pp 65–83
6. Epstein BS, Epstein JA, Jones MD: Lumbar spinal stenosis. In Radiol Clin North Am 15:227–239, 1977
7. Granit R, Leksel L, Skoglund GR: Fiber interaction in injured or compressed region of nerve. Brain 67:125–140, 1944
8. Hakelius A: Prognosis in sciatica. Acta Orthop Scand (Suppl) 129:6–71, 1970
9. Hochschuler SH: Diagnostic studies in clinical practice. Orthop Clin North Am 14:517–526, 1983
10. Hult L: Cervical, dorsal and lumbar spinal syndromes. Acta Orthop Scand (Suppl) 17:7–102, 1954
11. Hult L: The Munkfors investigation. Acta Orthop Scand (Suppl) 16:1–76, 1954
12. Johnson EW: Practical Electromyography. Baltimore, Williams & Wilkens, 1980
13. Johnson EW, Melvin JL: Value of electromyography in lumbar radiculopathy. Arch phys Med Rehabil 52:239–243, 1971
14. Jones DL, Moore T: The types of neuropathic bladder dysfunction associated with prolapsed lumbar intervertebral discs. Br J Urol 45:39–43, 1973
15. Kelsey JL: Idiopathic Low Back Pain: Magnitude of the Problem, In White II AA, Gordon SL (eds): Symposium on Idiopathic Low Back Pain, St. Louis, CV Mosby Co, 1982, pp 5–8
16. Khatri B, Barauh J, McQuillen MP: Correlation of electromyography with computed tomography and evaluation of low back pain. Arch Neurol 41:594–597, 1984
17. Kirkaldy-Willis WH: Pathology and Pathogenesis of Lumbar Spinal Stenosis, in Brown FW (ed): Symposium on the Lumbar Spine. St. Louis, CV Mosby Co, 1981, pp 16–20
18. Kirkaldy-Willis WH: The relationship of structural pathology to the nerve root. Spine 9:49–52, 1984
19. Kirkaldy-Willis WH, Farfan HF: Instability of the lumbar spine. Clin Orthop 165:110–123, 1982
20. Kirkaldy-Willis WH, Wedge JH, Yong-Hing K: Pathology and pathogenesis of lumbar spondylosis and stenosis. Spine 3:319–328, 1978
21. Klopsteg PE, Wilson PD (eds): Human Limbs and Their Substitutes. New York, McGraw-Hill Book Co, 1954

22. LaBan MM: "Vesper's curse" night pain-the bane of Hypnos. Arch Phys Med Rehab 65:501–504, 1984

23. LaBan MM: The Lumbosacral Pain Syndrome, in Kaplan PE (ed): The Practice of Physical Medicine. Springfield, Charles C Thomas, 1984, pp 107–160

24. LaBan MM, Meerschaert JR, Perez L, et al: Metastatic disease of the spine: Electromyographic and histopathologic correlation and early detection. Arch Phys Med Rehabil 58:491–494, 1977

25. LaBan MM, Meerschaert JR, Taylor RS: Symphyseal and sacroiliac joint pain associated with pubic symphysis instability. Arch Phys Med Rehabil 59:470–472, 1978

26. LaBan MM, Perrin JCS, Latimer FR: Pregnancy and the lumbar herniated disc. Arch Phys Med Rehabil 64:319–321, 1983

27. Lehman JF: Gait Analysis: Diagnosis and Management, in Kottke FJ, Stillwell GK, Lehman JF (eds): Krusen's Handbook of Physical Medicine and Rehabilitation, Philadelphia, WB Saunders, 1982, pp 86–101

28. MacNab I: Spondylolisthesis with an intact neural arch. The so-called pseudospondylolisthesis. J Bone Joint Surg 32B:325–333, 1950

29. Mixter JW, Barr JS: Rupture of the intervertebral disc with involvement of the spinal canal. N Engl J Med 211:210–215, 1934

30. Mooney V: The syndromes of low back disease. Ortho Clin North Am 14:505–515, 1983

31. Mooney V, Robertson J: The facet syndrome. Clin Orthop 115:149–156, 1976

32. Morris A, Randolph JW: Back rehabilitation programs speed recovery of injured workers. 53:53–68, 1984

33. Nachemson A: The load on the lumbar disk in different positions of the body. Clin Orthop 45:107–122, 1966

34. Nachemson A: The lumbar spine. An orthopedic challenge. Spine 1:59–71, 1976

35. Nachemson A, Morris JM: In vivo measurements of intradiscal pressure: Discometry, a method for determination of pressure in the lower lumbar disc. J Bone Joint Surg 46A:1077–1092, 1964

36. Nagi SA, Riley LE, Newby LG: A social epidemiology of back pain in a general population. J Chron Dis 26:769–799, 1973

37. National Center for Health Statistics. Surgical operations in short-stay hospitals, United States, 1975. Series 13, no. 34, 1978

38. Rothman RH, Simeome FA: The Spine, Philadelphia, WB Saunders, 1982

39. Roy R: Pain clinics: Reassessment of objectives and outcomes. Arch Phys Med Rehabil 65:448–451, 1984

40. Rydevik B, Brown MD, Lundborg G: Pathoanatomy and Pathophysiology of nerve root compression. Spine 9:7–15, 1984

41. Sashin D: A critical analysis of the anatomy and the pathologic changes of the sacroiliac joints. J Bone Joint Surg 12:891–910, 1930

42. Spangfort EV: The lumbar disc herniation. A computer-aided analysis of 2,504 operations. Acta Orthop Scan (Suppl) 142: pp 1–94, 1972

43. Steinberg GG: Epidemiology of Low Back Pain, M Stanton-Hicks, Boas R (eds): Chronic Low Back Pain, New York, Raven Press, 1982, pp 1–13

44. Sunderland S: Nerves and Nerve Injuries. Baltimore, Williams & Wilkins, 1968

45. Tile M: The role of surgery in nerve root compression. Spine 9:57–64, 1984

46. Verbiest H: Further experience on the pathological influences of a developmental narrowness of the bony lumbar canal. J Bon Joint Surg 37-B:576–583, 1955

47. Waddell G, Kummel EG, Lotto WN, et al: Failed lumbar disc surgery following industrial injuries. J Bone Joint Surg 61:201–207, 1979

48. Williams RC: Examination and conservative treatment for disc lesions of the lower spine. Clin Orthop 5:28–38, 1955

49. Wynn Parry CB: The 1981 Philip Nichols memorial lecture. Int Rehabil Med 4:59–65, 1982

50. Zachussen M: The Low Back School. Danderyd's Hospital, Danderyd, Sweden, 1972

Richard H. White

14

The Painful Shoulder

Pain in the region of the shoulder is a common complaint that can almost always be accurately diagnosed and effectively treated. The problem of shoulder pain spans all ages with young athletes, middle-aged workers, and more sedentary elderly individuals coming to physicians complaining of pain with or without restricted motion. Causes of shoulder discomfort are extremely diverse, ranging from local inflammatory arthritides in the glenohumeral joint to distant processes in the neck or abdomen that cause referred pain to the shoulder. Fortunately, a careful history and physical examination will pinpoint the major sites of pathology in most patients. Once a diagnosis is made, specific treatment and rehabilitation modalities can be initiated that greatly benefit the majority of patients.

ANATOMY

An understanding of the complex anatomy and function of the shoulder is essential when evaluating pain in this region.[16] The motion of the shoulder unit is the result of movement of three diarthrodial joints; the glenohumeral, the acromioclavicular (A-C), and the sternoclavicular, as well as two functional joints: the scapulothroacic and the subacromial or "secondary glenohumeral" joint (see Fig. 14-1). During complicated motions, such as throwing or circumduction, coordinated movement of each of these joints takes place. As a corollary, disease affecting any one of these joints may effect abnormal shoulder motion. Interestingly, dysfunction of the subacromial apparatus and acromioclavicular joint are implicated in the vast majority of patients with shoulder pain, the glenohumeral and sternoclavicular being less commonly affected by disease processes.

The center of the shoulder joint is made up of the glenoid fossa and the surrounding fibrocartilagenous labrum (see Fig. 14-2); the roof is made up of the acromion, the tough coracoacromial ligament, and the coracoid process of the scapula (see Fig. 14-3). In addition to the articular surface, the humeral head has three important landmarks; the greater and lesser tuberosities, to which the four rotator cuff tendons insert, and the intertubercular groove, through which the long head of the biceps tendon passes before inserting on the superior rim of the glenoid (see Fig. 14-3).

PRINCIPLES OF PHYSICAL MEDICINE AND REHABILITATION
IN THE MUSCULOSKELETAL DISEASES

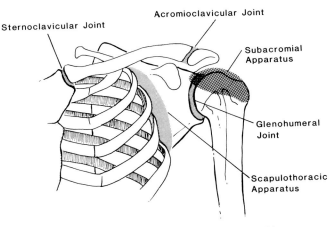

Fig. 14-1. Functional anatomy of the shoulder.

At rest, the humeral head is held firmly against the glenoid fossa by the joint capsule/ligamentous complex. During motion, the musculotendenous rotator cuff stabilizes and "sets" the humeral head. The major long muscles responsible for shoulder motion (deltoid, pectoralis major, latissimus dorsi, etc.) cannot function effectively without the critically important rotator cuff muscles. The four muscles that make up the rotator cuff (see Fig. 14-4 and 14-5) are: First, the subscapularis, which originates from the undersurface of the scapula and inserts along the lesser tuberosity. It internally rotates the humerus and provides anterior stability. Second, the supraspinatus, which originates on the superior aspect of the scapula, passes underneath the acromion and inserts superiorly on the greater tuberosity. It is the most important cuff muscle since it holds the humerus in the

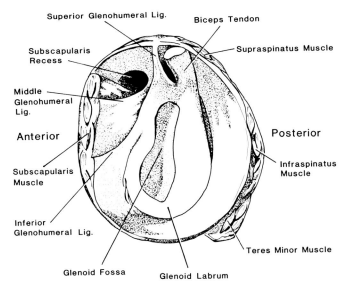

Fig. 14-2. Anatomy of the glenoid and surrounding structures viewed from a lateral projection.

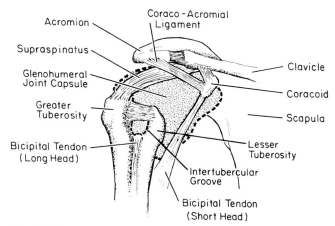

Fig. 14-3. Anterior view of the shoulder showing the important bony landmarks, the glenohumeral joint capsule, and the position of the most superior rotator cuff muscle, the supraspinatus.

glenoid fossa during abduction, allowing the deltoid a firm fulcrum for elevation. Third, the infraspinatus, which originates beneath the scapular spine and inserts on the posterior aspect of the greater tuberosity. Fourth, the teres minor, which originates even more inferiorly on the scapula and also inserts on the posterior aspect of the greater tuberosity.

Although rotation of the scapula during arm elevation tilts the acromion upward and medially, the rotator cuff tendons still become closely opposed to the undersurface of the acromium and coracoacromial ligament, particularly between 60° and 120° of flexion or abduction (see Fig. 14-6). Friction in this very tight space between the humeral head and the coracoacromial arch is minimized by the interposed slick subacromial bursa. This bursa essentially acts as a cushioning joint space. Any process that significantly narrows

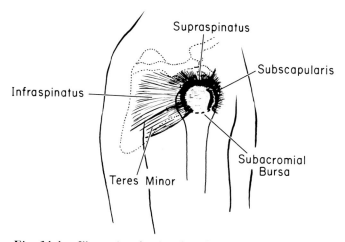

Fig. 14-4. Illustration showing the relative areas of insertion of the rotator cuff muscles on the humerus and the overlying subacromial bursa.

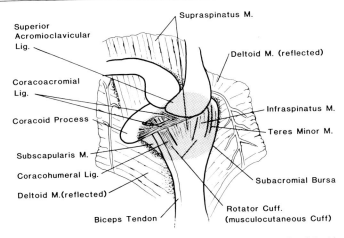

Fig. 14-5. Superior-lateral view of the shoulder with the deltoid muscle reflected showing the relative position of the subacromial bursa under the acromion and coracoacromial ligament.

the distance between the greater tuberosity and the coracoacromial arch will cause the rotator cuff to impinge on the bony/ligamentous roof, causing pain and abnormal shoulder motion. For example, degenerative osteophytes on the anterior undersurface of the acromion and the undersurface of the A-C joint may impinge on the rotator cuff and be responsible for chronic shoulder pain (see Fig. 14-7).

It is important to know that the vascular supply to portions of the rotator cuff is quite tenuous.[53] In particular, the area of the supraspinatus tendon just medial to its point of insertion is not well vascularized (see Fig. 14-6). The vascularity of this region appears to be most compromised when the humerus is in the resting position with the arm at the side. Since this portion of the tendon is the same "critical" region that impinges against the coracoacromial arch during abduction, microtrauma and the poor blood supply may explain why this area is prone to inflammation, degeneration, and rupture. This is also the area in which heterotopic calcification is most frequently noted.

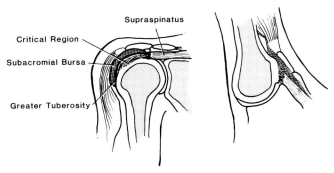

Fig. 14-6. Schematic cross-section of an anterior view of the shoulder showing the subacromial bursa and close proximity of the greater tuberosity to the undersurface of the acromion.

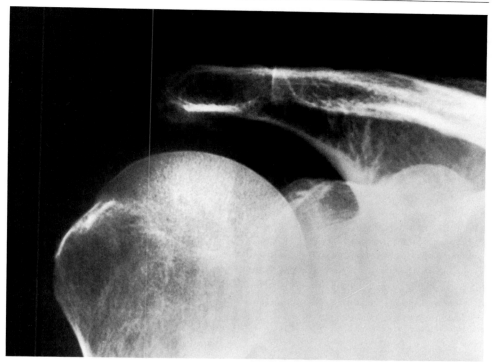

Fig. 14-7. Radiograph of a shoulder showing a large spur on the undersurface of the acromion. By narrowing the subacromial space, such spurs contribute to chronic inpingement.

EVALUATION OF THE PATIENT

History

Just as in the evaluation of a patient with severe chest pain or abdominal pain, a thorough and complete history must be obtained from every patient who complains of shoulder pain. Remote historical information, including shoulder trauma, dislocation, or systemic arthritis may point to a particular diagnosis. The rapidity of onset may be helpful, since massive rotator cuff tears, acute clacific tendinitis, and gout generally produce acute pain. The location of the pain is very important. Pain limited to the midtrapezius suggest a trigger point; pain over the acromioclavicular joint usually signifies local joint disease; pain over the region of the midhumerus at the insertion of the deltoid suggests referred pain from a rotator cuff disorder; and pain radiating down the arm in the C5 dermatome suggests either chronic shoulder pain or perhaps a cervical radiculopathy.[6] While most patients complain of a sharp or aching pain in the shoulder, the character of the pain may aid in making a diagnosis. Reduced motion with minimal pain suggests a frozen shoulder, pain made worse by elevating the arm suggests rotator cuff or A-C joint disease, and paresthesias suggest a radiculopathy or brachioplexus neuropathy. Associated systemic symptoms may point to a specific diagnosis: fever and chills may suggest a septic arthritis, vague abdominal pain or gastrointestinal symptoms may point to gallbladder or subdiaphragmatic disease, and polyarthritis suggests a systemic arthritide.

Physical Examination

The physical examination is the single most important part of the evaluation of shoulder pain. Every patient must be examined with both shoulders and arms fully exposed in order to compare findings. Inspection may reveal local swelling or erythema over the shoulder, as seen in cases of trauma, acute arthritis, or acute calcific bursitis. Changes in the hands may suggest a systemic form of arthritis, a reflex sympathetic dystrophy, or the thoracic outlet syndrome. Atrophy of the deltoid is seen in cases of chronic shoulder pain. Palpation of the shoulder region may reveal: local tenderness over the A-C joint in cases of advanced degenerative arthritis, swelling just lateral to the coracoid process when a glenohumeral effusion is present, local tenderness over the greater tuberosity in cases of bursitis or rotator cuff lesions, or exquisite tenderness over the bicipital groove in patients with bicipital tendinitis (see Fig. 14-8). When palpating the bicipital groove with the thumb, one should not press on the tendon sheath in an overly vigorous fashion since this structure is quite sensitive in normal individuals.

Assessment of active range of motion requires observing the patient perform five separate maneuvers (see Fig. 14-9 a-e).

Abduction. With both arms at the side and the thumbs pointing out, have the patient lift both arms away from the body until the thumbs touch over the head (Fig. 14-9a). This motion should be observed from the front and, more importantly, from the back. If the patient is unable to fully abduct one arm, one usually sees what is called abnormal "scapulothoracic rhythm."[6] Instead of the slow smooth outward rotation of the scapular tip above 30° abduction, one sees lifting of the entire shoulder apparatus—a shrugging motion. When measuring the arc of abduction with a goniometer, it is important to be sure that the torso is in an upright position and not tilted, as so often happens in patients who have to shrug the shoulder in order to lift the arm.

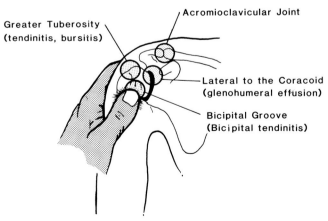

Fig. 14-8.   Important areas to palpate when examining the shoulder.

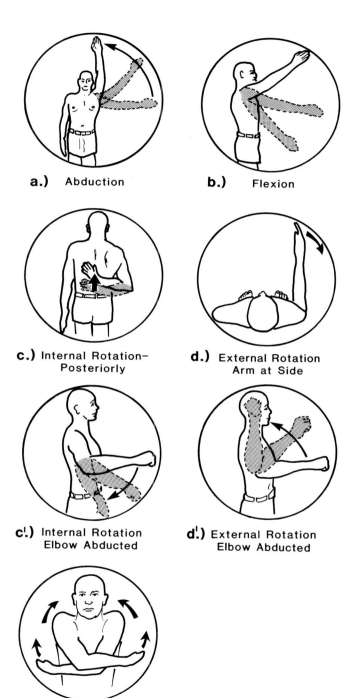

a.) Abduction

b.) Flexion

c.) Internal Rotation–
Posteriorly

d.) External Rotation
Arm at Side

c¹.) Internal Rotation
Elbow Abducted

d¹.) External Rotation
Elbow Abducted

e.) Shrugging

Fig. 14-9. Maneuvers suggested to assess shoulder range of motion.

Flexion. Have the patient slowly lift both extended arms forward until the hands touch overhead. Again, it is important to look for reduced range of motion and abnormal scapulothroacic rhythm (Fig 14-9b).

Internal rotation. Have the patient reach to touch the low back (this motion also includes some abduction) (Fig. 14-9c). As another measure of internal rotation, have the patient point his forearm forward with the elbow flexed to 90° and the arm abducted as close to 90° as possible. Have him rotate the forearm down as far as possible (Fig. 14-9c¹).

External rotation. Keeping the elbows at the side and flexed at 90 degrees, have the patient rotate each hand out as far as possible (Fig. 14-9d). Another measure of external rotation can be made with the forearm pointing forward, the elbow flexed at 90° and abducted as close to 90° as possible. Ask the patient to rotate the forearm upward as far as possible (Fig. 14-9d¹).

Shrugging. Ask the patient to shrug both shoulders while pulling each arm in opposite directions across the front of the chest (Fig. 14-9e).

Each of the above maneuvers should be repeated passively by the examiner (see Fig. 14-10). Another useful test to measure passive arm elevation is to have the patient bend forward and toward the side of the painful shoulder as far as possible, dangling the affected arm in a "gravity traction" (see Fig. 14-11). The examiner or patient should then hold the arm in the same position relative to the shoulder and have the patient stand straight up. This technique minimizes muscle spasm, which may limit the standard testing of abduction and flexion.

Eliciting pain against resistance is an important part of the physical exam. Localization of the major site of shoulder pathology may be helped in some cases by having the patient contract specific muscle groups against resistance. Forced abduction of an elbow that is held at 30° abduction tests the supraspinatus muscle. With the examiner holding the patient's elbow at the side, forced external rotation against resistance tests the infraspinatus and teres minor. Internal rotation with the elbow fixed at the side tests the subscapularis. Forced supination of the forearm and hand with the elbow flexed at 90° tests the biceps (see Fig. 14-12).

A full sensory and motor neurologic examination, including reflexes, should always be

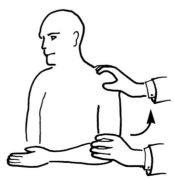

Fig. 14-10.   Passive abduction of the shoulder.

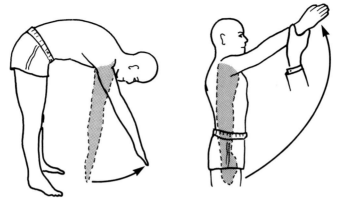

Gravity Traction   **Passive Abduction**

Fig. 14-11. Technique to measure passive abduction/flexion. First, have the patient dangle the arm, bending over as far as possible in gravity traction. Next, have him lift the arm as far out (or forward) as possible. Hold the arm in the same position relative to the torso and have the patient stand upright.

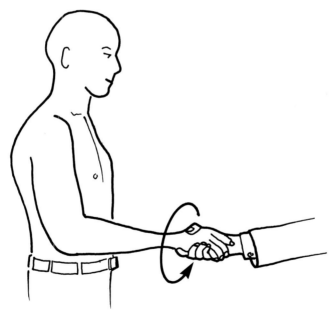

Fig. 14-12. Forced supination of the forearm against resistance often exacerbates isolated bicipital tendinitis.

343

performed to rule out neurologic disease at the level of the neck, brachial plexus, and upper arm. Additional testing for signs of vascular compromise may be necessary in patients with suspected thoracic outlet syndrome.

Radiologic Examination

In the majority of cases, the etiology of the shoulder pain can be diagnosed clinically, plain radiographs adding minimal information. In specific cases or in patients with recurrent episodes of shoulder pain, however, plain radiographs may be very helpful.[51] Patients with acute calcific tendinitis will show a large "fluffy" calcific mass (see Fig. 14-13). In cases of chronic rotator cuff tendinitis, one may see osteophyte formation on the undersurface of the acromion or A-C joint, small calcific deposits in the rotator cuff tendons, and/or degenerative changes, including osteopenia and cyst formation in the humeral head (see Fig. 14-14).[9] Fluroscopic evaluation in these cases may reveal direct contact between the undersurface of the acromion and the greater tuberosity when the arm is abducted. In cases of complete rotator cuff tears, one may see the acromiohumeral space narrowed to less than 0.6 centimeters. Subacromial bursography may reveal signs of chronic impingement, but the exact role of this procedure in the diagnosis and management of shoulder pain is unclear.[56] Arthrography can be diagnostic in suspected complete rotator cuff tears since contrast material injected into the glenohumeral joint will flow through the rent into the subacromial space (see Fig. 14-15). In patients with a frozen shoulder, arthrography

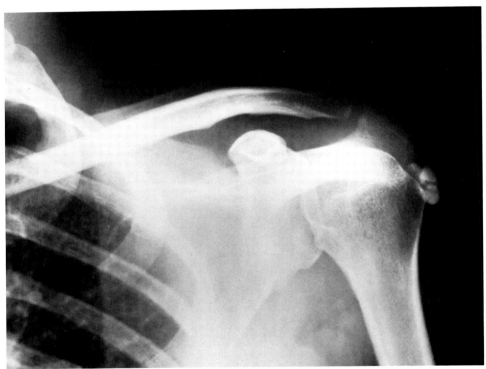

Fig. 14-13. Radiography demonstrating a large area of calcification in the region of the supraspinatus tendon—consistent with calcific periarthritis.

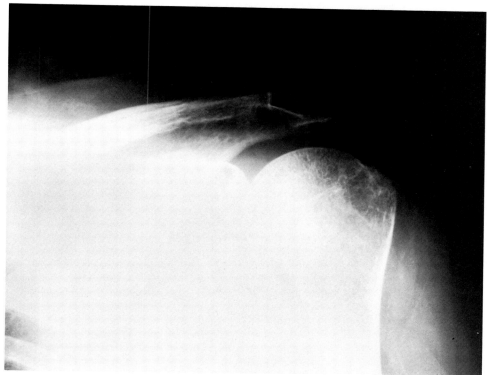

Fig. 14-14. Radiograph showing marked degenerative cystic changes in the humeral head with irregularities over the lateral aspect of the greater tuberosity. A small subacromial spur is also present.

may not only be helpful diagnostically—the joint space being small and contracted—but also therapeutically (see Fig. 14-16). Distention or "brisement" of the joint space at the time of arthrography with 50 milliliters of contrast material or saline has been reported to help this condition. Plain radiographs may also show evidence of more rare causes of shoulder pain, including chondrocalcinosis, "Milwaukee shoulder," aseptic necrosis, and metastatic tumor.

SPECIFIC SHOULDER DISORDERS

The multiple causes of shoulder pain can be readily classified as either extrinsic or intrinsic to the shoulder. Diagnosing each case can, however, be much more difficult. The most common extrinsic causes of shoulder pain are listed in Table 14-1, and the most common intrinsic causes of shoulder pain are listed in Table 14-2.

Rotator Cuff Lesions

The literature describing rotator cuff lesions is somewhat confusing since different authors use different criteria to define specific disorders. Still, there appear to be three basic clinical syndromes resulting from distinctly different pathologic processes in the

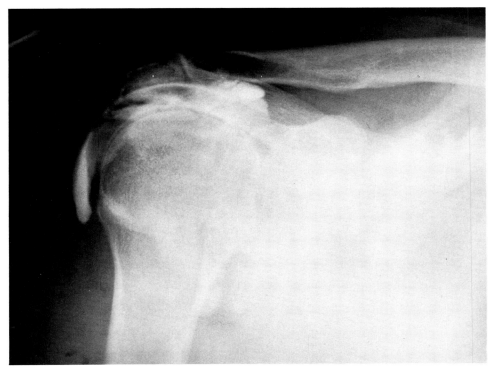

Fig. 14-15. Arthrogram of the glenohumeral joint showing opacification of the subacromial bursa, indicative of a complete tear in the rotator cuff.

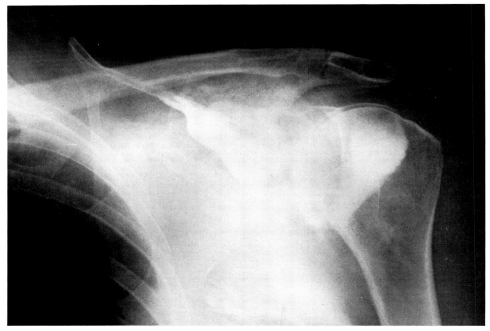

Fig. 14-16. Arthrogram of the shoulder of a patient with clinical evidence of a frozen shoulder. The capacity of the glenohumeral capsule is reduced with only a remnant of the axillary recess. Irregularity of the capsular insertion is also present.

346

Table 14-1

Extrinsic Causes of Shoulder Pain

Neurologic Disorders
  Cervical Radiculopathy
  Acute Brachial Neuritis
  Specific Nerve Lesions (long thoracic nerve, suprascapular nerve)
  Brachial Plexus Disease (trauma, pancoast tumor, etc.)
Vascular Disorders
  Thoracic Outlet Syndrome(s)
  Other Vascular Syndromes (Aortic Arch, Axillary Vein Thrombosis, etc.)
Myofascial Pain Syndromes
  Trigger Points
  Fibromyalgia
Tumor
  Primary Bone Tumors
  Metastatic Disease
Referred Pain
  Gallbladder Disease
  Myocardial Infarction
  Subdiaphragmatic Abscess
  Pleuropulmonary Disease

rotator cuff: first, inflammation and degeneration of the rotator cuff and subacromial bursa, second, acute massive rotator cuff tears, and third, acute calcific tendinitis.

Subacromial Inflammation/Degeneration (Rotator Cuff Tendinitis)

Diagnosis. The recent work by Neer[41] and by Kessel and Watson[28] has clarified the spectrum of clinical and pathologic findings associated with subacute lesions in the rotator cuff. A spectrum of changes in the rotator cuff ranging from inflammation with mild hemorrhage to chronic degenerative changes including cuff tears are felt to be the result of acute and chronic injury to the "critical" portion of the cuff that impinges on the coracoacromial arch during abduction (see Fig. 14-6).[16] When the tendons become inflamed, the overlying bursa also becomes inflamed. The descriptive terms *impingement syndrome* and *painful arc syndrome* that are used by these authors convey the appropriate clinical picture. Individuals who use their shoulders excessively appear to be at increased risk for developing shoulder pain. Specific risk factors include: participation in sporting activities that require circumduction of the humerus (tennis, pitching, swimming, etc.), chronic occupational trauma, and degenerative disease on the undersurface of the acromion or acromioclavicular joint, which narrows the coracohumeral distance.

Neer has proposed different "stages" in rotator cuff pathology from: Stage I, mild edema and hemorrhage, usually in young athletes less than 25 years of age; to Stage II, fibrosis and tendinitis with thickening of the subacromial bursa, usually in older athletes age 25–40 years; to Stage III, tendon degeneration, bony changes, and tendon rupture, seen in individuals over the age of 40 years.[43] While more extensive degenerative changes are seen in individuals over the age of 50 years, any of these stages of rotator cuff disease can be seen at any age.

Clinically, patients complain of a nagging, aching pain over the lateral midhumerus at the level of the insertion of the deltoid. The pain is often quite severe at night and it is

Table 14-2
Intrinsic Causes of Shoulder Pain

Rotator Cuff Lesions
    Subacromial Inflammation/Degeneration (The Painful Arc Syndrome, Subacromial
        Impingement, Rotator Cuff Tendinitis, Supraspinatus Tenditis, Subacromial Bursitis)
    Partial Rotator Cuff Tears
    Complete Rotator Cuff Tears
    Calcific Tendinitis/Bursitis
Biceps Tendon (Long Head) Lesions
    Tendinitis/Tenosynovitis
    Rupture
    Dislocation
Frozen Shoulder or Adhesive Capsulitis
    Idiopathic
    Secondary to Immobilization/Injury
Reflex Sympathetic Dystrophy
Arthritis
    Osteoarthritis
        Acromioclavicular Joint
        Glenohumeral Joint
    Systemic Arthritis (Rheumatoid Arthritis, Ankylosing Spondylitis, Psoriatic Arthritis, etc.)
    Crystal Induced Arthritis
        Gout
        Chondrocalcinosis or Calcium Pyrophosphate Deposition Disease.
    Other
        Septic Arthritis
        Polymyalgia Rheumatica
        The Milwaukee Shoulder Syndrome
        Amyloid Arthropathy
        Neuropathic Joint Disease
Aseptic Necrosis and Osteochondritis Dessicans
Acute Orthopedic Injury
    Dislocation
    Fracture
    Avulsion of Rotator Cuff
Shoulder Instability

provoked when the arm is actively lifted between 60° and 120° of abduction (see Fig. 14-17).[28] There is often point tenderness over the greater tuberosity where the supraspinatus tendon inserts and abduction against resistance often worsens the pain. Passive elevation of the arm may elicit the "impingement sign," which is pain associated with a painful grimace as the greater tuberosity is juxtaposed under the anterior aspect of the acromion (see Fig. 14-18). Patients with rotator cuff tendinitis often have tenderness over the bicipital groove in addition to tenderness over the greater tuberosity. This common finding usually signifies more extensive disease. Acute swelling, erythema, and joint effusion are not features of rotator cuff tendinitis, nor is true muscle weakness. Table 14-3 summarizes the most common clinical features associated with rotator cuff tendinitis.

    Local injection of 3–8 milliliters of 1 percent lidocaine into the subacromial bursa can be very useful in helping to make a diagnosis of rotator cuff tendinitis. this procedure ameliorates the pain of tendinitis/bursitis in almost all patients with inflammatory cuff

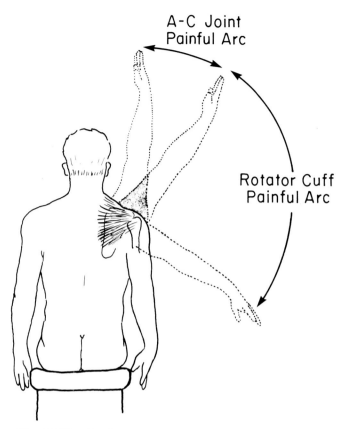

Fig. 14-17. Tendinitis of the rotator cuff classically causes a painful arc of abduction between 60° and 120° while pain due to degenerative disease in the acromioclavicular joint usually causes a high painful arc of abduction between 120° to 180°.

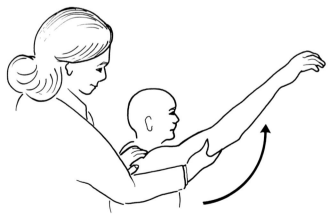

Fig. 14-18. Eliciting the "impingement sign." Forced elevation of the humerus causes the inflamed rotator cuff to impinge against the coracoacromial arch.

Table 14-3

Clinical Features of Rotator Cuff Tendinitis

1. Ill-defined pain over upper arm in the region where the deltoid inserts.
2. Night pain prominent.
3. Tenderness over the rotator cuff.
4. Painful arc of abduction between 60–120°.
5. Relief of pain, improved motion after injecting the subacromial bursa with
   3–8 ml of 1% lidocaine.

lesions, and it allows accurate assessment of the true range of shoulder motion. While some individuals with rotator cuff inflammation have a full range of motion prior to the injection of the local anesthetic, most have limited abduction and flexion secondary to pain. Ten to fifteen minutes after administration of lidocaine, active or passive range of motion should be greater than 130° of abduction. When passive range of motion is less than 90° abduction, particularly when testing passive range of motion using the gravity-traction technique, a partial frozen shoulder is likely to be present.

Kessel has suggested that abolishment of pain after injection of a small amount of lidocaine into the most tender area of the rotator cuff pinpoints the exact site of disease.[28] For example, tenderness over the posterior aspect of the greater tuberosity that is relieved by an injection signifies an infraspinatus lesion. Other authors feel that this method cannot reliably locate the major site of disease.[16] Regardless, there is near universal agreement that the most significant and serious changes occur over the superior portion of the cuff in the supraspinatus tendon where blood supply is limited and where close opposition to the coracoacromial arch occurs during arm elevation (see Fig. 14-6)

Based on the clinical examination alone, it is difficult to predict either the extent of pathologic changes in the rotator cuff or the response of a given patient to medical therapy. Different individuals with identical examinations may have very different pathology; one having mild swelling and inflammation and one having chronic degenerative changes with a small, complete rotator cuff tear.[15,22] While more advanced age, a history of multiple prior episodes of shoulder pain, atrophy of the infraspinatus and supraspinatus muscles, and degenerative changes in the greater tuberosity suggest more advanced pathology, many of these patients respond dramatically to a conservative treatment program. Thus, regardless of the historical or physical findings, all patients with the painful arc syndrome deserve a trial of medical therapy.

Therapy. Treatment of rotator cuff tendinitis generally includes: (1) reduction or discontinuation of any activity that traumatizes the shoulder (eg, stop throwing, lifting, etc.), (2) institution of a physical-rehabilitative exercise program to maintain range of motion and prevent the development of a frozen shoulder, (3) judicious use of analgesics, if needed, and (4) anti-inflammatory therapy using either local injection of a depocorticosteroid preparation into the subacromial bursa or an oral nonsteroidal anti-inflammatory agent.[16,29,58] Surgery to "decompress" the coricoacromial arch is recommended only in patients who have pain and disability after the protracted course of conservative treatment.[41] An arthrogram should be considered only in those patients who do not respond to conservative therapy and who are surgical candidates.

Although there have been no large, well-designed studies comparing physical rehabilitation modalities alone to various anti-inflammatory drug treatment plans, most physicians who treat shoulder pain feel that rest and physiotherapy are the most beneficial parts of any therapeutic regimen.[16,22,29,43] Avoidance of all shoulder motions that provoke pain is an obvious first step in any treatment, since active exercise tends to provoke further microtrauma, pain, and spasm. In the case of young athletes, specific alterations in shoulder motion can often be recommended that allow continuation of a modified training program.[49] Pain can often be dramatically reduced by application of ice, or, in other cases, moist heat. Ultrasound treatment for 7–10 days (1.2–1.5 w/cm for 5 minutes/ day to the supraspinatus region) is often beneficial. Transcutaneous nerve stimulation has been successfully used in some younger individuals with sporting injuries.

Rotator cuff strength and tone should be maintained or improved using isokinetic exercises or, more simply, by performing the Codman exercises (see Fig. 14-19). The patient bends forward and laterally at the waist, letting the arm of the affected shoulder fall vertically towards the floor in a "gravity-traction." Slowly and gently the arm is swung back and forth along the side and then across the front of the body with a small weight (5– 10 pounds) held in the hand. The rotator cuff muscles will gain tone and strength in proportion to the work that they perform, ie, the weight that is carried. Range of motion can also be preserved by doing finger-up-the-wall exercises. Standing an arm's length away from a wall, either facing the wall or standing 90° to the wall, the patient should "walk" two fingers up and down the wall as high as possible (see Fig. 14-20). Other exercise, including wand exercises, pulley exercises, rotation exercises and active shoulder flexion and abduction can also be used. Short wave diathermy is losing favor by most physiatrists, since application of too much heat can actually cause injury and overall worsening in the patient's condition.[29] A variant, pulse electromagnetic field therapy, may be a safer, albeit more cumbersome, method of delivering heat.[5] Other modalities that have been advocated include acupuncture and DMSO therapy.[17]

The efficacy of locally injected, long-acting corticosteroid preparations in the treatment of subacromial tendinitis/degeneration is not clear. Uncontrolled observations suggest that local injection of corticosteroids into the subacromial bursa or "region of

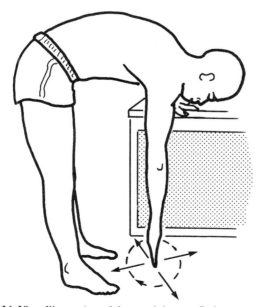

Fig. 14-19.   Illustration of the pendulum or Codman exercises.

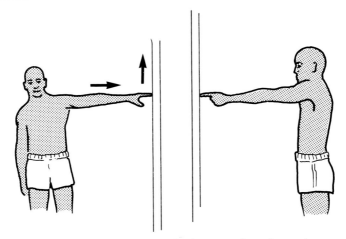

Fig. 14-20.   Illustration of the finger-up-the-wall exercise.

greatest tenderness" greatly benefits 60–80 percent of patients treated, at least over a short period of follow-up.[12,25] However, in an early study of 51 patients with shoulder pain who were treated with either 25 milligrams of hydrocortisone (equivalent to 5 milligrams of methylprednisolone) injected into the subacromial bursa or 5 milliliters of 2 percent lidocaine injected locally, both groups of patients improved equally with respect to pain and range of abduction.[40] In another study that compared local injection of 25 milligrams of prednisolone acetate to local injection of saline alone, a greater degree of improvement in range of motion was noted in the steroid group.[52] Unfortunately, no baseline data was given, and the study was neither blinded nor randomized. In a more recent study, Darlington and Coomes studied 40 patients with shoulder pain who had a painful arc of abduction and painful resisted abduction but who still had full range of motion.[15] They arbitrarily divided patients into 2 groups and treated half with a single injection of 40 milligrams of methylprednisolone acetate plus 1 milliliter of 2 percent lidocaine into the region of greatest tenderness, and the other half was treated with only 1 milliliter of 2 percent lidocaine. Overall, there was no significant difference in pain parameters or the percent of patients with a persistent painful arc after 6 weeks. Interestingly, 37 of the 40 patients in this study had an arthrogram and 27 (73 percent) had a complete cuff tear! This finding only underscores the point that patients may have full range of motion with a small capsular tear and that, clinically, they appear identical to patients who do not have capsular tears. In another small, single-blinded study, Berry and his colleagues compared local injection of 40 milligrams of methylprednisolone acetate plus 2 milliliters of 2 percent lidocaine with: (1) local corticosteroid injection plus nonsteroidal anti-inflammatory therapy with tolmetin, 1200 milligrams per day, (2) acupuncture alone, (3) physiotherapy with ultrasound treatments, and (4) placebo ultrasound plus placebo tolmetin.[4] Twelve patients were randomized into each group, and after 4 weeks there was no statistically significant difference in pain or range of motion in any of the groups. However, subsequent injection of "failures" with local corticosteroid injection plus lidocaine lead to "success" in 20 of 29 cases.

    Based on the clinical studies published to date, there is surprisingly little data to support the notion that local injection(s) of a long-acting corticosteroid preparation is more beneficial than a conservative approach using only rest and physiotherapy. Since injection of local corticosteroid into tendons has been shown to cause disruption of collagen structure and to be associated with subsequent tendon rupture in some cases, many physicians proscribe the use of local corticosteroid therapy in treating painful shoulders.[21,22,27] Still, early injection of a long-acting corticosteroid is advocated by many authorities in the field, including some sports medicine experts.[16,28,43,49] Kessel's results, for example, suggest that local steroids may be the only treatment required in patients with a painful arc syndrome who have tenderness confined to the area over the infraspinatus or subscapularis tendons.[28] If local corticosteroid injection is contemplated, there is evidence that the site of injection should be the region of the subacromial bursa immediately adjacent to the most significantly inflamed tendon, as determined by the clinical examination. Injection of the most tender area of the shoulder, which may be over the supraspinatus or deltoid muscles in some cases, is significantly less effective.[26]

The combination of physiotherapy plus treatment with an oral nonsteroidal anti-inflammatory agent is frequently recommended as the initial treatment for rotator cuff tendinitis.[6,29,49] However, the relative efficacy of this regimen has never been compared to local corticosteroid therapy. We recently completed a prospective, randomized, double-blind, double-dummy, study of 30 patients with the painful arc syndrome. In this study we compared subacromial injection of 40 milligrams of methylprednisolone acetate plus home physical therapy to treatment with 100 mg/day of indomethacin plus home physical therapy. In order to enter the study, each patient had to have a painful arc syndrome for less than 12 weeks duration and had to have a passive range of abduction greater than 90° after bursal injection of 2–3 milliliters of 1 percent lidocaine. This insured that we were not dealing with patients with a frozen shoulder. After the local lidocaine injection, patients were randomized to receive either placebo saline (injected with an opaque syringe) plus unmarked indomethacin, or active corticosteroid plus identical placebo indomethacin. Injection of the subacromial bursa was made using the lateral approach (see fig. 14-21). Range of motion was measured using a goniometer as well as a four-point grading system. Pain was measured using a 10 centimeter visual analog scale for both day

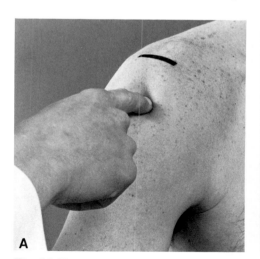
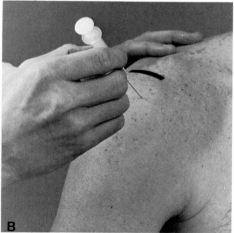

Fig. 14-21. Photo illustrating how to inject the subacromial bursa using the lateral approach. The black tape runs along the top of the acromium. (A) Placing an index finger somewhat anterior to the midline and 2–3 cm below the top of the acromion, one palpates the space between the lower surface of the acromion and the humeral head by passively abducting the humerus and feeling the deltoid dimple inward. (B) At this spot, one inserts the needle at a 45° angle and injects just as the needle tip meets resistance, after passing through the deltoid muscle.

Table 14-4

Comparison of Local Injection of Methylprednisolone Acetate Versus
Indomethacin in the Treatment of Rotator Cuff
Tendinitis/Degeneration.

	Indomethacin (N = 15)	Local Steroid (N = 15)
Men/Women	3/12	7/8
Age (years)	57 ± 15	56 ± 15
Painful Arc of Abduction (degrees ± SD)		
Initial	64° ± 18°	72° ± 27°
6 weeks	106° ± 46°	120° ± 46°
Maximal Arc of Abduction (degrees ± SD)		
Initial	104° ± 44°	104° ± 35°
6 weeks	119° ± 39°	138° ± 38°
Patient Pain Score (cm ± SD)		
(sum of day + night scores)		
Initial	12.2 cm ± 4.8	11.2 cm ± 2.8
6 week	6.1 cm ± 6.8	6.2 cm ± 5.5
Number Improved		
Significantly	8	6
Modestly	2	3
Minimally	5	6

and night pain. Patients were followed up at 3 weeks and given a second injection and refill of medication if they complained of "moderate" pain or if the examining physician noted "moderately" reduced range of motion. There was no difference in any motion or pain parameters between the groups initially. Results of the findings after 6 weeks are outlined in Table 14-4. Although there was a greater degree of improvement in the maximal arc of abduction in the corticosteroid-treated group, both groups showed similar degrees of improvement with respect to pain and the arc of initial pain during abduction. Overall, there were no significant differences between the groups either before therapy or after 6 weeks of therapy.

Taken together with the results of studies that have compared local corticosteroids to local lidocaine alone, our findings suggest that the most prudent initial treatment program should include: (1) local injection of a local anesthetic such as lidocaine (approximately 3–8 milliliters of 1 percent lidocaine) into the subacromial bursa as a useful diagnostic and, possibly, therapeutic maneuver; (2) temporary discontinuation of shoulder motions that provoke pain (especially true for athletes); (3) physiotherapy (ice or moist heat, ultrasound) aimed at minimizing pain while maintaining range of motion and rotator cuff muscle tone; and (4) drug therapy with a nonsteroidal anti-inflammatory agent to minimize pain and, possibly, inflammation (see Table 14-5). If this therapy does not lead to improvement in 6–8 weeks, 1 or 2 injections of a long-acting corticosteroid preparation spaced 3–4 weeks apart may lead to diminution of pain and, possibly, improved motion. Patients who fail this program and remain symptomatic 2 months following the injections can be considered as treatment failures and referred to an orthopedic surgeon for consideration of operative relief of subacromial impingement. Most series suggest that only a small proportion of patients eventually require surgery.[16,28]

Surgery for the painful arc syndrome is designed to relieve the impingement that occurs when the greater tuberosity and rotator cuff tendons meet the coracoacromial arch

Table 14-5

Treatment of Rotator Cuff Tendinitis

1. Local injection of 3–8 ml 1% lidocaine into the subacromial bursa
   (helpful diagnostically and, potentially, therapeutically).
2. Discontinuation of shoulder motions that aggravate pain.
3. Physiotherapy with ultrasound and isokinetic exercises.
4. Nonsteroidal anti-inflammatory drug therapy, such as indomethacin 100–150 mg/day and
   additional analgesia as needed.
5. If no improvement in 4–6 weeks, local injection of the equivalent of
   40 mg of methylprednisolone acetate into the subacromial bursa.

during abduction.[41] The Neer technique is generally felt to be the operation of choice.[2] The operation includes anterior acromioplasty to remove any subacromial spurs, resection of the coracoacromial ligament, and excision of the distal one centimeter of the clavicle if any degenerative spurs are present in this joint. If a rotator cuff tear is present, this is repaired, and if significant degenerative changes are noted on the undersurface of the acromioclavicular joint, this is excised. Surgery can be expected to alleviate pain, but it may not lead to improved range of motion.[48,57]

Rotator Cuff Tears

Rotator cuff tears are classified in two ways: acute versus chronic, depending on the way in which the patient presents, and according to size, gradations running from small (less than 2 centimeters), to medium, to large, to massive (greater than 5 centimeters). Most tears affect the supraspinatus tendon and extend, in some cases, into the subscapularis anteriorly or the infraspinatus posteriorly.[16,20,54] Lesions are either longitudinal or L-shaped, originating in the "critical" area of the supraspinatus tendon that is poorly vascularized. Large tears lead to significant shoulder dysfunction while small tears usually go undiagnosed and often heal without surgical intervention.

Patients with rotator cuff tears present clinically in two very different fashions: as an acute shoulder injury and as subacute shoulder pain, the latter mimicking the painful arc syndrome. Patients who present in the subacute fashion often give a history of occupational stress to the shoulder, as well as symptoms consistent with prior episodes of subacromial impingement. In these cases, the stress of very minor trauma to a rotator cuff with degenerative changes leads to a small full thickness rupture. As pointed out by Darlington and Coomes,[15] patients with small tears often have full range of motion and respond to conservative therapy.

Major tears of the rotator cuff usually occur in men over the age of 40 years following a fall or after lifting a heavy object. In younger individuals the tendons of the rotator cuff are so strong that the injury (eg, anterior dislocation) is usually associated with fracture and avulsion of the greater tuberosity. Individuals complain of acute shoulder pain and inability to abduct the shoulder beyond 30–40°. Examination reveals spasm of the deltoid and, in large tears, a tender depression just above the greater tuberosity where the supraspinatus tendon normally inserts. Injection of 8–10 milliliters of 1 percent lidocaine locally into the subacromial bursa relieves much of the pain and allows a more complete examination, which usually reveals marked weakness of the cuff muscles. Passive range of motion is normal, but the patient cannot maintain the arm at 90° abduction against gravity or minimal downward pressure. The most common clinical features of rotator cuff tears are outlined in Table 14-6.

Table 14-6
Clinical Features of
Rotator Cuff Tears

Small Tears
    Mimic rotator cuff tendinitis.
    Treat as rotator cuff tendinitis.
Large Tears
    Generally follow an acute injury.
    Spasm of the deltoid prominent.
    Inability to abduct above 40°
    Normal passive range of motion.
    Arthrogram makes the diagnosis.

All patients with suspected acute rotator cuff tears who are potential operative candidates should have an arthrogram performed. The diagnostic finding of direct communication between the glenohumeral joint and the subacromial bursa makes the diagnosis[51] (see Fig. 14-15). A small defect on the undersurface of a rotator cuff tendon suggests an incomplete tear. In a few cases, plain radiographs alone will reveal upward subluxation of the humeral head (normal acromiohumeral distance is greater than 0.6 centimeter), a specific but insensitive finding for a major rotator cuff tear. The role of arthroscopy in the diagnosis and management of cuff tears is not well defined.[20]

Surgical repairs should be performed expeditiously in all patients with acute tears who have no contraindication for surgery.[3] In some cases where large rotator cuff tears are not surgically corrected, a severe cuff-tear arthropathy,[45] which may be identical to "Milwaukee" shoulder, may develop with sclerosis of the glenoid and humeral head, periarticular calcifications, and synovial chondromatosis.

Acute Calcific Tendinitis

Radiographic evidence of calcium deposition in the rotator cuff is present in as many as 8 percent of persons over the age of 30 years.[7] In the majority of cases there is a small, sharply defined area of calcification near the point of insertion of the rotator cuff tendons (usually the supraspinatus tendon). Most patients with this finding give a history of shoulder pain, and the calcification very likely develops as a consequence of chronic tendinitis and degenerative changes in the cuff. However, in other totally asymptomatic patients, large areas of calcification can be seen in the "critical" zone of the rotator cuff tendon (see Fig. 14-13). This finding suggests a process very similar to calcific periarthritis, which can develop adjacent to other joints.[35] The exact reason(s) that the calcific material, which chemically is calcium hydroxyapatite, builds up in tendons is not known. Presumably, either local changes in the tendon structure or genetic influences play a major role. Regardless, it is in this group of patients that a syndrome may occur that is properly called acute tendinitis or bursitis.

Patients with acute calcific tendinitis present with a history of the sudden onset of excruciating shoulder pain and tenderness, much like a patient with acute gout.[29,55] While they may give a history of minor shoulder trauma, there is no history of severe trauma that would suggest a major rotator cuff tear or any history to suggest septic arthritis. Based on the operative findings in a few cases of chalk-like or "toothpaste-like" material in the tendon and bursa, it is likely that the acute syndrome represents an acute inflammatory response to the crystaline material that ruptures into the subacromial space (see Fig. 14-22).[37]

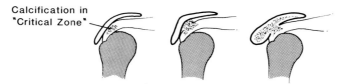

Fig. 14-22. Acute calcific tendinitis occurs when calcium hydroxyapatite crystals that build up in the critical region become hydrated, expand and burst into the subacromial bursa.

On examination, the patient splints the affected shoulder, preventing practically all motion. The area over the rotator cuff is often red, swollen, and warm; it is invariably tender. Shoulder flexion and abduction provoke such severe pain that range of motion is severely limited. Plain radiographs of the shoulder are helpful in making a diagnosis since they show a rather large, "fluffy" oval shaped area of calcification usually just above the greater tuberosity (see Fig. 14-13). If no calcific mass is seen on X-ray, other differential diagnostic possibilities should be seriously considered, including acute septic bursitis, septic arthritis, gout, pseudogout, or, in a patient who is unreliable or cannot give a clear history, a major traumatic injury.

Treatment of acute calcific tendinitis should begin with immobilization of the arm in a sling and administration of adequate analgesia to minimize the pain. Local ice and local injection of a long-acting local anesthetic agent also helps to minimize the pain. Although there have been no controlled trials, injection of a long-acting corticosteroid preparation into the subacromial bursa at the time of the initial examination is advised to treat acute inflammatory process.[55] In addition, during injection of the steroid, one can "needle" the calcific mass in an attempt to enhance the liberation of the material from the "calcium boil."[7]

As soon as the patient can tolerate modest shoulder motion, a physical therapy program that includes range of motion exercises should be instituted. Overall, the prognosis for rapid improvement in the first 4 weeks is excellent, although a second "needling" and steroid injection is sometimes necessary. In rare cases, more chronic pain persists, and surgery is necessary to remove the calcific material.

Bicipital Lesions

Tendinitis

The long head of the biceps tendon originates on the superior rim of the glenoid and passes anteriorly through the glenohumeral joint adjacent to ligamentous portions of the joint capsule before exiting out the intertubercular groove under the intertubercular ligament (see Figs. 14-2 and 14-3). The glenohumeral synovium, which surrounds the tendon as it passes in the groove between the tuberosities, acts as a tendon sheath to minimize the friction created from humeral motion relative to the more fixed tendon. if the intertubercular sulcus is shallow or if there is a prominent supratubercular ridge, the tendon tends to be traumatized by repeated use of the shoulder leading to inflammation and pain, and eventually even dislocation or rupture. In addition, because of the very close anatomical relationship between the rotator cuff tendons and the long head of the biceps, degenerative changes in the cuff, as seen in patient with chronic impingement, can also damage the biceps tendon.

Isolated bicipital tenosynovitis most often occurs in individuals over the age of 30 who traumatize the tendon using forced repetitive motion, most commonly overhead circumduction or forced extension (eg, pulling on slot machines or forcibly throwing objects backward).[46,55] The pain of bicipital tendinitis is felt in the anterior region of the shoulder and local tenderness over the intertubercular groove can be striking. While abduction against resistance is relatively painless, forced flexion against resistance and forced supination of the hand with the elbow flexed at 90° provoke intense pain over the groove (see Fig. 14-12). Even gentle palpation of the tendon as it exits the sulcus produces excruciating pain. A mildly painful arc of flexion and abduction is commonly noted since the inflamed tendon is pushed against the coracoacromial arch during arm elevation. The clinical features of bicipital tendinitis are listed in Table 14-7.

As noted previously, some bicipital tendon pain and local tenderness is frequently noted in patients with rotator cuff lesions. Indeed, numerous series have reported concomitant degenerative changes in both the biceps tendon and rotator cuff at necropsy or at the time of surgery to relieve chronic impingement.[10,46] However, it is distinctly unusual for rotator cuff impingement to present as isolated bicipital tendinitis. Patients with supraspinatus or subscapularis rotator cuff lesions will have painful resisted abduction but little pain on forced supination of the forearm and hand. Instillation of 5–8 milliliters of 1 percent lidocaine into the subacromial bursa substantially reduces the pain associated with rotator cuff disease but has negligible effect on bicipital tenosynovitis.

Treatment of an acute episode of bicipital tendinitis generally includes: (1) resting the shoulder and eliminating all motions that provoke pain, (2) applying local ice packs acutely or moist heat, (3) starting a nonsteroidal anti-inflammatory agent such as indomethacin 100–150 mg/day or phenylbutazone 400 mg/day for several days and, in resistant cases, (4) local injection of a long-acting corticosteroid preparation equivalent to approximately 5–10 milligrams of methylprednisolone into the tendon sheath together with 1 milliliter of 1 percent lidocaine. Since patients who develop bicipital tendinitis are prone to repeated episodes, they must be cautioned that continued use of the shoulder motion that provoked the initial attack may cause repeated flares. In rare cases of isolated chronic bicipital tendinitis, operative intervention may be necessary.[11]

Dislocation and Rupture

A shallow intertubercular groove or laxity/disruption of either the coracohumeral ligament or the transverse humeral ligament may lead to medial displacement of the long head of the biceps.[46] patients complain of anterior shoulder pain and the sensation of a clicking or "snap" as they externally rotate and abduct the arm, which forces the tendon to ride medially over the lesser tuberosity. An arthrogram with special views may reveal the displacement and make the diagnosis. In other cases, however, results are less clear, making it difficult to differentiate anterior subluxation of the shoulder from bicipital

Table 14-7
Clinical Features of Bicipital Tendinitis

1. Pain felt over the anterior aspect of the shoulder.
2. Bicipital tendon exquisitely tender to palpation.
3. Pain aggravated by forced flexion against resistance and forced supination of the hand against resistance.
4. Relief of pain after local injection of 2 ml of 1% lidocaine into the tendon sheath.

dislocation. Therapy for this problem is primarily surgical with various operative procedures advocated, depending on the findings at the time of surgery.

Frank rupture of the long head of the bicep is not an unusual problem in elderly individuals with chronic rotator cuff degeneration. Patients present with shoulder pain and a "Popeye the Sailor Man" appearance with a rather obvious, minimally contractile, lateral biceps muscle mass. Since most patients function quite well using only the short head of the biceps, treatment aside from analgesic therapy is usually not necessary. In evaluating each patient one should, however, exclude a major concomitant rotator cuff tear. Surgical repair of a ruptured tendon is necessary only in younger individuals who require the added strength that anchorage of the tendon will provide.

Frozen Shoulder

The term *frozen shoulder* was first coined by Codman and is aptly descriptive of the disorder that is characterized by mild to moderate shoulder pain and marked limitation of both active and passive range of motion of the glenohumeral joint.[8,29,39,55] Pathologically, the joint capsule is thickened and fibrotic with loss of elasticity. The other frequently used term, *adhesive capsulitis*, is a bit of a misnomer since adhesions are not a part of the pathologic process and synovial inflammation is not a common or major feature. The etiology of this disorder remains an enigma, but it is known to be associated with prolonged shoulder immobilization, particularly in association with a neurologic disorder such as subarachnoid hemorrhage and with rotator cuff injuries. However, most cases are idiopathic. Psychological factors have been suggested to play a role, but there is no solid evidence to support this contention.[59] The problem is unique to the shoulder joint and it usually causes significant disability for many months to several years. The most prominent clinical features associated with a frozen shoulder are listed in Table 14-8.

Patients with a frozen shoulder generally present with the insidious onset of vague shoulder pain and stiffness. In the majority of cases there is no history of major trauma or recent shoulder immobilization, only nagging shoulder discomfort and difficulty sleeping. On examination, the affected shoulder is held at the side. There may be rather obvious deltoid wasting and frequently there is some elevation, or shrugging, of the shoulder unit. Palpation may reveal mild tenderness over the rotator cuff, but the most striking finding is reduced shoulder motion in *all* planes, including internal and external rotation. More importantly, passive range of motion is no better than active range of motion, and local instillation of several milliliters of 1 percent lidocaine into the subacromial bursa fails to improve passive motion. While there are no universally accepted criteria for how limited shoulder motion must be before a frozen shoulder can be diagnosed, passive flexion less than 70°, passive abduction less than 70°, and passive external rotation less than 30° seem to be appropriate guidelines.

Table 14-8
Clinical Features of Frozen Shoulder

1. Insidious onset of pain and stiffness.
2. Atropy of the deltoid.
3. Reduced motion in all planes, including external rotation, before and after subacromial bursa injection of lidocaine.
4. Arthrogram shows a small shrunken capsule.

Plain radiographs are either normal or, in patients with symptoms lasting over several months, mildly abnormal with diffuse diffuse osteopenia of the humeral head. In chronic cases, arthrography usually shows a small shrunken capsule with loss of the subscapular and axillary recesses and irregularity of the capsular insertion (see Fig. 14-16). However, in other cases, arthrography is normal or shows evidence of a rotator cuff tear.[8] This latter finding has implications regarding treatment of the condition.

Any discussion of the treatment of a frozen shoulder must take into consideration the natural history of the disease. Retrospective and prospective studies suggest that the majority of the patients improve spontaneously, albeit slowly, over a 8–18 month period.[23,32,46] Grey reported that 24 of 25 frozen shoulders eventually resolved using analgesics alone.[19] Going along with the notion of spontaneous "thawing" of frozen shoulder, several controlled trials have suggested that simple home physiotherapy alone has the same long term benefit as local steroid injections into the glenohumeral joint or subacromial bursa.[33,46]

Some aggressive treatment regimens have been advocated, including infiltration brisement or joint distention,[1,47] manipulation under anesthesia[16] and direct surgical release of the subscapularis tendon with removal of the capsule.[55] The common end point for each of these procedures, and probably for physiotherapy as well, is rupture of the fibrotic capsule. It has been shown that improved motion is associated, arthrographically, with disruption of the capsule and subscapularis tendon.[1] The infiltration/distention method appears to work by tearing the capsule using hydrostatic pressure. Thirty to 50 milliliters of saline or contrast material, with or without a local anesthesic and a long acting corticosteroid preparation, is injected into the joint space under pressure. While proponents say that this procedure is safe, it has not been tested in any prospective randomized study.[29] Manipulation under anesthesia is a procedure that quickly improves range of motion, but it can be complicated by humeral fracture or brachial plexus injuries. More importantly, none of these more aggressive forms of therapy have been shown to shorten the overall course of the disease. Resolution of pain and disappearance of stiffness still require a number of months.

A rational treatment plan for a frozen shoulder should begin with an accurate diagnosis. Every patient should have active and passive range of motion tested before and after installation of several milliliters of 1 percent lidocaine into the subacromial bursa in order to rule out rotator cuff disease. If a frozen shoulder is present, the most sensible therapeutic plan appears to be an active physical therapy program with analgesia as required. Local injection of corticosteroids appears to offer little additional benefit.[8,23,32] Patients must be advised that the condition does not improve quickly but that the long term prognosis is excellent. In refractory cases, an arthogram seems advisable since a normal finding suggests that continued physical therapy is the only treatment necessary.[8] If major rotator cuff disease, such as a large tear, is present, specific surgical therapy may be necessary. Distention of the joint capsule at the time of the arthrogram may help those individuals who show only a tight shrunken capsule.[1,29]

Reflex Sympathetic Dystrophy

Reflex sympathetic dystrophy (RSD), or the "shoulder-hand-syndrome," is a rare, poorly understood condition characterized by pain and limited motion in the shoulder as well as changes in the forearm and hand.[29] The shoulder pain and dysfunction characteristic of this disorder is very similar to the clinical features of a frozen shoulder. The added findings that differentiate the RSD syndrome from a frozen shoulder include: pain and tenderness distally in the forearm and hand; signs and/or symptoms of vasomotor instability in the affected extremity, including vasodilatation, vasoconstriction, and hyperhydrosis; and swelling in the extremity with dystrophic skin changes, including hypertrichosis and nail changes. Radiographically there is usually evidence of extensive osteopenia in the shoulder and forearm.[30] Bone scintigraphy may show increased blood flow and enhanced periarticular radionuclide activity in the affected extremity.[30,31] Although the pathogenesis of this disorder is not known, it may be related to neuroregulatory dysfunction or changes in the autonomic innervation to the arm. Individuals over the age of 50 years, patients who are immobilized following stroke or myocardial infarction, patients with pulmonary tuberculosis and, interestingly, patients taking isoniazid, appear to be at increased risk for developing RSD. While treatment is controversial, intensive physical therapy should be initiated as soon as possible in order to preserve function and to prevent further deterioration. In the early stages of the disease, a short course of oral prednisone, starting with 40 milligrams twice a day and tapering over 4–6 weeks, appears to be very beneficial.[30,31]

Arthritic Disorders

Osteoarthritis of the Acromioclavicular Joint

The acromioclavicular (A-C) joint is diarthroidial with a thin intra-articular disc that usually degenerates by the time a person is 30 years old. Radiographic evidence of degenerative changes in the A-C joint is common in middle-aged and elderly individuals, the process usually secondary to either prior traumatic injury or generalized osteoarthritis.[16] Because the underside of the A-C joint is situated just above the supraspinatus tendon, an osteophytic spur on this side of the joint can distort the coracoacromial ligament and impinge on the rotator cuff (see Fig. 14-14).[9]

Clinically, degenerative disease in the A-C joint presents in two fashions. Most patients present with symptoms suggestive of rotator cuff disease, with a painful arc of abduction between 60° and 120° and radiographic evidence of a large spur on the underportion of the A-C joint. Other patients present with poorly localized shoulder pain that is aggravated when the arm is lifted between 120° and 180° of abduction.[28] This high painful arc causes compression to the acromion against the clavicle. Individuals presenting in this latter fashion typically have local tenderness over the A-C joint and local injection of 0.5 milliliters of 1 percent lidocaine into the joint space greatly reduces the pain.

Plain radiographs of the shoulder are useful in evaluating the A-C joint since narrowing and sclerotic changes as well as osteophytic changes on the undersurface can usually be seen quite clearly.[51] Osteophytes larger than 2.5 millimeters may be partially responsible for rotator cuff impingement in patients with the painful arc syndrome. It is important to remember, however, that many individuals who have advanced degenerative changes in the A-C joint are asymptomatic.

Treatment of A-C joint degeneration depends on the manner in which the patient presents. The presence of a degenerative spur in association with the painful arc syndrome should not modify initial medical therapy. If surgery is necessary in order to decompress the coracoacromial arch, most surgeons recommend removing the distal one inch of the clavicle if major degenerative spurs are present.[28,41] Symptoms of local A-C joint pain can be treated stepwise starting with elimination of motions that aggravate the pain and simple analgesic therapy. Injection of a small amount of a local long-acting corticosteroid preparation into the joint space can be tried if A-C joint pain continues to be a problem. In the most refractory cases, arthroplasty may be advisable.[16]

Glenohumeral Degenerative Arthritis

While primary osteoarthritis of the glenohumeral joint is unusual, it should be considered in any middle-aged or elderly individual who presents with shoulder pain.[16] Small anterior and inferior degenerative spurs off the glenoid fossa and inferior portion of the joint are common radiographic findings that are almost always asymptomatic. More advanced changes with marked narrowing of the joint space, subchondral cyst formation, and large osteophytes indicate significant degenerative disease (see Fig. 14-23).[51] Physical examination generally reveals decreased range of motion—particularly in abduction— some tenderness over the rotator cuff, and crepitus during passive and active movements. Local injection of 1 percent lidocaine into the region of the subacromial bursa does not significantly improve the pain or motion. Elderly individuals with degenerative arthritis can be managed quite well using a conservative treatment plan consisting of analgesics, local heat, and judicious use of locally injected corticosteroids. Younger individuals may benefit from total shoulder replacement if pain and disability indicate the need for surgery.

Rheumatoid Arthritis

The majority of patients with rheumatoid arthritis (RA) who develop significant shoulder pain and dysfunction are patients with advanced, progressive rheumatoid dis-

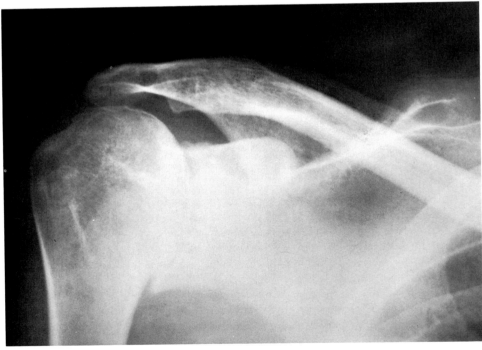

Fig. 14-23. Plain radiograph of the shoulder shows marked narrowing of the glenohumeral joint with subchondral sclerosis and cyst formation with hypertrophic new bone characteristic of degenerative joint disease.

ease. It is unusual for milder forms of RA to be manifest primarily in the shoulder region, but it has been reported.[13] Active inflammation in the shoulder region may cause a number of problems, including: (1) subacromial bursitis/rotator cuff tendinitis with striking proliferation of the bursal tissues; (2) glenohumeral synovitis, which may eventually lead to destruction of the joint; (3) bicipital tendinitis with or without tendon rupture; (4) acromioclavicular synovitis; and (5) sternoclavicular synovitis.[42]

Treatment of any of the shoulder manifestations of RA begins with adequate control of systemic inflammation using anti-inflammatory agents and the "disease-modifying" agents such as gold, penicillamine, or methotrexate. Range of motion exercises also play a central role in the therapy of RA. Maintenance of full motion in the shoulder is particularly critical, since immobilization can lead to a frozen shoulder. When assistive devices such as crutches are prescribed because of lower extremity disease, implications regarding stress on the shoulders must be considered.

Rotator cuff tendinitis/bursitis is the most common shoulder problem seen in patients with RA. Rheumatoid involvement is often confined to the subacromial bursa, causing a classic painful arc syndrome. Clinical findings are similar to other patients with subacromial impingement with the notable exception that bursal swelling and effusions can be a prominent feature in patients with RA. Conservative treatment using heat and ultrasound may greatly benefit some patients. Local injection of a long-acting corticosteroid preparation into the bursa usually produces striking benefit that may last for several months. Chronic recurrent pain with limitation of motion is an indication to consider bursectomy and decompression of the coracoaromial arch. If shoulder motion is compromised in the absence of advanced glenohumeral arthritis, Neer recommends release of the joint capsule and subscapularis tendon at the time of surgery.[42] Interestingly, rotator cuff tears are not a major problem in patients with rheumatoid arthritis, only 30 percent of the patients who require surgery for chronic impingement having this finding at the time of surgery.[44] Minor tears of the rotator cuff can be treated conservatively, while major tears are very difficult to repair since they generally occur in the setting of an active glenohumeral synovitis.

Synovitis involving the glenohumeral joint should be treated just like any other major joint: systemic inflammation must be controlled and disproportionate inflammation confined to the shoulder can be treated with local injection of a long-acting corticosteroid preparation, after infection has been ruled out by joint fluid aspiration with culture of the fluid. When glenohumeral disease is advanced, radiographic evidence of destructive changes can be striking, and clinical examination may reveal marked diminution of shoulder motion in all planes, suggesting a frozen shoulder. Aggressive local treatment at this stage is disappointing, and arthroplasty of the joint should be considered, particularly if there is unremitting pain.[42] Since poor hand or elbow function can compromise the results of shoulder arthroplasty, a thorough preoperative orthopedic assessment of the upper extremity including an arthrogram is mandatory. Results of Neer total shoulder replacement in selected patients are encouraging.[2] If the rotator cuff is damaged, a Kessel prosthesis may be indicated.

Since the bicipital tendon is surrounded by tenosynovium that is a direct extension of the glenohumeral synovium, it is easy to understand why bicipital tendinitis is a common finding in RA. Conservative treatment using local corticosteroid injections frequently reduces pain and improves motion. Bicipital rupture is, unfortunately, a common complication that usually does not require surgical intervention. Disease limited to the A-C joint or sternoclavicular joint can be treated in most cases with local measures. Surgery on these joints may be required in order to reduce pain.[16]

Crystal-Induced Arthritis

Both gout and calcium pyrophosphate deposition disease (CPPD), or pseudogout, may produce acute or subacute shoulder pain and inflammation. In both cases it is distinctly unusual for the shoulder to be the initial joint involved, and a careful history will usually elicit prior episodes of acute large toe, foot, ankle, or knee arthritis in the case of gout or knee and sometimes wrist involvement in the case of CPPD.[14] Aspiration of joint fluid to verify the presence of crystals is the only way to make a definitive diagnosis and to exclude the possibility of infection. Radiographic evidence of CPPD includes chondro-calcinosis of the articular cartilage and advanced degenerative changes of the glenohu-meral joint. Gout generally produces either no changes or joint space narrowing with sharply marginated erosions.[51]

Therapy of a gouty shoulder is the same as for acute gout involving any other major joint. Acute inflammation can be controlled using a nonsteroidal anti-inflammatory agent, such as indomethacin, 50 milligrams orally 3 times a day. Acute gout diagnosed in the first 24 hours after onset of symptoms can be treated with intravenous colchicine, 1 milligram intravenously over 1 minute with a second intravenous injection of 1 milligram 15–30 minutes later. Care must be taken to avoid extravasation of the colchicine into subcutane-ous tissues since this will lead to massive skin necrosis. Use of oral colchicine for an acute attack of gout is not advocated. Therapy designed to reduce the serum uric acid level is indicated in motivated patients who experience frequently recurring episodes of gout. Therapy for acute CPPD (pseudogout) begins with use of a standard nonsteroidal anti-inflammatory agent, such as indomethacin 100–150 milligrams a day in divided doses. Local injection of a long-acting corticosteroid preparation may be beneficial. For more chronic pain, therapy is the same as for osteoarthritis.

Infectious Arthritis

Acute nongonoccocal infectious arthritis involving the shoulder in not rare, most series reporting glenohumeral involvement in 5–15 percent of all cases of septic arthri-tis.[18,34] Since the rapidity with which one makes the diagnosis of acute infectious arthritis is a major factor affecting outcome, one must always consider the possibility of septic arthritis when evaluating a patient with shoulder pain. Historical features that should be sought include the presence of fever, chills, symptoms of infection elsewhere in the body such as the urinary tract or skin, prior arthritis in the glenohumeral joint, and recent antibiotic use. Examination of a septic shoulder usually reveals warmth and tenderness with a palpable glenohumeral effusion. Any motion of the joint provokes considerable pain.

Joint fluid must be aspirated in order to obtain a specimen for culture.[18] Staphlococci, streptococci, hemophilus influenza, and gram-negative organisms are responsible for most cases of nongonococcal septic arthritis. Synovial analysis generally shows: a positive Gram-stain, a white blood cell count greater than 50,000 cells/mm^3 (in most cases it is greater than 100,000 cells/mm^3) with a polymorphoneculear leukocyte predominance and low synovial fluid glucose (synovial/serum glucose less than 40 percent). Plain radiographs are usually normal early in disease but eventually show demineralization, joint space narrow-ing, and erosive changes.[50] An arthrogram may show synovial irregularity, extra-articular extension of the infection, and a tear in the rotator cuff.

Therapy for infectious arthritis is intravenous administration of an appropriate anti-biotic and repeated needle aspiration of the shoulder joint until no further fluid accumu-lates. Intravenous antibiotic therapy should be continued for at least 2 weeks for nongonococcal infection and therapy should be continued for an additional 2 weeks using oral antibiotics. Physical therapy should be initiated as soon as possible, since passive range of motion exercises may prevent significant long-term reduction in joint motion.

Rarely, unusual organisms such as tuberculosis or fungi cause infectious arthritis in the shoulder. If radiographic changes suggestive of an infectious process are noted and synovial fluid cultures are negative, biopsy and culture of the synovium may be necessary in order to make a diagnosis.

Polymyalgia Rheumatica

The diagnosis of polymyalgia rheumatica (PMR) should be considered in any patient over the age of 50 years who complains of vague bilateral, symmetrical shoulder girdle stiffness and pain.[24] Patients typically also complain of myalgias in the neck and pelvic region. Systemic symptoms are common, with fever, sweats, fatigue, anorexia, and weight loss being major features. Signs and symptoms of temporal arteritis are present in a substantial number of patients with PMR.[38] Clinically, muscles in the shoulder region are somewhat tender but frank synovitis of the glenohumeral joint is generally not present. Sternoclavicular joint swelling and tenderness may be present and the A-C joint may be tender. Radionucleotide studies may show signs of a mild symmetric synovitis involving the shoulders. The sedimentation rate is invariably above 50 mm/hour using the Westergren method, and a mild normochromic, normocytic anemia is also a common finding.

Diagnosis is usually made in a patient with classic clinical features and an elevated sedimentation rate.[24] If local features of temporal arteritis are present, such as unilateral headache, tender temporal artery, jaw claudication, or visual symptoms, a 2 centimeter temporal artery biopsy should be obtained to confirm the presence of giant cell arteritis. In the absence of local symptoms, a trial of low dose prednisone, 10–15 milligrams per day, should be instituted. Most patients respond dramatically with resolution of symptoms within several days and a fall in the sedimentation rate to within the normal range. The dose of steroid should be slowly tapered over several months, following the sedimentation rate closely. Some patients require prolonged treatment over a 1–2 year period in order to remain in remission. Patients with signs or symptoms of temporal arteritis generally require a higher initial dose of prednisone, on the order of 60 milligrams per day, in order to control symptoms and to effect a normalization of the sedimentation rate.

Milwaukee Shoulder

Recently a "new" clinical syndrome called "Milwaukee shoulder" has been described.[36] These patients have shoulder pain with evidence of glenohumeral joint degeneration, a rotator cuff tear, and noninflammatory joint fluid with evidence of hydroxyapatite crystals in spheroid-shaped masses as well as active collagenase and neutral protease activities. Some patients have evidence of osteochondromatosus on synovial biopsy. Whether this represents a truly unique problem or just represents more advanced degenerative arthritis in the setting of a rotator cuff tear is open to question.[45] Therapy for this condition is purely symptomatic.

REFERENCES

1. Andrein L, Lundberg BJ: Treatment of rigid shoulders by joint distention during arthrography. Acta Orthop Scand 36:45–53, 1965
2. Bade HA, Warren RF, Ranawat CS, et al: Long term results of Neer total shulder replacement, in Bateman JE, Welsh RP (eds): Surgery of the Shoulder, Philadelphia, B.C. Decker Inc., 1984, 294–302

3. Bassett RW, Cofield RH: Acute tears of the rotator cuff—the timing of surgical repair. Clin Orthop 175:18–24, 1983

4. Berry H, Fernandes L, Blood M, et al: Clinical study comparing acupuncture, physiotherapy, injection, and oral anti-inflammatory therapy in shoulder cuff lesions. Curr Med Res Opin 7:121–126, 1980

5. Binder A, Parr G, Hazleman B, et al: Pulsed electromagnetic field therapy of persistent rotator cuff tendinitis. Lancet 1:695–698, 1984

6. Bland JH, Merrit JA, Boushey DR: The painful shoulder. Semin Arthritis Rheum 7:21–47, 1977

7. Bosworth BM: Calcium deposits in the shoulder and subacromial bursitis. JAMA 116:2477–2482, 1941

8. Bulgen DY, Binder AI, Hazleman BL, et al: Frozen shoulder: Prospective clinical study with an evaluation of three treatment regimens. Ann Rheum Dis 43:353–360, 1984

9. Cone RO, Resnick D, Danzig L: Shoulder impingement syndrome: Radiographic evaluation. Radiology 150:29–33, 1984

10. Cotton RE, Rideout DF: Tears of the humeral rotator cuff. J Bone Joint Surg 46-B:314–328, 1964

11. Crenshaw AH, Kilgore WE: Surgical treatment of bicipital tenosynovitis. J Bone Joint Surg 48A:1496–1502, 1966

12. Crisp EJ, Kendall PH: Hydrocortisone in lesions of soft tissue. Lancet 1:476–479, 1955

13. Cruess RL, Mitchell NS: Surgery of rheumatoid arthritis. Philadelphia, JB Lippincott, pp 117–125, 1971

14. Curran JF, Ellman MH, Brown NL: Rheumatologic aspects of painful conditions affecting the shoulder. Clin Orthop 173:27–37, 1983

15. Darlington LG, Coomes EN: The effects of local steroid injection for supraspinatus tears. Rheum Rehabil 16:172–179, 1977

16. De Palma AF: Surgery of the shoulder. Philadelphia, JB Lippincott, 1983

17. Fernandes L, Berry H, Clark RH, et al: Clinical study comparing acupuncture, physiotherapy, injection and oral anti-inflammatory therapy in shoulder-cuff lesions. Lancet 1:208–209, 1980

18. Goldenberg DL, Cohen AS: Acute infectious arthritis. Am J Med 60:369–377, 1976

19. Grey RG: The natural history of "idiopathic" frozen shoulder. J Bone Joint Surg 60A:564, 1978

20. Ha'eri GB: Ruptures of the rotator cuff. Can Med Assoc J 123:620–627, 1980

21. Halpern AA, Horowitz BG, Nagel DA: Tendon ruptures associated with corticosteroid therapy. West J Med 127:378–382, 1977

22. Hawkins RJ, Kennedy JC: Impingement syndrome in athletes. Amer J Sports Med 8:151–158, 1980

23. Hazleman BL: The painful stiff shoulder. Rheum Phys Med 11:413–421, 1972

24. Healy LA, Wilske KR: Manifestations of giant cell arteritis. Med Clin N Am 61:261–270, 1977

25. Hollander JL: Intra-articular hydrocortisone in the treatment of arthritis. Ann Int Med 39:735–746, 1953

26. Hollingworth GR, Ellis RM, Hattersley TS: Comparison of injection techniques for shoulder pain: Results of a double blind, randomized study. Br Med J 287:1339–1341, 1983

27. Kennedy JC, Willis RB: The effects of local steroid injections on tendons: A biomechanical and microscopic correlative study. Am J Sports Med 4:11–21, 1976

28. Kessel L, Watson M: The painful arc syndrome. J Bone Joint Surg 59-B:166–172, 1977

29. Kozin F: Painful shoulder and the reflex sympathetic dystrophy syndrome, in McCarthy DJ (ed): Arthritis and Allied Conditions. Philadelphia, Lea & Febiger, 1979, pp. 1091–1120

30. Kozin F, McCarty DJ, Sims J, et al: The reflex sympathetic dystrophy syndrome. Amer J Med 60:321–331, 1976

31. Kozin F, Ryan LM, Carerra GF, et al: The reflex sympathetic dystrophy syndrome (RSDS). Am J Med 70:23–30, 1981

32. Lee M, Haq AMMM, Wright V, et al: Periarthritis of the shoulder: A controlled trial of physiotherapy. Physiotherapy 59:312–315, 1973

33. Lee PN, Lee L, Haq AMMM, et al: Periarthritis of the shoulder. Ann Rheum Dis 33:116–119, 1974

34. Master R, Weisman MH, Armbuster TG, et al: Septic arthritis of the glenohumeral joint. Arthritis Rheum 20:1500–1506, 1977

35. McCarty DJ, Gatter RA: Recurrent acute inflammation associated with focal apatite crystal deposition. Arthritis Rheum 9:804–819, 1966

36. McCarty DJ, Halverson PB, Carrera F, et al: "Milwaukee shoulder"—Association of microspheroids containing hydroxyapatite crystals, active collagenase, and neutral protease with rotator cuff defects. Arthritis Rheum 24:464–467, 1981

37. McKendry RJ, Uhthoff HK, Sarkar K, et al: Calcifying tendinitis of the shoulder: Prognostic value of clinical, histologic, and radiologic features in 57 surgically treated cases. J Rheum 9:75–80, 1982

38. Miller LD, Stevens MB: Skeletal manifestations of polymyalgia rheumatica. JAMA 240:27–29, 1978

39. Murnaghan JP: Adhesive capsulitis of the shoulder, in Bateman JE, Welsh RP (eds): Surgery of the Shoulder, Philadelphia, B.C. Decker Inc., 1984, pp 154–156

40. Murnaghan GF, McIntosh D: Hydrocortisone in painful shoulder. Lancet 2:789–800, 1955

41. Neer CS: Anterior acromioplasty for the chronic impingement syndrome in the shoulder. J Bone Joint Surgery 54A:41–50, 1972

42. Neer CS: Reconstructive surgery and rehabilitation of the shoulder, in Kelly WN, Harris ED, Ruddy S, et al (eds): Textbook of rheumatology. Philadelphia, WB Saunders, 1981, pp 1944–1959

43. Neer CS: Impingement lesions. Clin Orthop 173:70–77, 1983

44. Neer CS: Unconstrained shoulder arthroplasty, in Bateman JE, Welsh RP (eds): Surgery of the shoulder, Philadelphia, JB Lippincott, 1984, pp 240–245

45. Neer CS, Craig EV, Fukuda H: Cuff-tear arthropathy. J Bone Joint Surg 65A:1232–1244, 1983

46. Neviaser RJ, Neviaser TJ: Lesions of musculotendinous cuff of the shoulder: Diagnoses and management. Instr Course Lect 30:239–257, 1981

47. Older MWJ, McIntyre JL, Lloyd GJ: Distension arthrography of the shoulder joint. Canad J Surg 19:203–207, 1976

48. Packer NP, Calvert PT, Bayley JK, et al: Operative treatment of chronic ruptures of the rotator cuff of the shoulder. J Bone Joint Surg 65-B:171–175, 1983

49. Penny JN, Welsh RP: Shoulder impingement syndromes in athletes and their surgical management. Amer J Sports Med 9:11–15, 1981

50. Resnick D: Infectious arthritis. Sem Roentgenology 17:49–59, 1982

51. Resnick D: Shoulder pain. Orthop Clin N Amer 14:81–97, 1983

52. Richardson AT: The painful shoulder. Proc Roy Soc Med 68:731–736, 1975

53. Rothman RH, Parke WW: The vascular anatomy of the rotator cuff. Clin Orthop 41:176–186, 1965

54. Samilson RL, Binder WF: Symptomatic full thickness tears of the rotator cuff. Ortho Clin N Amer 6:449–466, 1975

55. Simon WH: Soft tissue disorders of the shoulder. Orthop Clin North Amer 6:521–539, 1975

56. Strizak AM, Danzig L, Jackson DW, et al: Subacromial bursography. J Bone Joint Surg 64-A:196–201, 1982

57. Watson M: The refractory painful arc syndrome. J Bone Joint Surg 60-B:544–546, 1978

58. White RH: Shoulder Pain. West J Med 137:340–345, 1982

59. Wright V, Haq AMMM: Periarthritis of the shoulder. Ann Rheum Dis 35:213–219, 1976

David Leffers
Thomas L. Greene
Bernard F. Germain

15

The Elbow

ANATOMY

The elbow is a complex of three joints: radio-capitellar, proximal radio-ulnar, and olecranon-trochlear (Fig. 15-1). The latter provides for essentially pure flexion and extension while the former two allow for rotation of the forearm. There is no significant medial-lateral mobility allowed.

Stability is provided primarily by the collateral ligaments, the medial complex being the most important (Fig. 15-2). The interlocking of the articular surfaces themselves provide for little inherent stability except for the locking of the olecranon process in the trochlear notch at full extension. Normal range of motion is from 0 to 5° of hyperextension to 150° of flexion. Pronation and supination are 80° each.[53]

The medial and lateral epicondyles serve as origins for major muscles of the forearm and are the sites of common inflammatory disorders. From the medial epicondyle originate the flexor-pronator group composed of the pronator teres, flexor carpi radialis, palmaris longus, and flexor carpi ulnaris (Fig. 15-3). From the lateral epicondyle originate the extensor carpi radialis brevis and the common extensor origin (Fig. 15-4). Flexion of the elbow is supplied primarily by the biceps and the brachialis, the former also acting as a strong supination force. The secondary flexors of the elbow are the brachioradialis, the radial wrist extensors and the flexor-pronator group.

The role of the elbow in the function of the upper extremity is to position the wrist and hand in space. Loss of various degrees of extension or pronation can be compensated for without a serious compromise to overall function, whereas severe loss of supination or especially flexion will produce considerable impairment.

Peripheral Neuropathies at the Elbow

Compression neuropathies about the elbow involving either the ulnar, median, or radial nerves produce signs and symptoms both at the elbow and more distally in the extremity. These three nerves cross the elbow and then enter the forearm through fibro-

PRINCIPLES OF PHYSICAL MEDICINE AND REHABILITATION
IN THE MUSCULOSKELETAL DISEASES

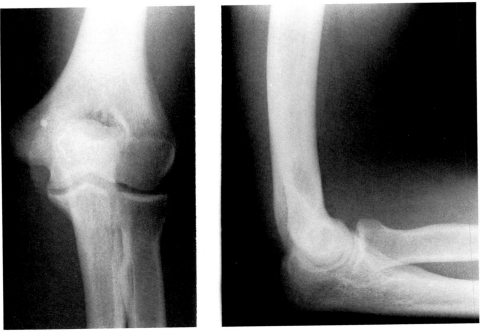

Fig. 15-1. An AP and lateral radiograph of the elbow. There are separate articular surfaces on the distal humerus for the proximal radius and ulna.

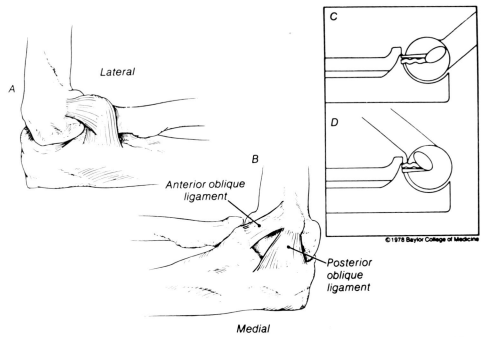

Fig. 15-2. The lateral (A) and medial (B) collateral ligaments of the elbow. The anterior oblique ligament is the most important for maintaining elbow stability. (Reprinted with permission from Schwab GH, et al: Biomechanics of Elbow Instability: The Role of the Medial Collateral Ligament, Clin Orthop Rel Res 146:42–51, 1980.)

370

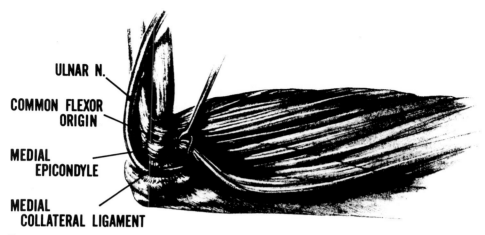

Fig. 15-3. The muscle attachments to the medial epicondyle. (Reprinted with permission from Green DP (ed): Operative hand surgery. New York, Churchill Livingstone, p. 1516, 1982.)

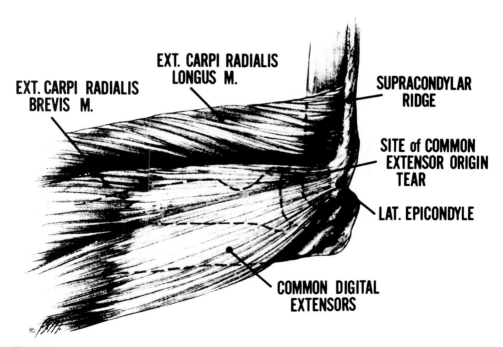

Fig. 15-4. The muscles originating from the lateral side of the elbow showing the site of pathology in tennis elbow. (Reprinted with permission from Green DP (ed): Operative hand surgery. New York, Churchill Livingstone, p. 1516, 1982.)

muscular arches formed by the origins of specific muscles; ulnar:flexor carpi ulnaris (Fig. 15-5), median:pronator teres (Fig. 15-6), radial:supinator (Fig. 15-7). It is at and about these arches that compression of these nerves is most likely to occur.

Ulnar Nerve

The ulnar nerve is most frequently entrapped as it passes behind the medial epicondyle and enters the forearm through the arch formed by the two heads of origin of the flexor carpi ulnaris muscle. Entrapment occurs at one or both of these sites. Although medial elbow pain is a frequent complaint, distal paresthesias and pain radiating into the hand often predominate the clinical picture. Local tenderness of the nerve at the elbow and a positive Tinel's sign with gentle percussion are typically found. Atrophy and sensory loss in the hand are signs of severe or long standing compression. Confusion may arise in early cases before distal symptoms occur in distinguishing this entity from medial epicondylitis. The precise localization of tenderness and response to stress of the flexor-pronator muscles originating from the epicondyle will serve to separate the two. An eighth cervical root impingement or a thoracic outlet syndrome should also be in the differential diagnosis of medial elbow pain of neurological origin.

Electromyography and nerve conduction studies will confirm the location and severity of the neuropathy. Treatment is usually operative for most cases but continuous splinting of the elbow in 30° or 45° of flexion, protection from local trauma to the nerve, and anti-inflammatory medications may relieve a neuropathy of short duration. Injections

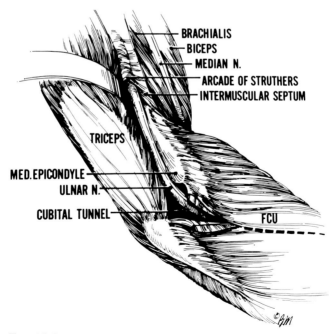

Fig. 15-5. The course of the ulnar nerve through the cubital tunnel. (Reprinted with permission from Green DP (ed): Operative hand surgery. New York, Churchill Livingstone, p. 978, 1982.)

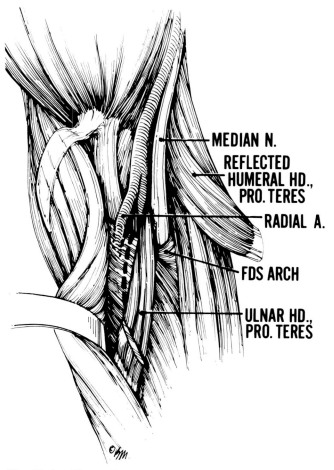

Fig. 15-6. The median nerve enters the forearm through the two heads of the pronator teres (humeral head reflected proximally). (Reprinted with permission from Green DP (ed): Operative hand surgery. New York, Churchill Livingstone, p. 963, 1982.)

Injections of steroid about the nerve are not recommended as intraneural injection is a distinct possibility.[15,35]

Median Nerve

The median nerve can become compressed as it courses across the elbow either at the lacertus fibrosis (aponeurosis of the biceps tendon), the pronator teres arch, or the flexor superficialis arch.

Symptoms of proximal forearm pain and paresthesias in the median nerve distribution predominate. The nerve exhibits tenderness and a positive Tinel's sign at the point of compression. Symptoms may be exacerbated by resisted pronation of the forearm. Compression at the carpal tunnel can coexist and confuse the clinical picture. Compression of

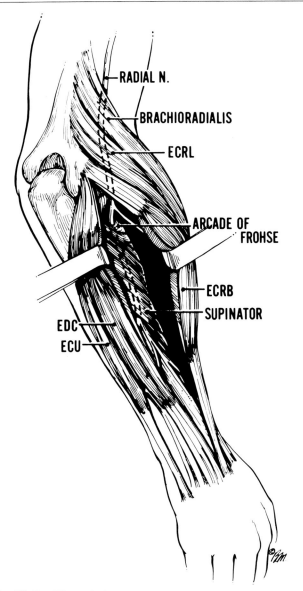

Fig. 15-7. The radial nerve enters the forearm between the superficial and deep head of the supinator on the dorsal surface of the radius. (Reprinted with permission from Green DP (ed): Operative hand surgery. New York, Churchill Livingstone, p. 988, 1982.)

the anterior interosseous nerve alone will produce weakness or paralysis of the flexor digitorium profundus of the index and middle fingers, flexor pollicus longus, and pronator quadratus. Sensory symptoms are not present with the anterior interosseous syndrome.

The localization and extent of the nerve entrapment may be confirmed by electromyography and nerve conduction studies. A period of immobilization of the elbow may relieve the symptoms. Avoidance of repetitive task requiring vigorous muscle contraction especially pronation and supnation is recommended. Lack of improvement after two or three months warrants surgical decompression.[30]

Radial Nerve

The posterior interosseous nerve, a major branch of the radial nerve, can become entrapped between the two heads of the supinator muscle in the proximal forearm (radial tunnel syndrome). This usually occurs at the proximal fibrous edge of the superficial head of the supinator, the arcade of Frohse, but compression can occur in any part of the muscle. The condition causes pain in the proximal forearm and lateral elbow and is commonly confused and sometimes coexistent with lateral epicondylitis. Maximum pain and tenderness are present over the supinator instead of the lateral epicondyle. Symptoms may be reproduced by resisted supination of the forearm or resisted extension of the fingers, particularly the middle finger. Injection of the lateral epicondyle with local anesthetic may be helpful in differentiating the source of the pain. Paresthesias in the distribution of the radial nerve on the dorsum of the hand are not present.

Immobilization of the wrist in 30° to 40° extension along with nonsteroidal antiinflammatory medications may abort an early radial tunnel syndrome. Lack of response to conservative care or severe symptoms requires surgical decompression of the nerve by sectioning of the superficial head of the supinator.

Radial tunnel syndrome should be considered in a patient with lateral elbow pain who presents with less than typical findings of lateral epicondylitis or who fails to respond to treatment, both operative and nonoperative.[36]

FRACTURES ABOUT THE ELBOW IN SPORTS

The overall incidence of fractures related to sports activity is low at all levels of competition when compared to strains, sprains, and contusions. In studies on high school sports injuries, fractures have accounted for 5–8 percent of all injuries.[16,58] Anatomically, these were widely distributed and often involved the small bones of the hand, wrist, or foot. Most were the result of a single traumatic episode, and not unexpectedly were most common in football.

Injuries to the elbow, apart from throwing and overuse injuries in baseball, are infrequent occurrences. Elbow trauma accounted for but 2.4 percent of all injuries in a large series of football injuries at the interscholastic level.[4] A similar percentage has been reported in professional football.[57] Statistics from other sports such as wrestling,[49] gymnastics,[61] basketball,[25] and skiing[10] show low incidence of elbow injury and fracture. This infrequency of sports related fractures belies their importance, as they are generally major injuries in terms of time lost from participation and are the most common injury requiring a physicians care.

Fractures of the elbow can be produced by indirect or direct trauma. Perhaps the most common mechanism in sports in indirect trauma, when the upper extremity, willfully or not, is placed in a position of weightbearing.

The outstretched arm "breaking" a fall can transmit significant longitudinal forces to the elbow and produce fractures.[45,46] The position of the forearm and contributing varus or valgus forces are additional determinants in the site and complexity of the injury pattern.

In falls, valgus forces often predominate, producing compression and shear fractures of the radial head or capitellum with concomitant medial tensile injury, manifested by medial collateral ligament injury in the adult or medial epicondylar avulsion in children and adolescents. This is but one scenario, and a myriad of fractures can be produced by indirect or direct trauma.[51]

A complete review of the various types of elbow fractures and their treatment is beyond the scope of this review. A general approach to these injuries will be pursued followed by a discussion of epiphyseal injuries.

In acute evaluation of a suspected or known elbow fracture, initial questioning and examination must first be concerned with the vascular integrity of the limb due to proximity of the brachial artery. The presence or absence of neurologic deficits must also be documented prior to and after institution of treatment. Although sports related fractures are low velocity when compared to motor vehicle and pedestrian trauma, exclusion of neurovascular injury is paramount. Deformity, soft tissue status, areas of tenderness, swelling, and ecchymosis should be noted. Standard frontal and lateral radiographs, with oblique views as necessary, suffice in most adults to visualize and classify injuries. Complex fractures and intraarticular fragments may require tomograms or CT scans to delineate pathology.

As with other fractures, the goals of treatment are restoration of anatomy and function. In general, with intra-articular fractures, such as those involving the capitellum, open reduction and internal fixation is appropriate if anatomy can be restored. However, the elbow tolerates incongruity poorly, and excision of fragments is preferable to their malreplacement.[9]

The method of treatment is often determined by elbow stability. One could not excise with impunity a comminuted radial head or olecranon fracture in the presence of medial collateral ligament insufficiency, as gross instability would result.[66] A gravity stress test or examination under anesthesia is indicated if coexistence of these injuries is presumed.

Although excision of the isolated, comminuted radial head fracture is satisfactory treatment,[47,51] the presence of valgus instability is one of the few indications for silastic replacement to restore a lateral buttress.[40]

In rehabilitation of the fractured elbow the key is early, protected active range of motion. This is dictated by the patient's discomfort, and may be as early as a few days in nondisplaced fractures of the radial head. In those fractures treated by debridement or secure internal fixation, active motion can generally be instituted by the time the skin incision has healed. When motion is restored and fracture union has occurred, strengthening exercises can be implemented. A return to one's activity or sport is allowed when the demands of that sport can be met. As with other injuries, the end results are often determined by the severity of the initial trauma, and consultation between physician and patient is important to allay fears or discuss possible limitations.

Epiphyseal Fractures

Epiphyseal fractures account for approximately 10 percent of skeletal trauma in childhood.[44] In one series of acute epiphyseal fractures, roughly 50 percent were sports or recreationally related, with football heading the list.[7] The importance of recognizing epiphyseal injury is that with physeal plate damage the potential exists for growth arrest and subsequent limb inequality or angular deformity. The epiphyses about the elbow contribute 20–25 percent to the longitudinal growth of upper extremity, and sequelae, when they occur, are usually of the angular variety. The likelihood of these complications is determined by the type of fracture, location, skeletal age and growth potential of the patient, associated soft tissue injury, and accuracy of reduction.[52]

As Rang has stated, children are not small adults.[48] Forces producing ligament tears or dislocations in adults will cause fractures in children due to the relative weakness of the physeal-metaphyseal junction compared to capsular, ligamentous, or tendinous insertions.

The peak incidence of sports related epiphyseal fractures is during the early adolescent growth spurt, ages 10–13 years in females and 12–15 years in boys.[7,44] In the upper extremity, injuries about the elbow occur less frequently than those to epiphyses in the distal forearm and hand. The mechanism of injury, as in the adult, can be indirect via a fall on the outstretched arm or from direct trauma. Avulsion fractures of the olecranon and medial epicondylar epiphysis can result from hard throws due to forceful contractions of the triceps and flexor-pronator muscles, respectfully.

The key to diagnosis is suspicion, and one should accept as untenable a diagnosis of elbow sprain in a youth prior to skeletal maturity. A neurovascular examination is requisite, and areas of tenderness should be localized. In interpreting radiographs, familiarity with the times of appearance, fusion, and normal variants in the secondary centers of ossification is helpful. Comparison views of the uninvolved elbow are useful to detect subtle differences. Signs such as the posterior fat pad sign or metaphyseal flake fracture are clues to epiphyseal injury.

Certain fractures warrant specific mention. Avulsion fractures of the medial epicondyle should be treated according to functional disability rather than specific displacement.[66] If valgus instability is present due to attachment of the medial collateral ligament to the fragment, open reduction and fixation is indicated.

Lateral condyle fractures are Salter-Harris Type-IV injuries and carry increased probability of growth disturbance. Nondisplaced fractures can be immobilized, but under close scrutiny for subsequent displacement. Initial displacement or subsequent change mandates open reduction and internal fixation. Growth arrest can lead to cubitus valgus and tardy ulnar nerve palsy.

Fracture of the proximal radius in children usually occurs through the radial neck.[48,62] Because the radial head epiphysis is completely covered by cartilage, vascular supply is attendant on metaphyseal vessels entering the neck. Fracture can, although not commonly, interrupt this supply and lead to avascular necrosis. Resection of the radial head, if significant growth potential remains, should be discouraged. Open reduction may be necessary in completely displaced fractures or in those that cannot be reduced to acceptable angulation (30°–40°) by closed means.[62] With correct diagnosis and treatment, actual growth disturbances are infrequent and results are good. Parents should be told from the outset of the potential dangers inherent in epiphyseal injuries, and even though their charge returns to normal activity, the final outcome is not determined until skeletal maturity and they must be followed until that time.

MUSCLE STRAINS ABOUT THE ELBOW

Including those muscles that act upon the wrist and hand, there are 24 muscles that cross the elbow joint. Strain can occur in any of these muscles, and knowledge of regional anatomy, sites of origin and insertion, and mechanism of injury aid in physical examination and diagnosis.

The majority of muscular strains about the elbow involve the common extensor and flexor-pronator musculotendinous units, exemplified by tennis and pitcher's elbow, respectively. These are generally "overuse" injuries and are discussed elsewhere in this chapter. Here we will be concerned with strains involving the prime movers of the elbow proper, the triceps, anconeus, brachialis, and biceps.

Muscle tears in the athletic setting generally occur when a stretching force is applied to a muscle already maximally contracting.[18] This force can be in the form of a severe resistance to a muscle's action or from vigorous, asynchronous contraction of its antagonist muscle. Less frequent causes of muscular tears in athletes are laceration and direct trauma. Anatomically, those muscles crossing two joints (ie, triceps, biceps) and short action muscles are said to be more susceptible to strain.[19] Other predisposing factors to muscular strain are a cold environment, localized and generalized muscular fatigue, inadequate conditioning, insufficient warm-up, and the presence of infective foci.[33]

The degree of muscular injury depends on the extent the muscle's elasticity and stability are exceeded. Muscular strains can be divided into three grades based on anatomical, clinical, and functional findings. Grade 1: a first degree strain with stretching of muscle fibers but no gross anatomical disruption, hence no soft tissue swelling or ecchymosis. Localized tenderness and discomfort with function of the musculoteninous unit are present. Grade 2: A second degree strain or partial tear with localized disruption of muscle bundles. Localized tenderness, spasm, swelling, and hematoma formation ensue, and a palpable softening or defect may be present. Functionally more limitation of active motion and increased pain with passive stretch are present. Grade 3: A third degree strain or complete muscle rupture, generally including investing fascia. Diffuse tenderness, soft tissue swelling, ecchymosis and a marked defect are the rule, along with loss of function.

About the elbow, stress induced strains are most commonly first and second degree in severity. Complete ruptures of the biceps and triceps have been reported,[3,6,18,55,56] but these have been associated with tendons damaged through attritional changes, systemic medical conditions predisposing to tendon rupture, or direct trauma.

Triceps

Occupying the posterior aspect of the arm, the triceps has the largest work capacity and potential contractile strength of all muscles acting on the elbow.[2] It is the prime elbow extensor and forearm propulsor. Comprised of three heads joining at the mid to distal arm, it inserts by a broad expanse onto the olecranon, contiguous with the fascia on the posterior forearm.

Strains can develop in throwers, particularly after a hard throw, in a cool or fatigued muscle. Weightlifters, boxers, and gymnasts are also susceptible.

Diagnosis can be made by localizing tenderness, usually at the confluence of the three heads distally. Pain can be elicited with resistance to elbow extension and passive elbow flexion. Complete ruptures are rare, as mentioned, and are manifested by inability or severe weakness in elbow extension against gravity.

Anconeus

The anconeus is a triangular shaped muscle taking origin from the posterior aspect of the lateral humeral epicondyle and inserting on the lateral aspect of the olecranon. It is an accessory elbow extensor and perhaps a dynamic lateral stabilizer of the elbow.[26] Strains must be differentiated from lateral epicondilitis, this by familiarity with its anatomic course.

Brachialis

The prime flexor of the elbow, the brachialis has almost the equivalent work capacity and contractile strength as the triceps. It blankets the anterior aspect of the elbow and inserts by a broad tendon into the lower portion of the coronoid process and tuberosity of the ulna. Strain can occur in weightlifters doing curls, hyperextension of the elbow, racket sport players mishitting a forehand or striking an immovable object (wall, net, etc.) Chronic strain can develop in throwers due to its deccelaratory function in the follow-through phase.

Pain is usually localized in the distal anterior aspect of the arm and antecubital fossa. Pain with passive elbow extension and active elbow flexion are present. This would not be affected by forearm supination, implicating strain of the biceps.

Complete rupture or avulsion of the brachialis is usually associated with posterior dislocation of the elbow or severe distal humeral fractures. The intimate relationship of the brachial artery and median nerve to the brachialis must be born in mind when treating these injuries. Also, the brachialis is the most common site about the elbow for myositis ossificans to develop, reflecting its injury in severe elbow trauma.

Biceps

The biceps occupies the most superficial portion of the anterior aspect of the arm. Narrow tendons, both proximally from the long head origin, and distally at the insertion into the radial tuberosity, make this muscle vulnerable to attrition and rupture. Muscle belly rupture is rare. A series has been reported in parachutists, resulting from what is basically a closed laceration from impact of the static line on the anterior arm.[24] The biceps functions as an accessory elbow flexor and an important forearm supinator. Pain with supination aids in differentiating biceps from brachialis strain. Ruptures, most common proximally, produce readily identifiable defects due to the superficial location of the muscle and retraction.

Treatment

Grade 1 muscle strains are self limiting injuries if treated. Acute application of ice, compression, and rest followed by physiotherapy and a strengthening and stretching program should return one to activity in a few days. "Working through" a pulled muscle can lead to partial tears.

Grade 2 injuries should also be managed first by measures to decrease pain, swelling, and inflammation. Thus ice, compression, and rest are customary, supplemented by analgesics and oral anti-inflammatory agents. Splinting may be necessary to ease muscular spasm and to approximate torn muscle bundles. Aspiration of a localized hematoma may be useful, usually in the biceps. In one to two days, active motion and physiotherapy (ultrasound, whirlpool) can be started, with progression to stretching and strengthening when full, painless motion is restored. One should guard against early passive motion or massage in the presence of pain, as these have been implicated as contributing factors in the development of myositis ossificans.[19] Full activity can generally be resumed at 3–4 weeks.

In Grade 3 injuries, or complete ruptures, the best chance for meaningful return to competitive sports is with surgical repair.[19,24,56]

Inherent in treatment is injury prevention, and measures should be taken to address those factors predisposing to strain. For the elbow and upper extremity this would include proper attire in cold weather, training to increase strength and endurance, and limitation of throwing, lifting, serving, etc., past points of fatigue.

THROWING INJURIES

The act of throwing has been found to be the most frequently used of the six fundamental movement categories in sports.[41] Unique stresses are developed in the throwing, serving, or swimming arm, and the ability of the athlete to adapt to and dissipate these stresses through conditioning and proper technique enhances performance and mitigates against injury. Improper or overzealous training and poor body mechanics, coupled with the repetitive use of the throwing mechanism in these various sports, can lead to acute and overuse injury.

Injury to the elbow in the baseball pitcher is almost endemic, prompting a majority of the clinical and research efforts present in the current literature. Similar injuries can be produced in the javelin thrower,[39] football passer, and racket sport athlete, but the baseball pitcher serves as a useful model in discussing injuries. Implicit in this discussion is an understanding of basic throwing mechanics.

Biomechanics of Throwing

Tullos and King[67] divided the pitching motion into the component phases of cocking, acceleration, and follow-through. To this may be added the wind-up, which precedes the cocking phase, is highly individualized, and lasts until the ball is removed from the gloved hand.

In the cocking phase, the ball is prepared for delivery, and is brought about by shoulder abduction and external rotation, and elbow flexion of approximately $40°–50°$.

The acceleration phase is a short, propulsive act that imparts velocity to the ball. The body rotates forward and the shoulder and arm accompany it with forceful internal humeral rotation. The elbow and hand follow, and through the latter stage of acceleration forceful propulsion of the forearm via elbow extension occurs. Acceleration culminates with ball release.

The follow-through phase is the tuner for ball control and is also responsible for dissipation of energy generated by the body and arm during acceleration. The shoulder adducts and moves across the body and elbow extension continues, accompanied by forearm pronation.

EMG analysis of the shoulder and arm musculature during pitching[29] has shown the major accelerators to be the pectoralis major, the latissimus dorsi, and the triceps. These muscles also serve as decelerators by eccentric contraction after ball release. The biceps and brachialis also serve in this capacity about the elbow, affording protection against hyperextension and impaction of the olecranon into its fossa.

Significant valgus forces are produced at the elbow during the acceleratory phase. These may be augmented by a more horizontal (side-arm) position of the pitching arm,[1] or by opening-up the lead shoulder.[1,38] The body rotates ahead of the pitching arm, increasing the valgus moment about the elbow.

Concomitant with the medial tension developed during throwing is lateral compressive forces.

Slocum classified throwing injuries in relation to stress distribution during the throwing act.[60] These are medial tension overload injuries, lateral compression injuries, and extensor overload injuries.

Medial Tension Overload Injuries

The medial supporting structures charged with absorbing the valgus-tensile stresses are the flexor-pronator musculotendinous unit and the medical (ulnar) collateral ligament. Acute Injury is generally due to inadequate warm-up, poor throwing mechanics, and occasionally to a particularly hard malthrow. The most common acute injuries are first and second degree strains and sprains of the flexor-pronator muscles and the medial collateral ligament, respectfully. Often pitchers can recall the exact pitch when injury occurred. Symptomatically, pain is present during activity and located over the site of soft tissue infraction. Soft tissue swelling and palpatory tenderness is also present. Differentiation between ligament or muscular injury is facilitated by the following tests. With muscular strain, pain is reproduced medially by resistance to wrist flexion. With ligament sprain, pain should be reproduced by applying valgus stress to the slightly flexed elbow. Fifteen to twenty degrees of flexion is necessary to unlock the olecranon from its inherently stable position within the olecranon fossa. No gross instability would be expected in first or second degree ligament sprains. Rarely, in the adult, radiographs may show a small cortical avulsion fracture from the medial epicondylar origin of the ligament. Treatment of these grade I and II injuries is largely symptomatic, with measures to reduce pain and inflammation. Undoubtedly the majority of these injuries go unreported to coaches, trainers, or physicians and are largely self-limiting. The problem lies in prevention, for they are apt to recur if caused by the reason aforementioned.

Isolated ruptures of either the flexor-pronator muscles or the medial collateral ligament are rare. Both would be severe injuries with inability to pitch. Muscle rupture would be associated with a palpatory defect and ligament rupture with valgus instability. Repair of grade III muscle ruptures have yielded poor results, with ligament repairs fairing somewhat better.[5]

Norwood reported on four cases of acute medial elbow ruptures.[42] None occurred during the throwing act, but resulted from a valgus producing blow to the forearm or in breaking a fall.

Chronic medial stress syndrome is the most common elbow malady affecting the baseball pitcher. It is a time and dose dependent result of the repetitive stress of throwing, which has several consequences. Attenuation of the medial supporting structures, primarily the medial collateral ligament, can produce an increased valgus carrying angle.[32] Increased valgus has also been attributed to trochlear hypertrophy, part of the generalized humeral hypertrophy seen in response to exercise.[31] Humeral hypertrophy is the most common generalized radiographic finding in baseball pitchers.[21] The uniaxial ulno-humeral joint has been described as a perfect hinge, with the carrying angle determined by the trochlear articulation, and instant centers of rotation centered about the arc formed by the trochlear sulcus.[37] One could anticipate with increase valgus secondary to ligament laxity and/or hypertrophy, a corresponding, joint incongruity resulting in adaptive changes over time in various areas of the joint. These changes are termed pathologic when they become symptomatic.

Chronic strain on the flexor-pronator muscle group can take the form of medial epicondylitis. Microtears and subsequent inflammatory response and fibrosis can lead to elbow flexion contracture, seen in approximately 50 percent of professional baseball pitchers.[32]

Tensile stresses on the medial collateral ligament induce traction spurs, most commonly emanating from the medial side of the coronoid tubercle. These spurs can cause local irritation, ulnar neuritis, and occasionally fracture.

The medial collateral ligament can become attentuated to the point of incompetency. This is a particularly disabling injury, as the primary stabilizer of the elbow is lost,[54] effectively terminating a pitcher's career unless surgical repair or reconstruction is undertaken. Chronic valgus laxity is also implicated in posterior and lateral compartment pathology. Traction stresses on the ulnar nerve can also induce neuropathy.

Clinically, apart from discomfort, many of the chronic medial lesions cause the pitcher to complain of early fatigue and inability to "let it go."

Radiographic findings may include the traction spurs and calcification within the ligament or muscles. Incompetency of the medial collateral ligament can be visualized by a gravity stress test.[69]

Treatment of these chronic injuries is initially conservative, and includes rest, oral anti-inflammatory agents, judicious use of local steroid injections, phonophoresis and other modalities, ice post activity, and a stretching and strengthening program. Surgery may be necessary for removal of traction spurs or calcific deposits, and in refractory cases, revision of the medial epicondyle, repair or reconstruction of the medial collateral ligament, and anterior transposition of the ulnar nerve.

Rehabilitation after surgery is variable but aimed first at restoring motion and strength, followed by gradual return of throwing activities.[28]

Lateral Compression Injuries

The radiocapitellar articulation bears the brunt of compressive forces generated laterally during pitching. This stress may be increased secondary to medial collateral ligament laxity and increased valgus deformity. In addition, shear stresses are introduced through the sliding motion between the articular surfaces of the radius and capitellum. Mediolateral shear stress has been demonstrated to be greatest in the extended, pronated forearm, the position normally attained at terminal acceleration and follow-through.

Lateral compression injuries are less common than medial side injuries, but their presence carries a poorer prognosis.

Acute osteochondral injury or capitellar fracture is rare in the adult, but may result from extreme valgus overload from contact or a particularly violent throw.

More commonly, laterial joint disease is manifested by marginal osteophyte formation, loose bodies, and degenerative changes. Symptomatic treatment is indicated, with surgery reserved for removal of osteophytes or loose bodies. Arthroscopy can be utilized for debridement and loose body removal in skilled hands.

Extensor Overload Injuries

The propulsion of the forearm during acceleration is accomplished by forceful contraction of the triceps. Acute and chronic strain in the triceps expansion can occur, along with stress induced fracture of the olecranon. The most common manifestation of the chronic traction stress is hypertrophy and osteophyte formation of the olecranon tip, with exfoliative changes and loose body production.[32] The posterior compartment is the most common site for loose body production and location in the pitching elbow and should be routinely inspected when loose bodies are encountered elsewhere in the joint during surgery.

An additional source of pain in the posterior compartment is the posteriomedial osteophyte, described by Wilson et al,[68] resulting from valgus-extension overload. The medial olecranon impinges in the posteriomedial fossa during early acceleration. True posterior impingement of the olecranon tip has not been seen in cineradiographs of the pitching arm.[32] Axial radiographs may be necessary to visualize these osteophytes. As with treatment of other spurs, symptomatic therapy can often alleviate discomfort periodically but refractory symptoms warrant their surgical removal. Corresponding chondromalacia and degenerative changes within the joint determine ultimate prognosis.

Less common causes of elbow pain in the pitcher are Bennet's facial compression syndrome[13] and anterior capsular or muscular injury. Forearm hypertrophy, primarily of the flexor-pronator group, accompanies the chronic stress of throwing. Muscle ischaemia may occur within tight facial compartments, manifested by burning pain, early fatigue, and weakness. Selective fasciotomy may be required if stretching, proper warm-up, and ice post activity do not suffice.

The anterior capsule, biceps, and brachialas may become inflamed from performing their deceleratory function during acceleration and follow-through. Rest and conservative therapy are usually all that is required.

In summary, injuries in the adult pitcher are common and result from the repetitive stress of throwing. Attention to proper conditioning and throwing techniques may avert injury. Prompt, accurate recognition is the key to treatment. Most injuries can be treated conservatively with good results. Surgical procedures are most successful when done for isolated problems such as a spur or loose body, or involve the medial or posterior compartment. Degenerative change in the lateral compartment is a poor prognostic sign. As Tullos has stated, however, all successful surgeries are merely palliative, because as long as they continue to pitch the problems will recur.[68]

Little Leaguer's Elbow

The term little leaguer's elbow was first coined by Brogdon[8] to describe clinical and radiographic findings in the medial epicondylar epiphysis of the immature throwing arm. The child and adolescent thrower is subject to the same elbow stresses generated by pitching as the adult. Manifestations of this repetitive stress vary according to soft tissue and skeletal maturity. Due to the relative ligamentous laxity in youth, the brunt of medial tensile stress is born by the flexor-pronator muscle group. The weak link in this defense is the epicondylar epiphysis, which first ossifies between the ages of 5 and 7 and is generally the last of the secondary center of ossification about the elbow to fuse, between the ages of 14 and 17, signifying elbow maturity.[59]

Chronic microtrauma can produce chondro-osseous injury, resulting clinically in tenderness and soft tissue swelling over the epicondyle, limitation of motion, and inability to perform. Ulnar nerve symptoms can also be induced,[20] although uncommonly. Radiographic changes may include enlargement, fragmentation, irregularity, beaking, and partial separation of the epiphysis.

The true incidence of little leaguer's elbow is unknown. In independent studies, Larson[34] reported elbow symptoms in 20 percent of pitchers aged 11 and 12, Gugenheim[23] reported 17 percent in those 9–13 years of age, Grana[22] reported 58 percent in those 14–19, and even a higher percentage by Torg[64] in a group ranging from 9–18. The majority of symptoms were referable to the medial side of the elbow, but rarely caused cessation in play. Also, no significant correlation between angular deformity, radiographic findings, pitching experience, or symptoms could be drawn.[22,33,34] Due to the plurality of contributing etiologic factors (age, skeletal maturity, individual susceptibility, geographic location, competitive level) it is difficult to make blanket statements about this syndrome. The throwing act or lesions induced by it, however, cannot be considered physiologic when clinical or asymmetric radiographic findings are present.

Treatment varies according to the severity of injury. In the usual case with epicondylar changes without separation, rest and measures to reduce discomfort (ice, aspirin) followed by return to limited throwing, not pitching, until sufficient strength and maturity are attained. Long term results from this injury are not known, but because the medial epicondylar epiphysis is extra articular and does not contribute to the longitudinal growth of the humerus,[59] disability would not be expected.

Medial tensile stress in the older adolescent can cause partial or segmental avulsion fractures of the epicondyle and lead to stress induced failure of union. Fractures, unless displaced, are treated conservatively with immobilization. Displaced fractures (greater than 1.0 cm) warrant open reduction.[69]

Lateral compression injuries occur in youth players, and, as is true with adults, carry a significantly poorer prognosis. Little leaguer's elbow implies a certain benignity to some and probably should not incorporate these injuries.

Apart from a familial tendency, there is implicated a causal relationship between compression and shear on the ossific nucleus of the capitellum and the development of osteochondritis dissecans.[43] This lesion typically presents in the 9–15 year age group with insiduous onset. The most common complaints are pain with throwing and loss of motion, primarily that of extension. Locking, clicking, and swelling may also occur. Clinically, the most common finding is elbow flexion contracture, followed by tenderness over the lateral joint line and crepitation.[63,70]

Radiographically, an island of subchondral bone in the superolateral portion of the capitellum, demarcated by a rarefied zone, is classical. In the latter stages of the disease, the fragment may separate and fragment, producing loose bodies. Flattening of the capitellum, enlargement of the radial head, and accelerated epiphyseal closure of the involved elbow may be present. Late stages of the disease would be reflected by degenerative changes.

Treatment, first and foremost, is rest and cessation of throwing. In those without fragment separation or loose bodies, surgery is unwarranted.[43] The osteochondritic lesion can be expected to revascularize and heal over a period of months. The presence of fragment detachment or loose bodies warrants their surgical removal. Results following pinning of undetached fragments, fixing a detached fragment, bone grafting, and drilling and/or curettage of the capitellar bed have been less than good.[63,70] Paramount in treatment is also counseling the parents, the involved youngster, and coaches. In those instances where surgery is not necessary, throwing should be halted until clinical and radiographic resolution of the lesion has occurred, and perhaps not until skeletal maturity has been reached. In those requiring surgery, a return to throwing sports should be discouraged.

Osteochondrosis, or aseptic necrosis, of the capitellum (Panner's Disease) occurs in younger aged boys (5–10 years of age) and has not been attributed to throwing.

Acute osteochondral fracture of the capitellum or radial head can occur following a hard or malthrow. Treatment depends on the size of the fragment and the amount of displacement. Tomography is often useful in delineating these lesions, and internal fixation may be necessary if size is significant. Failure of union would warrant loose body removal.

Posterior compartment pathology, apart from triceps strain, is rare in the youth pitcher. Adaptive changes in the olecranon and osteophytes have not had time to develop, and loose bodies, other than those developed in lateral compartment disease, are rare.

Acute and stress induced fracture of the olecranon,[65] as well as stress induced failure of union of its secondary ossification center can occur. These are treated by immobilization. Painful nonunion may require a bone grafting procedure.

An interesting but unusual injury is torsional fracture of the humerus caused by forceful internal humeral rotation during acceleration. The cortical hypertrophy seen in the conditioned adolescent or adult affords protection from this injury.

The overall approach to throwing injuries in youth players must include preventative measures. Varying etiologic factors, regional areas, levels of competition, and individual differences abound, but common ground can be approached through discussion with parents, players, and coaches as to conditioning, sensible throwing intervals and proper throwing mechanics, with emphasis on accuracy rather than velocity, and awareness of the possible injuries from throwing. They as well as physicians must be alerted to signs of injury, such as limitation of motion and flexion contracture, which portend a possible serious elbow abnormality.

Olecranon Bursitis

Olecranon bursitis may be due to trauma, eg, "miner's elbow," or may be associated with gout or rheumatoid arthritis (Fig. 15-8). Rheumatoid nodules can often be palpated in the olecranon bursae of patients with rheumatoid arthritis. Aspiration of the olecranon bursal fluid in patients with gout would be expected to yield needle-shaped urate crystals. Septic bursitis is an important consideration even in the absence of fever and a peripheral leukocytosis. The most frequent organism recovered from septic bursitis is Staphylococcus aureus.[11]

Lateral and Medial Epicondylitis

Lateral epicondylitis or tennis elbow is a common cause of elbow pain in tennis players and nontennis players. The wrist extensors, (the brachioradialis, the extensor carpi radialis longus, and the extensor carpi radialis brevis) originate from the lateral epicondyle of the humerus. Chronic or acute strain of the extensor apparatus causes microtears and resultant inflammation. Grasping, handshaking, and extending the wrist, or supernating the wrist causes pain. Extending the wrist against resistance will exacerbate the pain. On examination there is tenderness over the lateral epicondyle (Fig. 15-9). There is normal range-of-motion of the joint without pain and there is usually no heat or redness. Treatment consists of eliminating the aggravating activity that is causing the problem, resting the extremity, nonsteroidal anti-inflammatory drugs, and often a corticosteroid-lidocaine injection into the area of tenderness at the lateral epicondyle (Fig. 15-10). An exercise program to strengthen and stretch the extensor muscles can be helpful.

A similar syndrome may occur at the medial epicondyle of the humerus. The flexor-

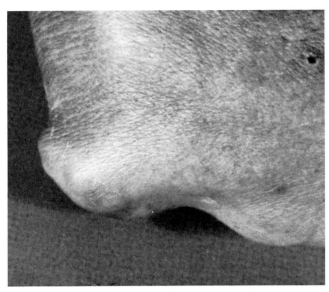

Fig. 15-8. Gouty tophi in the olecranon bursa. (Reprinted with permission from Germain BF (ed): Osteoarthritis and musculoskeletal pain syndromes. p. 115. Medical Examination Publishing Co., Inc.)

pronator apparatus is composed of the pronator teres, flexor carpi radialis, palmaris longus, and the flexor carpi ulnaris. Baseball players and golfers are prone to injury of the flexor-pronator apparatus. Treatment is similar to that of lateral epicondylitis.

SYSTEMIC DISEASES AFFECTING THE ELBOW

The elbow like other diarthrodial joints may be affected by various systemic diseases. Some are diseases that primarily affect the joints such as rheumatoid arthritis and gout; others may on occasion affect the joints, but the primary manifestations occur in other organ systems.

Rheumatoid Arthritis

Rheumatoid Arthritis is a disease of unknown etiology primarily affecting the peripheral joints. Synovial hypertrophy and inflammation lead to cartilage and subchondral bone destruction. The majority of patients with chronic rheumatoid arthritis have bilateral elbow involvement. Swollen synovium can be palpated on either side of the olecranon. Bilateral flexion contractures are not uncommon, but, in general, cause very little disability. In severe cases reduction of both extension and especially flexion can cause severe disability. Early extension and flexion of the elbow can be protected by using a posterior molded resting splint in 60° flexion with a program of active range-of-motion exercises several times a day. Supination and pronation exercises should be done with the elbow flexed at 90° and held to the side of the chest. Chronic painful synovitis can also be

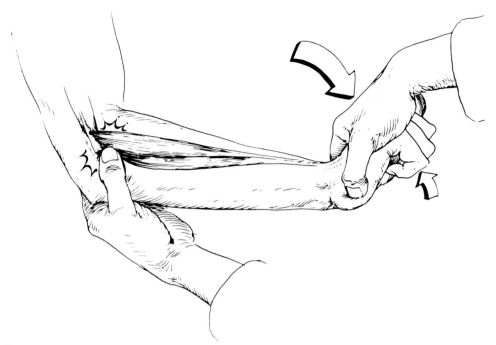

Fig. 15-9. Tennis elbow (lateral epicondylitis). (Reprinted with permission from Hoppenfield S (ed): Physical examination of the spine and extremities. p. 57, 1976, Appleton-Century-Croft.)

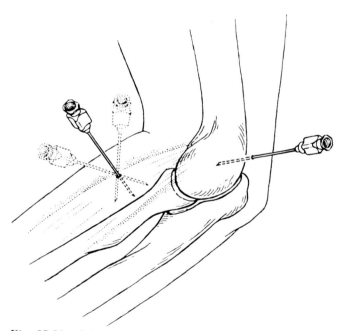

Fig. 15-10. Injection of the lateral epicondyle. (Reprinted with permission from Steinbrocker O, Neustadt D (eds): Aspiration and injection therapy in arthritis and musculoskeletal disorders. New York, Harper and Row, p. 55, 1972)

387

treated using intra-articular steroid preparations. The injection is made lateral to the olecranon and inferior to the lateral epicondyle.

Chronic synovitis may also lead to severe destruction at any of the three articulations of the elbow joint (Fig. 15-11). Synovectomy with radial head resection may be required if there is severe destruction at the proximal radioulnar joint and radiohumeral joint with pain during supination and pronation.[12]

Total elbow arthroplasty with or without use of a prosthesis may occasionally be necessary if there is severe destruction at the ulnohumeral joint.[14]

Synovial cysts may occur at the elbow especially in the antecubital fossa. They can dissect through tissue planes and cause median nerve or posterior interosseous nerve entrapment. Chronic swelling of the forearm may result from a large antecubital cyst; chronic cysts may also rupture.[17]

Chronic olecranon bursitis is also commonly found in patients with rheumatoid arthritis. Subcutaneous nodules in the olecranon bursa and along the extensor surface of the elbow are hallmarks of rheumatoid arthritis.

Osteoarthritis[27,50]

Symptomatic osteoarthritis of the elbow is unusual though postmortem examinations have shown osteoarthritis of the elbow to be common. Osteoarthritis of the elbow may occur in generalized osteoarthritis and in secondary osteoarthritis associated with several systemic diseases, ochronosis, hemochromatosis, Wilson's disease, hyperparathyroidism, acromegaly, Gaucher's disease, Ehlers-Danlos syndrome, other joint hyperlaxity syn-

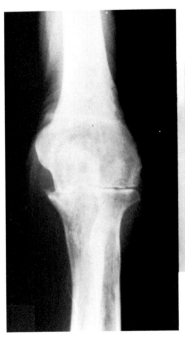
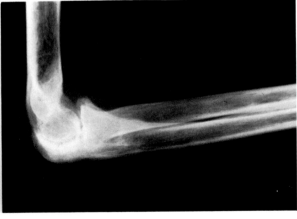

Fig. 15-11.   Rheumatoid Arthritis of the Elbow

dromes, and neuropathic joints. In particular syringomyelia or syphilis may be responsible for neuropathic joints at the elbow. More often osteoarthritis of the elbow is due to trauma, previous infection, or repeated hemarthroses. Chronic trauma may be due to previous fractures within the joint or occupations such as pneumatic tool operators, miners, and drillers.

Radiographic findings of osteoarthritis include loss of joint space, subchondral bony sclerosis, cyst formation, and osteophytes (Fig. 15-12). Olecranon spurs may be present. Olecranon spurs are also seen in DISH, diffuse idiopathic skeletal hyperostosis.

Infectious Arthritis

The elbow like other peripheral joints may be the site of septic arthritis (Fig. 15-13). The most common bacterial arthritis remains gonococcal arthritis, but Staphylococcus aureus and Pseudomonas organisms may be found especially in drug abusers. Hemophilus influenza arthritis is important in children, but not adults. The key to correct diagnosis remains synovial fluid aspiration with white cell count, blood/serum glucose differential, Gram stain, and appropriate cultures of the aspirated fluid. Arthritis may occur in association with hepatitis B infection, rubella, rubella vaccination, varicella, and has been reported in patients with infectious mononucleosis, Mycoplasma infection, and Herpes infection. Fungal and mycobacterial arthritis may also occur. Synovial biopsy may be required to confirm tuberculous arthritis.

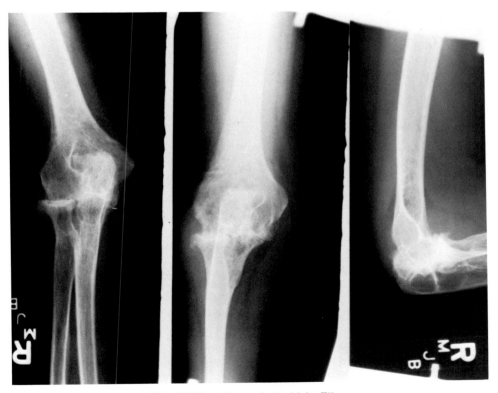

Fig. 15-12.   Osteoarthritis of the Elbow

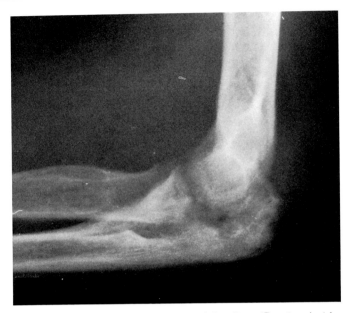

Fig. 15-13. Tuberculosis infection of the elbow. (Reprinted with permission from Germain BF (ed): Osteoarthritis and musculoskeletal pain syndromes. p. 119. Medical Examination Publishing Co., Inc.)

REFERENCES

1. Albright JA: Clinical study of baseball pitchers: Correlation of injury to the throwing arm with method of delivery. Am J Sports Med 6:15–21, 1978

2. An KN, Hui FC, Morrey BF: Muscles across the elbow joint: A biomechanical analysis. J Biomechs 14:659–669, 1981

3. Anzel SH, Covey KW, Weiner AD: Disruption of muscles and tendons. Surgery 45:406–414, 1959

4. Bachman DC (ed): Head-neck injuries and helmetry. New York, Reidel, Dordrecht, Nederlands, 1981

5. Barnes DA, Tullos HS: An analysis of 100 symptomatic baseball players. Am J Sports Med 6:62–67, 1978

6. Bennett BS: Triceps tendon rupture. JBJS 44-A:741–744, 1962

7. Benton J: Epiphyseal fractures in sports. Phys Sportsmed 10:62–71, 1982

8. Brogdon BG, Crow NE: Little leaguer's elbow. Am J Roentg 83: 671–675, 1980

9. Bryan RS: Fractures about the elbow in adults. In AAOS Instructional course lectures, Vol. XXX, 200–223, 1981

10. Carr D, Johnson RJ, Pope MH: Upper extremity injuries in skiing. Am J Sports Med 9:378–383, 1981

11. Carroso JJ, Sheckman PR: Septic subcutaneous bursitis: report of sixteen cases. J Rheumatol 6:96–102, 1979

12. Copeland SA, Taylor JG: Synovectomy of the elbow in rheumatoid arthritis: the place of excision of the head of the radius. J Bone Joint Surg 61-B:69–73, 1979

13. DeHaven KE, Evarts CM: Throwing injuries of the elbow in athletes. Ortho Cl North Am 4:801–808, 1973

14. Ewald FC, Scheinberg RD, Poss R, et al: Capitellocondylar total elbow arthroplasty. J Bone Joint Surg 62-A:1259–1262, 1980

15. Froimson AI, Zahrawi F: Treatment of compression neuropathy of the ulnar nerve at the elbow of epicondylectomy and neurolysis. J Hand Surg 5:391–395, 1980

16. Garrick JG, Requa R: Medical care and injury surveillance in the high school setting. Phys Sportsmed 9(2):115–120, 1981

17. Gerber NJ, St Dixon JA: Synovial cysts and

Juxta-articular bone cysts (Geodes). Semin Arth Rheum 3:323–348, 1974

18. Gilcreest EL, Albi P: Unusual lesions of muscles and tendons of the shoulder girdle and upper arm. Surg Gyn Obstet 68:903–917, 1939

19. Glick JM: Muscle strains: Prevention and treatment. Phys Sportsmed 8:73–77, 1980

20. Godshall RW, Hansen CA: Traumatic ulnar neuropathy in adolescent baseball pitchers. JBJS 53-A:359–361, 1971

21. Gore RM, Rogers LF, Bowerman J, et al: Osseous manifestations of elbow stress associated with sports activities. Am J Roentg 134:971–977, 1980

22. Grana WA, Rashkin A: Pitchers elbow in adolescents. Am J Sports Med 8:333–336, 1980

23. Gugenheim JJ, Stanley RF, Woods GW, et al: Little league survey: The Houston study. Am J Sports Med 4:189–200, 1976

24. Heckman JD, Levine MI: Traumatic closed transection of the biceps brachii in the military parachutist. JBJS 60-A:369–372, 1978

25. Henry JH, Lareau B, Neigut D: The injury rate in professional basketball. Am J Sports Med 10:16–18, 1982

26. Hollingshead WH: Anatomy for surgeons. Vol. 3. The back and limbs. New York, Harper & Row, 1969

27. Howell DS, Goldberg VM, Mankin HJ (eds): Osteoarthritis, diagnosis and management. Philadelphia, WB Saunders Company, 1984, pp. 377–387

28. Indelicato PA, Jobe FW, Kerlan RK, et al: Correctable elbow lesions in professional baseball players: A review of 25 cases. Am J Sports Med 7:72–75, 1979

29. Jobe FW, Moynes DR, Tibone JT: An EMG analysis of the shoulder in pitching. Am J Sports Med 12:218–220, 1984

30. Johnson RK, Spinner M, Shrewsbury MM: Median nerve entrapment syndrome in the proximal forearm. J Hand Surg 4:48–51, 1979

31. Jones HH, Priest JD, Hayes WC, et al: Humeral hypertrophy in response to exercise. JBJS 59-A:204–208, 1977

32. King JW, Brensford HJ, Tullos HS: Analysis of the pitching arm of the professional baseball pitcher. Clin Orthop 67:116–123, 1969

33. Krejci V, Koch P: Muscle and tendon injuries to athletes. Stuttgart, Georg Thieme, 1979

34. Larson RL, Singer KM, Bergstrom R, et al: Little league survey: The Eugene study. Am J Sports Med 4:201–209, 1976

35. Leffert RD: Anterior submuscular transposition of the ulnar nerve by the Learmonth technique. J Hand Surg 7:147–155, 1982

36. Lister GD, Belsole RB, Kleinert HE: The radial tunnel syndrome. J Hand Surg 4:52–59, 1979

37. London JT: Kinematics of the elbow. JBJS 63-A:529–535, 1981

38. Loomer RL: Elbow injuries in athletes. Can J Appl Spt Sci 7:164–166, 1982

39. Miller JE: Javelin throwers elbow. JBJS 42-B:788–792, 1960

40. Morley BF, Askew L, Chao EY: Silastic prosthetic replacement for the radial head. JBJS 63-A:454–458, 1981

41. Nicholas JS, Grossman RB, Hershman EB: The importance of a simplified classification of motion in sports in relation to performance. Orthop Clin North Am 8:499–532, 1977

42. Norwood LA, Shook JA, Andrews JR: Acute medial elbow ruptures. Am J Sports Med 9:16–19, 1981

43. Pappas AM: Elbow problems associated with baseball during childhood and adolescence. Clin Orthop 164:30–41, 1982

44. Pappas AM: Epiphyseal injuries in sports. Phys Sportsmed 11:140–148, 1983

45. Perlick PC, Kalveda DD, Wellman AS, et al: Roller skating injuries. Phys Sportsmed 10:76–80, 1982

46. Priest JD, Weise DJ: Elbow injury in women's gymnastics. Am J Sports Med 9:288–292, 1981

47. Radin EL, Riseborough EJ: Fractures of the radial head. JBJS 48-A:1055–1064, 1966

48. Rang M: Children's fractures. Philadelphia J.B. Lippincott, 1974

49. Requa R, Garrick JG: Injuries in interscholastic wrestling. Phys Sportsmed 4:44–51, 1981

50. Resnick D, Niwayama G: Degenerative disease of extraspinal locations, in Resnick D, Niwayama G (eds): Diagnosis of bone and joint disorders. Philadelphia, WB Saunders Company, 1981, pp. 1271–1368.

51. Rockwood CA, Green DP (eds): Fractures. Philadelphia J.B. Lippincott, 1975

52. Salter RB, Harris WR: Injuries involving the epiphyseal plate. JBJS 45-A:587–622, 1963.

53. Schwab GH, Bennett JB, Woods GW, et al: Biomechanics of elbow instability: The role of the medial collateral ligament. Clin Orthop Rel Res 146:42–52, 1980

54. Schwab GH, Bennett JB, Woods GW, et al: Biomechanics of elbow instability: The role of the medial collateral ligament. Clin Orthop 146:42–52, 1980

55. Searfoss R, Tripi J, Bowers W: Triceps brachii rupture. J Trauma 16:244–246, 1976

56. Sherman OH, Snyder SJ, Fox JM: Triceps tendon avulsion in a body builder. Am J Sportsmed 12:328–329, 1984

57. Shields CL, Zomar VD: Analysis of professional football injuries. Cont Orthop 4:90–95, 1982

58. Shively RA, Grana WA, Ellis D: High school

sports injuries. Phys Sportsmed 9(8):46–50, 1981

59. Silberstein MJ, Brodeur AE, Graviss ER, et al: Some vagaries of the medial epicondyle. JBJS 63-A:524–528, 1981

60. Slocum DB: Classification of elbow injuries from baseball pitching. Tex Med 64:48–53, 1968

61. Snook GA: Injuries in women's gymnastics. Am J Sports Med 4:242–244, 1979

62. Tibone JE, Stoltz M: Fractures of the radial head and neck in children. JBJS 63-A:100–107, 1981

63. Tivnon MC, Anzel SH, Waugh TR: Surgical management of osteochondritis dissecans of the capitellum. Am J Sports Med 4:121–128, 1976

64. Torg JS, Pollack H, Sweterlitsch P: The effect of competitive pitching on the shoulders and elbows of pre-adolescent baseball players. Pediatrics 4:267–272, 1972

65. Torg JS, Moyer RA: Non-union of a stress fracture through the olecranon epiphyseal plate osbsfrnfa in an adolescent baseball pitcher. JBJS 59-A:264–265, 1977

66. Tullos HS, Schwab G, Bennett JB, et al: Factors influencing elbow instability. In AAOS Instructional course lectures, Vol. XXX:185–199, 1981

67. Tullos HS, King JW: The throwing mechanism in sports. Orthop Clin North Am 4:709–720, 1973

68. Wilson FD, Andrews JR, Blackburn TA, et al: Valgus extension overload in the pitching elbow. Am J Sports Med 11:83–88, 1983

69. Woods GW, Tullos HS: Elbow instability and medial epicondyle fractures. Am J Sports Med 5:23–30, 1977

70. Woodward AH, Bianco AJ: Osteochondritis dissecans of the elbow. Clin Orthop 110:35–41, 1975

Stanley M. Naguwa
Kenneth S. O'Rourke
Linda B. Rosker

16

The Hand and Wrist

"Chiefly, the mold of a man's fortune is in his own hands." Francis Bacon.

The hand is used by man in many ways; whether for a powerful grip or a precise pinch, as emphasis of an expression or as tools of communication. Hands are finely tuned sensory receptors capable of supplementing or even replacing visual receptors. The vital role hands play in the ability to function cannot be minimized.

Sixteen million people sustain significant injuries to the upper extremity in the United States annually. These injuries account for 90 million days of restricted or lost activities and 16 million days of work loss, with an estimated cost of treatment in 1979 of 3 billion dollars.[3] When hands are diseased or injured the total damage is much more than physical. There is great psychological trauma associated with hand impairment. Loss of hand function may mean loss of work, play, or ability to care for one's self or family. Therefore, the task of caring for, repairing, and rehabilitating the traumatized hand is much more complex than might be imagined. The importance of close treatment coordination between physician or surgeon, hand therapist, and patient cannot be overemphasized.

While a gifted surgeon or a skillful therapist may contribute a tremendous amount of technical skill to the treatment of a dysfunctional hand, ultimately, the patient is the star of the treatment team. The patient must immediately appreciate the extent of the injury and the necessity of his or her dedication to the rehabilitative process. A cooperative, motivated patient has often meant the difference between a healthy, once again functional hand and a painful, chronically crippled appendage.

ANATOMY OF HAND AND WRIST

Bones of the Wrist

In general, the dorsal and palmar surfaces of the wrist bones are roughened for attachment of muscle, ligaments, and tendons. The remaining surfaces are smooth for articulation. The bones can be grouped into proximal and distal rows of four bones each (Fig. 16-1).

PRINCIPLES OF PHYSICAL MEDICINE AND REHABILITATION
IN THE MUSCULOSKELETAL DISEASES

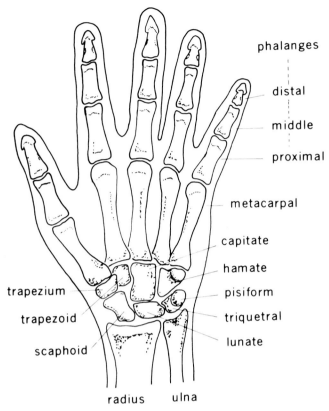

Fig. 16-1. Bones of the hand and wrist.

Proximal Row

Beginning at the radial side, the bones are the scaphoid (or navicular), lunate, triquetral, and the pisiform. The scaphoid (navicular) is the largest bone of the proximal row; the lunate has a deep dorsal cavity; the pisiform is anterolateral to the triquetral and is the smallest of the wrist bones. The scaphoid is the most frequently fractured, whereas the lunate is most susceptible to osteonecrosis.

Distal Row

Again, beginning radially, the bones are the trapezium, trapezoid, capitate, and the hamate. The capitate is the largest bone of the wrist; the hamate has a "hook" on the palmar aspect.

Bones of the Hand

The metacarpal bones are long with a flared and concave proximal end that articulates with the carpal bones and a smooth rounded distal end that articulates with the proximal phalanges. The phalanges are similar in structure but are progressively shorter as one proceeds distally. The distal phalanges have a "tuft" at their terminus.

Bony overgrowth or osteophytes may form at the dorsomedial and dorsolateral aspects with osteoarthritis. Osteophytes at the distal interphalangeal joint are called Heberden's nodes, and when formed at the proximal interphalangeal joint, Bouchard's nodes.

Joints and Ligaments

Wrist

The wrist joint is complex, with a condylar joint between the radius-ulna and the proximal row of the carpal bones; gliding joints with limited movement occur between the carpal bones themselves. Various ligaments stabilize the joints and form part of the joint capsule. The joint spaces are synovial lined and interconnect in most instances.

The second to fourth carpometacarpal joints (CMC) are also gliding joints with synovial linings that communicate with the carpal joint spaces. The second and third joints have flexion-extension motion but have relatively little abduction-adduction at full flexion. The third and fourth joints have greater motion that aid in grasping.

The first carpometacarpal joint is different. It is a saddle joint that permits a greater motion of the thumb, with flexion-extension, abduction-adduction and circumduction, which allows opposition of the thumb and digits.

Three large ligaments are found in the wrist (Fig. 16-2, Table 16-1). The palmar carpal ligament and the transverse carpal ligament form the flexor retinaculum, which keeps the flexor tendons close to the skeletal structure. The extensor retinaculum serves a similar purpose on the dorsum of the wrist. Unfortunately, while providing a necessary biomechanical function, these ligaments form confined spaces or compartments in the wrist that may be detrimental to the patient with an intercompartmental process, the most common of which is the carpal tunnel syndrome. The median nerve courses through the "tunnel" created by the flexor retinaculum and the bones (Fig. 16-3). It can be compressed by any process that swells the other structures that share the tunnel such as inflammatory arthritis, or hypothyroidism. A similar process can affect the ulnar nerve in Guyon's tunnel, between the hook of the hamate, pisiform, and the transverse carpal ligament. However, there is no tenosynovium and thus the ulnar nerve is less likely to be impinged upon.

The wrist joints are commonly affected in inflammatory arthritis while the first CMC joint is most affected by osteoarthritis.

Fingers

The metacarpophalangeal (MCP) joints are condyloid except for the first MCP. These joints have flexion-extension, abduction-adduction, and circumduction motion. The first MCP joint has fewer options and is more like a hinge joint. The joints are stabilized by strong palmar and collateral ligaments as well as a transverse ligament uniting the second through fifth MCP joints. The joints are synovial lined and may be afflicted in inflammatory arthropathies.

The proximal interphalangeal (PIP) joints are hinge joints with significant ability to flex and limited ability to extend. They are stabilized by palmar and collateral ligaments and the extensor tendons. They are synovial lined, with the PIP joint involved in both inflammatory/degenerative disorders, and the DIP joint more commonly involved in degenerative joint disease.

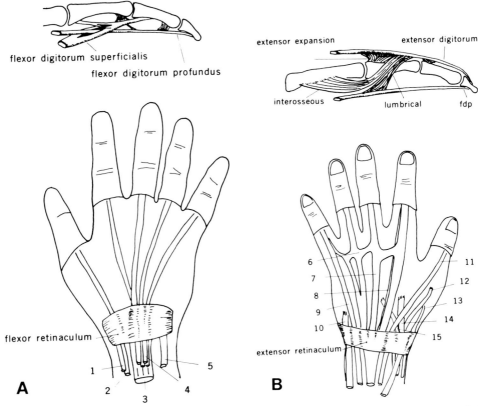

Fig. 16-2. (A) Flexor tendons (1) flexor carpi radialis, (2) flexor pollicis longus, (3) flexor digitorum profundus, (4) flexor digitorum superficialis, (5) flexor carpi ulnaris. (B) Extensor tendons (6) intertendinous band, (7) extensor digitorum, (8) extensor indicis, (9) extensor digiti minimi, (10) extensor carpi ulnaris, (11) extensor pollicis longus, (12) extensor pollicis brevis, (13) abductor pollicis longus, (14) extensor carpi radialis longus, (15), extensor carpi radialis brevis.

Arteries, Muscles, and Nerves

The radial and ulnar arteries enter the wrist at their respective anterolateral borders. The arteries anastomose and form the deep palmar arch, superficial palmar arch, and the dorsal carpal system (Fig. 16-4). The radial artery primarily forms the deep palmar arch and anastomoses with a small deep palmar branch of the ulnar artery. The ulnar artery primarily forms the superficial arch anastomosing with a small superficial branch of the radial artery. Both the radial and ulnar arteries send dorsal carpal branches that anastomose.

Each arch/system sends branches distally that anastomose to form the proper digital arteries that then course along the lateral aspect of the fingers.

The muscles, tendons, and nerves of the hand are tabulated and diagrammed for easy reference (Tables 16-2, 16-3, Figs. 16-5, 16-6).

Table 16-1
Tendons

	Insertion	Function
Dorsal group		
Extensor digitorium communis	Intermediate slip-base of middle phalanges	Extends digits
	Collateral slip-base of distal phalanges	
Extensor carpi radialis, longus	Base of 2nd metacarpal	Extends, abducts hand
Extensor carpi radialis, brevis	Base of 3rd metacarpal	
Extensor carpi ulnaris	Base of 5th metacarpal	Extends, adducts hand
Extensor digiti minimi	Joints extensor digitorium tendon	Extends 5th digit
Extensor pollicis, brevis	Base of 1st proximal phalanx	Extends thumb
Abductors pollicis longus	Base of 1st metacarpal	Abducts thumb
Palmar group		
Flexor digitorium, profundus	Base of digital phalanges	Flexes digits
Flexor digitorium, sublimis	Middle phalanges	Flexes digits
Flexor carpi, radialis	Base of 2nd and 3rd metacarpals	Flexes hand
Flexor carpi, ulnaris	Pisiform, hamate, 5th metacarpal	Flexes, adducts hand
Flexor pollicis longus	Base of 1st distal phalanx	Flexes thumb
Palmaris longus	Flexor retinaculum, palmar aponeurosis	Flexes hand

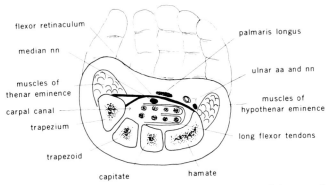

Fig. 16-3. Cross section of the hand, and outline of the carpal canal (tunnel).

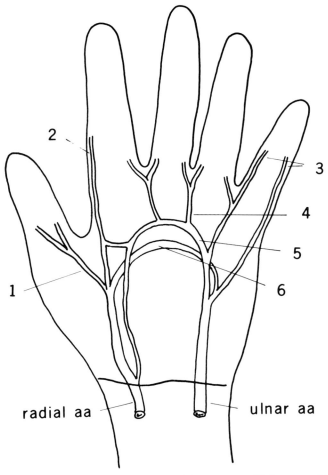

Fig. 16-4. Arteries of the hand, (1) princeps pollicis artery, (2) radialis indicis, (3) proper palmar digital artery, (4) common palmar digital artery, (5) superficial palmar arch, (6) deep palmar arch.

Table 16-2
Muscles

Muscles	Origin	Insertion	Function
Thenar group			
Abductor pollicis brevis	Transverse carpal ligament, navicular	Base of 1st phalanx	Abduction of thumb*
Opponens pollicis	Flexor retinaculum	1st metacarpal	Opposition of thumb by rotation, flexion and abduction
	Trapezium		
Flexor pollicis brevis	Flexor retinaculum	Base of 1st proximal phalanx	Flex† and adduction of thumb
	Trapezium		
Abductor pollicis	3rd metacarpal, capitate	Base of 1st proximal phalanx	Abducts thumb
	Tendon of flexor carpi ulnaris		
Hypothenar group			
Abductor digiti	Pisiform	Base of 5th proximal phalanx	Abducts, flexes 5th digit
Opponens digiti minimi	Flexor retinaculum	5th metacarpal phalanx	Opposition of 5th digit by rotation, flexion, and abduction
	Hamate		
Flexor digiti minimi brevis	Flexor retinaculum	Base of 5th proximal phalanx	Flexes 5th digit
	Hamate		
Palmaris brevis	Transverse carpal ligament	Cutaneous tissue of palm	"Adducts" skin
	Palmar aponeurosis		
Interossei	Metacarpals	Base of proximal phalanx	Adducts digits
Lumbricals	Tendons of the flexor digitiorum profundus	Tendinous expansion of the extensor digitorium	Flexes digits

*Adduction, abduction of the thumb is in a plane perpendicular to palmar surface. Adduction, abduction of fingers is in the plane of the palmar surface. Flexion, extension of the fingers is in a plane perpendicular to the palmar surface.
†Flexion, extension of the thumb is in the plane of the palmar surface. Flexion, extension of the thumb is in a plane perpendicular to the palmar surface.

Table 16-3

Nerves

	Course	Motor	Sensory
Ulnar nerve	Enters wrist deep to palmar carpal ligament and superficial to the ligament between the pisiform and hook of the hamate (Guyon's tunnel), divides into a superficial and deep branch	Palmaris brevis interossei 3rd, 4th lumbricals Adductor pollicis Flexor pollicus brevis	Ulnar 1/3 of palm; 5th digit; ulnar half of 4th finger
Median nerve	Enters at the palmar midline of the wrist deep to the flexor retinoculum in the carpal tunnel and subsequently, dividers	Abductor pollicis brevis Opponens pollicis 1st, 2nd lumbricals	Radial 2/3 palmar and distal 2/3 of dorsum of 1st, 2nd, 3rd fingers; radial 1/2 of 4th finger
Radial nerve	Enters at the radial aspect of the wrist anterior to the Lister's tubercle		Radial 2/3 of dorsum of hand and proximal 1/3 of fingers

PRINCIPLES OF REHABILITATION

Evaluation

To provide proper rehabilitative treatment of the arthritic hand, the hand therapist must have a sound knowledge of hand anatomy and function. A thorough history, a physical examination of the involved extremity, and an understanding of the disease process affecting the dysfunctional hand are required.

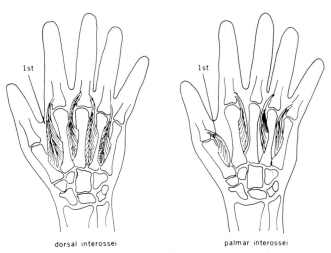

dorsal interossei   palmar interossei

Fig. 16-5. Palmar and dorsal interosseous muscles.

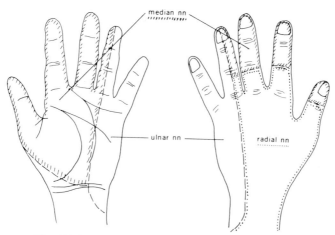

Fig. 16-6. Cutaneous nerve distribution in the hand.

Upon initial evaluation of a patient, the therapist must begin documentation. This information must be clear and concise. Range of motion may be charted on a graph or in an organized chart. Sensation may be illustrated with a drawing of the hand shaded to indicate degrees of sensation (Fig. 16-6). However the therapist chooses to record information, it must be easily interpreted and accurate.

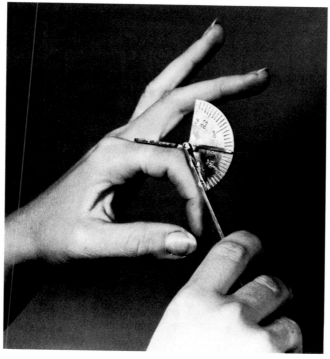

Fig. 16-7. Measurement of joint range of motion.

History

The history should include the patient's age, hand dominance, length of disease process, and any prior medical treatment. Past injuries, surgeries, therapies, and results should be recorded. The patient's occupation, vocation, and hobbies as well as a brief description of his or her family are noted. It is very important to ask the patient what arthritis is preventing him or her from doing and to request the patient to describe the nature of the pain. When does it hurt? What are the patient's expectation of therapy? Will therapy cause problems in terms of taking time off from work? Does the patient seem motivated and willing to follow the therapeutic program? Would the patient follow a home program?

An examination of the medical record is also important both to get information about relevant past surgeries and to examine general physical condition and identify any chronic disease that may affect therapy.

Physical Examination

The physical examination should include more than an assessment of the affected hand. The entire limb should be assessed from the shoulder distally. How the patient moves and holds the extremity may determine placement of the hand. Comparison of the involved and uninvolved extremity is very useful.

Range of Motion

Range of motion is measured both actively and passively if a discrepancy between the two exists. The goniometer is used to determine these measurements. Goniometers come in a variety of sizes and should be used according to size of the joint being measured (Fig. 16-7). Wrists are measured for flexion, extension (dorsiflexion), ulnar deviation, radial deviation, pronation and supination. Thumb flexion, extension, abduction, adduction, opposition, carpometacarpal extension, and abduction are all measured and recorded. Distance of fingertip to distal palmar crease is measured using a ruler, often part of the goniometer (Fig. 16-8). All active and passive motions are accurately measured and recorded.

Muscle testing may involve the entire extremity from the shoulder to the fingertips or the hand exclusively, depending on the nature of the dysfunction. Strength is graded from 0 to 5 with 0, no sign of muscle contraction and 5, normal strength. If there is an uninvolved extremity, it should be used to determine normal strength. In the hand, intrinsic muscle strength is evaluated separately from the extrinsic muscles and flexors apart from extensors.

Grip and pinch are measured using the grip dynamometer and the pinch gauge, respectively. The average of three tries is usually determined. The dynamometer has five adjustable settings, and after the patient is instructed in how to grasp the dynamometer with arm at side, elbow flexed 90° and wrist straight (Fig. 16-9), grip strength is measured at each setting alternating between the left and right hands. The patient is instructed to apply maximal force and these measurements are recorded. According to Beckol the difference in grip strength between the dominant and nondominant hand ranges from 5 to 10 percent.[6]

The three basic types of pinch are then examined; lateral (Fig. 16-10) or key pinch, tip

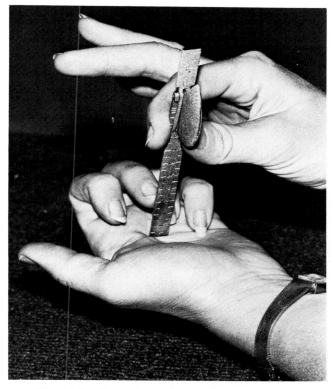

Fig. 16-8.   Fingertip-to-palmar crease measurement.

to tip pinch (Fig. 16-11), and jaw check (Fig. 16-12). The pinch gauge is used to measure these strengths (Fig. 16-13).

Sensation

Without sensation, the hand is blind.[14] Without accurate sensory testing the hand therapist does not have a complete picture of the hand injury and functional implications.

While the distribution of sensory nerves in the hand differs individually, the classic conception of radial, ulnar, and median nerves is represented in Figure 16-6. There are many sensory tests used today and there continues to be controversy regarding the most functional applicability. Moberg's "picking up test" (Fig. 16-14), Webers "two-point discrimination" test, von Frey filaments, Sedon's coin test, and Dellon's moving two-point discrimination test are a few of the tests used to assess sensibility.[5]

Commonly, two-point discrimination (2PD) along with careful skin examination is sufficient for practical purposes of sensory evaluation. A simple device made of paper clips and splinting material as described by the Loma Linda Hand Center (Fig. 16-15) may be used to evaluate 2PD.[47] The normal threshold for 2PD on a fingertip is 3–6 mm in adults and 2–3 mm for children; areas of unsatisfactory recovery can be easily determined.[35] This test is administered by seating the patient with the hand supine and slightly flexed at the wrist. The hand is cradled in the examiner's and with the patient's eyes closed, the

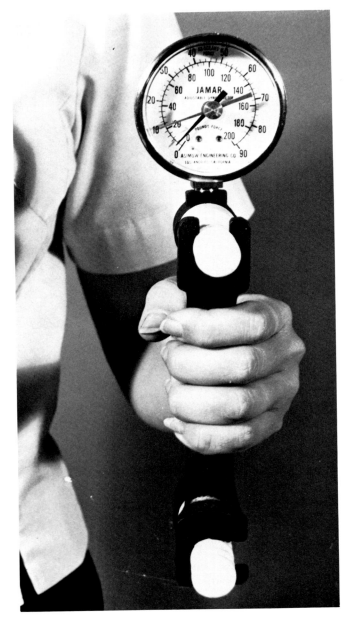

Fig. 16-9. Grip dynamometer.

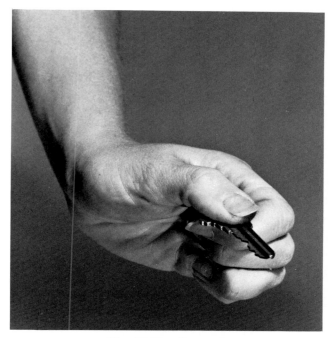

Fig. 16-10.   Key pinch.

examiner places the pressure in a longitudinal direction touching the skin lightly, just to the point of blanching the skin. The patient is asked whether he feels one point or two.

Functional Exam

Evaluation of motion, strength, and sensation is of little consequence if function is not assessed. There are several well documented, standardized tests that provide consistent information regarding hand function. Each seems to have positive and negative

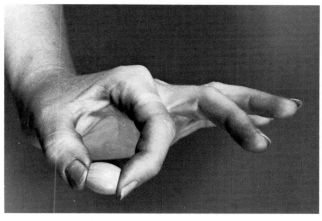

Fig. 16-11.   Tip-to-tip pinch.

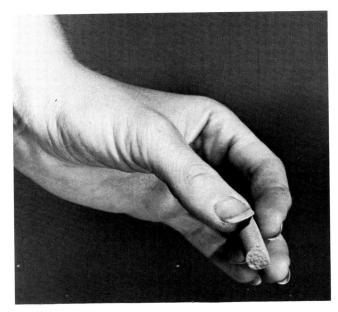

Fig. 16-12. Jaw check.

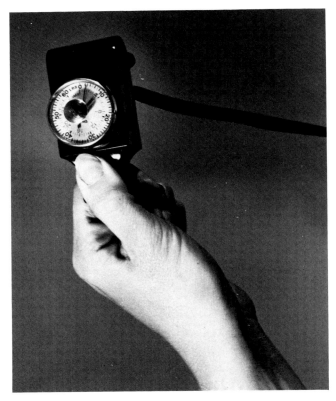

Fig. 16-13. Pinch gauge.

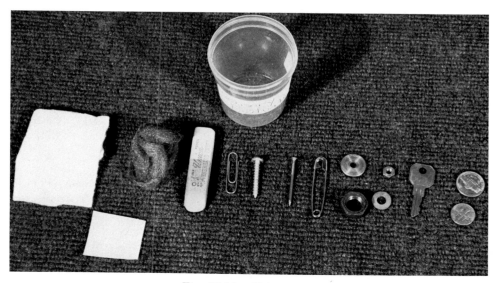

Fig. 16-14. Pick-up test.

attributes. The Jebson-Taylor Test of Hand Function, the Minnesota Rate of Manipulation Test, and the Purdue Pegboard Test are a few of the most commonly used assessments.

The Jebson-Taylor Test of Hand Function is an example of a test that assesses unilateral functional hand skills.[22] The items tested include writing, turning over cards, picking up small common objects, stacking checkers, simulated eating, and moving empty and weighted (#1) cans. Performance times are recorded and both hands are tested. This test takes about 15 minutes and can be easily assembled with minimal expense. A disadvantage of the test is that it does not assess bilateral hand function and poor prehension is not a consideration as performance speed is the basis of each score.

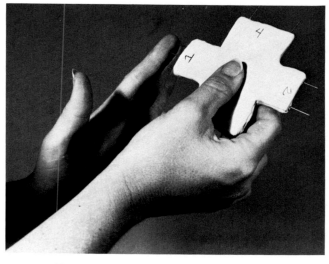

Fig. 16-15. Two-point discrimination test.

By contrast, the Purdue Pegboard Test assesses unilateral and bilateral function. To administer this test, the test board represented in Figure 16-16 and a stopwatch and test manual are required. This test focuses on prehension and sensory problems in the thumb or fingertips. It is also relatively easy to administer and takes about 15 minutes to complete.

Frequently, by utilizing more than one functional test, such as the Jebson and the Purdue Pegboard, a more accurate assessment of the patient's functional ability can be obtained.

Dysfunction

As previously stated, the hand is an integral part of man's ability to function in most activities and because of this exposure, the hand is subject to frequent injury and disease. A thorough review of therapeutic implications for the great variety of specific hand and wrist injuries and disease processes would be voluminous.

In this section the most commonly treated hand problems and rehabilitative techniques will be reviewed. These include arthritis flexor and extensor hand tendon injuries, fractures of the hand and wrist, nerve injuries, and burns. A discussion of splinting techniques will be included.

Splinting

Splinting has been discussed as a therapeutic modality for a variety of hand problems. Hand splinting may be done to increase function by protecting weak muscles or diseased joints. Splinting may assist weakened muscles (as in tenodesis splints for brachial plexus injuries); may stabilize by preventing unwanted motion (ulnar drift) and provide proper joint alignment; may be supportive to maintain or increase range of motion while preventing or decreasing deformity (radial/median nerve palsy wrist and impextension

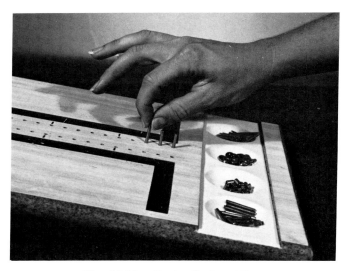

Fig. 16-16.   Purdue Pegboard Test.

splint); may act to transfer power from one joint to another or one finger to another (simple finger tap). Dynamic splinting can strengthen muscles through resistive exercise.

Comfort can be increased through splinting by promoting circulation, decreasing edema, or relieving compression (e.g., simple cock-up splint for carpal tunnel syndrome) (Fig. 16-17).

In addition, a splint can improve cosmesis and improve the patient's psychological acceptance of a deformed hand and therein, improve function.

Splints may be static, having no movable parts and holding the involved part in a functional, immobilized position,[31] or dynamic, with movable parts to provide low amplitude of force over a prolonged period to influence the synthesis of new tissues.[48] There is no "cook book" solution to splinting pathologic conditions of the hand. As Elaine Fess states, "splints must be individually created to meet the unique needs of each patient, as evidenced by designs that incorporate the variable factors of anatomy, kinesiology, pathology, rehabilitation goals, occupation, and psychological status."[17]

There are general principles to consider in splint fabrication including mechanics, fit, design, and construction.

Splint design must consider basic mechanical principles such as optimal length needed to stabilize a joint and contouring of the splint to give it strength.

Fit principles include anatomic considerations such as dual obliquity, the progressive decrease in the length of the metacarpals from the second to the fifth digits and the immobility of the second and third metacarpals compared to the first, fourth and fifth, arches of the hand, and usual joint motion.

The principles of design take the individual patient qualities into account. Ease in application and removal, cosmesis, functional limitations, and length of wear all affect design, as well as specific pathology and goals of splinting.

The principle of construction can be considered once the splint has been designed and a pattern made. There are a variety of materials that can be used in splint fabrication, each with different temperature and forming properties. Once a material has been selected, these properties must be respected. Padding and straps must be properly placed and secured. Corners must be rounded and edges smoothed. Joined surfaces must be stabilized and ventilation provided as required. Commonly used hand splints include the resting hand splint (Fig. 16-18), which covers the volar two-thirds of the forearm and hand, extending to the fingertips and is useful in providing joint and tendon rest in various arthritic conditions. A cock-up splint (Fig. 16-17) supports the wrist in a neutral or slightly

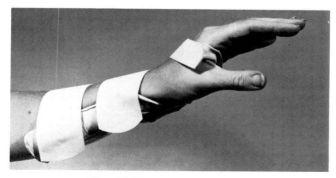

Fig. 16-17. Cock-up splint.

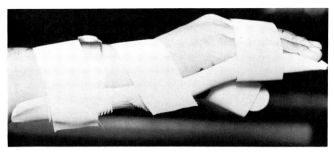

Fig. 16-18. Resting hand splint.

extended position is used in arthritis of the joint as well as in carpal tunnel syndrome. A thumb spica (Fig. 16-19) stabilizes the carpometacarpal joint which is frequently involved in osteoarthritis and in DeQuervain's tenosynovitis. An ulnar drift splint attempts to prevent or correct the ulnar drift of the digits as a result of inflammatory arthritis of the MCP joints, a common problem in rheumatoid arthritis and lupus.

There are numerous dangers inherent in a poorly conceived splint. They are summarized in Table 16-4.

MEDICAL CONDITIONS AFFECTING THE HAND

Disorders of the hand are common, and because of its functional significance, the potential for disability is high. Many systemic diseases have characteristic manifestations in the hand, or may present with hand findings, therefore early recognition of these signs and symptoms can lead to institution of appropriate therapy and may avert long-term complications. There is a great number and variety of medical conditions that affect the hand (Table 16-5). In this section these conditions will be summarized, with special emphasis placed on the more common diseases.

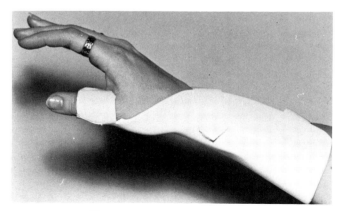

Fig. 16-19. Thumb spica splint.

Table 16-4

Dangers in splinting

Improper wearing schedule
Wearing the splint when no longer required
Failure to alter splints with change of conditions
Improper tension of rubber bands
Improper positioning of joints
Poor fit (note edema, redness, soreness, indentations)
Excessive pressure on bony prominences
Stiffness from prolonged static splinting
Pressure atrophy over articular cartilage from prolonged dynamic splinting
Prolonged pressure over denervated areas
Wound contamination by neglect of aseptic techniques
Failure of follow-up in splint management
Rejection of the splint by the patient
Splint shifts or falls off limbs when there is uncontrolled muscle activity (brain injury)
Patient or staff becomes so impressed with a good splint that old-fashioned exercise is neglected

Diffuse Connective Tissue Diseases

Rheumatoid Arthritis.

This chronic, relapsing, potentially disabling disease can affect the synovium, cartilage, tendon, bone, nerves, and vessels. The arthritis, by which it is known, is inflammatory, bilateral and symmetric, and can involve any diarthrodial joint, but characteristically
the PIP and MCP joints. Early in the course of the hand disease, acute synovitis causes a
fusiform shape to the fingers. There is pain, stiffness (including morning stiffness), and
decreased range of motion. With continued inflammation and progression, typical deformities are seen. Synovitis leads to erosion of the volar stabilizing elements, causing dorsal
displacement of the extensor apparatus. This, together with muscle and tendon shortening
from repetitive tenosynovitis leads to hyperextension of the PIP joints and flexion of the
DIP, and MCP joints: the swan-neck deformity. Disruption of the extensor mechanism over

Table 16-5

Medical Conditions Affecting
the Hand

Diffuse connective tissue diseases
The spondyloarthropathies
Osteoarthritis
Arthritis associated with infectious agents
Crystal-induced rheumatic diseases
Endocrine diseases
Arthritis associated with liver disease
Hematologic disorders
Neoplasm
Neuropathic disorders
Bone and cartilage disorders
Nonarticular rheumatism
Miscellaneous disorders

the PIP joint causes flexion there and extension of the DIP joints, leading to the boutonniere deformity. Other common deformities include ulnar deviation of the fingers, volar subluxation of proximal phalanges, and those listed in Table 16-6. Tenosynovitis of the tendon sheaths, both extensor and flexor, leads to swelling and decreased hand strength with progressive inflammation contributing to contraction abnormalities. Formation of rheumatoid nodules within sheaths causes trigger finger and locked-in fingers. Extensor tendon rupture can also occur with resultant predictable loss of function.

In the wrist, tenosynovitis causes a boggy texture to the dorsal surface, while inflammation along the volar aspect, together with synovial hypertrophy, can lead to median nerve entrapment and carpal tunnel syndrome, with secondary atrophy of the thenareminence. With time, progressive disease can lead to radial deviation of the wrist, volar subluxation, joint space loss with foreshortening of the carpus secondary to bony compaction, and eventually bony and fibrous ankylosis, which can involve the radiocarpal, intercarpal, and carpometacarpal joints.

Skin changes include palmar erythema, Raynaud's phenomenon (seen in 10 percent of patients), and changes secondary to vasculitis, including: skin necrosis, digital ulceration and skin infarcts, particularly near the nail bed. The degree of vasculitis, though, may not correlate with articular disease. Rheumatoid nodules are round or oval masses seen in the subcutaneous tissue, mainly over the extensor surface, and vary in consistency from soft and gelatinous to firm, rubbery masses. Pulmonary fibrosis can lead to clubbing of the distal phalanges.

Rheumatoid arthritis (RA) poses many therapeutic problems because unlike traumatic conditions in the hand, it is unpredictable, constantly changes, and is systemic, affecting many joints.[11] Treatment of the hand is but one facet of the total care of the patient with RA. The extent to which function may be affected depends on many factors: the systemic extent of the disease; other contiguous joints of the upper extremity involved; the psychological make-up of the patient and his or her reaction to the disease, as well as the social and domestic background of the patient.

Care of the rheumatoid hand varies from early care of the acutely inflamed hand to rehabilitation of the severely afflicted hand. Each patient must be treated individually and periodic reassessment is necessary as no patient presents the same problem for any long period of time.

Table 16-6
Common Deformities of the Rheumatoid Hand

Deformity	Description
Mallet finger	PIP neutral, DIP flexed
Intrinsic plus	MCP flexed, PIP extended
Intrinsic minus	MCP extended, PIP flexed
Main en lorganette (opera-glass hand)	Gross dislocation of all small joints telescoping of joints
Maine en griffe (claw hand)	MCPs hyperextended PIPs hyperflexed Flexion contracture of wrist
Trigger finger	Acute inability to extend PIP joint

Adapted from Kelley WN, Harris ED Jr, Ruddy S, et al: Textbook of Rheumatology, Philadelphia, Saunders, 1981.

A hand rehabilitation program should include the following.[32]

1. Patient education regarding causes of deformity as a result of the disease
2. Exercise instruction, according to the stage of the development and if the disease is active or in remission
3. Appropriate splinting
4. Principles of joint protection
5. Provision of self-help and to aid the patient in activities of daily living (ADLs)
6. Home assessments and recommended modifications for ease in living considering joint protection principles.

In general, the rehabilitation program for the rheumatoid hand aims at maintaining function and therein, the ability to grasp, manipulate, and hold objects of varying size. Problems encountered include joint instability, flexor/extensor imbalance resulting in flexion contractures, collateral ligament contractures, intrinsic muscle contractures, thumb immobility and deformity, wrist instability, ulnar drift, swan neck, and boutonniere deformities, singly or frequently in multiple.

Exercise is aimed at maintaining range of motion and muscle strength, preserving arches and decreasing developing deformities, and increasing joint stability. These exercises may involve use of light objects such as sponges, isometric contractions, and cautious passive motion followed by active or active assisted motion.

Sessions should be short and frequent and carefully monitored for discomfort versus persistent pain. If persistent pain is noted, the program must be modified.

Splinting can be just as harmful to the rheumatoid hand patient as it can be helpful if used improperly. The function of the splints must be considered to aid in function, to rest inflamed joints, to stabilize points, or to correct deformities. Patients often need more than one type of splint depending on the stage of the disease, e.g., resting wrist splint, ulnar drift splint. A fundamental principle of splinting the rheumatoid hand is to make the patient as comfortable and pain free as possible while accomplishing the purpose of the splint.

A joint protection program serves to minimize the stresses on a joint to reduce pain, preserve joint structures, and conserve energy. While the first two goals are obvious, the third may require explanation that many arthritis conditions are systemic in nature and that the increased effort to overcome a disability may result in local and overall fatigue.

Pain must be respected as a symptom of dysfunction with efforts directed to minimize *while* preserving joint structure and function. Rest must be balanced by work in ROM exercise to preserve motion and strength. The position of rest is critical as the least painful position may not be the best functional one.

While ADLs may be accomplished in various manners, an arthritic hand should be used with efforts to use the largest joint in its most stable position for the shortest periods of time. For example an object should be grasped with the whole hand with wrist in a neutral position instead of with fingers alone as in drinking from a cup. Those activities that cannot be easily stopped should not be undertaken, e.g., carrying a large water-filled vase from kitchen to living room.

Essential ADL may be preserved with the use of assistive/adaptive equipment such as handles that may be modified to permit use of a greater area of the hand, e.g., faucet, eating utensils, scissors, brushes. Many electrically operated appliances are available, for example, scissors, tooth brushes, can opener, shavers. Keys may be adapted to provide a larger grasping area. Velcro fasters may be substituted for buttons. A mechanical assistive device to open car doors is available. Catalogues for such devices are available from commercial sources as well as the Arthritis Foundation.

Local heat and cold may reduce painful swelling while increasing mobility. Application can take many forms such as the paraffin bath, which provides long lasting, even distribution of warmth to the hands.

Occasionally, medical measures are insufficient to control the pain in RA, particularly if it originates in a joint with secondary degenerative joint disease and surgery may be necessary. Synovectomy may be useful to treat a joint whose activity is more severe than others, perhaps permitting less systemic medications to be used. Persistent (more than six months), unremitting tenosynovitis at the dorsum of the wrist should be operated to prevent tendon rupture. The rupture of tendons must be urgently undertaken to best recover functions. With progressive deformity, timing of the reconstructive surgery is critical as the goal is to improve function. If destruction is too advanced, the surgery may not be feasible; too early, it may not significantly improve function with a prospect of a future surgery with prosthesis failure.

In summary, sample rehabilitation programs are outlined:

Early RA, no deformities
    Education in joint protection and energy conservation
    ROM, muscle strengthening exercise
    Resting splints
Moderate RA, early deformities:
    Do above plus
    Active assisted stretching exercises
    Muscle strengthening with sponges
    Transverse arch preserving exercise, e.g., squeezing a sponge ball
    Functional splints
    Adaptive/assistive equipment
    Dorsal tenosynovectomy
Advanced RA, advanced deformities:
    As above plus
    Passive stretching exercise
    Reconstructive surgery
Carpal Tunnel Syndrome in RA
    Resting splint
    Change of systemic medication if other joints are flaring
    Local steroid injection into the carpal tunnel
    Surgical decompression with failure of above symptoms or with clinical evidence of malar involvement

Chronic Arthritis and Rheumatic Diseases of Childhood

The list of rheumatic diseases affecting children closely approximates that seen in adults, including (juvenile) arthritis, systemic lupus erythematosus, scleroderma, the spondyloarthropathies, and others. There may be, however, varying presentations and manifestations when compared with disease in the adult, as exemplified by juvenile rheumatoid arthritis,[10] and the reader should consult texts of pediatric rheumatology, as this material exeeds the scope of this presentation. A few diseases will be mentioned.

The adult presentation of systemic-onset juvenile rheumatoid arthritis, or Still's disease is becoming a more frequently recognized entity. Still's disease in adults[15] is a

seronegative polyarthritis, associated with typical constitutional and extra-articular manifestations. Median age of presentation is approximately 30 years, but age greater than 50
years is also seen. The synovitis is often mild, but may also lead to progressive chronic
joint disease with erosions and bony ankylosis. The wrist is often most severely involved.

Involvement of the hands and wrists in sickle cell disease is not limited to bone pain
secondary to sickle cell crisis. The hand-foot syndrome is a characteristic finding in
children, and is frequently the presenting complaint. There is diffuse swelling and tenderness of the hands, accompanied by warmth and erythema. The dactylitis is due to periostitis of the metacarpals and proximal phalanges. Effusions of the large joints are seen,
usually of noninflammatory character on synovial fluid analysis. These affect one or two
joints at a time, and occasionally can progress to chronic synovitis with cartilage destruction or erosion.

Hemophilic arthropathy is less frequent in the hands than in the wrists and large
joints. The arthropathy is the result of hemarthroses, which cause a warm, swollen, tender
joint. Repeated episodes lead to hemosiderosis of the synovium, causing synovial proliferation, collagenase production, and degeneration of articular cartilage. Radiographically
there is irregular narrowing or total loss of joint space, and sclerosis of subchondral bone
with areas of cystic lucency.

The child with arthritis may require more intensive rehabilitation than an adult as
they may react to their disease either with overuse of a mildly affected joint or assumption
of a totally antalgic posture in a more severely affected one. The former may require
protective splinting and the latter local heat for pain relief and to increase mobility prior
to ROM exercises. Loss of motion is often a problem after the arthritis has been controlled. While the pattern of joint involvement is similar to RA, children may have a
problem with radial deviation as opposed to ulnar drift.[13]

Systemic Lupus Erythematosus

Articular symptoms are the most common manifestation, and frequently the presenting symptom in systemic lupus erythematosus (SLE),[29] with either arthritis or arthalgia
seen in 95 percent of patients. Arthritis is seen in approximately 75 percent of patients.
Typically, this is symmetric arthritis, most commonly involving the PIPs, MCPs, and the
wrist. Tenosynovitis is seen in approximately 10 percent of patients. Erosion of bone and
cartilage is rare, although joint deformities can be seen. A largely reducible swan neck
deformity of the phalanges occurs, which is caused by capsular laxity and both tendonous
and ligamentous involvement, which leads to partial subluxation. Jaccoud's syndrome,
ulnar deviation of the fingers and subluxation of the MCP joints secondary to repeated
synovitis and similar to that seen in rheumatic fever, is also described.[10]

Mixed Connective Tissue Disease

This disease is characterized by a combination of clinical signs and symptoms seen in
SLE, progressive systemic sclerosis and polymyositis. Findings include Raynaud's phenomenon (85 percent), a sausagelike puffiness to the fingers, erythematous papules over
the knuckles, and periungual telangiectasias. Diffuse sclerodermatous changes and fingertip ulcerations, though, are infrequently seen.

The arthritis of mixed connective tissue disease (MCTD) is a symmetric polyarthritis
that may mimic early RA.[8] There is synovitis and joint effusions, with noninflammatory
synovial fluid on aspiration. The wrists, PIP, and MCP joints are most commonly involved.
Potential joint deformities include: ulnar deviation of the fingers, swan-neck deformity,

and subluxation of the MCP joints. A mutilans-like arthopathy has also been described.[1] Asymmetric bone erosions are most characteristic radiographically. Distal tuft erosion and periarticular calcification is also seen.

The cartilage in patients with SLE and MCTD is less often involved and the potential for rehabilitation perhaps greater, unlike in patients with RA. Range of motion exercises (active, active-assisted, passive) will lessen muscle-tendon-ligament shortening and preserve joint motion and abnormal forces about the joint. Resistive exercises to maintain normal hand arches will likewise keep the muscle forces about the joint as near normal as possible, hopefully to forestall aforementioned deformities from occurring.

When deformities do appear stabilization by splints may be useful. At that point, careful instruction on joint protection (see RA) is important as improper use of the involved joint, digit, hand, may cause progression of the deformity.

Progressive Systemic Sclerosis

Progressive systemic sclerosis (PSS), or scleroderma, is a progressive degenerative disease of the connective tissue. Its characteristic changes in the hand can be seen in both diffuse scleroderma, and in the CREST syndrome (calcinosis cutis, Raynaud's phenomenon, esophageal dysmotility, sclerodactyly, and telangiectasia). The skin disease begins as progressive, diffuse, pitting edema, that is painless and symmetric, giving the fingers a "sausage" appearance. These signs may last from weeks to several months. Following this, the indurative phase occurs, with a thickening and progressive hardening of the skin that clings tightly to the underlying tissues. This phase may last for years; in some patients the skin softens and may revert to normal, but more commonly contraction deformities may occur.

Other skin manifestations include subcutaneous calcifications in the fingers (calcinosis circumscripta) and macular telangiectasias. Raynaud's phenomenon is almost universal, and may precede the development of other manifestations of PSS by many years.[9] Secondary digital ulceration and loss of distal pulp occurs.

Arthralgia and distal polyarthritis occurs, with mild erosive arthritis and effusions occurring in a few patients. Tendon sheath inflammation and deposition of fibrinous material on tendons and joints contribute to decreased range of motion and produce friction rubs, principally over such larger joints as the wrist.

Calcinosis of the soft tissues and soft tissue atrophy is seen radiologically. Tufts of the terminal phalanges can be resorbed, and progress to complete resorption of the terminal and rarely of the middle phalanges. Resorption of bone in the distal portions of the radius and ulnar occurs. Therapy should include intensive education on provocative factors, warming measures, and the local care of ulcerations. The loss of ROM may be treated with passive ROM exercises and dynamic splinting after careful preparation with application of heat and emollients.

Polymyositis and Dermatomyositis

These nonsuppurative inflammatory diseases of the muscle commonly involve the hand. Articular manifestations occur in approximately 35 percent of patients,[41] and the skin changes are characteristic. In the skin, erythematous papules develop over the dorsal aspects of the interphalangeal and MCP joints. Called Gottron's papules, these lesions develop into atrophic plaques with telangiectasias. Telangiectasias commonly occur over the nail folds. Calcification of the soft tissues and muscles is rarely seen in the fingers, unless the disease is associated with progressive systemic sclerosis. Raynaud's phenomenon occurs in 15 to 45 percent of cases.

Arthritis and arthralgia can antedate the development of myositis. The arthritis is usually mildly inflammatory, nonerosive, and transitory, and coincides with the early manifestations of the disease. It usually involves the wrists, PIP, or MCP joints. Mild erosive changes occur uncommonly. In one series,[41] there was a high correlation of arthritis and pulmonary manifestations (fibrosis, or decreased diffusing capacity). Symptoms usually resolve with steroid treatment of the systemic disorder.

The Spondyloarthropathies

This group of diseases includes: ankylosing spondylitis, psoriatic arthritis, Reiter's syndrome and reactive arthritis, and the arthritis associated with chronic inflammatory bowel disease. Their common features[49] are listed in Table 16-7. There are, however, significant differences and unique characteristics in the manner in which they affect the hand.

Ankylosing Spondylitis

Although this disease principally involves the axial skeleton, a peripheral polyarthritis can be seen in up to 55 percent of patients.[18] In the distal upper extremity, the wrist and the MCP joints are most frequently involved, in a pattern resembling that of rheumatoid arthritis. The synovitis resembles that of rheumatoid arthritis, but is less erosive. There is more asymmetry and less periarticular demineralization radiographically than in rheumatoid arthritis and there is a propensity for ankylosis.

Psoriatic Arthritis

Psoriasis not only affects the skin of the hand and produces characteristic changes in the nails, but 7 to 10 percent of patients with psoriasis develop arthritis as well. Psoriasis usually predates the onset of arthritis by 2–11 years, but occasionally the arthritis appears first. The clinical presentations of psoriatic arthritis have been divided into five groups, which are not mutually exclusive.[23,33] The most common is the oligoarticular presentation (70 percent), in which scattered PIP, DIP, and MCP joints are involved. The next most common (15 percent) is a symmetric polyarthritis that may mimic rheumatoid arthritis. The so-called "classic form" (5 percent), is asymmetric and can affect any joint, especially the DIPs. Nail changes are frequent in this type. Psoriatic spondyloarthritis (5 percent) affects the axial skeleton, with 40 percent of patients HLA-B27 positive. Arthritis multilans

Table 16-7
Features Common to the Spondyloarthropathies

Seronegativity
Male predominance
Common genetic predisposition, reflected in the strong HLA-B27 association.
Frequent sacroiliac and lower spinal involvement
Characteristic radiographic features (periostitis, proliferative erosions)
Enthesopathy
Extra-articular manifestations not typical of rheumatoid arthritis (uveitis, psoriasiform skin lesions, mucocutaneous ulceration, aortic insufficiency)
Absence of extra-articular manifestations typical of rheumatoid arthritis (subcutaneous nodules, pleuropericarditis, Sjogren's syndrome, Felty's syndrome, vasculitis)

Reprinted by permission of the Western Journal of Medicine: Wofsy D: Seronegative Spondyloarthritis—Medical Staff Conference, UCSF. West J Med 134:134–140, 1981.

(5 percent) is a particularly disruptive and disabling form, causing osteolysis of joints. In general, the arthritis is of insidious onset, with painful synovitis as well as tenosynovitis and periostitis, which lead to sausage-shaped fingers. Severity tends to parallel the skin disease. Pitting of the nails is common, and while onycholysis is seen in only 20 to 30 percent of patients with psoriasis alone, it is found in 80 percent of patients with psoriatic arthritis. Typical psoriatic skin changes can be seen, including pustular psoriasis.

Radiographs of the hand show an erosive arthritis, with predilection for the DIP joints. There may be predominant involvement of the joints in a single ray, often only affecting one hand. Progressive erosion causes resorption of the terminal tufts, pencil-in-cup deformity (usually of the DIPs), and potentially bony ankylosis. Unlike rheumatoid arthritis, there is no periarticular osteoporosis.

Arthritis Associated with Chronic Inflammatory Bowel Disease

Peripheral arthritis can be a feature of both ulcerative colitis (UC), and Crohn's disease.[34] The peripheral arthritis tends to occur during active phases of bowel disease. It is usually acute and oligoarticular, but can be polyarticular. Peripheral joint disease occurs in 11 percent of patients with ulcerative colitis, but infrequently in the hand. Arthritis tends not to recur after colectomy. In Crohn's disease a peripheral arthritis affects up to 20 percent of patients, with the wrist and MCPs involved. As this disease may involve the entire gastrointestinal tract, patients may have recurrence after gastrointestinal surgery, as resection is usually limited. Remaining intestine can thus become inflamed, and lead to recurrent arthritis. Radiographically, both UC and Crohn's disease rarely produce bony changes peripherally.

Reiter's Syndrome and Reactive Arthritis

The triad of arthritis, conjunctivitis, and either urethritis or enteric infection constitutes Reiter's syndrome. The etiology is unknown, but the occurrence of arthritis after genitourinary or enteric infection, without the presence of the organism in the joint, suggests an inflammatory (perhaps immune-mediated) mechanism in a susceptible host. There are patients, though, with similar symptoms, (oligoarthritis, enthesopathy, sacroilitis), in which no evidence of overt infection can be found.[24]

As mentioned, the arthritis of Reiter's syndrome is oligoarticular, often with abrupt onset, usually within 30 days of infection. Large joints, e.g., the wrist, tend to be affected, but even the small joints of the hand can be involved, generally asymmetrically. Bouts of arthritis may last from weeks to years, usually with good recovery. Unlike psoriatic arthritis, there is no predilection for the DIP joints, or joints of a single ray. Characteristically, though, there is marked enthesopathy: inflammation at the sites of tendon attachment to bone.

Acute rheumatic fever, caused by a beta-hemolytic streptococci, has as its most frequent manifestation polyarthritis (75 percent of patients). The arthritis is transient, migratory, and can be abrupt. It is usually within five weeks of the initial infection and coincident with the rise of Antistreptolysin-O titers. In the hand the MCP joints are most commonly involved. Bursitis and tendonitis can also occur. Repeat attacks of synovitis can lead to Jaccoud's syndrome (chronic postrheumatic fever arthropathy: painless ulnar deviation and subluxation of the MCP joints without swelling) as in SLE.

Finally, arthritis is reported in up to 40 percent of patients undergoing intestinal bypass surgery (jejunocolostomy, or jejunoileostomy). An erosive, symmetric arthritis that can mimic rheumatoid arthritis[12] can be seen, but more commonly the distribution is similar to that found in colitic arthritis: oligoarticular, affecting the larger joints of the body including the wrist. Inflammation of tendons also occurs. Symptoms can remit spontaneously but relapse is common.

Management, in general, involves joint protection and preservation of ROM, eg, cock-up wrist splint and ROM exercises of the wrist until spontaneous or therapy-induced remission for post-bypass wrist arthritis. In those cases resembling RA, all rehabilitation measures applicable to RA may be necessary.

Osteoarthritis

Osteoarthritis (OA), or degenerative joint disease, is the most prevalent arthopathy. The disease is characterized by destruction of cartilage and reactive new bone formation. Osteoarthritis is classified into primary, or secondary types, the latter if an etiology is found. The list of secondary causes is lengthy[2] (Table 16-8), hence this discussion will concentrate on primary OA.

The most common form of OA is Heberden's nodes, and is due to osteophyte formation, and cartilagenous, synovial, and capsular enlargement of the DIP joints. These nodes develop gradually over months to years. Progressive cartilage destruction leads to flexion, lateral deviations, and subluxations of the joints. Similar changes occurring at the PIP joints are called Bouchard's nodes. These changes occur more commonly in women. Disability results from restricted motion, and the pain from the loss of articular cartilage and joint space.

Primary generalized OA in the hand involves the PIP and DIP joints, and the first carpometacarpal (CMC) joint of the wrist. First, CMC joint disease gives the hand a "squared-off" appearance. Trapezioscaphoid involvement is also seen. The disease is seen mainly in middle-aged females, and is inherited: dominant in women, recessive in men.

Table 16-8
Causes of Secondary Osteoarthritis

Posttraumatic
Congenital or developmental diseases
Hip diseases, e.g., leg-calfe-Perthes, congenital hip dislocation, slipped capital femoral epiphysis, shallow acetabulum
Bone dysplasias, e.g., epiphyseal dysplasia, spondyloepiphyseal dysplasia, osteonychrondystophy
Other bone and joint disorders, e.g., avascular necrosis, rheumatoid arthritis, gouty arthritis, septic arthritis, Paget's disease, osteoporosis, osteochondritis
Other diseases
Metabolic diseases, e.g., hemachromatosis, ochronosis, Gaucher's disease, hemaglobinopathy, Ehler's Danlos
Endocrine diseases, e.g., diabetes mellitus, acromegaly, hypothyroidism, hyperparathyroidism
Neuropathic arthropathy
Mechanical and local factors, e.g., obesity (?), unequal lower extremity length, extreme valgus varus deformity
Miscellaneous, e.g., frostbite, Kashin-Beck disease, Caisson's disease

Adapted from Altman RD, Hochberg MC: Degenerative joint disease. Clin Rheum Dis 9:681–693, 1983.

Symptoms of an acute inflammatory arthritis occur, but are episodic. Roentgenographic findings often exceed clinical signs.

Erosive OA is the term applied to the severe, painful inflammatory disease of the interphalangeal joints of the hand. Repeated episodes of acute inflammation lead to erosion, severe bony proliferation, cartilage destruction with synovitis, and eventually joint deformity and ankylosis.[44] Synovial fluid analysis is noninflammatory or mildly inflammatory.

Radiographic criteria for diagnosis of OA are well defined, and include: (a) osteophyte formation of joint margins or ligamentous attachments, (b) cystic areas within subchondral bone, (c) joint space narrowing, typically segmental with sclerosis of subchondral bone, (d) altered shapes of bone ends, (e) periarticular ossicles, mainly in DIP and PIP joints. In erosive OA, articular soft tissue swelling and subchondral bone destruction are prominent, especially in DIP joints. In contrast to rheumatoid arthritis, periarticular demineralization is not present.

Significant pain relief can be obtained with appropriate application of heat and cold, with improvement of stiffness an additional benefit of heat. Splints will prevent motion, which aggravates pain, e.g., resting hand splint for DIPs, PIPs, thumb spica for the first CMC joint. Education is most important in this usually slowly progressive disease, particularly adaptive use of the hands in the activities of daily living (ADL), e.g., hand grasp versus pinch grasp, and the use of assistive devices, e.g., beverage tool for "pop top" beverage cans. In the former, a large grasping unit (hand versus two fingers) is used and in the latter, a tool providing mechanical advantage is used to decrease the force on the joints.

Tenosynovitis of the flexor tendons with nodule formation may result in a trigger finger, and of the abductor/extensor pollicus tendon, a De Quervain's tenosynovitis. Definitive therapy may require surgery though the process may respond to local steroid injections with active or active-assisted range of motion exercises with the use of extension or thumb spica splints especially at night.

Arthritis Associated with Infectious Agents

The majority of hand infections occurs secondary to local trauma or puncture. Hematologic spread is uncommon.[26] In blood-borne infection, joints affected by pre-existing arthritis, and large joints such as the wrist and knee are more likely to be involved. Virtually any organism is a potential causative agent, including: bacterial, spirochetal, mycobacterial, fungal, and viral; examples to follow.

Hematogenous spread of *Neisseria gonorrhoeae* can cause septic arthritis of multiple joints, tendonitis, and give rise to pustules on the skin. The small joints of the fingers, wrists, and knees are often affected.

The hand and wrist are involved in less than 10 percent of cases of adult skeletal tuberculosis. Tendonitis, synovitis, and bony involvement can occur, and certain radiographic criteria have been defined.[7]

Joint protection by splinting and ROM exercises early will prevent the sequela of loss of joint range of motion that occurs as the joint is held in an antalgic posture. The ROM exercise should begin with passive ROM progressing to active assisted ROM and to active ROM exercise according to the clinical improvement of the patient.

Crystal-Induced Rheumatic Diseases

Gout. Gout is characterized by the release of monosodium urate crystals into the joint cavity, causing acute inflammation. Along with recurrent attacks of arthritis, deposits of monosodium urate monohydrate (tophi) occur in tissues, chiefly around joints and in the kidneys.

The hands and the wrist are usually not the initial sites of involvement of acute gouty arthritis, but in time they can be affected. Chronic tophaceous gout in the hand and wrist is manifested by the presence of tophi over the joints, which lead to severe crippling and deformity from tendon and secondary bony erosion. The average time for the appearance of tophi is 10 years after the onset of disease.

The radiographic appearance of a joint affected by early gouty arthritis may be normal. With time, and progressive damage of cartilage and subchondral bone, marginal erosions may occur. Erosions are usually near tophi, and may be periarticular or intra-articular. They have a thin "overhanging margin," which is a segment of eroded cortex extending over the tophus. Occasionally, there is a subperiosteal bone apposition in the metacarpals.

Tophi may require special consideration but usual (as in RA) rehabilitation measures apply.

Calcium pyrophosphate deposition disease.   The deposition of calcium pyrophosphate dihydrate (CPPD) crystals can occur in cartilage, synovial tissue, tendons, bursae, joint capsules, and soft tissues. The acute inflammatory arthritis caused by CPPD crystal deposition in joints is called pseudogout, while the radiologic appearance of calcified cartilage is termed chondrocalcinosis. CPPD may be hereditary, sporadic (idiopathic), or associated with other metabolic conditions (hyperparathyroidism, hemochromatosis, hypothryroidism, gout, hypomagnesemia, hypophosphatasia, aging).

Pseudogout can potentially involve all synovial joints. There are a number of common presentations in the hand and wrist. Isolated pseudogout is an oligoarticular arthritis seen in 25 percent of cases. It is acute or subacute, often as severe as gout, with seemingly contiguous spread from a large joint (eg, the wrist), to smaller daughter joints. Acute attacks are often provoked by surgery or medical illness. A pseudorheumatoid arthritis pattern occurs, with morning stiffness, fatigue, and proliferative synovitis that affects approximately 5 percent of patients. Multiple, symmetric joint involvement is seen, with low grade inflammation that may last weeks to months. Pseudo-osteoarthritis may occur both with and without superimposed acute attacks. Disease is chronic over months to years, affecting the wrists and the MCP joints in a bilaterally symmetric pattern. Flexion contractures and osteophyte formation are common. Overall, approximately 50 percent of patients afflicted experience progressive degeneration of multiple joints, with the wrists and the MCP joints commonly involved.

On plain radiographs, the linear or punctate deposition of CPPD crystals is unique, and in the upper extremity occurs most commonly in the triangular cartilage of the wrist. Crystal deposition and arthopathy, though, need not coexist.[39] Other radiographic changes include: joint space narrowing, subchondral sclerosis, osteophyte formation, and widespread discrete rarefactions in subchondral regions, all of which resemble osteoarthritis.

Apatite crystal deposition disease.   Apatite is the normal storage form of calcium in bone. It is becoming recognized as a cause of crystal deposition disease. Syndromes described include an acute, recurrent or chronic periarthritis, and acute or erosive arthritis. The periarthritis commonly affects the fingers and wrists, with severe pain, swelling and erythema over the superficial deposits. The arthritis is mono- or oligo-articular, (although polyarthritis is possible), and is also common in the fingers and wrists. Radiographs may show calcification (different from the linear deposition in CPPD disease) in soft tissue in or around joints, and erosions.

Hemochromatosis. A characteristic distal arthropathy occurs in 40–50 percent of patients with this disease,[4] and may be the presenting symptom. Iron deposits in the synovial lining cells causes synovial inflammation and proliferation. Typically the PIP and the MCP joints are involved, with the second and third MCP joints classically affected. Joints are enlarged, mildly tender, and stiff, but without morning stiffness. Attacks may also be due to pseudogout. On radiographs there is joint space narrowing and irregularity, mild subluxation, cystic subchondral lesions and bony sclerosis.

Neuropathic Disorders

Reflex symmetric dystrophy (RSD), once known as shoulder-hand syndrome, is a disease of excessive or abnormal response of the sympathetic nervous system in a limb to a traumatic injury or medical condition. The most common cause is trauma, but other conditions affecting the limbs (eg, left arm pain from myocardial infarction, hemiplegia) may be the cause. A precipitating agent, though, can only be remembered by the patient in two-thirds of cases. Most commonly there is a painful disability of the shoulder, which may preceed, accompany, or follow a painful condition with vasomotor and dystrophic changes in the hand. The initial presentation in the hand is edema and pain, followed by hair loss, decreased range of motion and bone rarefaction. With resolution of the vasomotor changes there is atrophy and contracture deformities. Radiographic features include patchy osteoporosis, and erosions of the MCP, DIP, and PIP joints. Osteoporosis and increased uptake on bone scan can be seen bilaterally, supporting the hypothesis that changes are mediated by a sympathetic reflex arc.

The main principle of therapy is to avoid aggravation of the pain, which would stimulate the sympathetic reflex arc. Splinting of the joint serves to protect, reduce pain, and prevent contractures. Heat will provide comfort, reduce swelling, and relieve muscle spasm. Exercises, both range of motion and resistive should be of short duration frequently, again avoiding pain. The exercise should be progressive corresponding to the decreasing level of pain. Later in the course of disease, the exercise program is important in the remineralization of osteopenic bone.

Nerve entrapment occurs not infrequently at the wrist as previously discussed with carpal tunnel syndrome, the most common clinical entity. Conservative treatment involves a neutral wrist splint with treatment of the underlying systemic process.

Bone and Connective Tissue Disorders

Hypertrophic osteoarthropathy. This syndrome is defined as (1) chronic proliferative periostitis of long bones, (2) clubbing of the fingers and/or toes, and (3) oligo or polysynovitis. Clubbing is defined as softening of the nail bed, loss of the normal angle between the nail and the cuticle, convexity of the nail, and clubbed appearance of the fingertips. This disease may be primary (often hereditary), or secondary to other conditions, most commonly associated with malignant, infectious, or cardiopulmonary disease.[25]

Clubbing may occur as an isolated condition, and is usually asymptomatic. However, dyesthesias of the fingers and stiffness of the hand may be associated. Articular complaints vary from mild arthralgia, to severe articular pain that is symmetrical and involves the wrist and MCP joints.

Dupuytren's contracture.   Dupuytren's contracture is a condition of unknown etiology characterized by hyperplasia and hypertrophy of the palmar fascia, and related structures, with nodule formation and contraction of the palmar fascia.[36] Nodules lie superficial to the palmar fascia, usually near the distal palmar flexion crease, and superficial to the affected digits. Most commonly the fourth and fifth fingers are involved. Secondary features include knuckle pads, and contracture of the longitudinal fibers in the fascia leading to flexion of the MCP, PIP, and less often, the DIP joints. Symptoms are usually mild and bilateral, and can include tenderness of the palmar nodules, and hypoesthesia and paresthesias of the involved digits.

Surgery may be necessary to definitively treat a Dupuytren's contracture followed by extension splinting, ROM exercises, and friction message of the scar. Primary conservative measures include local steroid injections with active or active-assisted range of motion exercises and the use of extension or thumb spica splints (Fig. 16-19) especially at night.

Systemic vasculitis.   In the hand the systemic vasculitides principally involve the small digital arteries. The necrotizing process leads to discrete infarcts, and progressive loss of soft tissue. Osteolysis of the distal phalanges occurs with severe disease. Arthralgia is more common than arthritis.

The involvement of the vaso nervorium presents most commonly as a mononeuritis multiplex. This significant problem is complex and therapy is directed along several lines (1) splinting for joint protection and prevention of deformities secondary to imbalance of muscle forces, (2) sensory retraining, (3) muscle conditioning during the recovery phase.

Tendon injuries.   Treatment and rehabilitation following tendon injury to the hand and wrist are subjects of much research and discussion. In March 1984, hand surgeons and hand therapists from around the world met in Philadelphia, Pennsylvania, for a symposium entitled "The Hand: Another Decade of Tendon Surgery." The most current surgical and rehabilitative approaches to hand tendon damage were presented. Nevertheless, as Dr. James Strickland, one of the featured speakers wrote in reference to flexor tendons, ". . . the return of satisfactory digital performance following tendon interruption remains as one of the most difficult and challenging problems for the hand surgeon . . . the problem is not so much how to achieve tendon repair and healing as how to decrease or eliminate the propensity for peritendinous scarring with the inevitable limitation of tendon gliding."[43]

This is the dilemma facing the hand therapist especially in relation to flexor tendon injuries. Flexor tendon injuries are considered according to the extent of the laceration and the level of injury. A modification of Verdan's zone system is commonly utilized to specify level of injury[46] (Fig. 16-20). Because of the frequency of injury and the anatomic configuration of the tendons, pulleys, and sheath in zone II known as "no man's land,"[45] this area presents the greatest challenge to hand therapists and will now be discussed.

Early motion is the key to success following most flexor tendon repairs to avoid adhesion formation and maintain a smoothly gliding mechanism.[21] Many techniques have been devised to allow early motion, prevent adhesion formation, and achieve a fine balance between motion and rupture of the repaired tendon. Duran and Houser used a method of controlled passive motion following repair of both tendons in zone II following injury and found that 3–5 mm of extension at the anastomosis in a passive exercise program is sufficient to prevent adhesions.[16] To allow early controlled motion, Kleinert and associates designed a dynamic splint consisting of a dorsal plaster "cobra" splint applied with wrist in flexion and the digit at zero degrees and a dynamic rubberband traction applied to the fingernail holding it in flexion but permitting active extension within the confines of the splint.[27]

A modification of the Kleinert orthosis adds a palmar pulley "to maximize flexor tendon excusions through full finger flexion, improve digital function with increased digit mobility, and demonstrate that advancement of the pulley in the palm of the hand does not over-stress the repair" (Fig. 16-21).[28] The hand is maintained in this splint 3–4.5 weeks. From day 1, the patients are instructed to actively extend the finger to the full limit of the splint and allow the rubberband to passively flex the finger 10 times an hour. Care is taken to watch for developing flexion contractures and take appropriate action in the form of additional exercises if this problem begins to occur.

At approximately 3–4.5 weeks the dorsal splint is usually removed and a wristlet with elastic band traction added. This allows active extension of interphalangeal (IP) and metacarpophalangeal (MP) joints with wrist in neutral position.

The wristlet is removed at 5–6 weeks and active flexion begins with isolated tendon gliding. Light ADL are also commenced. Vibration may also be utilized to decrease scar adhesions.

Mild resisted exercise begins at 8–10 weeks. This may involve putty exercises, crumbling newspaper or other light grasp activities. At 3 months, most heavy resisted activities are permitted.[20]

Injuries and tenosynovitis of the extensor tendons of the hand can also be devastating

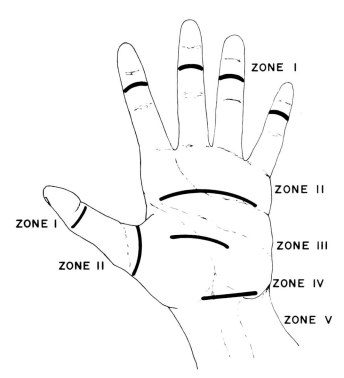

Fig. 16-20.   Zone classification of flexor tendon injuries.

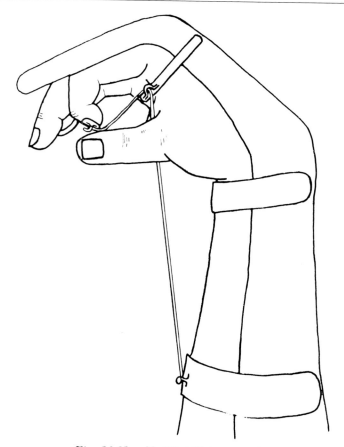

Fig. 16-21. Modified Kleinert traction.

and require the same degree of careful management and rehabilitation as the flexor tendon injuries.

Injuries to the dorsum of the wrist often involve the wrist extensor tendons. Generally, if the wrist extensors are the only tendons involved, after primary repair the hand is splinted in approximately 40° extension for 4 or more weeks while full finger motion is preserved. If adhesions are later noted, friction massage is utilized.

Extensor injuries to the fingers may result in a variety of common deformities including the mallet deformity and boutonniere deformity. The mallet finger results from injuries to the extensor tendon over the DIP joint and distal portion of the middle phalanx.

Successful treatment of a mallet finger involves splinting the joint either dorsally or volarly in slight hyperextension for 6 weeks, followed by night splinting for 4 more weeks. Flexion of the PIP joint is preserved throughout and DIP motion begins after 6 weeks.

The boutonniere deformity develops as lateral extension bands slide volarly and beneath the PIP joint. Closed injuries may be treated with splinting the PIP joint in extension for 1–6 weeks depending on the degree of injury and leaving the distal joint free for flexion. Open injuries require surgical repair, immobilization for 4–8 weeks and follow-up and therapy.

Injury to the common extensor tendon or extensor hood may be open or closed. If surgery is required, splinting the hand with slight (20–30°) wrist extension, MP extension, and slight finger flexion is required for 4 weeks. Gentle active flexion/extension exercises commence at 4 weeks and gradually the splint is removed more often allowing light functional activities.[30]

The key to rehabilitation following most extensor tendon injuries is carefully monitored splinting along with closely monitored motion. Each patient must be treated individually with the goal of increasing motion while preventing extensor lag.

Bone and joint injury. In light of the number of bones and joints in the hand combined with the high exposure to injury, fractures of the hand and wrist are more complicated than they superficially appear to be. Discussion of each type of hand fracture in terms of rehabilitation is beyond the scope of this chapter, thus, general rehabilitative principles will be discussed.

Edema is commonly the first problem encountered when dealing with fractures of the hand. Elevation, with the hand in a position so that each joint in a distal to proximal direction is higher than the next and each is elevated above the heart is useful.[19] Edema may be assessed using hand volumeter (Fig. 16-22).

To reduce edema, one or more techniques can be utilized. Active motion can assist the return of the fluid to the heart by the action of the muscle pump. External compression can be accomplished in many ways. String wrapping using heavy yarn or soft cord wrapped around each finger snugly, distally to proximally, until the entire hand is wrapped and is followed by elevation for 5 minutes is effective (Fig. 16-23). The patient then fists the hand 10 times after the string is removed.[19] External compression through use of surgical gloves, isotoner glovers, or coben finger wraps (Fig. 16-24) can also be utilized. These devices allow exercises while they are in place.

An intermittent compression pump may also be used for severe hand edema. A pneumatic sleeve is inflated under pressure and then deflated. Specific pressure and time of compression is adjusted according to each patient's diagnosis.

Retrograde massage, assists the return flow circulation of blood by milking the fluid from a distal to proximal direction.

Remobilization assists in the mobilization of edema fluid. Frequently neighboring joints also become stiff due to immobilization and it is important to immobilize hand fractures for the minimum period of time necessary and not to immobilize more fingers than is necessary. In the case of a wrist fracture, active motion of the uninjured joints must be begun immediately and done regularly and frequently.

Active motion is initiated with minimal force. Each joint is exercised independently and with proximal support. Pressure motion is utilized to maintain joint mobility and should not increase edema or cause undue pain.

Splinting or serial casting may be utilized to stretch and remodel joint tissue once the fracture is considered solid. Several types of dynamic splint can be utilized, such as the safety pin splint (Fig. 16-25) or the custom made Capener splint (Fig. 16-26) to gain either flexion or extension.

In addition, friction massage may be utilized to prevent or reduce adhesions while reducing swelling. Light activities are also extremely useful in regaining motion and returning patients to their preinjury occupational status (Fig. 16-27).

Nerve injury. The hand is supplied by three major nerves; the median, ulnar, and

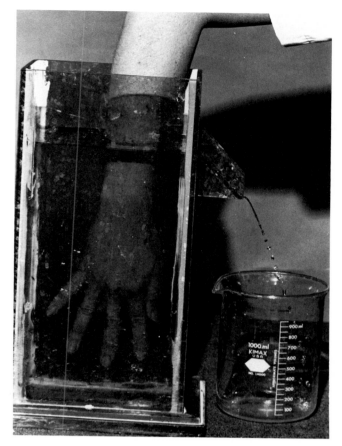

Fig. 16-22. Hand volumeter.

radial (Fig. 16-6, Table 16-3), each having motor and sensory function. Injury to any or all of these nerves constitutes major disability by "blinding" part or all of the hand.

Severance of a nerve (or nerves) in the hand requires prompt surgical intervention either by primary, delayed, or secondary repair. Rehabilitative concerns encountered postoperatively include edema control, minimizing scar adhesions, desensitization, sensory re-education, functional splinting, and protective sensory education. Desensitization can be accomplished using various textures and a program of vibration to raise the threshold for sensory input. At the Hand Rehabilitation Center in Philadelphia, Callahan differentiates patients who are candidates for protective sensory re-education from those who are candidates for discriminative sensory re-education.[12] Patients whose protective sensation is either lacking or severely decreased as evidenced by their inability to perceive such stimuli as pinprick, hot, cold, and deep pressure are candidates for protective sensory re-education. These patients are taught to compensate for the lack of protective sensory input. The pain or discomfort that would be perceived by a normally sensing hand does not occur and the patient is taught to avoid exposure to various elements, observe carefully for signs of stress, and care for skin daily to preserve moisture.

Patients who are able to perceive the previously noted stimuli but cannot perceive

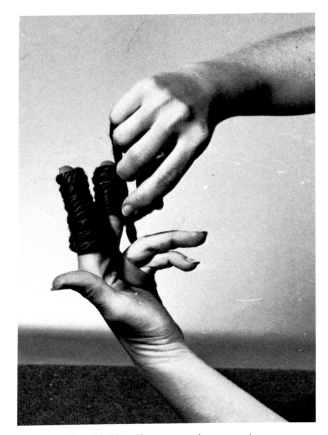

Fig. 16-23. Yarn external compression.

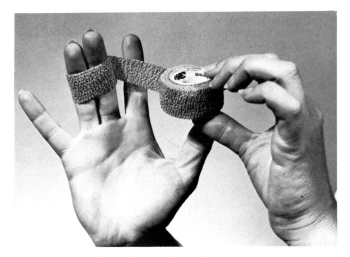

Fig. 16-24. Coben finger wrap.

428

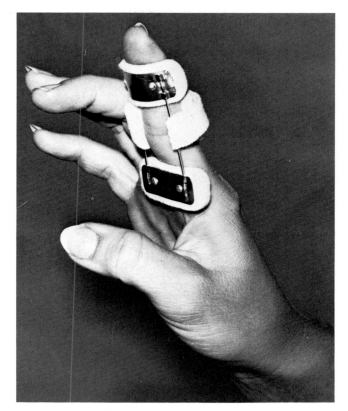

Fig. 16-25. Safety pin splint.

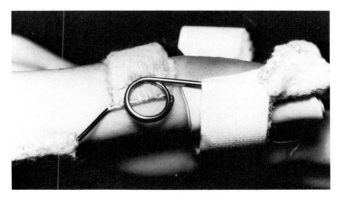

Fig. 16-26. Capener splint.

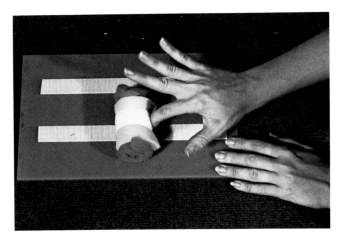

Fig. 16-27.   Light exercise.

discriminative sensation (2PD, stereognosis, localization) receive discriminative sensation. A pencil eraser can be used for constant and moving touch. Differing everyday objects with various textures, materials and shapes can all be utilized for varying degrees of discrimination. The selection of the exact activities must be based on baseline evaluations.

Splinting the nerve injured hand can be done for three purposes (1) to restore suppleness with full passive motion and assist in restoring active motion and strength in muscles not affected by nerve injury, (2) to prevent deformities caused by muscle imbalance, and (3) to provide function position for the hand.[38] Following initial treatment, which frequently involves casting for 3–4 weeks, static splints may be used to hold the wrist in more functional positions.

When a muscle loses its nerve supply, its antagonist unopposedly pulls the joint into its most shortened position. Splinting is necessary to maintain the balance between the two muscles.

There is a variety of functional splints that can be fabricated according to the nerve or nerves injured. In ulnar nerve palsy, the splint must prevent hyperextension of the MP joints while allowing functional hand use. A radial nerve palsy results in wrist drop but this may not necessitate splinting. If the wrist drop is problematic and painful to the patient, a wrist mobilization splint may be fabricated with dynamic extension assist. In the case of a median nerve injury, the thumb is unable to oppose. Splinting with a C-Bar, or thumb-post splint may provide the stability needed to increase function. In the case of multiple nerve damage, a combination of principles in splinting can be utilized to increase function.

Compression of the nerves of the hand are common and result in specific symptoms and disability. Compression of the median nerve at the transverse carpal ligament or carpal tunnel syndrome is often treated conservatively by splinting the wrist in a neutral to slightly dorsiflexed position day and night.

The median nerve can also be compressed at the elbow as it passes through the two heads of the pronator terses muscle. Splinting to prevent pronation is the conservative treatment often used in conjunction with steroids and procaine.[37]

This is by no means a complete review of all hand pathology and rehabilitation. Congenital deformities, burns, amputations, hemiplegia, and replantations all catastrophically affect hand function, and thereby become rehabilitative concerns.

Whatever the disability, rehabilitation must be highly individualized and closely monitored. The patient must understand that the problem with his or her hand is primarily his or hers, not the physician's nor the therapist's, and the patient is largely responsible for the result. The patient must be taught about his or her hand and its treatment from the initial visit and throughout the course of treatment.

Based on these principles, the patient becomes the "self-therapist" and the hand therapist assumes the role of the educator, evaluator, coach, cheerleader, and coordinator of the treatment program.

REFERENCES

1. Alarcon-Segovia D, Uribe-Uribe O: Mutilans-like arthropathy in mixed connective tissue disease. Arth Rheum 22:1013–1018, 1979
2. Altman RD, Hochberg MC: Degenerative joint disease. Clin Rheum Dis 9:681–693, 1983
3. American Academy of Orthopaedic Surgery: Musculoskeletal Research. A.A.O.S. Publication TFR-81
4. Askari AD, Muir WA, Rosner IA, et al: Arthritis of hemochromatosis. Am J Med 75:957–965, 1983
5. Avlicino P, DuPuy TE: Clinical examination of the hand. In: Hunter J (ed): Rehabilitation of the Hand. St. Louis, The C.V. Mosby Co., 1984, p. 45
6. Bechol C: Griptest: The use of the dynamometer with adjustable hand spacings. J Bone Joint Surg 36A:800–824 and 832, 1954
7. Benkeddache Y, Gottesman H: Skeletal tuberculosis of the wrist and hand: A study of 27 cases. J Hand Surg 7:593:600, 1982
8. Bennett RM, O'Connell DJ: The arthritis of mixed connective tissue disease. Ann Rheum Dis 37:397–403, 1978
9. Blunt RJ, Porter JM: Raynaud Syndrome. Semin Arth Rheum 10:282–308, 1981
10. Bywaters EGL: Jaccoud's syndrome, a sequel to the joint involvement in systemic lupus erythematosus. Clin Rheum Dis 1:125–148, 1975
11. Cailliet R: Hand Pain and Impairment, Philadelphia, F.A. Davis Co., pp. 68–83, 1974
12. Callahan AD: Methods of compensation and re-education for sensory dysfunction, in Hunter J, Schneider LH, Macklin EJ, et al (eds): Rehabilitation of the Hand, St. Louis, C.V. Mosby Co., 1984, pp. 432–442
13. Cassidy JT: Juvenile rheumatoid arthritis, in Kelly WN, Harris ED, Ruddy S, Sledge CB (eds): Textbook of Rheumatology (2nd Ed), Philadelphia, Saunders, p. 1247–1277, 1985
14. Dellon A, Curtis RM, Edgerton M: Reeducation of sensation in the hand after nerve injury and repair. Plastic Reconstruc Surg 53:297–305, 1974
15. Del Paine DW, Leek JC: Still's arthritis in adults: disease or syndrome? J Rheumatol 10:758–762, 1983
16. Duran RJ, Houser RG: Controlled pressure motion following flexor tendon repair in zones two and three. A.A.O.S. Symposium on Tendon Surgery of the Hand. St. Louis, C.V. Mosby Co., 1975, pp. 105–114
17. Fess EE: Principles and methods of splinting for mobilization of joints, in Hunter J, Schneider LH, Macklin EJ, et al (eds): Rehabilitation of the Hand, St. Louis, C.V. Mosby Co., pp. 853–861, 1984
18. Ginsburg WW, Cohen MD: Peripheral arthritis in ankylosing spondylitis. Mayo Clin Proc 58:593–596, 1983
19. Hunter JM, Macklin EJ: Edema and bandaging, in Hunter JM, Schneider LH, Macklin EJ, et al (eds): Rehabilitation of the Hand, St. Louis, C.V. Mosby Co., 1984, pp. 146–154
20. Jaeger SH, Macklin EJ: Primary care of flexor tendon injuries, in Hunter JM, Schneider LH, Macklin EJ, et al (eds): Rehabilitation of the Hand, St. Louis, C.V. Mosby Co., 1974, pp. 268–269
21. Jaeger SH, Macklin EJ: Primary care of flexor tendon injuries, in Hunter J, Schneider LH, Macklin EJ, et al (eds): Rehabilitation of the Hand. St. Louis, C.V. Mosby Co., 1984, p. 261
22. Jebson, RH, Taylor N, Trieschmann RB, Trotter MJ, Howard LA: An objective and standardized test of hand function. Arch Phys Med 50:311–19, 1969
23. Kammer GM, Soter NA, Gibson DJ, et al: Psoriatic arthritis: A clinical, immunologic and HLA study of 100 patients. Semin Arth Rheum 9:75–97, 1979
24. Keat A: Reiter's syndrome and reactive arthritis in perspective. N Engl J Med 309:1606–1615, 1983
25. Kelley WN, Harris ED, Jr, Ruddy S, et al (eds): Textbook of Rheumatology, Philadelphia, Saunders, 1981, p. 1648
26. Kilgore ES: Hand infections. J Hand Surg 8:2:723–726, 1983
27. Kleinert HE, Kutz JE, Atasoy E, et al: Primary repair of flexor tendons. Orthop Clin North Am 4:865–876, 1973

28. Kouba SH, Milnor WH, Thomas LJ: A modified flexor tendon dynamic postoperative rehabilitative orthosis. Report presented to the Society of Military Surgeons, Nov. 1982, El Paso, TX, as cited by Lopez MS, Hanley, KF: Splint Modifications for Flexor Tendon Repairs. Am J Occ Ther 6:398–403, 1984

29. Labowitz R, Schumacher R: Articular manifestations of systemic lupus erythematosus. Ann Intern Med 74:911–921, 1971

30. Lovett WL, McCalla MA: Management and Rehabilitation of Extensor Tendon Injuries. Orthop Clin North Am 14:811–826, 1983

31. Malick MH, Manual on Static Hand Splinting. Harmonville, PA: Harmonville Rehabilitation Center, 1972

32. Masur-Grieve M: Methods of assessment and management of the rheumatoid hand at the Institute of Rheumatology, Warsaw, Poland, in Hunter J, Schneider LH, Macklin EJ, et al (eds): Rehabilitation of the Hand, St. Louis, C.V. Mosby Co., 1984, pp. 651–662

33. Moll JMH, Wright V: Psoriatic arthritis. Arth Rheum 3:55–78, 1978

34. Neumann V, Wright V: Arthritis associated with bowel disease. Clin Gastroenterol 12:767–795, 1983

35. Onne L: Sensibility of the hand. Orthopedic Surgery: Recovery of sensibility and pseudomotor activity of the hand after nerve suture. Acta Chir Scand (Suppl) 300, pp. 5–69, 1962

36. Paletta FX: Dupuytren's contracture. Am Fam Phys May 1981, p. 85

37. Parry CBW: Rehabilitation of the Hand, London, Butterworths, 1981, pp. 355–373

38. Pearson SO. Splinting the nerve-injured hand, in Hunter J, Schneider LH, Macklin EJ, et al (eds): Rehabilitation of the Hand, St. Louis, C.V. Mosby Co., 1984, pp. 452–456

39. Resnik CS: Hand and wrist involvement in calcium pyrophosphate dihydrate crystal deposition disease. J Hand Surg 8:856–863, 1983

40. Schaller JG: Chronic arthritis in children. Clin Orth Rel Res 182:79–89, 1984

41. Schumacher RH, Schimmer B, Gordon GV, et al: Articular manifestations of polymyositis and dermatomyositis. Am J Med 67:287–292, 1979

42. Stein HB: The intestinal bypass arthritis-dermatitis syndrome. Arth Rheum 24:684–690, 1981

43. Strickland W: Management of Acute Flexor Tendon Injuries. The Orthopedic Clinic of North America, Rehabilitation After Reconstructive Hand Surgery, October 1983, 827

44. Utsinger PD, Resnick D, Shapiro RF, et al: Roentgenologic, immunologic, and therapeutic study of erosive (inflammatory) osteoarthritis. Arch Intern Med 138:693–697, 1978

45. Verdan C, Michon J: Latraitment desplaies des tendons fleschisseurs des doights. Rev Chir Orthop 47:285, 1961

46. Verdan C: Reparative surgery of flexor tendons in the digits, in Verdon C (ed): Tendon Surgery of the Hand. London, Churchill Livingstone, 1979, pp. 57–66

47. Wayle H, Janet G (eds): Hand Rehabilitation Center Procedure Manual and Teaching Syllabus. Loma Linda University, 1980, pp. 148–160

48. Weeks P, Wray RC: Management of Acute Hand Injuries. St. Louis, C.V. Mosby Co., 1973

49. Wofsy D: Seronegative Spondyloarthritis-Medical Staff Conference, UCSF. West J Med 134:134–140, 1981

Richard F. Santore
Vernon C. Nickel
Richard D. Coutts

17

Reconstructive Surgery and Rehabilitation of the Arthritic Hip

Reconstructive surgery of the hip encompasses a spectrum of technically demanding procedures, the most celebrated of these being total joint arthroplasty. Since its introduction into this country in 1969, the reliability and efficacy of the surgical management of advanced hip disease has dramatically improved. Approximately 100,000 total hip replacements are now performed annually in the United States.[1]

Increasingly, the longevity of the result is looming as the most important variable.[2] Not only is the average lifespan of the population increasing but also the physical activities of the elderly are as apt to include tennis, golf, or skiing as they are to include more sedentary interests. Additionally, in the rheumatoid population, and certain other exceptional circumstances, the age of the patient at time of surgery is quite young.[3]

These considerations help to explain the reason for the explosive pace of research in the area of component design and fixation to the human skeleton. Great interest currently is focused on the concept of direct fixation of artificial implants to bone, either by permitting direct growth of bone into specially fabricated surface topographies (so-called porous ingrowth or bony ingrowth prostheses) or press fitting a geometrically compatible implant into bone similar to the technique used for the Moore prosthesis for many years.

The success of these efforts has important implications for the future, since the loosening of prostheses years after insertion has emerged as the most important long-term problem of total joint replacement surgery.

This chapter reviews the relevant options in advanced arthritis of the hip, and the principles and specifics of rehabilitation in both surgical and nonsurgical management.

HISTORICAL PERSPECTIVE

The vast majority of prostheses heretofore, has been secured to bone with the use of polymethylmethacrylate ("cement"), which is mixed in the operating room. In the early years a radiolucent acrylic resulted after polymerization. Barium sulfate was eventually

PRINCIPLES OF PHYSICAL MEDICINE AND REHABILITATION
IN THE MUSCULOSKELETAL DISEASES

added to the mixture to permit radiologic visualization of the cement layer on follow-up x-rays. The methacrylate functions as a space filling cement and results in secure fit of prosthesis to bone. This permits immediate weight bearing without pain.

The marriage of this material with prosthetic components that substitute for the acetabulum (acetabular component) and femoral head (femoral component) of the hip joint was pioneered by John Charnley of England in the early 1960s.[4] A true revolution in the quality of the results of major reconstructive hip surgery ensued.

Prior to the emergence of the total hip procedure, cup arthroplasty was the principal option. The cup arthroplasty was introduced by Smith-Petersen of Boston in 1923, and popularized by Otto Aufranc who succeeded him at the Massachusetts General Hospital.[5] A landmark paper in which 1000 consecutive cases were reviewed was published in 1967.[6] Only four percent of the patients had excellent results at followup. The majority of patients were much improved over their preoperative results but persistent limps, short-ened limbs, activity-related aches or pain and permanent crutch or cane dependency often compromised the results. This procedure was largely abandoned once total hip arthro-plasty had been introduced.

The Charnley prosthesis consisted of a stainless steel femoral component and an acetabular component made of high molecular weight polyethylene. The early years were not without their frustrations. The original acetabular component was fabricated from a teflon-like plastic material. Several hundred operations had been performed before the early cases began to fail after only a short period of time due to extremely poor mechanical wear characteristics of the teflon-like material. It was thus not without some historical precedent that the wear characteristics of the polyethylene were a subject of great concern in the early years of its use. Theoretical wear rates of up to 1 mm per year were widely circulated in the literature in the late 1960s and early 1970s. The wear rate actually has proven to be only a fraction of the speculated rate, and only seldom the cause of a problem of clinical concern.

The stainless steel femoral component resulted in a significant rate of failure due to bending of the shaft from fatigue of the base metal (stainless steel). Importantly, however, the work of Charnley established the feasibility and reproducibility of the procedure. He continued to make valuable contributions to the field until his death in 1982. His follow-up studies helped to identify the principal long term consequence of total hip replacement—loosening of the fixation of the components to bone.[8]

Many prosthetic designs emerged over the two and a half decades following the first successful Charnley implantation. Variables operative in the design considerations include nature of base metal or alloy, gross configuration, surface topography, stem length, stem width, proportionality between length and width, angle between head and shaft, diameter of head, to name a few. Some principles common to the vast majority of contemporary designs have emerged. "Super alloys" of cobalt-chrome or titanium-aluminum-vanadium, specially fabricated for enhanced fatigue strength are the metals of choice for the femoral stems.

An *unlinked articulation* between the femoral and acetabular components is common to all current designs. Linked prostheses for the hip were advocated as they were in the knee and implanted in the early years, though never in large numbers.

A *metal-on-plastic* articulation is nearly universal. Metal-on-metal designs were in use for a number of years, i.e., Ring prosthesis, and are under serious consideration for reintroduction in Europe. Ceramic components have also been used because of their excellent biocompatibility.

In hemi-arthroplasty of the hip joint the acetabulum is preserved and the prosthetic head diameter corresponds to the diameter of the resected femoral head. In this circumstance, direct articulation between metal and human articular cartilage takes place. The most frequent indication is in displaced fractures of the femoral neck in elderly patients. The prototype prostheses were the Moore and Thompson implants. More recently bipolar designs have become widespread. The term bipolar denotes the fact that a double articulation transpires between femur and pelvis. A femoral stem common to a total hip system is either cemented or inserted cementless into the femur. A small femoral head diameter is used, either 22 or 26 mm. A large, metal component that corresponds in diameter to that of the resected femoral head is then snap-fitted on to the femoral head of the femoral component. Motion then takes place both at the site of attachment of the large head to the femoral stem and between the large head and the articular cartilage of the acetabulum (Fig. 17-1).

X-ray studies have shown that the major portion of the motion arc occurs at the former site, with motion between the prosthetic units and the articular cartilage reserved for the more extreme limits of the motion arc.[9] This prosthesis has gained wide acceptance in recent years.

Surface replacement of the hip was heralded as a "conservative" form of total hip replacement in the late 1970s. This device consisted of a metal or ceramic, large diameter surface covering of the femoral head, fixed by cement. A thin plastic cup was then cemented to the acetabular side. A high failure rate was reported in both Europe and the United States after a few years, largely due to acetabular failures attributed to the thinness of the cup wall. Cracks in the cement mantle around the cup developed that led to loosening and failure. This technique has largely been abandoned by the mainstream of orthopedic surgeons. Serious work has continued in several research centers.

Amstutz of the University of California at Los Angeles reports encouraging results with the use of a metal backing of the acetabular cup that compensates for the thinness of the plastic shell. The goals of preservation of the femoral neck and intramedullary cancellous architecture of the proximal femur motivate the continuation of this important work.

SURGICAL CONSIDERATIONS IN THE RHEUMATOID PATIENT

The human hip joint is a modified ball-in-socket articulation composed of the acetabulum (socket) of the pelvis and the head of the femur (ball) within it. The joint is inherently stable, even in the face of fulminant destruction by arthritic disease. The metacarpophalangeal joints of the hand and the elbow joint, in contradistinction, experience frequent subluxation, even frank dislocation, as a manifestation of the arthritic process.

The hip joint is subject to intense pain and disabling stiffness, which combines to markedly restrict functional capabilities. This is greatly magnified when the process is bilateral, as is so often the case in rheumatoid arthritis.

Once radiologic evidence of joint destruction has become manifest, the control of pain by nonsurgical means becomes largely ineffective. The timing of surgical intervention is based on duration of symptoms and their severity.

SYNOVECTOMY

Synovectomy has not been clearly established as an effective modality in the hip, though it is effectively and frequently employed in early arthritis of the wrist and knee. Because of the deep location of the hip joint, an open synovectomy requires extensive

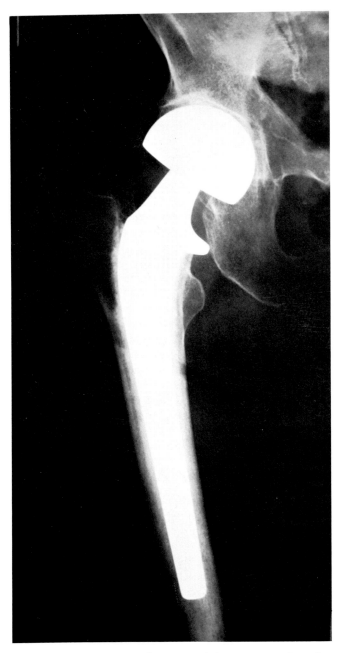

Fig. 17-1. A bipolar implant is used for reconstruction of a femoral neck fracture. The stem is identical to that for a full total hip replacement. The outer metal shell articulates with acetabular cartilage via a snap fit articulation with the ball of the femoral component. Immediate weight bearing is possible for rapid rehabilitation of elderly patients.

surgical exposure. The theoretical risk of osteonecrosis of the femoral head due to intraoperative dislocation is of some concern, though documentation of osteonecrosis secondary to such maneuvers of short duration is virtually unreported in the literature. Great care must be taken to protect the vasculature located along the posterior aspect of the femoral neck. It is not possible to perform a thorough synovectomy without intertrochanteric osteotomy or dislocation of the femoral head, and arthroscopy poses too great a risk of damage to the articular cartilage surface, as well as formidable technical difficulties.

Some European orthopedic surgeons advocate a more aggressive attitude toward early hip synovectomy than is presently practiced in this country. Gschwend of Switzerland reports the use of simultaneous intertrochanteric osteotomy and total synovectomy.[10] In the German literature, Meuli has also reported favorable results with early synovectomy in rheumatoid patients.[11]

The rehabilitation of patients after open synovectomy is enhanced by the use of continuous passive motion begun immediately after surgery in the recovery room. Prevention of stiffness after such an extensive procedure is the major goal of this modality. The device is well tolerated and is used in an adjunctive role with intensive physical therapy rehabilitative exercises.

Radioisotope synovectomy is currently undergoing intensive human clinical investigation in macroaggregate form via direct intra-articular administration. Because the hip joint is not a multiloculated joint like the wrist, it would be potentially well-suited for this method. Its use in young patients still poses considerable theoretical concerns.

Age, per se, is no contraindication to surgery in rheumatoid arthritis. In osteoarthritis, conversely, every effort is made to postpone total joint replacement either by effective use of nonsurgical therapy or alternative surgical procedures. Arthrodesis of the hip or intertrochanteric osteotomy are not viable options in the rheumatoid population.

The principal goal of surgery is the relief of pain. Among surgical procedures, total hip arthroplasty is extraordinarily successful in this regard, in the absence of infection. It is the procedure of choice for rheumatoid hip involvement.

Influence of Other Joints

In the rheumatoid population, hip symptoms are infrequently among the early manifestations of the disease. Hand and foot involvement generally occur earlier in the evolution of the disease and in a much higher percentage of cases. This involvement has important implications regarding both the rehabilitation potential of the patient and the ability of the hip surgery to favorably alter functional abilities.

Feet

A painful foot may tarnish the outcome of otherwise successful hip surgery. Before hip surgery the feet must be carefully assessed. In some cases the provision of appropriate orthotics and footwear will suffice. If surgery is required this should be performed prior to anticipated hip surgery, since persistent pain will impede the postsurgical ambulation activities. Additionally, the rheumatoid foot is susceptible to impaired wound healing and infection after corrective surgery.

Hands

The hands and proximal joints of the upper extremities require careful assessment prior to hip surgery because of the need to provide a period of protected weight bearing for the operated hip. Splinting or surgery of the hands or wrists might be indicated.

Traditional axillary crutches are most often inappropriate. Platform crutches that off-weight the wrist and hand or modified walkers with attached bilateral platforms for the forearms are often required.

Appropriate management of the upper extremities highlights the advantages of the multidisciplinary team approach to the rheumatoid patient with severe involvement. Skilled hand surgeons compliment a team that includes the hip surgeon, rheumatologist, occupational therapist, orthotist, physical therapist, podiatrist, social worker, and recreational therapist. Dedicated units devoted to the acute care and rehabilitation of these challenging patients are particularly valuable. A successful surgical outcome demands much more than skillful surgery alone.

When surgery of the hand and wrist is contemplated, a trade-off is often necessary between pain and deformity on the one hand and strength on the other. For the wrist, arthrodesis offers the attractions of being able to relieve pain, correct deformity and improve strength. For these reasons, it is often the procedure of choice when surgery is indicated.

Arthroplasty of the smaller joints of the hand is capable of relieving pain, preserving or restoring motion and correcting deformity, but loss of strength is not unusual.

It is important to emphasize that surgery of the hand be delegated to a surgeon dedicated and specifically trained in the particularly complex anatomical and functional challenges of the rheumatoid hand.

BILATERAL INVOLVEMENT

Bilateral involvement of rheumatoid hips is common (Fig. 17-2). Wide spacing between procedures is to be avoided since the unoperated hip is poorly suited to bear the brunt of additional weight bearing loads during the recuperation of the operated side. The practice of performing the second operation two weeks after the first, during the same hospitalization, is well-suited to the rehabilitation needs of the rheumatoid patients. However, socio-economic pressures against prolonged hospitalization work against this timetable.

Same day, consecutive bilateral arthroplasties can be successfully performed.[12] We caution against the use of the side-lying position on the operating room table, since the fragile rheumatoid skin is exposed to direct gravity pressure on a fresh operative wound during the second procedure. The use of a modified Watson-Jones approach permits the procedures to be performed in the supine position on an egg-crate mattress.

A single procedure for both hips offers several distinct advantages. In patients with significant cervical spine involvement, awake intubation or other special anesthetic techniques might be required to protect the vulnerable cervical cord during intubation and throughout the procedure. Avoidance of a second anesthetic is the most apparent advantage.

Blood replacement needs also affect the decision. Two procedures done back-to-back render a blood loss recovery-replacement device effective. This permits readministration of spent blood cells to the patient and dramatically reduces the volume of transfusions required. When this advantage is coupled with the practice of obtaining autologous (patient's own) blood prior to hospitalization, the risks associated with transfusion can be minimized.

The rehabilitation of consecutive, same day bilateral hip replacement procedures is not as arduous as might be anticipated. Pain is so reliable and immediately reduced by the

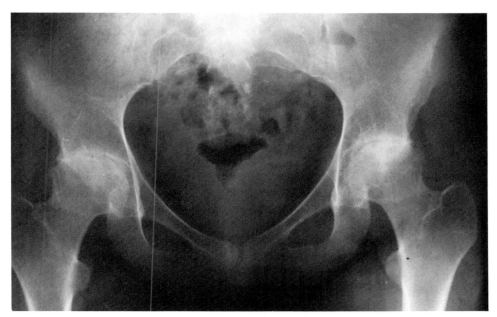

Fig. 17-2. Bilateral rheumatoid arthritis of the hips with characteristic findings of joint space narrowing, sclerosis and cyst formation.

arthroplasties that ambulation can be resumed usually within 48 hours of surgery. Good strength and function of the upper extremities is particularly helpful in the recovery from a bilateral procedure.

CONTRAINDICATIONS

Active infection is an absolute contraindication to arthroplasty. Infection must always be considered in the evaluation of acute exacerbation of hip pain in the rheumatoid. Many patients are on chronic systemic steroids and have had multiple intraarticular injections of corticosteroids. A low threshold for diagnostic hip aspiration under strict sterile conditions is warranted. Should infection be proved, aggressive treatment is indicated.

In the case of previously infected hips, major advances in recent years now permit successful replacement surgery in selected cases. The methyl methacrylate powder can be mixed with one or more appropriate antibiotics in powder form. Antibiotics that have been used successfully include gentamycin, tobramycin, colistin, and erythromycin, among others. Factory-mixed cement powder containing gentamycin has been available for more than a decade in Western Europe. It is not yet approved for sale in this country by the Food and Drug Administration.

The admixture of antibiotics into the cement results in significant weakening of the cement in laboratory studies of fatigue properties. How much weakening is too much is the subject of debate and conjecture. Because of this concern antibiotics are not used on a routine basis, and are reserved for cases associated with previous infection and in certain revision cases. In addition to the antibiotics in the cement, perioperative, high-dose parenteral antibiotics and long-term oral suppression antibiotics are used.

Lack of motivation or cooperation, advanced concurrent medical illness, senility, or neuromuscular disease represent other relative contraindications.

PREOPERATIVE CONSIDERATIONS

All patients about to undergo major implant surgery of the hip deserve a careful inspection of the mouth and current dental history. Any anticipated dental work should be completed prior to surgery. The same holds true for genitourinary problems. If a history of obstructive uropathy is elicited, consultation is indicated. Prostatectomy is best performed some months prior to admission to the hospital. Occasionally it is suggested that this be done during the same hospitalization. We urge against this approach because of the need for indwelling urinary catheterization.

Up until a few years ago it was common practice to admit patients to the hospital 36 or even 48 hours before surgery for execution of preoperative assessments and laboratory studies. This preparation is now completed on an outpatient basis in anticipation of admission. It is imperative for cooperation to exist between rheumatologist or internist and surgeon to ensure that all relevant preadmission studies have been performed and reviewed.

All of our patients are urged to donate their own blood prior to surgery. The exclusive use of autologous blood for operative and postoperative blood replacement has virtually eliminated the specter of serious transfusion-related problems.

For single hips three units are obtained. For bilateral and revision cases, four or more units are obtained. In rheumatoid patients baseline hemoglobin counts are routinely quite low. Single units can be donated and frozen to permit wide spacing between donations. Fresh units can be refrigerated for up to 35 days. Frozen units can be stored for years.

When substantial blood loss is anticipated, the cell saver is used to recover spent blood, cleanse the erythrocytes and readminister them intraoperatively. The presence of metal, plastic or cement debris or the use of antibiotic irrigation does not interfere with the use of the cell saver technology.

Prior to surgery a total body pHisoderm shower is ordered. Immediately before transport to the operation room a clip shave or depilatory cream is used to remove hair from the operative field. The skin is painted with betadine solution. Special care is taken in the handling of the skin of rheumatoid patients, particularly those on parenteral steroids.

Preoperative intravenous cephalosporins are administered upon arrival in the operating room. In our institution all joint replacement procedures are performed in the laminar air flow room with all operating room personnel gowned in space suits. The use of these three modalities (laminar air flow, i.v. antibiotics, and space suits) in combination has been shown in the British Multicenter Study to have resulted in the lowest rate of postoperative infections, less than one half of one percent.

Ultraviolet light is an acceptable alternative since ambiant, air-borne bacteria are virtually eliminated. Drawbacks include the need to protect the skin and eyes of patients and all operating room personnel from direct exposure, and risk of direct contamination of the wound by members of the surgical team who are not gowned in space suits. Major positive features include the relatively low cost of installation and maintenance and its proven effectiveness.

In the weeks immediately preceding the operation all patients participate in a teaching session for orientation to the hospital, physical therapy routines, and goals and hospital personnel.

Many patients are invited to participate in various clinical research projects and are given detailed information packets to permit informed consent documents to be signed prior to admission to the hospital.

Egg-crate mattresses are ordered for all rheumatoid patients. Careful handling in transfer is stressed.

Radiographic assessment of the cervical spine is obtained as part of the preoperative preparation. If fusion is indicated this takes precedence over the hip procedure. Careful handling of the neck by the attending anesthesiologist cannot be overemphasized.

All patients on chronic steroid regimens or those with a history of recent use of steroids are given intravenous hydrocortisone before, during surgery, and in the recovery room to preclude the onset of addisonian crisis.

All patients receive prophylactic measures for deep vein thrombosis (DVT) prevention prior to surgery. Most receive aspirin, which is continued until discharge. Those with prior history of phlebitis or embolization or with a history of peptic ulcer disease or aspirin intolerance receive warfarin.

A randomized, prospective study is currently in progress to assess the efficacy of continuous passive motion in the prophylaxis of DVT in hip surgery patients. Half of the patients are placed in the device and half in a balanced suspension. All receive pharmacologic DVT prophylaxis and all wear thromboembolic stockings (Fig. 17-3).

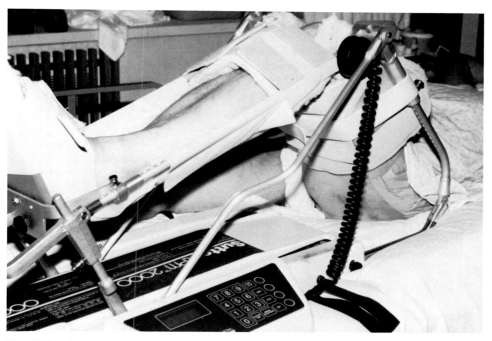

Fig. 17-3. The continuous passive motion machine is very helpful in the post-operative rehabilitation of previously stiff hips, as well as in special circumstances such as fracture-dislocations of the hip. Its potential use is deep vein thrombosis prevention is currently under investigation. Machine shown is manufactured by Sutter Biomedical.

SURGICAL TECHNIQUE

Our preference for surgical exposure is a straight lateral skin incision with anterior dislocation of the hip. We use a modified Watson-Jones approach, which is commonplace in Europe but less widely used in this country. The more commonly used Gibson or posterior approach requires division of the external rotator muscles and division or resection of the posterior capsule. This enhances the risk for posterior dislocation. The anterior approach affords superior visualization of the acetabulum and easy access to the proximal femur. It is technically slightly more difficult than the posterior approach. Additional advantages are that the procedure can be done equally as well in the supine and semilateral positions.

For cemented arthroplasties we currently use a femoral stem precoated with a thin layer of polymethymethacrylate to enhance bonding to cement. The component has a modular neck that can be used with head units of different diameters, different lengths and can be adapted to hemi-arthroplasties or bipolar configurations. Cement is centrifuged to minimize air voids, which act as stress risers. The cement is inserted retrograde with a cement gun and then pressurized against a femoral canal plug. The acetabular component is metal backed. Though not yet convincingly shown to be clinically efficacious, finite element analysis studies have demonstrated a beneficial effect of metal backing in terms of damping of the load transmitted to the cement. We preserve the subchondral bone plate whenever possible and place bone graft along the superolateral aspect of the acetabulum if incomplete coverage of the component is seen.

We are engaged in clinical research using cementless prostheses in both rheumatoid and osteoarthritic patients (Fig. 17-4). The benefits of avoidance of cement on the acetabular side have been demonstrated in Europe where experience with these devices is approaching 10 years. On the femoral side clinical experience is more controversial. Careful clinical research will be required before the safety and efficacy are clearly established.

We inform all of our patients that the use of cementless devices is experimental.

Biomechanical Considerations

Biomechanical concepts figure prominently in the rationale for reconstructive surgical procedures and the rehabilitative maneuvers that support and complement them. Pauwels of Germany is credited with popularizing the conceptualization of the forces about the hip as analogous to a simple lever arm system in which the center of rotation of the femoral head is considered the balance point.[13] (Fig. 17-5)

If one imagines an individual standing on one leg, the forces of the abductors and the iliotibial band lateral to this balance point must offset or counterbalance the gravity force of the body weight on the medial or opposite side of the balance point. The length of the lever arm for the body weight is approximately three times that of the abductor lever arm. The abductors therefore must generate a force nearly three times the body weight to maintain the pelvis in a level position relative to the ground.

The total force on the femoral head and hip joint includes the magnitude of the body weight (minus the weight of the supporting limb) and the forces generated by the abductors. Forces at the hip joint regularly reach magnitudes that are multiples of body weight.

Several elegant theoretical biomechanical works have been published in which forces generated in normal activities of daily living have been studied. Normal walking generates

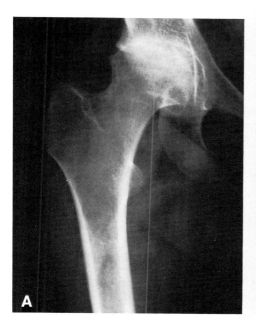

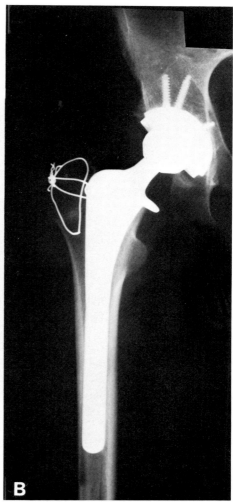

Fig. 17-4. The pre and post-op x-rays of a total hip replacement in a 30 year old patient with rheumatoid arthritis are shown. A cementless device (Zimmer Corp.) is shown in place.

forces 1.5 times body weight. The force used for running is capable of generating multiples of five times body weight or more.

The impact of body weight in excess of normal is readily apparent. An individual 50 pounds overweight can generate forces 200 pounds or more in excess of normal with certain activities. The theoretical consequences of this load on the finite articular cartilage surface area is sobering. The surface area available for load transmission is anatomically fixed. Load per unit area must increase in response to added weight burden. How much is too much remains an unanswered question.

Other factors that contribute to the magnitude of the load in addition to activity level and body weight include the nature of the interactive surface (i.e., concrete versus thick carpet), type of footwear (hard, thin soles versus rubber soles and heels) and the integrity

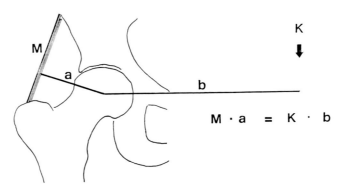

Fig. 17-5. The simple lever arm system of forces about the human hip.

of the compensatory mechanisms of the locomotor apparatus (heel pad, knee flexion, absorptive capabilities of the soft tissues and cartilage surfaces of the foot and leg).

BIOMECHANICAL CONCERNS IN TOTAL JOINT REPLACEMENT SURGERY

For some years deliberate medial displacement of the acetabular cup was advocated to reduce the length of the body weight lever arm and thereby reduce the forces on the artificial joint. This was done at the expense of bone mass, which was resected in order to place the component medially. The stout subchondral bone plate was sacrificed.

Follow-up studies of patients from around the world 10 years or more past the time of surgery have highlighted the problems of loosening of the components.[2,14,15] The failure rate on the acetabular side was particularly worrisome since it was shown to increase in a nearly vertical fashion after eight years.[14] The need to deliberately displace medially has been reassessed. Great effort is now taken to preserve the critical subchondral plate whenever possible and to restore the biomechanical lever arms to physiologic levels.

Protrusio, or medial displacement of the acetabulum is recognized on preoperative x-rays in up to 30 percent of rheumatoid patients. Weakening of the abductors can often be demonstrated by checking the Trendelenburg sign and observing the gait pattern. Reestablishment of the acetabulum in its physiologic position at the time of surgery results in strengthening of the abductors and correction of the abnormal gait pattern.

When deliberate medialization of the acetabular cup is performed, weakening of the abductors can be avoided by trochanteric osteotomy and distal and lateral transfer of the greater trochanter.

INSTRUMENTED PROSTHESES

With rare exception[17,18] all biomechanical values have been calculated on the basis of theoretical values or values indirectly obtained by Electromyogram and gait analysis studies.

Within the past year information has been obtained from two research centers where instrumented prostheses have been inserted into consenting human subjects. Hodge and Harris of Boston have inserted an endoprosthesis (similar to a Moore prosthesis) with multiple transducers on the load bearing surface of the prosthesis. An electronic telemetry system engineered by co-workers Fijan and Mann of the Massachusetts Institute of Technology monitors strain gauge deflection.

Results of studies during the first four days after implantation were reported in January of 1985.[19] Bed rest in balanced suspension or abduction splint resulted in peak forces up to 390 psi. Walking partial weight bearing with a walker resulted in loads of up to 635 psi. Sitting on the edge of the bed rated 490 psi and moving onto a bed pan caused forces of up to 500 psi. Brown et al. at Case Western Reserve have inserted a telemetrized total hip prosthesis in a 67-year-old woman who weighed 125 pounds.[20] Preliminary data indicate directly measured forces of 2.19 times body weight with crutch walking. Data reflecting more normal activities of daily activity are planned and are awaited with keen interest.

SURGICAL RESULTS OF TOTAL HIP REPLACEMENT IN RHEUMATOID ARTHRITIS

The immediate result of total hip replacement is exceptionally good. It is not unusual for a patient to emerge from anesthesia more comfortable than before surgery. Preservation of this gratifying early result over time has proved to be more elusive.

Stauffer, in reporting the 10-year results of 300 consecutive total hip replacements at the Mayo Clinic, disclosed a 12 percent incidence of loosening of the femoral component and 35 percent incidence of acetabular cup loosening in the 17 rheumatoid hips included in the study.[14] This incidence of acetabular loosening was fivefold greater than that among the osteoarthritic patients in the same series. The incidence of protrusio in this rheumatoid group was not specifically noted. However, at the time these operations were performed (1969–1970), the importance of bone grafting for acetabular protrusio was not recognized, nor was reestablishment of the center of rotation of the femoral head in a lateralized physiologic position practiced. In 1985, Bayley et al., from the Robert Brigham Hospital reported that bone grafting of the medial acetabulum had a protective effect, whereas use of cement alone resulted in a 19 percent incidence of acetabular migration by x-ray criteria and a 13 percent revision rate at a mean follow-up time of 7.5 years.[21]

Colville and Raunio of Finland reported on the follow-up of 378 arthroplasties of the hip for rheumatoid arthritis at the Rheumatism Foundation Hospital in Finland.[22] The average age at surgery was 39 years. The follow-up time was short, with a mean of 2.5 years and range of from one to six years postoperation. At follow-up 95 percent were reported to be pain free and 98.5 percent had improved functional capabilities. Radiographic evidence of loosening was reported in 3.4 percent of cases. Though 40 percent of the patients were on chronic steroids, the overall infection rate was 0.7 percent, which compares favorably with that reported in other nonrheumatoid series.[23]

Poss et al. have contended that the infection rate for total hip arthroplasty in rheumatoids is comparable to that seen in large osteoarthritic series.[24] Revision surgery is the variable associated with the greatest risk for deep infection.

Other than sudden death, the development of infection is the single most serious postoperative complication. Some of the techniques available to deal with prior infection have been discussed earlier in this chapter. Aggressive wound exploration, soft tissue debridement, large volume, pulsative lavage with antibiotic solutions and primary wound closure are capable of salvaging some early infections. Once established, surgical treatment may require removal of prostheses and all cement, a long convalescence in traction followed by several months of observation off all antibiotics prior to reimplantation with antibiotic-containing cement. Permanent resection arthroplasty is required in many cases, and death directly related to this complication has been reported in 23 of 135 infected hips by Hunter and Dandy of Canada.[25]

REHABILITATION OF THE HIP

Close cooperation between the primary physician and an orthopedic surgeon is invaluable. A painful hip is a serious matter. Errors in diagnosis or management can lead to lifelong disability.

For example, an adolescent who develops a limp, or begins to complain of pain, should be referred without delay for orthopedic evaluation. During the rapid phase of skeletal growth, the growth plates of the proximal femora are uniquely susceptible to an affliction known as slipped capital femoral epiphysis or epiphysiolysis. A disruption occurs through the growth plate that alters the anatomical alignment between the portions of the femoral heads on either side of the growth plate. If promptly and correctly treated, irreversible damage can be avoided in most cases. Surgery is often required.

The immediate treatment should include the use of crutches and mild analgesics, pending orthopedic assessment. Failure to protect the hip from weight-bearing loads can lead to progression of the malalignment.

One should be aware that a painful hip may present as an ache in the anterior knee region. The evaluation of a painful knee, particularly in the absence of athletic or other injury, should always include a careful and gentle documentation of the range of motion of the hip. A reduction in the ability to passively internally rotate the leg may be the first clue in inflammation of the hip joint.

If gentle internal rotation causes pain or results in asymmetrical limitation of hip motion, emergency consultation is indicated. Infection must be considered in the differential. Documentation of temperature is indicated. Stress fracture must be considered.

The diagnosis of 'tendonitis' is abused and overused. The institution of an exercise therapy program or other rehabilitative modalities in the absence of a clear diagnosis can lead to disastrous results.

Special care in the interpretation of x-rays is needed and specific views often necessary.

The most effective way to protect the hip in the face of the sudden onset of pain is with two crutches and touch-down weight bearing on the affected side. There are few indications for total nonweight-bearing since muscle forces are required to off-set the gravity drag of the suspended limb. Analgesics should be chosen that do not function as antipyretics since the masking of a fever may impede accurate diagnosis. Care should be taken to titrate dosage so that significant impairment of psychomotor skills does not result.

The guiding principle is the need to establish an accurate diagnosis. In the meanwhile, effective protection of the hip is imperative.

CONSERVATIVE MANAGEMENT OF THE ARTHRITIC HIP

Several effective modalities are available in the conservative (nonsurgical) treatment of the patient with early osteoarthritis of the hip. Included in this category are many individuals who were active in contact and collision sports in their early years, and many individuals who are overweight.

A great fallacy is to equate the concept of conservative treatment with passive involvement with the patient. Time, wit, patience, and empathy are required in varying proportions to achieve a stable equilibrium. Realistic goals must be outlined. The complete relief of pain with a return to unrestricted athletic activities is an unrealistic, though unfortunately common, expectation.

The adverse theoretical effects of excessive body weight were discussed earlier in the chapter. Sustained weight reduction is thus a key goal. It is unwise and ineffective to simply tell a patient that he or she must lose weight. There is perhaps no easier way to destroy one's rapport with a patient. Patient's will be reluctant to return to the office to have their "failure" dutifully recorded by the office nurse. Moreover, the presence of the hip pain has invariably brought on unwanted reductions in exercise tolerance.

An excellent way to gain the patient's confidence and appreciation is to give appropriate guidance outlining ways in which exercise can be performed that is not harmful to the hip. Indoor pools in which the water temperature is kept warm are particularly useful. Pool exercises are encouraged since water suspension reduces the gravity force of body weight. In our community a network of swimming pools has been organized by the Arthritis Foundation. The water temperature is maintained at 90 degrees or more. Range of motion and endurance exercises are supervised by trained volunteers or regular staff members of the participating institutions.

Stationary exercise bicycles are relatively inexpensive and invaluable. Fancy gadgets are unnecessary. Essentials include a comfortable seat with adjustable height and adjustable friction on the wheel. Even patients with relatively stiff hips can successfully use the bicycles with the seat elevated.

Floor calisthenics that do not include jumping activities are helpful. Range of motion exercise should be designed to preserve motion. Passive exercises to increase motion in arthritic hips are invariably unsuccessful, contribute to increased pain, and should be discouraged.

All activities that involve high impact loading of the legs or subject the hips to sudden twisting or torque movements should be eliminated. Jogging, volleyball, tennis, and basketball, among others, fall into these categories.

A serious effort at weight reduction includes a rational program of exercise with a tolerable, sustainable reduction in caloric intake. The organization of the dietary component is best delegated to an experienced, interested, and well-trained professional. This not only brings in welcome expertise, but provides an important psychological buffer. Dietary fads, crash diets, and most appetite suppressant pharmaceuticals are to be condemned. It benefits patient and doctor little to achieve a dramatic reduction in body weight over three months only to see the shed weight reappear over the next year.

The next most effective mechanism for reduction of forces in the hip joint is the use of a cane. Bombelli and others have carefully studied the biomechanics of the use of a cane.[26] For the hip joint the cane should always be used on the opposite side of the involved hip. For most patients this comes intuitively. Certain patients assume that the cane should be used on the side of the pain and never experiment with the cane in the opposite side. These patients are invariably very grateful when the proper use of the cane is explained and demonstrated to them. The use of the cane on the same side as the pain results in heavy loads on the arm with fatigue and pain in the hand and wrist and much less effective non-weighting of the painful hip.

Many patients have quite strong emotional prejudices against using a cane. Empathy and salesmanship on the part of the treating doctor can go a long way in overcoming these unfortunate, but understandable, attitudes.

Appropriate footwear is an often overlooked asset in the overall management of the patient. Shoes with soft soles and wide heels are advisable. Inserts are helpful. Heel or full sole designs are available. These function to reduce the peak loads sustained at heel strike.

The home environment should not be neglected. Well installed carpet is preferable to hardwood or other hard surfaces. In kitchen areas rubber mats can be placed at the sink, in front of the stove and at other sites of frequent daily activities.

When selecting an automobile consideration should be given to the ease of entry and exit and the comfort of the seat. Few car manufacturers have given serious consideration to the sitting biomechanics in seat design and ease of entry. Volvo corporation is the exception and deserves special mention for the exceptional design of their seats.

ANTI-INFLAMMATORY MEDICATION

The pharmacology of the nonsteroidal anti-inflammatory medications lies outside the scope of this chapter. The medications have proven to be extremely useful in reduction of pain in many arthritic conditions about the hip. They are invaluable in the initial treatment of most patients. Indefinite administration raises concerns regarding long term safety. Additionally, most are quite expensive and share some of the short term side-effects commonplace with aspirin therapy.

It is prudent to become familiar with at least one drug in each of the three major pharmacological categories with regard to side-effects, dosage levels, and cost.

Patients need to be informed that the effectiveness of these medications depends upon regular ingestion. Many will intuitively stop taking the medications when they begin to feel better, as they are accustomed to doing with simple analgesics.

Efforts at long-term conservative control are best directed in the areas of weight reduction, exercise, and the other methods of force reduction as outlined above. Pharmaceuticals are best looked upon as adjunctive. This is not to impune their importance, but to place their usage in perspective.

REHABILITATION OF THE POSTOPERATIVE PATIENT

The most frequently performed surgical procedure for arthritis of the hip is total replacement arthroplasty (total hip). (Fig. 17-6) The immediate postoperative treatment protocol is under the control of the orthopedic surgeon and physical therapist.

The rate by which patients achieve functional goals is quite variable. Therefore, arbitrary rules regarding rest periods and target days for certain activities are not advisable. Patients are best progressed as rapidly as their pain thresholds will permit.

It is not uncommon for some patients to begin standing on the first day after surgery.

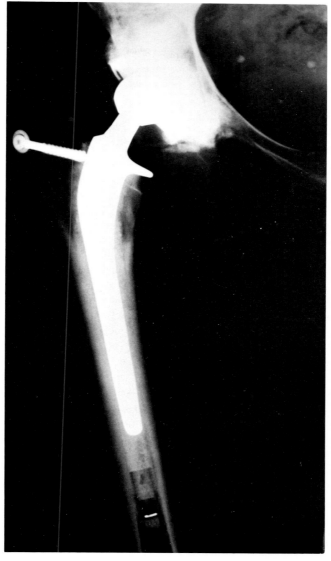

Fig. 17-6. A conventional total hip replacement is shown in a 79 year old woman with osteoarthritis.

Before discharge from the hospital it is important for the patient to be independent in transfers in and out of bed and a chair, to be capable of walking up stairs, to be able to use bathroom facilities, and to understand the precautions necessary to avoid dislocation of the prosthesis. The first six weeks are the period of maximum vulnerability for dislocation of the prosthesis.

Active dorsiflexion and plantar flexion of the ankle are stressed on a regular basis beginning on the day of surgery. Prevention of deep vein thrombosis and subsequent pulmonary embolization is one of the major goals of the program of rapid postoperative rehabilitation.

Patients with rheumatoid arthritis require more time and patience in the early postoperative phase, and benefit greatly from the input of occupational therapy for assistive devices for the upper extremities and exercises for the arms and hands. Special walking aids are most helpful, particularly a walker fitted with bilateral forearm supports.

In nonrheumatoid cases, discharge from the hospital in one week or less from the date of surgery is becoming commonplace.

Assistive devices useful during the early phase of recuperation include an elevated chair for sitting, an elevated toilet seat for use in the bathroom, an abduction pillow to keep the legs separated in bed and crutches or a walker. A pick-up walker with coasters is usually appropriate.

Long-term rehabilitation goals include the recovery of normal muscle strength of the abductors, adductors, flexors and extensors of the hip, improvement of range of motion of the hip and gradual increase in weight bearing tolerances.

In cemented total hip replacement, partial weight bearing is permitted immediately. Two crutches or a walker are used for six weeks followed by a variable period for use of a cane. Once the patient is capable of walking without a limp and without pain the cane may be discarded.

In cementless replacements, three months or more of minimal weight bearing is commonly recommended to protect the fragile zone between prosthesis and bone. Again, some assistive device, i.e., crutch or cane, is recommended until the patient is capable of walking without a limp or pain.

Once the period of cane dependency is passed, rehabilitative guidelines include maintenance of a regular exercise program, avoidance of any shock producing activities, the use of soft shoes and inserts to cushion the blows of normal walking and maintenance of as normal a body weight as possible.

Rehabilitation centers with divisions for arthritis patients can play an important role in the comprehensive care of arthritis patients. They are uniquely suited to bring together in a coordinated fashion the assets of multiple disciplines such as physical and occupational therapy, social service, pharmacology, chaplaincy, and recreational therapy, in addition to the supervising surgeon and other treating or consulting physicians. They can function as focal points for preoperative education as well as the site for the second phase of acute postoperative care.

REFERENCES

1. Hori RY, Lewis JL, Zimmerman JR, Compere, CL: The number of total joint replacements in the United States. Clin Ortho 132:46–52, 1978

2. Stauffer RN: Ten-year follow-up study of total hip replacement. J Bone Joint Surg 64-A:983–990, 1982

3. Scott RD, Sarokhan AJ, Dalziel R: Total hip and total knee arthroplasty in juvenile rheumatoid arthritis. Clin Orthop 182:90–98, 1984

4. Charnley J: Arthroplasty of the hip. A new operation. Lancet 1:1129–1133, 1961

5. Smith-Petersen MN: Arthroplasty of the hip: a new method. J Bone Joint Surg 21(2):269–288, 1939

6. Aufranc OE: Constructive hip surgery with the Vitallium mold. A report on 1,000 cases of arthroplasty of the hip over a fifteen year period. J Bone Joint Surg 39A:237–248, 1957

7. Charnley J, Halley OK: Rate of wear in total hip replacement. Clin Orthop 121:126–142, 1976

8. Charnley J: Low Friction Arthroplasty of the Hip. Springer-Verlag, Berlin-New York, 1979

9. Drinker H, Mall JC: Radiologic aspects of new universal proximal femoral hip prosthesis. Am J Roentgenol 129:531-533, 1977

10. Gschwend N: Synovectomy. In Kelly WN, Harris ED, Ruddy S, et al. (eds), Textbook of Rheumatology, pp 1824-1899, WB Saunders Company, Philadelphia, 1981

11. Meuli HC: Zur operativen behandlung der polyarthritschen hufte. Deutsch Med Wschr 91:1779-1787, 1966

12. Salvati EA, Hughes P, Lachiewicz P: Bilateral total hip replacement arthroplasty in one stage. J Bone Joint Surg 60A:640-644, 1978

13. Pauwels F: Atlas zur Biomechanik der Gesunden und Kranken Hufte. Springer, Berlin-New York, 1973

14. Sutherland CJ, Wilde AH, Borden LS, Marks KE: A ten-year follow-up of one hundred consecutive Muller curved stem total hip replacement arthroplasties. J Bone Joint Surg 64A:970-982, 1982

15. Salvati EA, Wilson PD Jr, Jolley MN, et al: A ten-year follow-up study of our first one hundred consecutive Charnley total hip replacements. J Bone Joint Surg 63A:753-767, 1981

16. Poss R, Maloney JP, Ewald F, et al: Six to 11-year results of total hip arthroplasty in rheumatoid arthritis. Clin Ortho 182:109-116, 1982

17. Rydell N: Intra-vital measurements of forces active on the hip joint. In Evans FG (ed), Studies on the Anatomy and Function of Bone and Joints, pp 52-68, Springer-Verlag, New York, 1966

18. English TA, Kilvington M: In vivo records of hip loads using a femoral implant with telemetric output (a preliminary report). J Biomed Eng 1:111-115, 1979

19. Hodge WA, Fijan R, Mann RW, et al: Preliminary in vivo pressure measurements in a human acetabulum. (abstract) In Transactions of the 31st Annual Meeting, Orthopaedic Research Society 10:284, 1985

20. Brown RH, Davy OT, Heiple KG, et al: In vivo load measurements on a total hip prosthesis. (abstract) In Transactions of the 31st Annual Meeting, Orthopaedic Research Society 10:283, 1985

21. Bayley JC, Christie MJ, Ewald FC, et al: Results of total hip arthroplasty in protrusio acetabuli. Presented at 52nd Annual Meeting, Am Acad Ortho Surg, Paper No. 131, Las Vegas, 1985

22. Colville J, Raunio P: Charnley low-friction arthroplasties of the hip on rheumatoid arthritis. J Bone Joint Surg 60B:498-503, 1978

23. Poss R, Thornhill TS, Ewald FC, et al: Factors influencing the incidence and outcome of infection following total joint arthroplasty. Clin Ortho 182:117-126, 1984

24. Poss R, Ewald FC, Thomas WH, et al: Complications of total hip replacement arthroplasty in patients with rheumatoid arthritis. J Bone Joint Surg 58A:1130-1133, 1976

25. Hunter G, Dandy O: The natural history of the patient with an infected total hip replacement. J Bone Joint Surg 59B:293-297, 1977

26. Bombelli R: Osteoarthritis of the Hip. Springer-Verlag, Berlin-New York, 1983

F. Richard Convery
Martha Minteer-Convery

18

The Knee

ANATOMY AND BIOMECHANICS

The knee is a diarthrodial (freely moving), three-compartment joint. The articulating surfaces of the femur and tibia make up the medial and lateral compartments and the patellar-femoral articulation is the third. The joint is surrounded by a capsule and ligamentous complex that is richly innervated by pain fibers and is exquisitely sensitive to stretch. The synovial membrane deep to the capsule is normally only one to two cells thick, is poorly innervated by neural fibers, but is very responsive to irritation or inflammation. The synovial membrane extends proximally to attach to the patella and, in disease states, may extend even more proximally (Fig. 18-1). The extension proximally is occasionally referred to as the "suprapatellar bursa," a misnomer in that this area is a contiguous portion of the joint itself. Inserting into the upper pole of the synovial membrane is a small muscle arising from the anterior surface of the femur, the articularis genu, which is said to pull the membrane proximally in terminal extension to prevent impingment of the membrane by the patella.

Ligamentous Support

The knee, unlike the hip, has no inherent stability but is entirely dependent upon soft tissue-supporting structures to maintain alignment and control motion. Ligamentous support on the lateral side of the joint is arranged in three layers, as described by Seebacher.[40] Superficially are the iliotibial tract and its anterior expansion inserting onto the tibia at Gerdy's tubercle and the tendon of the biceps femoris inserting onto the proximal fibula. The middle layer is formed anteriorly by the retinaculum of the quadriceps descending to insert on the tibia. In the midportion is the lateral collateral (fibular collateral) ligament and posteriorly the proximal and distal patellofemoral ligaments. The deep layer is the lateral part of the joint capsule, which attaches to the lateral meniscus via the coronary ligaments. The tendon of the popliteus muscle (which arises from the posterior aspect of the tibia) passes through a hiatus in the coronary ligaments at the posterior-lateral corner

PRINCIPLES OF PHYSICAL MEDICINE AND REHABILITATION
IN THE MUSCULOSKELETAL DISEASES

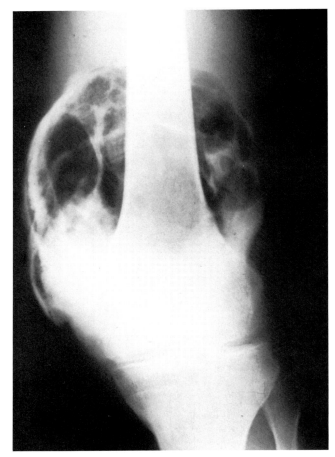

Fig. 18-1. A double contrast arthrogram demonstrating the sometimes massive size and proximal extension distended joint capsule. The multiloculated appearance is due to a very proliferative synovitis.

and inserts onto the femur beneath the lateral collateral ligament. Posteriorly, the capsule divides into two laminae. The more superficial portion ends at the variable fabellofibular ligament. The deep portion attaches to the posteriorly placed y-shaped arcuate ligament (which spans the popliteus muscle) as it crosses the backside of the lateral aspect of the joint running from the fibula to the femur. The fibular collateral ligament is tight in extension, relaxed in flexion and further tightened by rotation.

The medial side of the knee, as described by Warren and Marshall,[43] is also best visualized in three layers. Superficial is the deep investing fascia that surrounds the tendious portion of the sartorius. The sartorius, unlike the other two muscles of the pes anserinus immediately below, inserts into a network of fascial fibers. The gracilis and semitendinosus insert directly onto the tibia. The middle layer contains the superficial layer of the medial (tibial collateral) ligament and posteriorly blends with the fibrous sheath of the semimembranous muscle. The tendon of the semimembranous inserts directly onto the tibia at the posterior medial corner but the fibers of the tendon sheath extend proximally and laterally, to cover the posterior aspect of femoral condyle and insert into the lateral condyle, thus forming the oblique popliteal ligament. The deep layer contains the joint capsule and the deep portion of the medial (tibial collateral) ligament. The deep portion, especially its posterior portion, is firmly attached to the medial meniscus as well as to the tibia and femur. Anteriorly, the capsule does not exist but the supporting structures consist of the quadriceps and its tendon, the patella, the patellar ligament and the retinacular extension from the quadriceps to the tibia.

Cruciate Ligaments and Menisci

The cruciate ligaments, anterior and posterior, are named for their tibial attachments and lie within the joint capsule. Surrounded by synovium, they are extrasynovial but still intracapsular. The anterior cruciate ligament arises from the anterior intercondylar area of the tibia, extends posteriorly, superiorly, and laterally to attach into the medial aspect of the lateral condyle of the femur. The posterior cruciate arises from the posterior intercondylar area of the tibia, extends more vertically to attach into the lateral aspect of the medial condyle. The femoral attachment of the posterior cruciate is thus more anterior than that of the anterior cruciate.

The menisci, medial and lateral, are wedge-shaped and cup the femoral condyle to provide additional stability to the joint. The medial meniscus is somewhat incomplete, shaped like a comma and firmly attached in its midportion to the deep medial ligament. This firm attachment is often implicated to explain the greater frequency of injury to the medial as compared to the lateral meniscus. In addition, the lateral meniscus is, from its posterior surface, attached to the femur by the menisco femoral ligaments of Humphry and Wrisberg. Because of these ligaments the lateral meniscus is more closely related to femoral motion and thereby less susceptible to injury.

Movements of the Knee

The movements of the knee joint are flexion, extension, internal rotation, external rotation, and if there is any ligament looseness, some varus and valgus motion. As the knee moves from a position of flexion to extension, the first limitation to further extension is a tightening of the anterior cruciate ligament. Extension of the lateral condyle of the femur stops when the anterior cruciate becomes taut. Further extension of the knee occurs by anterior rotation of the lateral condyle around the pivot of the anterior cruciate. At the same time, the medial condyle slides posteriorly to complete extension of the knee. The internal rotation of the femur tightens the posterior cruciate for maximum stability of the joint in terminal extension.[26] The preceding is usually referred to as the "screw-home" mechanism.

Flexion from a position of full extension is initiated by the popliteus muscle, which externally rotates the femur to unwind the cruciates and allow the hamstring muscles to flex the knee. Maximum rotation of the joint occurs in flexion with the cruciate ligaments unwound. In this respect, the knee is analogous to the hip in that maximum stability is provided in extension for ambulation and maximum mobility in flexion for activities of daily living.

The Patella

The function of the patella is twofold. First, it functions as a linkage between the quadriceps tendon and the tibia via the patellar ligament. Secondly, it maintains the quadriceps moment arm, which is the perpendicular distance from the patellar ligament (tendon) to the axis of joint motion, which in the knee is not constant but moves along a circular path in the posterior femoral condyle.[13,24] The patella contributes to the quadriceps moment arm throughout the full range of motion but is least in flexion and maximal in full extension.[24] In full flexion, the patella drops into the intracondylar area of the femur thus reducing the length of the moment. With progressive extension, the patella rides up the patellar groove, gradually increasing the moment, to lie, in full extension, on the anterior surface of the femur at which point the moment is at its greatest for maximal quadriceps strength. The effect of patellectomy has been demonstrated in cadavers where 15–30 percent more force on the quadriceps tendon was required to fully extend the knee than when the patella was in place.[24]

The Quadriceps

The function of the quadriceps muscle is to extend the knee. The specific contribution of the component parts has been appreciably clarified by Leib and Perry.[28] The vastus intermedius was found to be the most effective extensor of the knee but more important was the force necessary to achieve full extension. Nearly twice as much force on the quadriceps was required to produce full extension as compared to extending the knee from 90–15 degrees of flexion. These studies also demonstrated the failure of the vastus medialis to produce terminal extension, a long-held belief. They concluded that the only selective function of the vastus medialis was to maintain patellar alignment and that the often seen atrophy of the medialis and loss of terminal extension were indicative only of generalized quadriceps weakness rather than a specific deficiency of the medialis.

Perry et al. later demonstrated the magnitude of force needed to stabilize the knee during flexed knee stance.[34] The force required was 75 percent of the load on the femoral head at 15 degrees of flexion, 210 percent at 30 degrees, and 410 percent at 60 degrees. The effect of a flexion deformity, according to this data, not only increases the load across the knee joint but forces the quadriceps to function at a mechanical disadvantage.

Joint Lubrication

Standard machine bearings are lubricated by hydrodynamic lubrication in which a wedge of lubricant forms at the leading edge of bearing contact. Machine bearings usually rotate continuously at high speed, which maintains the wedge of lubricant. It has been long known that such a mechanism was rarely possible in animal joints because maintenance of the wedge of fluid depends on a continuous motion of the two surfaces.[6] Animal joints oscillate slowly and reverse motion constantly, which effectively prevents hydrodynamic lubricating conditions, ie, the wedge cannot be maintained.

Two major mechanisms function to lubricate articular cartilage depending upon the load and motion conditions imposed.[35] In low load circumstances, boundary lubrication is predominant and under high load and speed, a self-pressurized hydrostatic mechanism called weeping lubrication becomes predominant.[36] In boundary lubrication, molecules of proteoglycans attach themselves to the articular cartilage and create a motion interface between the molecules that is less resistant to shear than the articular cartilage. In animal joints, the boundary mechanism does not function at high loads as the boundary layer is too fragile to withstand the high shear forces applied.

A self-pressurized hydrostatic mechanism called weeping lubrication seems to be the prevalant lubricating mode in joints under high loads and speed.[36] As a joint is loaded, interstitial fluid is squeezed out of the cartilage at the leading edge of contact. As the joint slides, a film of interstitial fluid is added to the synovial fluid to separate the cartilage surfaces. At the completion of loading, the interstitial fluid is restored to the cartilage at the trailing edge by osmotic pressure. The combined interstitial and synovial fluid lubricant is referred to as the squeeze film. The squeeze film concept is often used to explain why the coefficient of friction in animal joints decreases with increasing load.[23] In addition to these lubricating mechanisms, there is some deformation of the cartilage in response to applied load, which flattens the surface and may decrease the frictional resistance. This is usually referred to as the elastohydrodynamic effect. From the above, it is clear that lubrication of joints utilizes several mechanical mechanisms in addition to the lubricant of soft tissue, which is thought to be facilitated by hyaluronate.

PAIN MECHANISMS

Articular cartilage has no neural tissue and the synovium is only sparsely innervated with fibers that are thought to be vasomotor in function.[14] The capsule of a joint is richly innervated with pain fibers and, like the gastrointestinal tract, is exquisitely sensitive to stretch as by distension. The relief of pain following aspiration of a tense effusion dramatically demonstrates this later point. The underlying bone is innervated but the pain perceived with bone involvement is a dull aching nauseating pain as distinct from the sharp acute pain caused by capsular stretching. Severe aching pain at rest has been attributed to impairment of venous drainage and elevation of intraosseous pressure in both the hip and knee.[2] In osteoarthritis of the knee, intraosseous pressures were low in the tibia but high in the femur.[3] An unexpected finding in the later study was the measurement of high intraosseous pressures in both the femur and tibia in patients with severe aching rest pain but no demonstrable evidence of osteoarthritis. The authors suggest that circulatory changes in the subchondral bone might be of etiological significance in osteoarthritis. Perception of pain in the knee is, accordingly, of two distinct types: an acute sharp pain caused by stretching or distension of the capsule as caused by instability or an effusion and a dull aching pain, especially at rest after activity, arising from bone and probably secondary to venous engorgement.

EXAMINATION OF THE KNEE

Soft Tissue

Swelling of the knee is either localized or diffuse. Localized swelling is usually related to involvement of one of the 12 bursae about the knee. A bursa is a potential space, lined with serosal tissue that lies over a bony prominence or between bone and tendinous attachments to bone. When irritated by repetitive minor trauma or infected, the swelling is well-defined and localized. Each bursa about the knee has the potential to become inflamed but the most commonly involved are the infrapatellar, prepatellar, and the anserine, (beneath the combined tendinous insertion of the sartorius, semitendinous and gracilis muscles, the pes anserinous).

Diffuse swelling of the knee (Fig. 18-2) may be interstitial edema fluid, an effusion or synovial hypertrophy, either separately or in combination. Synovial hypertrophy has a characteristic soft, doughy feeling whereas an effusion alone, as in a hemarthrosis or acute sepsis, has a tense tight feeling. In the presence of an effusion (Fig. 18-3), a fluid wave can be identified by compressing the suprapatellar pouch and tapping one side of the joint and the patella can be balloted.

Swelling in the posterior aspect of the knee is most usually a popliteal cyst (Fig. 18-4). In children, the cyst is usually congenital and will spontaneously resolve without treatment.[10] In adults, it is a manifestation of underlying disease of the knee joint. It is most commonly seen in rheumatoid arthritis but is not uncommon in degenerative arthritis and chronic internal derangements of the knee. Because of the "ball-valve" effect, synovial fluid flows into the cyst but cannot return.[22] Treatment of the cyst is treatment of the underlying joint disease and rarely is it necessary in either adults or children to address the cyst directly. Not infrequently, especially in the patient with rheumatoid arthritis, a popliteal cyst will rupture. The clinical presentation suggests acute thrombophlebitis, usually occurs spontaneously and causes severe pain and swelling in the calf. Since the patient with rheumatoid arthritis is relatively privileged with respect to thrombophlebitis, an arthrogram is usually the first diagnostic step, and if positive, treatment is directed toward the inflammation of the knee rather than the inflammation of the calf.

Diarthrodial joints have a position of maximum capacity, at which the intra-articular pressure is the least.[12] In the knee, this position is between 30 and 60 degrees of flexion.

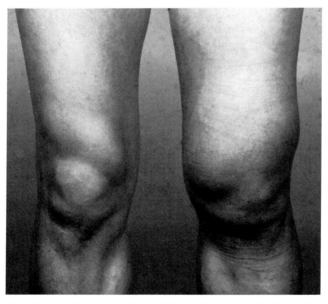

Fig. 18-2. Diffuse swelling of the left knee with distension medially and laterally.

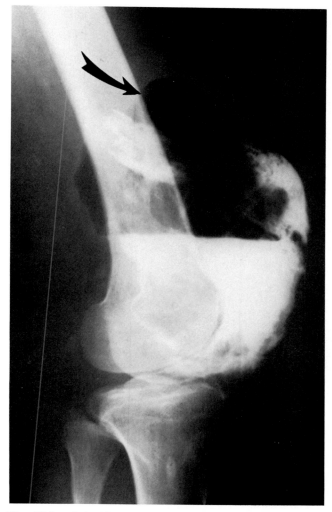

Fig. 18-3. A double contrast arthrogram demonstrating an air-fluid level and the proximal extension of the joint (arrow)

Both extension and flexion beyond these points will increase the intra-articular pressure. Accordingly, the patient will place the knee in this position to minimize pain. De Andrade et al. have shown that distension of the knee (as by either an effusion or synovial hypertrophy) will weaken the quadriceps and as the intra-articular pressure increases, the ability to perform straight leg raising decreases to the point of failure.[18] In this same study, electromyographic activity in the quadriceps decreased as the intra-articular pressure was increased, indicating that the loss of function was due to quadriceps weakness, probably on a reflex basis and not due to a mechanical disadvantage because of the distension. It is thus suggested that a distended knee leads to quadriceps atrophy and further, that attempts to strengthen the quadriceps in a distended knee will not only increase pain but be also ineffectual.

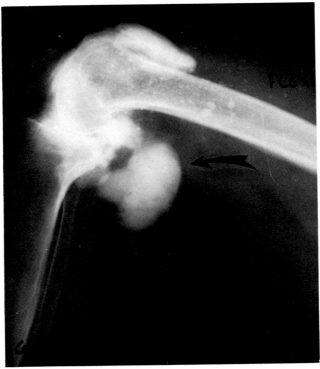

Fig. 18-4. An arthrogram demonstrating a popliteal cyst (arrow), but which in this patient has not ruptured.

Deformities

A normal knee is centered on and perpendicular to the mechanical axis of the limb. The mechanical axis of the limb is a straight line from the center of the femoral head to the center of the ankle (Fig. 18-5). The line of action of the body weight is a line from the center of gravity, just anterior to the second sacral vertebra, which converges with the mechanical axis at the center of the ankle. The long axis of the femur intersects with the long axis of the tibia at the center of the knee to form a valgus angle of five to seven degrees, males having a slightly smaller angle than females. Since the horizontal plane of the knee joint is perpendicular to the mechanical axis and the center of the ankle, valgus of the knee is determined by the shape of the femur as the long axis of the femoral shaft intersects with the mechanical axis. A femoral-tibial angle of greater than seven degrees is a valgus deformity and an angle of less than five degrees is a varus deformity. In all joint deformities, valgus orientation is lateral and varus orientation is medial. It must be emphasized that the point of reference is not the joint but the distal limb of the angle. For example, in bow legs, genu varum, the knee is lateral to the mechanical axis but the distal limb is directed medially; hence, a varus deformity. A "windswept" deformity, in which the right knee is in valgus and the left in varus is shown (Fig. 18-6). Valgus deformities tend to predominate in the patients with rheumatoid arthritis and are frequently associated with an external rotation deformity, whereas varus deformities are more commonly seen in noninflammatory joint disease.

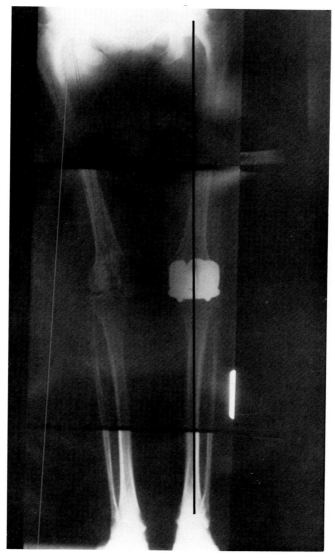

Fig. 18-5. The mechanical axis of the limb. In this patient, the knee replacement was properly centered on the mechanical axis and is parallel with the ground.

A fixed inability to extend the knee is a flexion deformity or a flexion contracture (Fig. 18-7). A greater than normal amount of extension is logically hyperextension or a recurvation deformity (Fig. 18-8). An extensor lag is the difference between active and passive extension. Internal rotation deformities, because of joint disease of the knee, are rarely present. The explanation for this is not clear but most likely the externally oriented axis of motion in the ankle joint and the predilection for hip disease to produce external rotation deformities would seem to be important.

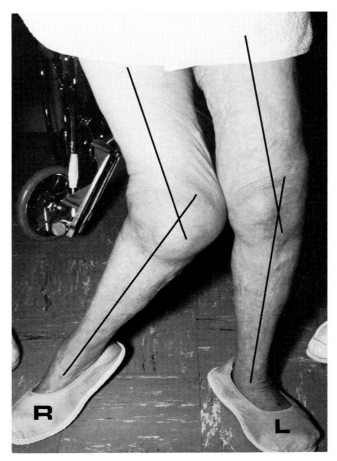

Fig. 18-6. A "windswept" deformity with marked valgus angulation on the right and a varus deformity on the left. The valgus deformity appears to be more severe but since physiologic valgus angulation is approximately seven degrees, this is added to the varus and subtracted from the valgus angulation to describe the degree of displacement from normal.

Patella alta and patella infra are terms used to designate the relative height of the patella with respect to the insertion of the patellar tendor into the tibial tubercle. A high riding patella (patella alta) is thought to be significant in the etiology of chondromalacia of the patella and recurrent subluxation, which may lead to chondromalacia patellae. A low riding patella (patella infra) has been related to Osgood-Schlatter's disease. In some patients, the diagnosis is quite clear but in more subtle cases and in surgical realignment precise measurements are needed. Blumensaat's line was long the standard method of measurement. Blumensaat's method[4] requires a lateral radiograph of the knee in 30° of flexion. A line is projected anteriorly from the intercondylor notch and in a normal knee this line should intercept the lower pole of the patella. Exact positioning is hard to achieve in most clinical centers, but in addition the method is not accurate.[20] Insall and Salvati

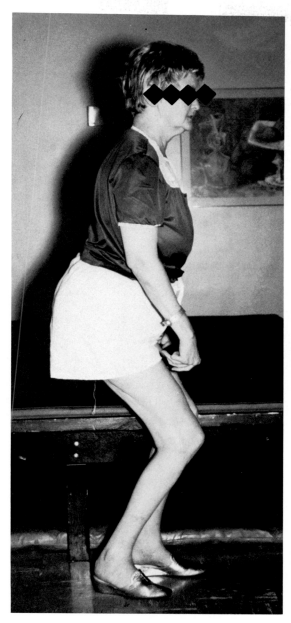

Fig. 18-7. Bilateral fixed flexion deformities of the hips and knees. The patient is unable to walk because of a precarious balance and mechanical disadvantage requiring more quadriceps strength than she can generate.

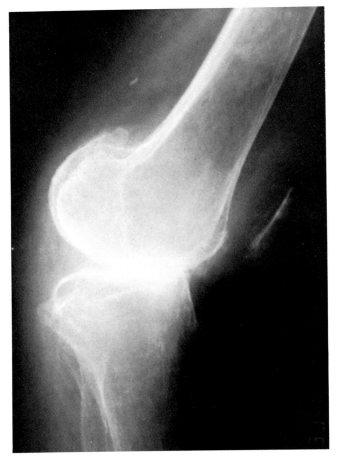

Fig. 18-8.   A recurvatum deformity resulting from long-standing rheumatoid arthritis and quadriceps weakness.

have demonstrated that the length of the patella is approximately equal to the length of the ligamentum patellae (patellar tendon) regardless of the size of the patient.[19] To account for variations in size, the measurements are expressed as a ratio of the length of the patellar tendon to that of the patella as an index of patellar height. A ratio of greater than 1.0 indicates an abnormally high patella (patella alta) and a low ratio, a low riding patella (patella infra). In their measurements, the average value of the ratio LT:LP was 1.02 with a mean standard deviation of 0.13 (Fig. 18-9).

The Q angle is the angle formed by two lines overlying the patellar tendon and the shaft of the femur, which intersect at the patella. Exact figures for normal are not available because of the difficulty in establishing precise landmarks but it is a relative relationship that influences patellar tracking in the supracondylar groove. A low Q angle is rarely of clinical significance but a high Q angle is associated with recurrent subluxation of the patella and is frequently seen in the patient with rheumatoid arthritis in which valgus, external rotation deformities, are quite common. It is a particularly important concept in total knee replacements in that failure to recognize the effect of a high Q angle on patellar

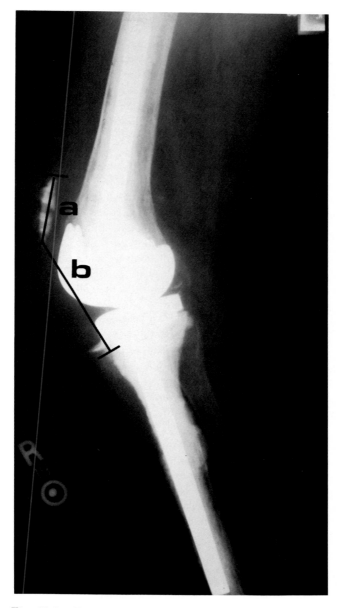

Fig. 18-9. Patella alta after total knee replacement causing a large extensor lag. The length of the patella tendon (B) is greater than the length of the patella (A). The tendon:patella ratio is 3.5:1.8 = 1.94.

tracking and, hence, failure to do an adequate lateral release of the quadriceps mechanism will result in dislocation of the patella or, at a minimum, subluxation (Fig. 18-10).

The patellar inhibition test is a useful way to assess the status of the patellofemoral joint particularly in chondromalacia and degenerative joint disease but less so in the rheumatoid patient. In this test (PIT), the quadriceps is relaxed, the patella moved distally between the thumb and index finger but not forced against the femur. The patient is then instructed to contract the quadriceps. Normally, the patient will be able to pull the patella through the examiner's light grasp. Immediate relaxation of the quadriceps or a series of quick ineffectual contractions is indicative of disease of the patellofemoral articulation.

Instability

Instability of the knee is due to a deficiency of the ligament supporting structures, to loss of hard tissue (cartilage and bone) or to a combination of both. Stability on the medial side of the knee is provided primarily by the tibial collateral ligament, which if deficient, will allow increased valgus motion to stress. Likewise, a loss of bone and cartilage in the lateral compartment will allow increased valgus motion. In a similar manner, the fibular collateral ligament, along with the iliotibial band, provides lateral stability to stress, directed medially. Increased medial motion will result from a loss of bone and cartilage in the medial compartment as well as to a deficiency of the lateral soft tissue structures.

In joint disease, in contrast of traumatic injuries, the collateral ligaments are rarely completely destroyed but are elongated due to chronic stretch. the anterior cruciate ligament is the exception to this generalization. The anterior cruciate ligament is frequently absent in advanced rheumatoid disease but less so in the degenerative knee. The diagnostic distinction between hard and soft tissue instability is sometimes difficult but by palpation of the ligaments when stressing the joint, one can usually detect a tightness of the ligament at the physiologic position and then detect a further increase in the deformity as the knee "falls into a hole." Anterior cruciate instability is usually quite apparent when doing an anterior drawer test, the tibia is drawn forward with the knee flexed. Classically, this maneuver has been done at 90° of flexion. Recently, Lachman has shown that a position of 30° of flexion, when looking for anterior cruciate deficiency, is more accurate and reproducible.

Posterior subluxation of the tibia on the femur is a deformity particularly common in juvenile rheumatoid arthritis (JRA) and hemophiliac arthritis (Fig. 18-11). Although the mechanism is not exactly clear, it is well known that inflammation about an open epiphyseal plate (the physis) alters the size and shape of the epiphysis of the distal femur and proximal tibia. Since JRA and hemophiliac arthropathy are the two major nonseptic joint diseases in the growing child with open physis, it seems likely that the effect of chronic inflammation on the physis plays a role. Posterior tibial subluxation in the adult is usually a manifestation of a long standing flexion deformity. It is difficult to identify posterior tibial subluxation with the knee flexed and it usually is not apparent until the deformity is passively corrected or at the time of arthroplasty when it becomes necessary to extensively release the posterior capsule and cruciate ligament to provide full extension. In an uncontrolled, unpublished study, 20 normal knee joints were x-rayed at a position of 30° to 60° of flexion (unpublished data). A line was drawn along the posterior border of the tibia and extended proximally across the femoral condyles. In these 20 knees, this line as 10–20 mm anterior to the most posterior portion of the femoral condyle. A line less than 10mm anterior to the posterior border of the femoral condyle is thought to represent subluxation (Fig. 18-12).

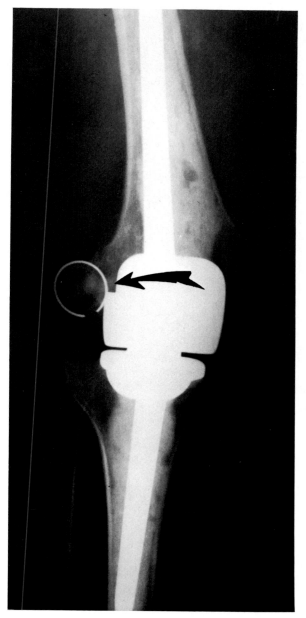

Fig. 18-10. Lateral dislocation of the patella following inadequate lateral release when the knee was replaced. The metal ring is a marker wire incorporated in the polyethylene patellar button.

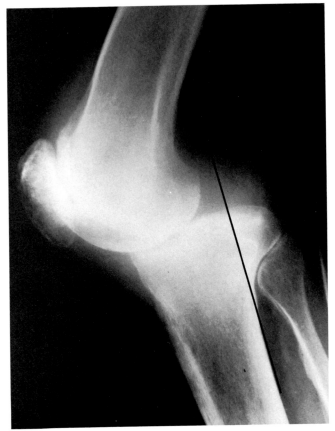

Fig. 18-11. Posterior subluxation of the tibia that is readily apparent radiographically.

DIAGNOSIS AND TREATMENT

Noninflammatory Joint Disease

Osteoarthritis

The causes of osteoarthritis are multiple but can be summarized as an imbalance between the stress applied and the ability of the joint to successfully tolerate this stress. In many patients, the inciting event is quite clear. Malalignment of fractures and childhood deformities will shift the mechanical axis of the limb to cause asymmetric loading which, in time, leads to cartilage failure on the overloaded side. In others, the precipitating cause is more direct, such as cartilage damage caused by a torn meniscus or an osteochondral fracture, while in many patients no apparent cause can be found.

The diagnosis of osteoarthritis is based on the history, characteristic physical findings and confirmed radiographically. The onset is usually slow and intermittent with good days and bad, followed by an unpredictable rate of progression in which pain increases and

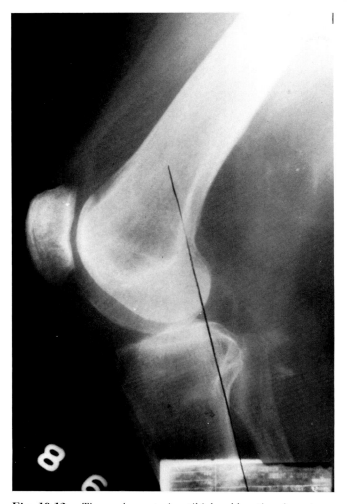

Fig. 18-12. The early posterior tibial subluxation is not so apparent on this radiograph. The reference line drawn along the posterior cortex of the tibia lies posterior to its usual ten to twenty millimeters anterior to the posterior-most aspect of the femoral condyle.

function decreases. Pain occurs primarily with weight-bearing and is usually relieved by rest. Early in the course of the disease, the patient will relate increased pain and stiffness after excessive activity such as in the evening or the next day. Later, activities are curtailed in an effort to avoid pain and a meaningful assessment can be obtained by ascertaining what activities are avoided because of anticipation of pain. Stiffness in the morning and after rest, as in sitting in a theater, is characteristic, but distinctly different than the morning stiffness of rheumatoid arthritis. The patient with osteoarthritis has stiffness in the specific joint rather than the total limb or body stiffness of the rheumatoid patient. In addition, the stiffness is relatively brief, i.e., 15–20 minutes, as compared with rheumatoid stiffness, which lasts one to three hours, depending upon the degree of disease activity. A

brief period of exercise or a hot shower usually is sufficient to "loosen up" an osteoarthritic knee.

Angulatory deformities also tend to be disease specific. Osteoarthritic knees are more likely to have a varus deformity, whereas in the rheumatoid patient, valgus deformities, combined with fixed external rotation, are more common. Early in the course of the disease, effusions are common and, at times, quite large. The synovial fluid is clear but exhibits a variable amount of particulate debris (Fig. 18-13). The total white blood cell count will usually be between one and three thousand cells per cubic millimeter and will be predominantly monocytes. the synovial fluid glucose will be approximately equal to the serum level.

Synovial hypertrophy is not marked but popliteal cysts are frequent. As in rheumatoid arthritis, the presence of a popliteal cyst is not an isolated phenomenon but is a secondary manifestation of the underlying joint disease. Instability, most usually an opening medially to valgus stress, is frequently present. Patellofemoral involvement is quite common and is identified by painful crepitation and often a positive patellar inhibition test. Crepitation at the patellar femoral joint itself is not necessarily indicative of degenerative disease as it is often seen in completely asymptomatic joints.

The radiographic findings in osteoarthritis can be summarized as hypertrophic with narrowing of the joint space the earliest change seen. Weight-bearing radiographs are essential to identify subtle narrowing and the presence of a flexion deformity invalidates an assessment of narrowing. The x-ray beam must be aligned parallel to the joint space to adequately assess joint space narrowing. Most technicians do not make this adjustment in the presence of a flexion deformity. In addition to narrowing, sclerosis or increased density of the subchondral bone is an early manifestation. Later in the natural progression, osteophytes and cysts appear. Osteophytes, which are an attempt at repair, develop at the chondro-osseous junction. Articular cartilage is unable, or at best poorly able, to repair itself. Hypertrophic new bone (osteophytes), subchondral sclerosis, and capsular thickening will lead to a progressive loss of motion with complete ankylosis the ultimate goal. Nature's way to relieve the pain of joint disease is to eliminate the joint rather than to repair the damage. Intraosseous cysts develop in the weight-bearing portions of the joint. Whether these cysts are due to failure of the subchondral plate and subsequent intrusion of synovial fluid into the bone or are secondary to an osseous mechanism, perhaps intraosseous venous hypertension is a question for debate. They are, however, a manifesta-

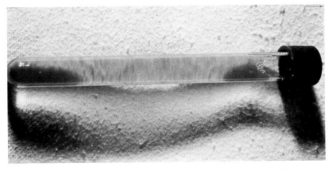

Fig. 18-13. Synovial fluid obtained from an osteoarthritic knee. Abnormal because of the amount of debris present but still essentially clear.

tion of advanced disease and, if extensive, lead to collapse of subchondral bone, which magnifies both pain and deformity.

The treatment of osteoarthritis of the knee is either operative or nonoperative and the indications for surgical treatment are based primarily on the response to medical management. Salicylates and nonsteroidal anti-inflammatory medication are the mainstays of medical management and the response to these drugs is poorly correlated with the initial radiographic appearance of the joint. Early in the natural history of the disease, symptoms are usually quite moderate for a considerable length of time (three to five years or more) and many patients will treat themselves with over-the-counter medications on a sporadic basis. Later, when symptoms and disability become more constant, a regular dosage schedule is needed. Intra-articular corticosteriods are especially helpful in selected cases, but there is no place for treatment with systemic corticosteriods. The knee that responds well to intra-articular steroids has a significant inflammatory component. Inflammation of the knee, as by increased warmth and swelling, an effusion and possible a popliteal cyst, will initially become quite quiescent after a single steroid injection.

The use of intra-articular steroids requires further comment. It has been well-demonstrated that corticosteriods adversely affect the metabolism of articular cartilage. The syntheses of glycosaminoglycans as well as collagen is impaired. In addition, injudicious use has clinically led to accelerated joint destruction, which has been labeled steroid or Charcot-like arthropathy. These considerations, however, do not mean that intra-articular steroids should be avoided. In the patient who is still symptomatic despite regular medication and in whom operative treatment is the only alternative, the use of intra-articular steroids may well maintain function and relieve pain for a considerable period.

The indications for operative treatment are based on a lack of response to medical management in a patient in whom the expected benefits are appreciably outweighed by the risks, complications, and long-term results of the surgical procedure. The specific procedure elected is primarily a function of the severity of the joint destruction. The possibilities in order of increasing magnitude and of surgical complexity are: arthroscopic lavage and chondral abrasion; osteotomy of the proximal tibia; total knee replacement; and arthrodesis.

Arthroscopic abrasion arthroplasty is a relatively new tool in the operative treatment of osteoarthritis. It has been long suspected that lavage of an arthritic joint will provide transient although sometimes prolonged relief of symptoms. An early review of a series of diagnostic arthroscopies has shown that approximately 50 percent of patients will be improved following a diagnostic arthroscopic examination in which lavage with two to three liters of saline is routine.[21] Abrasion arthroplasty is an extension but a distinctly different concept than the previously performed open debridement and drilling of subchondral bone first suggested by Pridie. Debridement and drilling, although done occasionally in selected patients, rarely achieved sufficient improvement to make this a widely popular procedure. This procedure was based on the concept that drilling (opening up) the subchondral bone stimulates the formation of a fibrocartilagenous "resurfacing." This concept has been demonstrated experimentally and clinically, but rarely has it resulted in lasting relief of symptoms (Fig. 18-14A,B).

Abrasion arthroplasty, as now proposed via the arthroscope, is a distinctly different concept. In this procedure, exposed eburnated bone, is "abraded" to expose and facilitate expansion of the intraosseous blood supply, which is said to resurface the areas of bone denuded of cartilage. Despite the seemingly physiologic paradox in which experimental

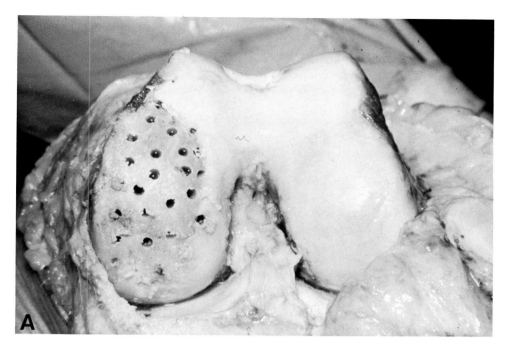

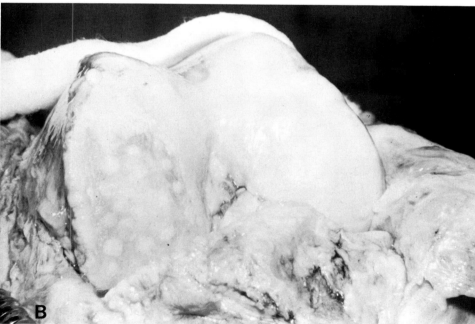

Fig. 18-14. (A) Debridement of localized osteoarthritis of the medial femoral condyle and drilling of the subchondral plate. (B) One year later at that time of knee replacement. Soft fibrocartilage, but not hyaline cartilage, has filled in the drilled defects but has not resulted in a complete resurfacing.

work in animals suggests that no benefit would be derived from such a procedure, early clinical series are reporting quite excellent relief of pain. The long term value of abrasion arthroplasty is, however, still to be demonstrated and whether this procedure will become an established procedure for early disease or fall by the wayside remains to be determined.

Osteotomy of the tibia between the proximal joint surface of the tibia and the tibial tubercle is a well-established procedure. The clinical results are, however, heavily dependent upon two factors: patient selection and surgical skill in obtaining precise realignment. In high tibial osteotomy (HTO), a triangular wedge of bone is excised with the base opposite the direction of the tibial deformity or a dome-shaped osteotomy is done without removing bone. The distal tibia is then realigned perpendicular to the tibial surface and immobilized until union occurs. The margin of error is small and the ease by which undercorrection or overcorrection can be produced is well recognized.

Equally, or perhaps more important than surgical precision, is the need to properly select patients for this procedure rather than the alternative, which is joint replacement. The ideal patient for an HTO is young, has joint disease confined to the medial compartment (with a varus deformity) and does not have an inflammatory component. Older patients do poorly because of the immobilization and patients with valgus deformities rarely obtain a satisfactory result. The indications for osteotomy in the patient with rheumatoid arthritis are extremely rare and are based on factors not relating to the joint disease.

Total knee replacement is by far the most common procedure done for osteoarthritis. Over the past 14 years since its inception, there have been multiple improvements in design, cement technique and surgical skill to the point that a success rate of 80–90 percent is predictable. The most serious early complications are postoperative sepsis and deep vein thrombosis and, late, the risk of bone cement interface failure, which leads to loosening. The surgery is elective and is undertaken when, in the view of both the surgeon and the patient, the expected benefits outweigh the risks. A prerequisite to a surgical decision is the demonstrated failure of nonoperative management.

The recent introduction of cementless fixation has stimulated a great deal of interest and enthusiasm in the orthopedic community. Cementless fixation is by biologic fixation, whether bone or fibrous tissue, is still controversial. Multiple metal beads or titanium mesh is sintered onto the surface of the implants to create a porous surface into which bone and/or fibrous tissue grows to provide a biologic fixation. There has been extensive experimental work done over the past 15 years that supports this concept, and early clinical results are quite excellent. The ideal patient is the young, large, active individual in whom the risk of loosening with conventional cement technique is unduly high. There are two very significant concerns that have not yet been clarified but must be resolved before this technique receives widespread acceptance. The technical process of applying the beads or mesh requires that the prosthesis be heated almost to the melting point. This process markedly reduces the fatigue life of the implant and fatigue fractures of the prosthesis are a real threat. The large surface area produced by placing the mesh or beads on the implant raises again the spector of metal sensitivity due to a marked increase in metal ion release. Whether either or both of these concerns become significant is yet to be demonstrated.

Arthrodesis of the knee, in view of the success rates of knee replacement that are well known by the lay public, is rarely done as a primary procedure but is frequently indicated as a salvage procedure. The most common indication is sepsis following knee replacement. In some circumstances, a two-stage procedure is necessary. That is, an initial debridement followed by the definitive arthrodesis but in most cases a one-stage procedure is feasible. Success rates of arthrodesis following knee replacement are directly proportional to the amount of bone stock remaining. The less bone sacrificed at the time of the initial surgery, the greater the rate of union.

Calcium Pyrophosphate Deposition Disease

Calcium pyrophosphate deposition disease (CPDD), or pseudogout is a particular type of crystal synovitis that is associated with a high incidence of osteoarthritic changes. The radiographic changes are sometimes severe enough to suggest a neuropathic joint. Although a crystal synovitis that simulates classic gout in the early stages, CPDD may present initially as characteristic osteoarthritis and the diagnosis is only made secondarily. The entity is suggested by chondrocalcinosis and severe degenerative changes radiographically. Calcification in the meniscus and articular cartilage is suggestive and is also seen in the symphysis pubis and triangular cartilage of the wrist. It must be kept in mind that calcification in articular cartilage is frequently seen in patients with diabetes and hyperparathyroidism in the absence of CPDD. The definitive diagnostic test is the identification of calcium pyrophosphate crystals in the synovial fluid, which are rhomboid in shape and are weakly positively birefringent when viewed with ultraviolet light. Uric acid crystals of classic gout are long needle-shaped crystals that are negatively birefringent.

The treatment of CPDD is essentially the same as for the osteoarthritic patient except that these patients seem to respond uniquely well to aspiration and intra-articular steroids. Frequently, aspiration alone will provide relief of pain and inflammation. Nonsteroidal, anti-inflammatory medication is also effective and should be tried despite the presence of advanced radiographic changes. It is not uncommon to achieve excellent relief of pain with nonsteriodal medication in these patients. The indications for knee replacement are the same as listed above. Because CPDD is a multicompartment disease, osteotomy is not indicated and because the need for surgical treatment tends to occur in older patients, arthrodesis is more rarely indicated than in the usual patient with osteoarthritis.

Neuropathic Arthropathy

The loss of proprioceptive and deep pain sensation in the knee as caused by tabes dorsalis, long-standing diabetes, and other chronic neurologic disorders is thought to produce the neuropathic or "Charcot" joint. The clinical presentation is quite distinctive. Pain is not severe and may be absent or insignificant. The knee is usually enlarged due to osseous overgrowth and synovial hypertrophy due to incorporation of bone and cartilage fragments. Large effusions are characteristic but inflammation is minimal or nonexistent. Instability and weight-bearing deformities, secondary to the instability, are the usual presenting complaints.

The radiographic appearance is striking and quite characteristic. Old subchondral fractures with repair are frequently seen. Much loss of articular bone but with marked osteophytic new bone and intracapsular bone are the usual radiographic features. The physical findings and radiographic changes in the absence of appreciable pain are suggestive. These findings combined with evidence of a neurologic deficit are sufficient to establish the diagnosis. It is not uncommon that the underlying neurologic deficit has not been previously recognized and the joint disease is the initial presentation that leads to the neurologic diagnosis. Neuropathic arthropathy secondary to diabetic neuropathy is much more common in the foot but does occur, usually as a late manifestation, in the knee.

Since instability rather than pain is the primary problem and also because of the frequently unsatisfactory results of surgical intervention, nonoperative treatment is preferred. The instability is usually correctable and orthotic management successful. A double upright orthosis is required because of activity unrestrained by pain. If surgical intervention becomes necessary, because of a failure of orthotic management, knee replacement is contraindicated. Acute sepsis and a Charcot joint are the two absolute contraindications for knee replacement. In almost all early series of knee replacement, one or two patients are included with neuropathic arthropathy and almost uniformly, the procedures failed. Recurrent instability, periprosthetic fracture, implant fracture, and premature loosening occurred. Accordingly, if surgical treatment is undertaken, arthrodesis with its attendant limitations, is the procedure of choice. In the past, the frequency of union after arthrodesis was considerably less than after arthrodesis for nonneuropathic disorders. With the use of contemporary methods of external fixation, the frequency of union should be improved but caution, with respect to outcome, is still advisable.

Osteonecrosis

Osteonecrosis, or as sometimes labeled avascular necrosis, occurs in either femoral condyle as well as the tibial plateau. Most of the recognized systemic causes, specifically, systemic corticosteroids, systemic lupus erythematosus, Caisson's disease, and the hemoglobinopathies, which are more likely to cause osteonecrosis of the femoral head, also affect the knee. The femoral condyles are most frequently involved but similar lesions have been reported in the tibial plateau (Fig. 18-15).

A new syndrome recently has been identified and labeled "spontaneous osteonecrosis of the knee" by Ahlback et al.[1] This syndrome occurs primarily in elderly patients and, in the great majority of cases, the lesion is localized in the central portion of the medial femoral condyle. Radiographically, the lesion is similar to the adolescent-occurring osteochondritis dessicans, which occurs, however, not in the central portion but in the lateral (intercondylar notch) portion of the medial femoral condyle and is widely believed to be traumatic in origin (Fig. 18-16). Spontaneous osteonecrosis (SON) is unique to older patients with an average age in the mid-sixties, has a characteristic presentation, and is easily overlooked.

The onset is quite acute, spontaneous in nature, and not associated with trauma. In contrast to the intermittent onset of osteoarthritis, the patient with SON remembers specifically the time and place of onset. The pain is perceived medially and there is tenderness along the medial joint line or the medial femoral condyle. If seen at the time of the onset, the knee will be swollen, acutely tender and lack a full range of motion, especially a limitation of terminal extension that might suggest a locked meniscus. Radiographs are initially normal or demonstrate early osteoarthritic changes, which in both cases would lead to an erroneous diagnosis. Autopsy studies have shown that degenerative tears of the medial meniscus are quite common in this age group, presumably most of them are asymptomatic, and acute meniscal tears are most usually secondary to recognized indirect trauma.[33] The radiographic findings of early osteoarthritis does not exclude the diagnosis and the clinical presentation is distinctly different.

There are two essential considerations necessary to establish a diagnosis. The first and most important is a high incidence of suspicion and secondly, the need to obtain a radionuclide scan. The acute onset and physical findings suggest a torn meniscus, which may be further implied by negative radiographs, but the age of the patient and the

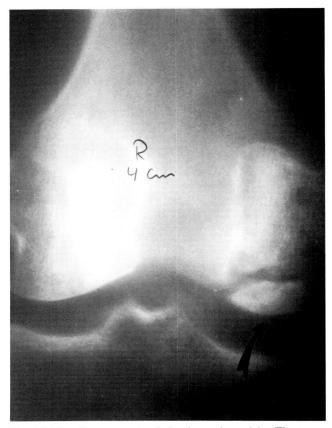

Fig. 18-15. Osteonecrosis of the femoral condyle. The tomogram shows the separated necrotic fragment (arrow). This patient had undergone a renal transplant and received high doses of corticosteriods. She also had ostenoecrosis of the opposite knee and both femoral heads.

mechanism of onset should immediately raise the question. Radionuclide imaging with technetium 99-labeled EHDP will show increased uptake over the affected condyle early in the course of the disease and before there are any radiographic findings.

Initial treatment is conservative and in six months approximately two thirds of the patients will be much improved, but still symptomatic with an occasional but persistent dull ache. Most of these patients will eventually demonstrate a radiographic defect and approximately one third will develop or show progressive changes of osteoarthritis.[38]

Conservative management consists of aspiration of the effusion, protected and restricted weight-bearing, anti-inflammatory agents and analgesics. Resistive isometric quadriceps exercises are commonly employed and thought to be beneficial but the rationale is not apparent. Approximately one third of patients, especially those with larger radiographic lesions will have persistent symptoms for more than six months and as further collapse occurs, are likely to develop angulatory deformities, mostly varus. These patients may require surgical treatment.

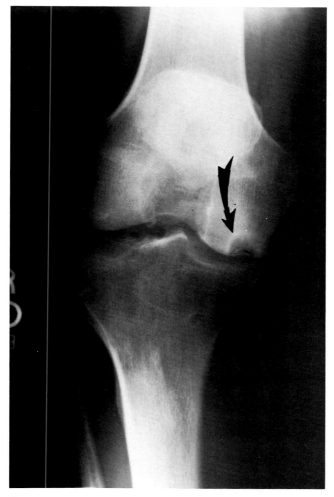

Fig. 18-16. Spontaneous osteonecrosis of the medial femoral condyle in a 78-year-old male. An arthroscopic debridement was done for early osteoarthritis before the lesion was apparent radiographically. A scan was not done.

The surgical options have been narrowed to two procedures.[25,38] High tibial osteotomy combined with an arthrotomy to remove possible loose fragments and drilling of the osteonecrotic crater is preferable in the young, more active patient. In the older, less active patient, complete knee replacement is the procedure of choice. Arthrotomy and drilling without osteotomy does not alter the natural course of the disease and unicondylar replacement has, until just recently, fallen into disfavor for unicompartmental disease.

A third alternative, which is conceptually attractive but still experimental may prove, in the future, to be beneficial for these patients. Osteochondral allografting is now technically feasible and may be suitable for the younger patients before the onset of an angulatory deformity. If the results of allografting warrant, it may be appropriate to shorten the time of conservative treatment in that the long-term expectations in the younger patients are much less optimistic when treated conservatively than in the more elderly sedentary patient.

Hemophilic Arthropathy

Joint destruction secondary to repeated intra-articular bleeding in childhood and adolescence is the most common and most disabling aspect of hemophilia in the adult. The mechanism of the joint destruction is not completely understood but at least three mechanisms have been implicated. It has been demonstrated that synovial cells isolated from hemophilic synovium release a neutral proteinase capable of degrading the protein core of the glycosaminoglycans of articular cartilage. In addition, these cells also released collagenase in quantities comparable to similar studies of rheumatoid synovium.[29] The mechanical factors relating to the joint destruction are thought to be a combination of the destructive effects of intra-articular blood and the collapse of subchondral cysts, which develop after intraosseous bleeding.[7,17] In addition, growth deformities of the epiphysis occur secondary to repeated bleeding, which results in synovitis causing increased blood flow around the physis during growth (Fig. 18-17). Ankylosis is frequent in the adult, but this is more usually a manifestation of treatment in childhood than the natural course of the disease. In the days before frozen cryoprecipitate and Factor VIII availability, it was common practice to treat intra-articular bleeding with splints and casts and deformities with traction and hinged casts. Frequently, these practices led to ankylosis of the joint.

Hemophilic arthropathy is most frequently seen in the knee although any diarthrodial joint may be subject to spontaneous bleeding. Prevention or immediate treatment, usually

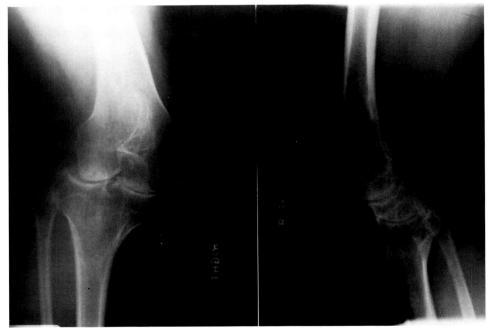

Fig. 18-17.   Hemophilic arthropathy in an adult. The joint space narrowing, posterior and lateral subluxation and deformity, secondary to growth distrubance, are well demonstrated.

self-administered, with Factor VIII concentrate is effective and aspiration of an acute hemarthrosis is rarely indicated. Physical measures are still important but serial casting and splinting, if necessary, should be minimized and combined with a regular exercise regime designed to maintain the range of motion. As in all knee disorders, the whole quadriceps muscle is at risk of disuse atrophy. Resistive isometric quadriceps exercises in maximum extension are essential.

In the adult, recurrent intra-articular bleeding as a result of proliferative synovitis or advanced joint destruction is much more common than that of trauma or spontaneous occurrence and may require large doses of Factor VIII for control. If the articular surface is well preserved, angulatory deformities have not developed and there is a good range of motion, spnovectomy will markedly reduce the number of bleeding episodes.[30,41] Factor VIII coverage is required in the perioperative period and it is our practice to maintain factor levels at 100 percent for approximately 10 to 14 days postoperatively and longer if aggressive physical therapy is continued or manipulation undertaken.

In the face of severe artricular damage, contractural deformities, and limited motion, a synovectomy is not indicated as recurrent synovitis and loss of motion can be antici- pated. These knees are best managed by knee replacement.[15] In the past, arthrodesis of severely destroyed knees was the common practice and, in some patients, may still be appropriate. These patients are usually relatively young, i.e., 20 to 60 years and the long- term success of conventional knee replacement with cement fixation is still a major concern, particularly with respect to loosening. Conversely, hemophilic arthropathy is not usually a monoarticular disease but involves also the joints adjacent to the knee most commonly the contralateral knee, the ankles and, occasionally, the hips. In this setting, arthrodesis, which transmits forces normally absorbed by the movable knee to the adja- cent joints, can be expected to accelerate the destruction of these adjacent joints.[11]

INFLAMMATORY JOINT DISEASE

Rheumatoid Arthritis

Pathogenesis of Joint Destruction

The immunopathology and enzymatic mechanisms responsible for joint destruction in rheumatoid arthritis is a highly complex and constantly changing subject due to the tremendous amount of investigative work that has occurred in recent years and continued at present. A simplified account is presented in the belief that one interested in the field should have a rudimentary understanding of the process.

The etiologic agent or agents responsible for the disease is unknown. It is commonly believed that synovium produces IgG, an immunoglobulin, in response to an unknown antigenic stimulus. Rheumatoid factor (IgM) combines with IgG to form an insoluble immune complex. This activates the complement system, causing increased vascular per- meability and reduced levels of complement in the synovial fluid. Polymorphonuclear leukocytes ingest the immune complex causing the release of lysosomal enzymes and other mediators of inflammation. The rheumatoid synovial tissue also releases large quantities of collagenase. These enzymes, in themselves, provoke an inflammatory reaction and are destructive to the cartilage by degrading collagen and splitting the proteoglycan mole- cules. Synovitis occurs in response to the antigenic stimulus and extends over the surface of the articular cartilage to erode both cartilage and bone at the periphery. As the synovial panus progresses over the articular surface and the lysosomal enzymes disrupt the proteoglycans, erosions occur at the osteochondral junction and the weakened articular cartilage can no longer withstand the stresses of normal use and is destroyed (Fig. 18-18).

The diagnosis of rheumatoid arthritis is based on the history, physical findings in the peripheral joints, characteristic serological tests, and radiographic findings. By the time the patient presents with knee problems the diagnosis is usually well established. The two major exceptions to this generalization are in the adolescent, who most frequently is a female, with monoarticular juvenile rheumatoid arthritis (JRA) and septic arthritis. In both situations, an analysis of the synovial fluid is essential.

Monoarticular JRA, a benign disease that rarely progresses to characteristic polyarticular rheumatoid arthritis in the adult, is usually a self-limited process that responds well to medical management and rarely results in long-term joint destruction. The importance, however, of establishing an accurate diagnosis cannot be overestimated. The need for an accurate diagnosis is not so much to assure appropriate treatment but, conversely, to avoid inappropriate treatment. These patients present with none of the historical symptoms of rheumatoid arthritis. They have no physical findings in the peripheral joints and are young, usually active adolescents. In this setting, a traumatic injury is much more commonly seen and an inflammatory disease less frequently considered. The patient presents with swelling, an effusion, mild inflammation, and can usually relate the symptoms to

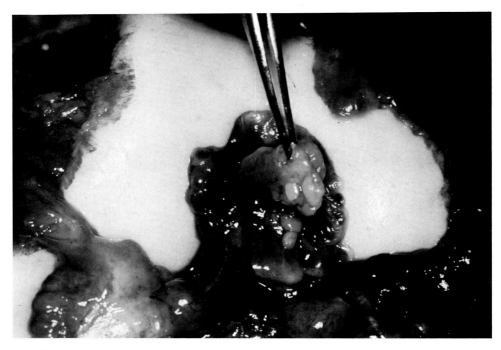

Fig. 18-18. Hypertrophic synovitis in rheumatoid arthtiris. Panus is seen creeping over the articular cartilage at the osteochondral junction. The villonodular features of the synovial hypertrophy are seen in the intracondylar notch. The forceps are picking up the necrotic nodules that have outgrown their blood supply and will drop off into the joint to become known as rice bodies.

some minor traumatic event. Furthermore, the initial complaint will frequently be a "sprained or twisted" knee, and the initial diagnosis may well be a sprained or partially torn collateral ligament, overuse syndrome a torn meniscus, or even septic arthritis. Radiographs will be negative except for soft tissue swelling. Once started in this misguided direction, plaster immobilization, arthroscopy and even meniscectomy or surgical drainage are likely to follow. Aspiration of the effusion and synovial fluid analysis will show an increased leukocyte count with more than normal polynuclear cells, perhaps a lowered glucose level, and negative cultures. This information should lead to an accurate diagnosis and avoid the mistakes of inappropriate treatment.

Treatment of the adult rheumatoid knee is initially systemic with anti-inflammatory medication supplemented by local measures such as splinting, prophylactic exercises, and instruction in joint protection. The response to systemic management dictates the course of further intervention. If the patient responds poorly or incompletely, specific treatment for the knee is initiated. The judicious use of intra-articular corticosteroids, in addition to systemic management, frequently is a valuable adjunct and may in many patients delay the need for more aggressive intervention. The reluctance to use intra-articular steroids when surgical intervention is the alternative seems overemphasized. Conversely, repeated injections in the face of a limited or short-term response is equally inappropriate and, at this point, surgical management should be considered.

The indications for operative intervention are relative and based on a consideration of the previous response to medical management, the degree and disabling nature of the knee pain, the degree of functional loss due to limited motion, instability or deformity, and the needs of the patient. In the patient with polyarticular joint disease, the effect of the knee disease on the adjacent joints and the possible need for multiple joint procedures must be considered.

Synovectomy has been a favored, very popular procedure in Europe for the past 40 years. In the United States, the procedure was frequently undertaken in the 1950s and 1960s. For the past 10 to 12 years, however, synovectomy of the knee has been done only rarely in the United States. The two primary reasons for the decline in interest in this procedure are the availability and ability of the rheumatologist to control inflammation until the joint destruction is beyond that in which a synovectomy can be successfully done and the steadily improving reliability of knee replacement. Recently, there has been a renewed interest in synovectomy with arthroscopic techniques. The results are preliminary and a small number of patients have undergone the procedure. Open synovectomy requires intensive postoperative rehabilitation, 10–20 days of hospitalization, and a loss of motion frequently occurs. If arthroscopic synovectomy and outpatient physical therapy can achieve short-term results comparable to those obtained with open synovectomy, the procedure will undoubtedly be done in greater numbers.

In the presence of advanced joint destruction, instability and deformity, knee replacement is the procedure of choice as compared to the alternative arthrodesis. Because of the forces transmitted to adjacent joints following arthrodesis and the presence of future polyarticular disability in rheumatoid arthritis, arthrodesis is rarely indicated. In the presence of septic destruction, however, knee replacement is contraindicated and even in the rheumatoid patient arthrodesis may be necessary.

Postoperative management of a knee replacement consists of early range of motion, both active and passive, quadriceps rehabilitation, and quadriceps protection by splinting. Active motion is started within one to two days of surgery and, in many institutions, continuous passive motion is begun in the recovery room. Quadriceps setting is started immediately and resistive isometric exercise is begun as soon as the patient is able. The knee is protected with a posterior splint until good quadriceps control is achieved.

The initiation of weight bearing is highly variable among different institutions. There is some evidence that bone cement increases in strength for up to 48 hours after placement. Beyond this point, weight bearing to tolerance is allowed with appropriate quadriceps protection. If an uncemented technique is used, it is probably desirable to prevent weight bearing for three to six weeks after surgery. It is likely that earlier weight bearing will be allowed as more experience with uncemented knee replacement is obtained.

The question is often raised in the patient with polyarticular destruction in the lower extremities as to whether the hip or knee should be replaced first. In general, most surgeons recommend that the hip be done initially, although individual patient needs may dictate otherwise. The postoperative rehabilitation needs following hip replacement are minimal, whereas intense and prolonged physical therapy is required for a successful knee replacement. This intensive patient involvement is difficult to achieve in the presence of a painful hip and full knee extension during gait cannot be achieved until hip flexion contractures are corrected. Finally, patient motivation is critically important after knee replacement, but minimally important following hip replacement. Experience with the particular patient following replacement of the hip may be most helpful when knee replacement is a consideration.

Septic Arthritis

The superimposition of septic arthritis in a patient with established rheumatoid arthritis is not uncommon, frequently missed, and sometimes a difficult distinction to make. Patients with rheumatoid arthritis are especially susceptible to septic complications. The patient and the physician are accustomed to flares of the disease activity in isolated joints and they are treated with anti-inflammatory medication. All of these factors contribute to a clinical setting in which the possibility of sepsis is overlooked with disasterous effects on the joint and the patient. Avoidance of this pitfall requires a high index of suspicion in the presence of monoarticular flares and aggressive aspiration and synovial fluid analysis.

The total leukocyte count in a very active rheumatoid joint can be a high as 75,000 to 80,000 cells and a septic joint will usually have more than 100,000. In both, the polymorphonuclear cells will be close to 100 percent. The synovial fluid glucose in a septic joint will be zero or very low and it is unusual for the low glucose in a very active rheumatoid joint to be this low. There is, however, considerable overlap and a distinction cannot be made until cultures are completed. It should also be remembered that false negative cultures are not uncommon in septic arthritis. In these situations, i.e., when the synovial fluid analysis indicates a septic process before the culture results are available and when the cultures are returned as negative, treatment must be aggressive. Appropriate intravenous antibiotic and adequate drainage are imperative.

Pigmented Villonodular Synovitis

Pigmented villonodular synovitis is a monoarticular, or disease of marked synovial proliferation and, frequently, bone destruction. The extra-articular form may arise from the underlying joint or directly from the synovial lining of the tendon sheaths. The knee is, by far, the most commonly involved joint with the hip, and the ankle the next most frequently affected.

The synovial fluid is a dark chocolate brown, similar in color to chocolate agar used in microbiology. In addition, the large amount (100–300 cc) of fluid that can be aspirated is, in itself, quite characteristic. Arthrograms are also characteristic, demonstrating a very multiloculated appearance and a large effusion (Figs. 18-1 and 18-3). The synovium is very hypertrophic and is usually a dark chocolate brown much like the color of the synovial fluid (Fig. 18-19). The synovium is hypercellular with intra- and extracellular hemosiderin deposits and giant cells. The presence of giant cells is the primary distinguishing feature that separates this entity from hemophilic arthropathy.

The radiographic presence of bone destruction, which can be extensive, is frequently a diagnostic aid. The symptoms are usually mild and intermittent for some time before medical assistance is sought, but once osseous changes occur pain and disability rapidly increase and the radiographic changes progress more rapidly than in the more common inflammatory joint disease.

There is no medical treatment of any value and synovectomy is the preferred method of management. Synovectomy is, however, complicated by a recurrence rate of 16–48 percent.[5] Recurrent synovitis is usually treated by a repeat synovectomy although low dose radiation (1500–3000 r) has been used for recurrence in some cases.

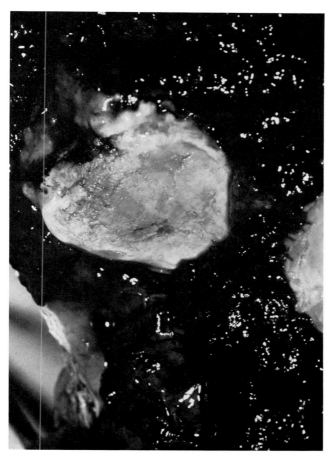

Fig. 18-19.   The synovium of pigmented villonodular synovitis surrounding the cruiate ligaments in the intercondylor notch.

TREATMENT MODALITIES

Rest and exercise are major treatment modalities for arthritis that have been used for several centuries. Rest and exercise predate modern drug therapy.

The major goals of conservative treatment of the knee are pain reduction or elimination and the prevention or reduction of deformity during the various stages of arthritis of the knee through the use of rest, exercise, and heat. The ability to eliminate pain and deformity depend on the diagnosis and will be more successful in some diagnoses than others. Examples are rheumatoid arthritis were damage to one or both knee joints is probably the most important causes of pain and disability as compared with pseudogout, which is less destructive but very painful.

Arthritis management can be subdivided into three main phases or stages; acute, subacute, and chronic. Conservative treatment varies more by phase than by diagnosis. Physical treatment of infectious arthritis is the same as that of acute rheumatoid arthritis with the addition of the appropriate antibiotic therapy. Rheumatoid arthritis and other inflammatory arthritis have frequent acute and subacute stages, whereas osteoarthritis is a slow progressive disease without acute exacerbation unless there has been superimposed trauma. The pain and symptoms of osteoarthritis tend to be nonacute or chronic.

The acute stage of any type of arthritis is treated with rest and maintenance of good knee alignment done by splinting of the knee in almost complete extension. Splints are made from plaster of Paris or lightweight molded plastic material, the latter tend to be more comfortable and washable. During the acute stage, the most comfortable position of the inflamed knee joint is in flexion, this position is to be avoided as the patient quickly develops knee flexion contractures from shortening of the hamstring and gastrocnemius muscle and the posterior capsule of the knee joint.

Knee joint mobility is maintained even during the acute stage by daily gentle range-of-motion exercises. The leg is supported by the therapist and the knee gently ranged with the therapist eliminating gravity and assisting the patient throughout the comfortable range of knee motion. This exercise is called active assisted exercise. After range of motion is completed, the knee is returned to the resting splint.

The physical therapist instructs the patient in the isometric exercises for the quadriceps and hamstring muscles to prevent muscle atrophy, which occurs quickly in muscles placed at rest. Isometric exercises are exercises performed by contracting a muscle without moving the joints to which the muscle is attached, i.e., no knee joint movement. This is an ideal form of exercise in arthritis as the strength around the joint is maintained or increased. This form of exercise differs from isotonic or isokinetic exercises where there is movement in the associated joint or body part. The patient is taught to perform the isometric contractions for 3–5 minutes each hour to prevent atrophy.

Heat is not applied to an inflamed swollen joint; cold may be tried as the patient tolerates. The major modes of treatment in the acute stage are rest, immobilization, gentle active assistive range-of-motion exercises to maintain range and isometric exercises.

The subacute phase is a transition period between the acute and chronic stages. The major goal in this phase is to increase mobility of the knee joint and progressively ambulate the patient without increasing knee joint pain and symptoms. Progression must be gradual to avoid a relapse.

Frequent assessment of the knee joint is done during treatment and problems relating to range-of-motion, strength, and deformity are noted. If the patient did develop knee flexion contractures during the acute phase, then serial casting is a consideration. With serial casting the knee is casted in maximum extension and the splint or cast changed

Margaret M. Portwood

19

The Foot and Ankle in Rheumatic Disorders

The joints of the foot and ankle are affected in most patients who suffer from a rheumato-logic disorder. The actual percentage of people affected is determined by the type of the disease. In Vainio's study of 1000 patients with rheumatoid arthritis foot and/or ankle involvement was found in 85 percent of men, 91 percent of women, and 69 percent of children,[27] while 50 percent of Reiter's patients diagnosed and studied by Chand et al. were found to have foot and/or ankle involvement.[4] Ankylosing spondylitis usually affects the axial skeleton but Achilles bursitis or inflammation of the small joints of the foot may occur. Acute gouty arthritis will affect the great toe in 90 percent of patients at some time during the course of the disease.[28] Other joints of the foot and the ankle joint will also be affected but less frequently. As there is a difference in incidence of involvement of the foot and ankle among the various disorders there is also a difference in trend of specific joint and soft tissue involvement.

FUNCTIONAL ANATOMY

To understand the effect of rhematologic disorders on the foot and thereby on function, it is necessary to have familiarity with the structural components of the foot.

The ankle-foot complex is a specialized structure in bipedal man as compared to the more generalized functional unit, the wrist and hand. Only the gorilla shows a similar specialization of structure. The structural unit provides a strong, stable platform that can bear the total weight of the body during standing and ambulation and also provides a base for propulsion during the latter activity. In order to accomodate a variety of terrain, the structure must also be flexible. These requirements are satisfied by the medial and lateral longitudinal arches and the transverse arch. These arches are maintained through intact bony structure and soft tissue support. Derangement of either component will weaken stability and flexibility of the foot causing abnormal gait patterns and/or pain.

For simplification the ankle-foot complex can be divided into four major components; ankle, hindfoot, midfoot and forefoot (Fig. 19-1). The ankle is formed by the articulating surfaces of the distal tibia, the lateral malleolar portion of the fibula, and the talus. The

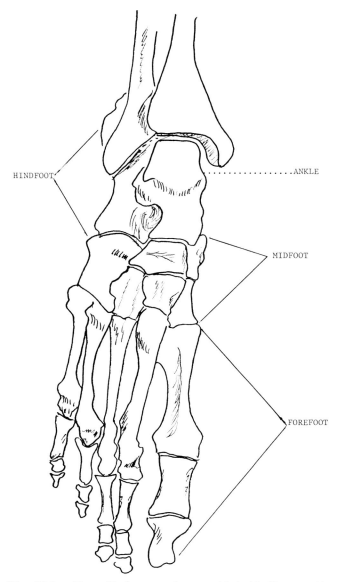

Fig. 19-1.   The ankle foot complex: a. ankle b. hindfoot c. midfoot d. forefoot

hindfoot consists of the talus, the calcaneus and the synovial joints between them and the
bones of the midfoot. The midfoot is made of the navicula, the cuboid, and the medial,
middle, and lateral cuneiform with their respective joints. The five metatarsals, two
sesamoids and the phalanges make up the forefoot.

The ankle joint is a deep-set hinge joint that allows dorsiflexion and plantar flexion
only, as contrasted to the wrist, which accomodates a greater variety of positions necessary
for hand activities. Because the talus is wedged shaped with the wider portion anterior,
and the narrower portion posterior, plantar flexion brings the narrow part of the talus into

the functional ankle joint. This allows for more lateral movement within the joint space, which with the relatively slack lateral ligaments accounts for the greater instability of the ankle in plantar flexion. The opposite is true for dorsiflexion when the joint space is narrower and the ligaments are tighter causing a more stable position. The weight of the body is transmitted through the tibial portion of the joint to the underlying talus and from there to the midfoot and forefoot.

The hindfoot accepts the weight of the body during the touch-down phase of ambulation and transmits the weight forward to the midfoot and forefoot. According to Hamilton and Ziemer, the intertarsal joints; the posterior talocalcaneal, the talocalcaneonavicular and the transverse tarsal joint, provide for inversion-eversion and pronation-supination of the foot. These accommodate the terrain and lock or unlock the tarsal bones for provision of a stable platform or a resilient lever.[10]

Inversion-eversion describes changes of the shape and position of the nonweight-bearing foot relative to the talus.[10] Inversion causes the foot to move upward on its medial border, while eversion moves the foot upward on its lateral border. Pronation-supination are terms defining the relationship of the mid- and forefoot to the hindfoot when the foot is weightbearing. During pronation the medial portion of the foot moves closer to the ground. Supination is the downward movement of the lateral portion of the mid- and forefoot.[10] The normal foot is slightly pronated during stance.

The midfoot consists of the navicula, the cuboid, and the cuneiform bones. These are wedge-shaped forming longitudinal and transverse arches, which provide for the structural stability of the foot. The intertarsal joints of the midfoot provide gliding and rotation contributing to the suppleness of the foot, allowing it to withstand the stresses of vigorous activity.[10]

The forefoot has limited mobility in the tarsal-metatarsal joints because they are planar, so there is no opposition here as there is in the hand. The metatarsals themselves are wedge shaped as are the tarsal bones. This allows continuation of the longitudinal arches, which start in the hind foot, into the forefoot. The medial arch is the highest and maintains an arch even during weight bearing. It starts at the calcaneus and ends at the first metatarsal head. The lateral arch also starts at the calcaneus but ends at the fifth metatarsal head. It is not as well developed as the medial arch and may collapse when bearing weight. The first and fifth metatarsal heads and the necks of the second, third and fourth metatarsal form the transverse arch, which blends with the two longitudinal arches to form a spring-like platform for weight bearing and propulsion.

The first metatarsal, the strongest, is important in propulsion and weight bearing. The two sesamoids articulate with it on its plantar surface and assist with weight bearing. The second metatarsal is the longest and the most stable of the five metatarsals. It contributes to the longitudinal arch and is a pivotal point to define adduction and abduction of the forefoot (Fig. 19-2). The metatarsal heads are important for weight bearing during ambulation. The weight is transmitted forward from the calcaneus through the medial and lateral longitudinal arches to the metatarsal heads, first through the fifth metatarsal head progressing to the first before toe-off. The first metatarsal-phalangeal joint and the great toe are important for propulsion during the toe-off phase of ambulation.

All the joints of the ankle and foot, including the joints between the sesamoids and the first metatarsal are synovial lined so that in inflammatory conditions affecting synovium, the foot and ankle may show dramatic changes clinically, radiographically, and pathologically.

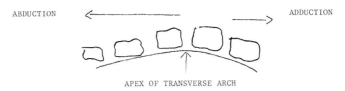

ABDUCTION ←———————   ———————→ ADDUCTION

APEX OF TRANSVERSE ARCH

Fig. 19-2. The second metatarsal forms the apex of the transverse arch. It is also the reference point that defines abduction and adduction in the foot.

SPECIFIC DISEASES AFFECTING THE FOOT

Rheumatoid Arthritis

Rheumatoid arthritis (RA) is an inflammatory condition of unknown etiology that primarily affects the synovial lining of joints, tendons, and bursae. Secondarily, it may cause destruction to cartilage, bone, ligaments, and other soft tissue. Most people with RA have foot and/or ankle involvement. Short stated that the joints of the feet are initially involved more often than the joints of the hands.[22] Vainio showed that greater than 88 percent of adults and 69 percent of children have involvement of the feet during some phase of the disease.[27] In RA the ankle joint and the joints of the feet are not affected with equal frequency. Because many of the changes seen in the rheumatoid foot are similar to those in other arthridities, the rheumatoid foot will be discussed in detail. The foot in other disorders will be compared to it.

Guerra states that the earliest sign of rheumatoid arthritis is congestion of the synovial membranes with edema.[9] As the synovial inflammatory tissue and fluid within the joint accumulate, there is soft tissue swelling, and decreased range of motion of the joint. The inflamed synovium adjacent to the marginal bare areas causes destruction of bone, resulting in the typical marginal bony erosions. Because the inflamed synovium, the pannus, also proliferates, expansion occurs over the cartilage. It destroys the cartilage through enzymatic action, producing symmetrical joint space narrowing. The pannus may also penetrate the unprotected bare bone and cause destruction of the cartilage from the marrow side. The reactive hyperemia, part of the inflammatory process, is implicated in the periarticular osteoporosis and the discontinuity of the subchondral bony plate.[9]

Similar inflammation of the sheaths of tendons occur that weaken the tendons and allow rupture, though this phenomenon is not as common in the foot as in the hand. The inflammatory process of the tendon sheaths and the ligaments may extend to the adjacent bones and causes local inflammatory changes of the bones. Such is seen when the inflammatory process of the peroneal tendons causes involvement of accessory bones. Joint destruction and deformities occur and become fixed as the weakened support structure of the ankles and foot gives way to the normal mechanical stresses placed upon it; changes in alignment of joints allow muscles, tendons, and ligaments that cross the joints to exert different forces and joint stiffness and pain prevent mobility.

Because RA does not affect the joints of the ankle and foot with the same severity and incidence, it is easier to remember the changes if the component parts of the ankle-foot complex are examined individually.

Ankle

Ankle involvement in RA is not as common as involvement of other foot joints.[25] Initially, four percent of patients with rheumatoid arthritis have involvement of the ankle. Thomas states that in a survey 48 percent of people admitted to a "rheumatic disease unit" had disability because of ankle pain.[24] He does not state whether people with diagnoses other than rheumatoid arthritis are included, nor does he define the extent of the disability. It seems, that more than four percent of patients with rheumatoid arthritis do have involvement of this joint. This concurs with the work of Spiegel et al. who found ankle synovitis in 63 percent of 50 patients who had rheumatoid arthritis for less than 10 years, and in 37 percent of patients who had the disease for greater than 40 years.[23] Ankle range of motion, that is dorsiflexion and plantar flexion, is decreased by greater than 25 percent in 25 percent of the patients. Tillman reports complete loss of range of motion (ROM) in 10 percent of his patients.[25]

Physical examination of the ankle. Physical examination of the ankle joint may only reveal subtle changes and careful examination is needed to differentiate ankle pain from subtalar joint pain. Actual palpation of the synovitis is difficult, but objective findings include increased warmth over the anterior aspect of the ankle, a subtle bulge, again on the anterior aspect just lateral to the medial malleolus, and a decrease in dorsiflexion or plantar flexion. Tenosynovitis of the retromalleolar tendons may account for some of the pain and stiffness of the ankle joint. A fullness of the tendons in the retromalleolar area associated with warmth suggests that the synovium of these structures is also involved.

Radiologic appearance. Radiologic changes in the ankle are subtle early in the disease process. Vainio says that ankle views are of little diagnostic help since the only major change is that of soft tissue swelling.[27] The effusion and synovial thickening cause protrusion of the pericapsular fat streaks.[25] Later in the disease process there may be discrete symmetrical radiolucencies in the intra-articular bone. The joint space may be narrowed. Small erosion of the articular surfaces of the malleoli and talus herald the joint destruction.[25] The erosions may develop sclerotic borders. If these erosions are asymmetric with respect to the joint, a varus or valgus deformity may result. Bony ankylosis of the ankle joint is rare in adult rheumatoid arthritis.

Hindfoot

Unlike the ankle, the hindfoot is often affected early in rheumatoid arthritis. Spiegel notes that 30 percent of patients having rheumatoid arthritis for less than five years demonstrate synovitis of the subtalar joint.[23] Vainio reports involvement of hindfoot joints in 71.4 percent of women and 58.2 percent of men.[27] In a study of 59 feet of patients referred for surgery, Tillman found the talocalcaneal, the talonavicular, and the calcaneocuboidal joints to be affected in 44 percent, 58 percent, and 37.5 percent respectively.[25] Inflammation of these joints causes pain and decreased ROM, but in addition leads to specific hindfoot deformities.

The most common deformity of the hindfoot is that of pes planovalgus, or more simply, valgus of the hindfoot and flattening of the longitudinal arches. Different investigators have their own theories as to why this particular deformity dominates. The normal slight valgus position of the hindfoot is exaggerated by the weakening effects of inflammation of the tarsal joints and ligaments. Because of pain and inactivity, this cannot be compensated for by the muscles of the foot.[25] The effects of gravity, and possibly the osseous changes themselves allow a sliding forward of the talus. According to Spiegel this forward motion causes the foot to pronate and the muscles of the foot will distort their normal pull and increase the deformity.[23] This allows flattening of the arches. Tillman and Vahvanen implicate involvement of the talonavicular joint as the initial site of flattening of the longitudinal arch,[25,26] while Vainio suggests that the weakest point is at the cuneonavicular joint.[27] Tillman suggests that the tenosynovitis of the lateral tendons with extension of the inflammation to the lateral tarsal-metatarsal joints allows further flattening of the lateral longitudinal arch, an abduction of the forefoot and a valgus of the hindfoot.[25] Tenosynovitis in the foot is not thought to be as major an influence in deformity occurrence as it is in the hand.

Although the pes planovalgus is the most common deformity of the hindfoot, it is possible to have a cavus deformity, an excessive arch in of the longitudinal arches, or an equinus deformity, plantar flexion at the ankle joint, eversion at the subtalar joint, and flattening of the longitudinal arches. The latter is more common in bedridden patients who develop flexion contractures of the hips and knees. Tillman states that previous foot deformities play an important role in the development of foot deformities in rheumatologic disorders, but he also acknowledges the effects of extrinsic forces.[25] A varus position of the knee predisposes to the development of a valgus hindfoot, while a valgus knee position predisposes the hindfoot toward a varus deformity. If a slight valgus deformity of the hindfoot already exists, valgus forces at the knee exaggerate the hindfoot deformity. Both Tillman and Vainio feel that the resting foot position may help determine the eventual structural outcome.[25,27]

Physical examination of the hindfoot. Involvement of the hindfoot is often subtle and may escape cursory examination. Swelling with tenderness may be palpated over the talocalcaneal joint especially at the site of the sinus tarsi, which can best be examined when the foot is inverted. Either the patient or the examiner should place the foot through pronation and supination. Compression and pulling of the subtalar joints help elicit pain if joint involvement is suspected. The foot should be examined weight bearing and nonweight bearing. Active dorsiflexion and plantar flexion usually do not bother the patient with hindfoot dysfunction, however weight bearing should cause him or her to complain of severe pain. Examining the patient while weight bearing or nonweight bearing also helps to determine whether a valgus deformity is present since it is much more pronounced on weight bearing and may revert to a more neutral position with the loss of weight. Tenderness behind the os calcis at the insertion of the Archilles tendon suggest either inflammation of the tendon at this site, or a retrocalcaneal bursitis. Pain on the bottom of the heel while weight bearing suggests either a plantar calcaneal spur or plantar fasciitis. Because involvement of the hindfoot is not readily apparent on clinical examination, radiologic examination may provide more information.

Radiographic appearance. Unlike the ankle, the hindfoot demonstrates radiologic abnormalities early in the course of rheumatoid arthritis. Narrowing of the talonavicular joint is often the first sign of involvement of the tarsal joints,[7,27] although Vahannen describes isolated involvement of the cuneonavicular joint.[26] Eventually, all tarsal joints are uniformly destroyed and bony or fibrous ankylosis with loss of range of motion may result. Soft tissue swelling may be evident, followed by erosions. A periosteal reaction may be evident at the insertion of the plantar aponeurosis. Such an occurrence is usually inconspicuous as compared to similar changes in seronegative arthritidies, such as Reiter's syndrome. Dorsoplantar views show all the bones and joints of the hindfoot and midfoot, but weight bearing AP and laterals usually suffice.[6]

Midfoot

The midfoot tarsal joints develop inflammatory changes that contribute to the pes planovalgus deformity of the hindfoot and midfoot.[25] As mentioned previously the talonavicular joint is first involved, but with time all the tarsal bones seem to be equally involved causing loss of pronation/supination and malleability of the foot in general.

Physical examination of the midfoot. Examination reveals swelling over the dorsum of the foot, which is usually symmetrical. The patient usually complains of diffuse pain. Holding the calcaneus firm and pulling on the forefoot causes pain at the sight of the talar joints. Because of the dense soft tissue on the plantar aspect of the foot, examination of this area usually does not contribute information concerning the midfoot. On the lateral aspect of the midfoot, palpation may reveal swelling of the peroneal tendons.

Radiographic appearance. Radiologic examination by standard views initially shows soft tissue swelling, and symmetrical joint narrowing. As the disease progresses erosions may be seen and with continued destruction the tarsal bones dislocate and contribute to the flattening of the arch. Osteoporosis may be evident.[25] Narrowing of the tarsal-metatarsal joints occurs with the joints showing equal involvement. As in the rest of the midfoot, bony ankysosis is the end result.

Forefoot

The forefoot shows marked abnormalities on clinical and radiologic examination. The altered forces created by hindfoot and midfoot deformities act with the inflammatory process affecting the metatarsal-phalangeal, (MTP) joints and proximal interphalangeal, (PIP) joint to give the typical findings of hallux valgus, claw toes, abduction of the forefoot and splay foot. Involvement here as in other parts of the foot is symmetric and increases with disease duration.[25]

Synovitis of the metatarsal phalangeal joints is frequently the site of initial involvement of rheumatoid arthritis in the foot. Spiegel et al. reported involvement of the MTP joints in 65 percent of patients having the disease less than 5 years.[25] Unlike Tillman, who reports a greater incidence of involvement in the second and fifth metatarsals,[25] they report equal involvement of all the MTP joints. As the inflammatory process destroys cartilage, it also invades the joint capsules and ligaments, causing weakness of the joints.

The weakness of the MTP joint capsule is a major factor in the development of the claw toe, which is found in greater than 50 percent of the rheumatoid patients.[27] During the toe-off phase of ambulation, the forces are transmitted dorsally through the weakened joint, while the toes are passively dorsiflexed. The net effect is dorsal subluxaton of the proximal phalanges two through five. With time, as the subluxation increases, the strong toe flexors slip into valley between the metatarsal heads and become extensors of the MTP joint and the dorsal subluxation continues. The flexor tendons continue to act as flexors of the interphalangeal joint, while the intrinsic and extrinsic extensors of the toe have diminished effect. The claw toe deformity thus occurs. As the metatarsal heads become depressed the plantar fat pad moves distally. To accomodate the stress and friction that act at the site of the metatarsal heads, plantar callouses develop. Under these callouses are synovial-lined bursae that become inflamed and the patient develops a shuffling gait to avoid weight bearing on the painful metatarsal heads. If shoes are worn that do not allow room for the deformed toes, painful calluses develop over the dorsal aspect of the proximal interphalangeal joints.[24]

In the great toe, the joint laxity causes a bowstringing of the great toe extensors. The muscle imbalance allows the toe to drift laterally, even to the point of over- underiding the second toe. This deformity is hallux valgus and depending on length of the disease process and the criteria to define valgus, is found in 39 percent–80 percent of patients with rheumatoid arthritis.[23,25,27]

The splay foot deformity is also a result of the chronic joint synovitis, joint laxity, loss of longitudinal and horizontal arches, and depression of the metatarsal heads and weakening of the plantar aponeurosis. Vainio reports it in 40 percent of women and 19 percent of men whom he evaluated preoperatively.[27]

Physical examination of the forefoot.   Clinically, the patient complains of pain during weight bearing and the toe-off phase of ambulation. He or she walks with a shuffling gait. There is redness, swelling, and warmth to touch over the metatarsal heads. Lateral compression of the metatarsal heads increases the pain. The proximal interphalangeal joints may show the same signs, but rarely are the distal interphalangeal joints involved in rheumatoid arthritis. With time the painful callouses develop on the plantar aspect, under the depressed metatarsal heads, and on the toes as they assume a clawed position. If the deformity is passively correctable, it is incomplete. If the deformity cannot be passively corrected, then it is complete.[23]

Radiologic Appearance.   Radiologic changes occur early in the forefoot of a patient with rheumatoid arthritis. Again soft tissue swelling around the MTP and PIP joints is a prominent early finding. As an initial finding, the first MTP joint is affected about as frequently as all the other joints combined.[25,27] Because of joint effusion, occasionally joint widening may be seen. Eventually, there is symmetric joint narrowing because of the loss of cartilage. Subchondral osteoporosis near inflamed joints may be an early sign.[7] Marginal erosions appear on the medial borders of the metatarsal heads two through four, and on the lateral border of the fifth, at the site of ligamentous attachments. These erosions and the later occurring ones on the plantar surface of the metatarsal heads are irreversible.[15] As the destructive process continues large cysts are prominent at the joint space. Because the sesamoids articulate with the first metatarsal head and have a cartilage surface, the sesamoids may become eroded by pannus or by extension of the inflammatory process from adjacent tendon. Late in the course of the disease hypertrophic spurring and subchondral sclerosis appear at the onset of secondary osteoarthritis and even then tend to be minimal. Finally, the alignment of the joints can be examined radiologically. Tillman found hallux valgus in 80 percent of the feet of preoperative rheumatoid patients.[25] By defining a deviation of less than 15 degrees from the shaft of the metatarsal, Spiegel et al. attempted to account for the normal hallux valgus present in the population at large. They report an incidence of the hallux valgus of 6 percent in patients with the disease less than 3 years, and 39 percent in patients who had RA greater than 10 years. Lateral deviation is seen in toes one through four, with the great toe having the greatest inc..dence, 34 percent.[23]

Rheumatoid vasculitic involvement of the foot.   Rheumatoid vasculitis is a major complication of rheumatoid arthritis that may have manifestations in the ankle and foot. Specific abnormalities occur because of deposition of immune complex in vascular walls. The abnormalities include skin ulceration, ischemia progressing to frank gangrene of the toes, (secondary to involvement of the small digital arterioles), rheumatoid nodules, and peripheral neuropathy. Treatment should be based on clinical parameters.[23] Minor skin involvement should be protected from trauma, pressure, and shear forces. Speigel recommends elevation of the extremity. Digital gangrene should be treated conservatively, since the areas will demarcate and auto-amputate. If large areas of skin open, or the peripheral neuropathy is severe, treatment with corticosteroids or immunosuppressive medications should be considered.[23]

In summary, the rheumatoid foot is marked initially by soft tissue swelling, secondary to the synovitis, symmetric joint narrowing, marginal erosions, cyst development and destruction of the joints. Pes planovalgus deformity is seen in combination with hallux valgus, claw toes, and splaying of the forefoot. Bony fusion of the tarsal bones is common. Painful callouses with underlying bursae may be palpated under the metatarsal heads two through four or behind the os calcis.

Juvenile Rheumatoid Arthritis

Juvenile rheumatoid arthritis (JRA) is a disease that is similar to the adult form of rheumatoid arthritis in that the disease primarily affects the synovial linings of joints and tendons. However, JRA has different forms of presentation and because the disease affects growing tissue, the sequelae are sometimes different.

JRA affects girls approximately twice as often as boys and the peak incidence is between 1 and 3 years of age.[10] Presenting forms of the disease include: acute systemic, monoarticular, pauciarticular, and polyarticular. According to Rana, even though the primary involvement is often the large hip joints or the ankles, in monoarticular or pauciarticular forms of JRA, some patients show nontender swelling of the PIP joints of the toes a few weeks prior to the clinical onset of the disease. In the polyarticular form of the disease, the ankle and subtalar joints are frequently involved early. Although the foot may not be a major site of involvement in monoarticular or pauciarticular, (less than four joints affected), it is important to remember that iridocyclitis is a major complication of these forms of JRA, and slit lamp examination is recommended every 6 months.[18]

Because the inflammatory reaction affects maturing tissues, the deformities found in the feet of JRA patients reflect the modeling that occurs. Normal weight-bearing and shear forces affect the outcome but in addition the reactive hyperemia places a role. There may be overgrowth of epiphysis, or there may be premature fusion of the epiphysis, leading to shortened or smaller osseous tissue. Unlike the adult form of the disease, involvement of the ankle may lead to fusion. It is possible to have pronation of the foot with valgus of the hindfoot.[18] Tarsal bones frequently become fused leading to flattening of the arches. There may be hallux valgus with or without clawing of toes two through five. The end deformities are a product of disease severity and duration and intervention therapy.

Radiologic changes of JRA show similarities to the adult form of RA. Soft tissue swelling is present early as is osteoporosis near inflamed joints. Because the disease affects children, however, there are major differences. Linear periosteal new bone is very common in children but rare in adults.[7] Children have more abundant cartilage as compared to adults, so the subchondral bone changes and erosion indicate later and more severe

involvement than the same changes indicate on radiographs of adult feet.[18] Growth disturbances are a primary feature. Reactive hyperemia causes early epiphyseal closure, shortening of bones occurring. The fourth metatarsal seems particularly prone to this process.
According to Gold the early fusion of epiphysis may also occur in bones distal to an
inflamed knee or ankle so that the foot is smaller than normal even though the foot joints
are not primarily involved.[7]

Seronegative Spondyloarthropathies

The seronegative arthritides are ankylosing spondylitis, Reiter's snydrome and its
variants, and psoriatic arthritis. There are major differentiating points between these
forms of inflammation and that of rheumatoid arthritis. The inflammation is frequently
low-grade and indolent with a tendency to resolve through intense fibrosis.[3] The fibrotic
scar tissue has a greater tendency to calcify than that in rheumatoid arthritis. Capsules,
ligament-bone junctions, bone-cartilage interfaces, and the cartilage itself seem to be
targets for the inflammatory process in addition to the synovial tissue.[3] Certain of these
diseases seem to have a direct association with infectious agents. There also may be a
genetic predisposition to them as determined by the high frequency of HLA-B27 positive
markers in the syndromes.[3] Clinically, men outnumber women in the seronegative arthridities, while in rheumatoid arthritis the women to men ratio is 3:1. The subclinical incidence
of the seronegative arthritides suggest that they may be more prevalent than previously
suspected and that the incidence of men and women is equal.

Ankylosing Spondylitis

This form of arthritis has been recognized for centuries, but only recently has it been
determined that it is not a form of rheumatoid arthritis. Similarities to rheumatoid
arthritis include; synovitis with pannus formation, cartilage destruction from superficial
and deep erosions of the pannus, and marginal erosions.[3,19] The inflammatory process is
not as marked and the pannus formation less intense. In addition, there is subchondral
bone sclerosis and periosteal elevation, events that are more common in the seronegative
arthridities than rheumatoid arthritis. It is a disease that has a predilection for the axial
skeleton as opposed to the more peripheral joints. The early involvement of the sacroiliac,
(SI) joints and the progressive discitis and capsulitis of cartilagenous and synovial joints of
the spine that leads to the characteristic hunched appearance clinically and bamboo spine
radiologically, is well recognized. Peripheral manifestations of the disease do occur, however, and should not be overlooked since they also cause discomfort, pain, disability, and
loss of function. There seems to be more involvement of the feet as compared with the
hands, which in ankylosing spondylitis seem to be relatively spared.[3]

In the ankle and foot, retrocalcaneal bursitis is a major site of inflammation. It may
be acute or subacute and may or may not involve the ankle joint itself. The calcaneal
attachment of the plantar aponeurosis is frequently involved although not as frequent as
in Reiter's syndrome. The smaller distal joints of the foot may become involved, but the
clinical involvement of the spine overrides the foot symptomatology.[3]

Clinically, the patient will complain of tenderness behind the ankle and will decrease
the plantar flexion activities of gait. This is seen as a shuffling gait with emphasis on toe
walking. Palpation of the area reveals tenderness and swelling. Active plantar flexion may
increase the pain. On the plantar aspect of the heel, deep palpation may reveal tenderness,
which is intensified by weight bearing. Compression of the metatarsal joints occasionally
reveals involvement of the MTP joints.

Radiologically, most of the abnormalities are seen in the SI joints and the spine. Changes in 60 percent will demonstrate the peripheral joints that tend to be transient and mild.[7] In the ankle and foot, there may be soft tissue swelling and calcaneal erosions in the area of the retrocalcaneal bursa. Calcaneal spurs or a fluffy periosteal reaction may be evident on the plantar aspect of the calcaneus. These frequently are associated with erosions that tend to be smaller than in RA. Bone formation is seen at the peripheral capsular attachments in particular at the base of the fifth metatarsal and medial aspect of the tarsal navicular joint. In a few patients lateral deviation and dorsal subluxation of the toes may be seen.[9]

Reiter's Syndrome

Reiter's syndrome is a disease that seems to have an infectious etiology. Most cases occur after sexual activity or a bacterial gastroenteritis. It is most common in sexually active young men, and is usually an acute illness consisting of urethritis, conjunctivitis, and arthritis. Some authors now include the presence of skin lesions, balantitis circinata, keratodermia blennorrhagica, oral buccal lesions, or nail changes, as major constituents of the disease profile. The disease is self-limited in most of the patients, but 20 percent of patients will develop a chronic rheumatic disease developing findings similar to those of ankylosing spondylitis.[3] Like ankylosing spondylitis, there is a strong association with the HLA-B27 locus. The disease primarily affects the peripheral joints, especially those of the feet. Chand and Johnson report foot and ankle involvement in one-half of Reiter's patients.[4] According to various authors, almost any joint of the foot including the ankle could be involved. The actual incidence of involvement of the joints depends on the study. The most common areas of involvement according to Chand and Johnson, are the posterior calcaneus, the metatarsophalangeal joints, the phalangeal joints and the ankle. Rarely is there involvement of the subtalar or midfoot joints.[4] This is similar to the findings of Sholkoff et al. who report SI joint and tarsal joint involvement, but no inflammation of the phalangeal joints.[21] Pathologically, the findings are similar to those of ankylosing spondylitis. There is synovial inflammation and pannus formation, bony erosion with adjacent periostitis. Bony proliferation is common especially at the calcaneal insertion of the plantar aponeurosis.

Clinically, the symptoms of urethritis, conjunctivitis, arthritis, or skin lesions may not all be present at the same time. It is possible for the symptoms to wax and wane before a patient will seek medical attention. Pain is usually mild to moderate, as is erythema and swelling of the ankle and foot.[4] Subjective stiffness occurs in approximately 50 percent of cases. The typical "sausage digit" of one or more toes (Fig. 19-3), is present in six percent of patients in the Mayo study.[4] The persistent hindfoot pain is often the most severe problem causing significant disability in otherwise healthy individuals.

Radiologic studies indicate that there is no one specific change pathognomonic for Reiter's syndrome. Changes are similar to other seronegative processes. Chand and Johnson indicate that erosions and soft-tissue swelling dominate the forefoot, while spur formation and erosions are the major findings of the hindfoot.[4] The interphalangeal joint of the great toe and the MTP joint undergo extensive erosions. The first MTP joint may show involvement of the sesamoids with proliferation of new bone and erosive damages. Equal involvement of all the MTP joints is not a feature of Reiter's syndrome and if a comparison of right to left side is made, there is an asymmetry.[7] Generalized involvement of the distal interphalangeal joint is uncommon, although individual involvement is not. Bony ankylosing of the IP joint occurs in approximately 15 percent of patients. Erosions of

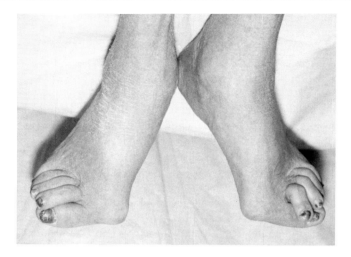

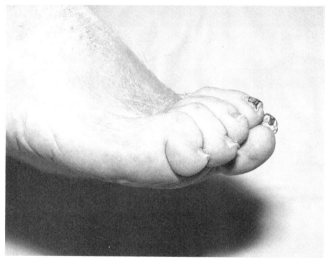

Fig. 19-3. Typical deformities in the foot affected by rheumatoid arthritis, hallux valgus and claw toes.

bone is less marked than in RA. Periosteal new bone formation may increase the width of the eroded bone causing further joint dysfunction. Subluxation may occur in advanced joint destruction. The periosteal reaction is particularly marked on the calcaneal insertion of the plantar aponeurosis. A large calcaneal spur at this site is common in Reiter's syndrome. The spur in RA tends to be inconspicuous compared to the other findings. Severe osteoporosis is not as common a feature in RA.

Psoriatic Arthritis

Although seemingly a simple term, psoriatic arthritis has yet to be defined. This is because it is now recognized that arthritis associated with psoriasis has different clinical pictures. Definitions that say it is "arthritis following long-standing uncontrolled psoriasis" or "arthritis confined to the distal interphalangeal joints" or other proposed definitions do not encompass the syndrome.[2] Bennett recognizes five clinical psoriatic syndromes: classic psoriatic arthritis involves primarily the distal interphalangeal joints and is associated with nail changes, arthritis mutilans causes resorption of the phalanges and metacarpals, symmetric arthritis is similar to rheumatoid arthritis, oligoarthritis usually asymmetrical involvement of interphalangeal joints, and ankylosing spondylitis associated with psoriatic arthritis.[2] Arthritis is more common in the seronegative patients and, like psoriasis in general, seems to have a genetic basis. The histopathologic changes in psoriatic arthritis are virtually indistinguishable from rheumatoid arthritis. Guerra states that the degree of cellular infiltration with lymphocytes and plasma cell is less marked in psoriatic arthritis than in rheumatoid arthritis and finds differences between the two diseases in pannus destruction of cartilage and bony proliferation.[9] It seems that comparisons of the two diseases is dependent on the type of psoriatic arthritis.

Arthritis precedes the skin and nail changes in 16% of patients with psoriatic arthritis.[2] The correct diagnosis is made when the typical skin changes appear. Classically, the arthritis affects the distal joints more than the proximal joints, and differing from Reiter's syndrome has a predilection for the hands with relative sparing of the feet. The interphalangeal joints are affected more often than the MTP joints. The distal joint involvement along with a tenosynovitis may cause significant soft tissue swelling of a digit, the "sausage digit," which can be seen in other seronegative arthridities. The great toe may be the first affected, clinically appearing like an acute gouty attack. Except for the particularly deforming arthritis mutilans, the course of the psoriatic arthritis is relatively benign in the majority of cases.

Radiologic findings of psoriatic arthritis in the feet are dependent on the duration and severity of the disease. They include asymmetric involvement of the interphalangeal joints with relative sparing of the metatarsalphalangeal joints, bony ankylosis of the small joints, terminal phalangeal tuft erosion, severe articular joint destruction, which is also known as "whittling," and periosteal new bone formation. The combination of the latter two findings is known as "pencil-in-cup" and may also be seen in Reiter's syndrome.[7] As in Reiter's syndrome, osteoporosis is not a major finding. Hindfoot and midfoot involvement is uncommon, but spur formation at the calcaneal insertion of the plantar aponeurosis is reported.

Gout

Gout is a true intermittent asymmetric inflammatory arthritis that is related to the presence of monosodium urate crystals in the synovial fluid. Gout is related to a disturbance of the metabolism of uric acid. Either there is overproduction or decreased renal clearance or a combination of the two. The presence of the needle-shaped crystals in joint fluid analysis is the major criteron for establishing the diagnosis of gout. In order to see the crystals, it is necessary to examine the synovial fluid under polarized light. They exhibit a strong negative birefringence and may be found in the fluid or in leukocytes.[38] The presence of the crystals in the fluid or soft tissue elicits a nonspecific inflammatory response. The release of superficial crystals from the synovium may initiate an acute attack of gout.

With time there may be progression of the disease to chronic tophaceous gout, especially if the serum levels of uric acid exceed 9 mg/100 ml.[17] Large tophi of urate crystals are deposited in articular cartilage, subchondral bone, synovial membranes, and capsules of the joints.[9] These tophi penetrate osseous, cartilagenous and soft tissues, causing joint destruction, and where the overlying soft tissue is thin, an open draining sore.

The garden variety type of gout can be diagnosed by history and clinical examination. The disease usually presents in mid-life, i.e., the 30s–50s. Men are 95 percent of its victims. It is rare to see the disease present itself in premenopausal women.[28] The first MTP joint is affected in 50 percent of cases and starts out as a dull ache that becomes an acute arthritis within 24 hours. The pain is excrutiating but usually subsides within 72–96 hours, although severe cases may last for weeks. Within a year, 60 percent of people will have a recurrence of the symptoms, either in the same joint or a different one. Occasionally, more than one joint may be clinically affected at a time. Emotional stress, indulgence in food or alcoholic beverages, certain medications, i.e., thiazides, or trauma may exacerbate a gouty attack.[28] Early in the disease course, the quiescent period is marked by freedom from symptoms. As the years continue, the repair process is incomplete, and a chronic aching arthritis develops.

Radiologically, erosions that have well demarcated sclerotic borders help define the disease. These are particularly present on the dorsum of the first MTP joint, but may be anywhere that tophi are present. The slow invasion of the subchondral bone by the tophi allows the sclerotic repair process to occur. At the margins there may be excess bone formation leading to the typical "overhanging edge"[7] of gout. There is preservation of joint space since only portions of the cartilage surface are destroyed by the gouty process. During a flare, there is marked soft tissue swelling. Occasionally, it is possible to delineate the actual tophi laying adjacent to the erosion, since calcium urate crystals are present and make the tophi appear slightly denser radiographically than normal sort tissue.

Osteoarthritis

Osteoarthritis is not a systemic inflammatory disease. Rather it is a polyfocal disease that is secondary to the wear and tear phenomena on joints. Dysruption of the cartilagenous matrix occurs as a result of enzymatic action. Large weight bearing joints of the body are particularly prone to dysfunction. The ankle joint and first MTP seem susceptible. Weight bearing, trauma, and footwear have all been implicated as causative agents.

Physical examination reveals enlargement of joint that seems to be bony in origin. This is because of the marginal osteophytes. There may be warmth to touch, but it is not the heat that is felt in the acute joint of rheumatologic disorders. Range of motion of the joint may be decreased. The great toe often demonstrates a hallux valgus deformity. Laboratory investigations are noncontributory.[7]

Radiologic examination reveals asymmetric joint space narrowing, the areas of stress demonstrating less interosseous space. There is irregular subchondral bone sclerosis and cyst formation. According to Guerra the etiology of the cysts is unknown.[9] Marginal osteophytes are present to a variable degree.

Other Systemic Disorders

Systemic Lupus Erythematosis

Of patients with systemic lupus erythematosis (SLE) 90 percent will have arthralgias during the course of their disease. Foot and ankle involvement is infrequent. In incidence the ankle joint predominates, while the midfoot and forefoot joints are rarely affected. Joint manifestations include: joint distention, osteoporosis, synovitis, and cartilage thinning. Erosions may be present but are minimal. Calcification of the joint capsule is occasionally seen.[7]

Progressive Systemic Sclerosis

Scleroderma (PSS) is a systemic disorder affecting the connective tissue of skin, synovium, arteris, and internal organs. Course of the disease is variable and joint changes are a minimal problem. According to Gold, the hands are the site of most of the changes seen in PSS, while the feet are less affected.[7] Changes include: resorption of the terminal tufts of the distal phalanges, development of flexion contractures of the toes because of involvement of the skin and joint capsule, and replacement of the fat pad by fibrous connective tissue. "Pressure and frictional forces result in thinning of the articular cartilage of the metatarsophalangeal joints, progressing to irregular destruction and sclerosis of the subchondral bone. Marginal erosions are usually absent."[7]

Treatment of Foot and Ankle Disorders in Rheumatologic Disorders

To treat a rheumatologic disorder of the ankle or foot it is necessary to understand the disease process and pathomechanics, examine the feet in detail and have a working knowledge of available treatment alternatives. The examination of the ankle-foot complex needs to include examination of the weight-bearing and nonweight-bearing foot, examination of gait patterns and examination of the shoes. The feet need to be inspected for active joint ROM, deformities, callous formation, skin and nail changes, and areas of swelling. Palpation assesses passive joint range of motion, contractures, areas of tenderness, joint temperature, and joint effusion. The shoe will reveal stress and weight-bearing patterns. After the physical examination is completed, therapeutic plans are formulated that take into account the specific problem(s), age, medical history, lifestyle and economics of the patient. For some patients medication or physical treatments alone may be sufficient. For others, the combined effects of anti-inflammatory medications and physical modalities may be necessary to provide relief of symptoms and increase function. Still in others surgery with or without the other two approaches may provide the most effective means of caring for the patient. The individualization of the therapeutic plan is important.

Physical modalities and treatment for the arthritic ankle and foot may provide sufficient relief by themselves if the deformities are not severe. They may be useful temporary supportive measures when a patient is not a good surgical candidate. Physical measures may enhance or support the surgical correction or may be the only measures available to treat disabling pain or deformities in a patient who will never be a surgical candidate. Physical modalities should not take the place of appropriate surgical intervention, when delaying the surgery only increases the misery and possibly the disability of the patient.

Thermotherapy and therapeutic exercises are important adjunct modalities, no matter what portion of the ankle-foot complex is affected by arthritis. In prescribing these modalities, especially if the treatment is carried out with a therapist, it is necessary to remember that the prescription is as legal a document as a medicine prescription. The diagnosis, condition to be treated, goals, precautions to therapy, need to be indicated as do the modalities to be used, dose if appropriate, and the frequency and duration of treatments. It is also appropriate to request feedback on the efficacy of treatment so the program can be altered to accommodate the patient's needs.

The application of heat and cold have been discussed in a previous chapter. Application of heat and or cold to the foot and ankle is accomplished in a variety of ways, depending on the goals of the heat treatment.

To help alleviate pain in the arthritic foot gentle, superficial heating is usually recommended. Techniques that are simple, readily available to the patient and inexpensive include: warm, wet towels wrapped in plastic wrap and covered with dry towels wrapped around the foot, heat packs or pads, and warm soaks in basins of water heated to not greater than 104 degrees Farenheit. If many joints of the lower extremities or body are involved immersion in a whirlpool tank may prove beneficial. The use of these heating methods can also precede therapeutic exercise. If vigorous heating is to be used in chronic arthritic conditions to improve ROM activities, deep heating is desirable. Ulrasound provides the deepest heat, is quickly and easily applied and can be used with metal implants. Because the effect of the ultrasound waves on methacrylate is not known, it is not recommended that ultrasound be used where the substance has been used to cement artificial joint components to the bony substrate. Cold treatment can easily be given by immersion in basins of combination ice and water, cold water alone (50 degrees Farenheit), use of an ice bag, or rubbing the affected area with ice popsicles. The latter can be made at home using tap water, paper cups, and small wooden sticks.

After the use of heat or cold or when the gel phenomenon is at its minimum therapeutic exercises can be carried out to preserve, maintain, or increase joint ROM and in relatively quiescent periods to increase strength and endurance. Joint ROM exercises should be active, in which the patient moves the joint through its range or active-assisted, in which the patient actively moves the joint but is assisted by himself or herself, or another person. The guideline for activity is pain in rheumatologic conditions and the patient is the one to determine this. Exacerbated pain caused by an exercise program should be gone within 2 hours or by the following day the pain should be no greater than at the onset of the exercise period. If the pain persists for longer periods, the exercise activity is too rigorous for the patient and the stage of the disease, and needs to be modified.

Achilles tendon stretching is done to preserve ankle mobility and prevent equinus deformities especially in children or in patients who are nonambulatory. Active-assisted dorsiflexion may be necessary to stretch the tendon or use of a tilt table in a more physically fit person does the same. If the person can tolerate active exercise, the stretching is accomplished by having the patient stand in front of a table, one leg extended with foot flat on the ground. The other leg is flexed at the knee. The patient leans toward the table, helping to support the body weight by using the arms. As he or she leans the Achilles tendon of the extended leg is stretched. It is desirable to have at least 5 degrees of dorsiflexion, but the ankle at neutral is a functional position.

Subtalar motion can be preserved by having the patient sit in a chair with the knees flexed. A diagram of concentric circles or a spiral is placed on the floor within reach of the toes. Starting with the smallest circle, and proceeding outward the patient traces the diagram. Flexion of the knees helps isolate ankle motion and prevents substitution of internal/external rotational movements of the hip. Since the rheumatoid foot often assumes an exaggerated pronation deformity, an exercise has been devised to counteract this position. Standing with feet wide apart, the patient points the toes in, then rolls on the lateral border of his or her feet. During this maneuver he or she actively flexes the toes.[1]

Other joints of the foot should have daily ROM to preserve function. The patient can be instructed by a therapist, and carry out the activities at home. If necessary a friend or family member may assist. If a family member is not available then a paraprofessional should assist. Maintenance of the range may be assisted by orthotic devices designed to support the lax joints.

Bardwick and Swezey recommend towel wrinkling and toe raises to strengthen the toe flexors.[1]

Children with rheumatoid disease require special attention. Usually the disease process makes it difficult for children to participate in normal play activities. Exercise therapy can take on the guise of play. This seems to help with compliance.

Treatment for specific areas.   Although thermotherapy and therapeutic exercises are integral parts of physical management of the arthritic ankle and foot, additional measures are usually necessary. Padding, orthotic devices, and shoe modifications provide additional means of treatment to decrease pain, preserve joint function, and increase function. Starting with the most simple, least conspicuous device and progressing to types that provide more support is a basic rule. This of course is modified depending on the pain, the deformity, and the goal.[8]

Ankle.   Pain on weight bearing and with plantar flexion or dorsiflexion are symptoms indicating ankle joint involvement. The pain needs to be differentiated from Achilles tendonitis, retrocalcaneal bursitis and subtalar joint involvement. Examination of each of these areas on the weight-bearing and nonweight-bearing foot will help differentiate the source of pain. Warmth or swelling may be palpated on the dorsum of the ankle where there is little tissue covering the joint. Methods of treatment should be designed to decrease weight-bearing, decrease ankle joint movement, or a combination of both.

Two orthotic braces designed to provide decreased weight-bearing on the ankle joint are the below the knee-bearing brace (BKBB), and the patellar tendon brace (PTB),[1] (Fig. 19-4). The first is a double-upright brace with a leather calf cuff. As the cuff is tightened weight is removed from the ankle joint. The ankle joint can either be free allowing movement at the ankle or dorsiflexion or plantar flexion stops can be added to limit motion of the ankle joint. This brace is attached to an orthopedic style shoe that has a long metal shank. The latter is necessary in a limited motion ankle to distribute the weight

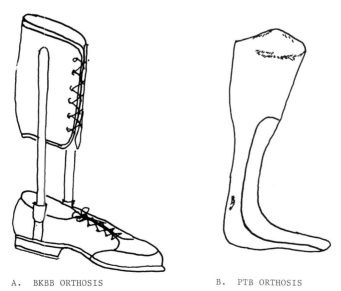

A. BKBB ORTHOSIS   B. PTB ORTHOSIS

Fig. 19-4.   The BKBB brace (a) and the PTB (b) brace decrease weight through the ankle. The weight is carried by the anterior tibial flares, and the muscle mass of the posterior portion. Imagine a cone supporting the leg.

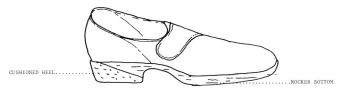

CUSHIONED HEEL............

...........ROCKER BOTTOM

Fig. 19-5. The cushioned heel of this shoe, acts as a shock absorber and decreases the need for plantar flexion during touchdown. The rocker portion of the sole is placed behind the metatarsal heads. This facilitates toe-off and propulsion with weight being transmitted to the metatarsal heads or necessitating MTP joint movement.

forward to the metatarsal heads. If the shank is weak the shoe "breaks" in the midsole area and if the shank is too short, it will wear through the insole and put pressure on the proximal portion of the forefoot.

The design of the PTB orthosis allows weight bearing over the relatively pressure-insensitive patellar tendon, anterior tibial flare, and the back of the calf. It is a custom made polypropylene orthosis, which can be worn with a variety of shoes as long as the shoes all have the same heel height. The ankle can be rigid or semi-flexible depending on the construction and trim at the ankle. Two ideas developed for prothesis, the soft ankle, cushioned heel (SACH), heel and a rocker bottom sole can be added if necessary to the shoe to mimic normal heel-toe walking (Fig. 19-5).

The latter two modifications are also beneficial when limited motion is desired at the ankle and forefoot. Another simple modification of shoe design is the shaving or cutting of the posterior portion of the heel at a 45-degree angle. This decreases the flexion forces at the knee with the end result being of decrease forces at the ankle (Fig. 19-6).

Hindfoot and Midfoot

Hindfoot pain and dysfunction have several etiologies, subtalar joint dysfunction, Achilles or peroneal tendonitis, retro-calcaneal bursitis, calcaneal spur formation, or plantar facsiitis. Subtalar joint involvement is marked by pain on weight bearing, pronation/supination, and inversion/eversion motions. Tenderness or effusion may be palpated over the sinus tarsi. The hindfoot may assume a valgus or more rarely a varus position and need

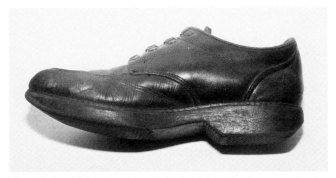

Fig. 19-6. This trimming of the heel in this shoe can also be seen in many sports shoes on the commercial market. This type of shoe is excellent for relief of heel pain and forefoot deformity. It is an inexpensive alternative to special orthopedic inserts or shoes.

support. Tendonitis, bursitis, spurs, and fasciitis show local swelling and/or tenderness at the affected sites. Plantar flexion may increase pain if the Archilles tendon, its insertion or the overlying retrocalcaneal bursae are inflamed. Tenderness behind the lateral malleolus that increases with eversion or inversion suggests lateral tendon involvement. Deep tenderness to pressure under the calcaneus, pain during weight bearing and the touch-down phase of gait indicate calcaneal spurs or plantar fasciitis. As in the ankle, there are several alternative treatments available.

Achilles' tendonitis and/or retrocalcaneal bursitis have several treatment options. The goals of treatment are to rest the inflamed area and prevent shear forces over it. The use of sandals or shoes that have release of the posterior seam relieve pressure. Felt or foam pads with cut-outs, or pressure redistributing pads such as the Spenco dermal pad (Spenco Spence Co., Waco, TX) decrease pressure over the area. To lessen motion in the area and provide rest, a higher heel shoe may help, but the SACH heel and rocker bottom sole, are more efficient in decreasing motion. These methods can be used by themselves or in conjunction with local steroid injections. Because of the complication of rupture of the Archilles tendon poststeroid injection, the use of steroid should be carried out as infrequently as possible and not more than two to three times per year.

Pain due to calcaneal inflammation or spurs respond to measures designed to redistribute weight away from the tender areas. Spenco inserts or a similar material is a simple effective solution for minor discomfort. The inner sole of the shoe can be excavated to relieve pressure area. Lipstick can be used to mark the painful area, the foot carefully placed in the shoe and then the area of the shoe marked by the lipstick trimmed. If necessary a compound such as Spenco foam, which distributes pressure can be used to fill in the depression. Commercial heel pads are available but care is needed to have the cut-out in the right position (Fig. 19-7). A heel cup is effective for heel pain as shown by

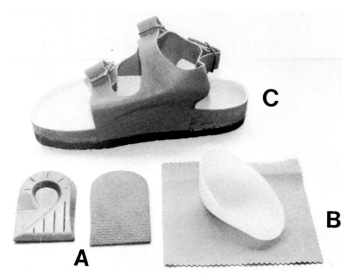

Fig. 19-7. Devices available to help decrease heel pain: a) heel pad with cutout which can be further modified to alleviate pressure under specific points. b) heel cup which acts as a buttress. c) recessed heel in commercial available sandal.

Katoh.[11] It acts either by redistributing pressure to the periphery by acting as a buttress, or shifting weight to the midfoot and forefoot. Katoh et al. report that contrary to popular belief, raising the heel did not improve painful heels. They recommend a flat heel made similar to the Earth shoe or Birkenstock-style shoe.[11]

Plantar fasciitis is effectively treated by either a simple longitudinal arch support or the University of California Biomechanics (UCB), orthosis (Fig. 19-8). These designs relax the tension on the plantar fascia and it supports the longitudinal arch. The insert is custom made from an impression made during partial weight bearing. The foot is slightly pronated and adducted and the leg is externally rotated. This position decreases the tension on the plantar fascia. It is worn until symptoms subside and reinstituted if symptoms recur.

Treatment of valgus of the hindfoot is dependent on its severity and if it is combined with other deformities. Alternatives range from simple inserts to ankle-foot orthosis (AFO) with T-strap. Heel cups that are inserted in the shoe, may keep the heel from assuming a valgus position. Wedging of the medial heel may also provide support and decrease the valgus deformity. The wedge is placed on the medial heel in the shoe, incorporated into a shoe insert or placed on the outside medial heel. Small wedges of a maximum depth of one-quarter inch may be placed in the medial aspect of the shoe. If more correction is necessary, the wedge is placed on the medial heel outside of the shoe. This can be combined with wedge modification of the lateral sole of the shoe. The net effect is one of correcting the valgus and pronation forces of the hindfoot. To stabilize the shoe and to counteract valgus forces, Cracchiolo recommends fiberglass lamination of the counters of the shoes.[5] Because of its construction, an orthopedic shoe easily allows these modifications. An insert requires a larger shoe size to accomodate it (Fig. 19-9).

Heel cups are placed in the shoe and act as a buttress to the heel pad, restricting the heel from assuming a valgus position.[13] This decreases subtalar and talonavicular motion and longitudinal arch strains. If valgus is pronounced, a double upright AFO is required. A medial T-strap is provided at the ankle to decrease the static and dynamic valgus forces. Some feel the above methods are ineffective in the treatment of heel valgus and have developed a medial buttress support (Fig. 19-10).

Since pronation of the mid and forefoot and loss of the longitudinal arches are often associated with a valgus deformity of the hindfoot, correction of the valgus position may include a system to help correct the other deformities. A shoe insert that combines the heel orthosis with an extension that supports the subtalar joints and longitudinal arches is

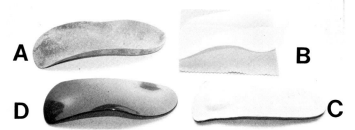

Fig. 19-8. An assortment of longitudinal arch supports available which support the arch and decrease strain on plantar fascia. Materials include: a) cork, b) polypropylene (UCBL orthosis), c) cushioned plastic, and d) plastics.

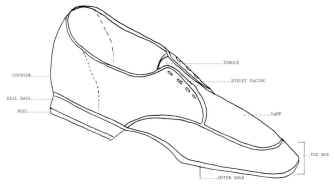

Fig. 19-9. This is the basic othopaedic shoe with the component parts listed. A long metal shank is placed in the sole of the shoe to provide support of the arch of the foot.

often recommended for mild to moderated valgus deformity with arch loss. The insert can be made of fiberglass in a fashion similar to the UCB orthosis. If necessary it may be lined with a Spenco type of material. To facilitate a heel-toe type of cadence, the SACH heel/ rocker bottom sole combination or a crepe-soled shoe can be used. According to Gould, this system is not effective for patients with severe collapse of the arch. The more severe deformities require consideration of Plastazote sandals or shoes (Bakelite Xglonite, Ltd., New York) custom made shoes, or surgical correction (Fig. 19-11).[8]

Forefoot

Forefoot deformities in the rheumatoid arthritic foot include calluses, bursitis under the metatarsal heads, depression of the metatarsal heads and loss of the horizontal arch, claw toes, hallux valgus, and splay foot. The principles in treatment of pain and deformity

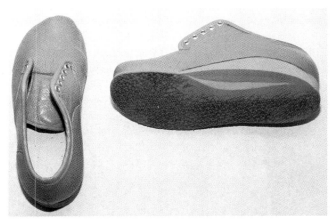

Fig. 19-10. The medial arch is supported by building up the medial sole. The contouring decreases pronation or valgus and supports the longitudinal arch. The contouring materials are high density foam and add little weight to the shoe. The shoe is made from plastazote. Note the accommodation for the hallux valgus deformity.

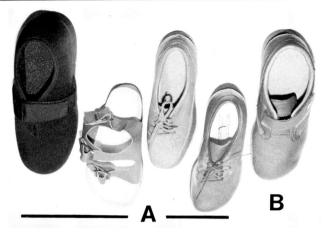

Fig. 19-11. Shoes available to treat moderate to severe deformities. (A) Shoes with extra-depth toe boxes. Various inserts and/or cushioning devices can be placed in the shoe to accommodate deformities if necessary, (B) Plastazote shoes that can be molded to accommodate deformities.

in forefoot are the same as treatment of the ankle hindfoot or midfoot. That is relief of pressure, distribution of pressure over greater areas and decreasing shear forces. As in the rest of the foot, the shoe and its modifications may determine the functional status of a patient.

Patients often complain of metatarsal head pain with or without callus development. The goal for this area is relief of pressure. This can be accomplished in a variety of ways. Shoe heel height should be low. If calluses are present, they should be softened by soaking in warm soapy water, then trimmed even with the skin line using a disposable #15 scapel.[5] The lesions should not be trimmed to the point of bleeding. Excavation of the sole of the shoe under the pressure points relieves stress and friction. The excavations may be filled with Spenco. Metatarsal pads (Fig. 19-12) insert into the shoe and cushion the area but are not very effective for relieving significant pressure. Milgram feels that these may be helpful for inflammation of the third and fourth metatarsals, less for inflammation of the second and worthless for relieving pressure under the first metatarsal head.[14] He customizes foam pads using a basic "L" shape to relieve pressure. The mechanics are similar to the metatarsal bar, which effectively relieves pressure on the plantar aspect of the metatarsal heads. The bar is placed on the outer sole just behind the metatarsal heads so that weight is transmitted from the hindfoot to the bar to the toes. A rigid rocker bottom sole performs similarly and decrease the motion necessary at the metatarsal-phalangeal joint during toe off, so that it can help rest painful joints. Use of a Plastazote liner in the shoe, with either of the two latter options redistributes pressure over the entire plantar surface and decreases shear forces.

Plastazote is heat-deformable polyethylene material that comes in different gradients. The lightweight one is pink, decreases friction, and rests against the foot. The next dense grade is white, provides better support, and does not loose form as easily as the pink. The most dense is black, and is cork-like in consistency. It is used for soles in sandals and shoes. The Plastazote is heated, an impression of the foot made and the insert applied to the shoe thus providing total contact for redistribution of weight and shear forces.

If the metatarsal head depression deformity is moderate to severe there are off-the-

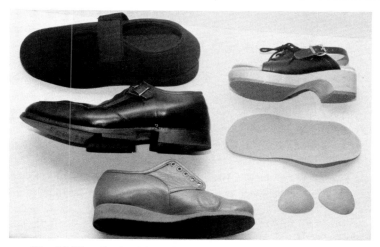

Fig. 19-12.   Devices/shoes for metatarsal head discomfort. (bottom right) Metatarsal pads, (middle right) foam insert, (top right) rocker bottom shoe, (top left) plastazote shoe, (middle left) shoe with metatarsal bar, (bottom left) plastazote shoe with modification for hallux valgus deformity.

shelf Plastazote shoes and sandals available that often decrease discomfort with weight bearing. If the person has a small or large foot and/or if the deformities are very severe, custom Space shoes are made from the impression of the foot. These can be used long term or postsurgery (Fig. 19-11 and 19-12).

The hallux deformity and the claw toes require modification of the type of shoes patients (especially women) wear. Large sports shoes with lacing extending over the dorsum of the shoe have room for the deformed toes and inserts provide further decrease shear or weight forces. Sandals help somewhat. Making a slit in the leather of the shoe by the great toe or an "x" over the clawed toes decreases pressure in these areas. Some shoes have extra-depth or width toe boxes (Fig. 19-11), which easily accommodate the toe deformities. The shoe should fit the forefoot since the heel is easily modified to fit by laminating the counters. Again, the stiffened sole or rocker bottom shoe may help. Bardwick recommends control of pronation forces of the hind and midfoot to help alleviate some of the forces causing the valgus deformity of the great toe. The arch support with reinforcement of the medial heel counter lessens these forces. The insert makes the extra-depth toe box necessary. If the deformities are severe the Plastazote shoe or sandal or the Space shoe may be required.

The combination of the extra-depth toe box and the molded arch support support the splay foot. Again with severe deformities the custom made shoe may be required. This is an expensive alternative but in nonoperative conditions, it may be the permanent solution (Fig. 19-11, 19-12, and 19-13).

Surgery

As more modifications are required the question of surgery inevitably arises. There are innumerable techniques to remove inflamed synovium, stabilize the ankle and hind-

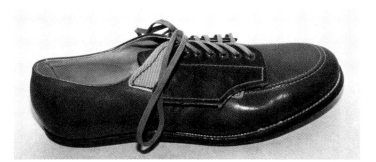

Fig. 19-13. Adding a Velcro closure to a shoe can be cosmetic, yet increase function in someone with involvement of the hands.

foot joints, resect the painful MTP joints and possibly replace them with prosthetic joints. Prosthetic joints are available for the ankle. When are these options appropriate?

Most authors agree that surgery for correction should not be attempted in the foot while there is still active inflammation because of the possibility of further deformity occurring that would require additional surgeries for corrections and revisions. If there is a relative quiescent disease and active inflammation of a joint has not occurred for greater than 5 months and the "conservative approaches" provide less than adequate function, then surgery should be considered. In children surgery should be postponed until skeletal maturation has occurred if possible. Arthrodesis of the ankle can be done at ages 10-12 years with fair to good results expected. Deformities of the metatarsophalangeal joints is usually asymptomatic in children. If necessary, excision/resection is done after fusion of the metatarsal and phalangeal epiphysis around 20 years. Soft tissue releases such as Achilles tendon releases and capsulotomies can be done much earlier.

REFERENCES

1. Bardwick PA, Swezey RL: Physical modalities for treating the foot affected by connective tissue diseases. Foot and Ankle 3 (1): 17-20, 1982
2. Bennett M: Psoriatic arthritis in McCarty DJ (ed): Arthritis and Allied Conditions, 9th edition: Philadelphia, Lea & Febiger, 1979, pp 642-655
3. Bluestone R: Collagen diseases affecting the foot. Foot and Ankle 2(6): 313-317, 1982
4. Chand Y, Johnson KA: Foot and ankle manifestations of Reiter's syndrome. Foot and Ankle 1(3): 169-172, 1980
5. Cracchiolo III, A: Office practice: footwear and orthotic therapy. Foot and Ankle 2(4): 242-248, 1982
6. Glass MK, Karno ML, Sella EJ, et al: An office-based orthotic system in treatment of the arthritic foot. Foot and Ankle, 3(1): 37-40, 1982
7. Gold RH, Bassett LW: Radiologic evaluation of the arthritic foot. Foot and Ankle 2(6): 332-41, 1982
8. Gould JS: Conservative management of the

hypersensitive foot in rheumatoid arthritis. Foot and Ankle 2(4): 224-229, 1982
9. Guerra J, Resnick D: Arthridities affecting the foot and ankle-pathology and treatment. The relationship between foot and ankle deformity and disease duration in 50 patients. Foot and Ankle 2(6): 325-331, 1982
10. Hamilton JJ, Ziemer LK: Functional anatomy of the human ankle and foot in Kiene RH, Johnson KA (eds). American Academy of Orthopedics Symposium on the Foot and Ankle. St. Louis, MO, 1983, pp 1-15
11. Katoh Y, Chao EYS, Morrey BF, et al: Objective technique for evaluating painful heel syndrome and its treatment. Foot and Ankle 3(4): 227-37, 1983
12. Keat A: Reiter's Syndrome and reactive arthritis in perspective. N Engl J Med 309(26): 1606-1615, 1983
13. Mann RA: Conservative treatment and office procedures, in Mann RA (ed): Durvies' Surgery of

the Foot, 4th Ed, St. Louis, MO, CV Mosby Co, 1978, pp 507-515

14. Milgram JE: Design and use of pads and strappings for office relief of the painful foot. American Academy of Orthopedics Symposium on the Foot and Ankle, St. Louis, MO, 1983, pp 89-123

15. Murray RO: Some current concepts in skeletal radiology, in McLaren JW (ed): Modern Trends in Diagnostic Radiology. London, Butterworths, 1970

16. Potter TA, Tesla NN: Painful feet in McCarty DJ (ed): Arthritis and Allied Conditions, 9th edition: Philadelphia, Lea & Febiger, 1979, pp 1009-1022

17. Rana NA: The foot in systemic disease, gout, in Jahss MH (ed): Disorders of the Foot, Philadelphia, Saunders, 1982, pp 1014-1023

18. Rana NA: Juvenile rheumatoid arthritis of the foot. Foot and Ankle 3 (1): 2-10, 1982

19. Rana NA: Rheumatoid arthritis, other collagen diseases, and psoriasis of the foot in Jahss MH (ed): Disorders of the Foot, Philadelphia, Saunders, 1982, pp 1024-1063

20. Rodan GP: Progressive systemic sclerosis (scleroderma) in McCarty DJ (ed): Arthritis and Allied Conditions, 9th Ed, Philadelphia, Lea & Febiger, 1979, pp 762-763

21. Sholcoff SD, Glickman HL, Steinbach HL: Roentgenology of Reiter's syndrome. Radiology 97: 497-503, 1970

22. Short CL, Bauer W, Reynolds WE: In Rheumatoid Arthritis, Harvard University Press, Cambridge, 1957, pp 194-195

23. Spiegel TM, Spiegel JS: Rheumatoid arthritis in the foot and ankle—diagnosis, pathology, and treatment. Foot and Ankle 2 (6): 318-324, 1982

24. Thomas WH: Correction of arthritic deformities in the lower extremity and spine: Part II ankle and foot in McCarty DJ (ed): Arthritis and Allied Conditions, 9th Ed, Philadelphia, Lea & Febiger, pp 590-581

25. Tillmann K: The Rheumatoid Foot: Diagnosis Pathomechanics and Treatment, Stuttgart, Georg Thieme Publishers, Boston, PSG Publishing Co, 1979, pp 3-61

26. Valvanen V: Rheumatoid arthritis in the pantalar joints. Acta Orthop Scand 107 (Suppl): 1-55, 1967.

27. Vainio K: The rheumatoid foot: A clinical study with pathologic and roentgenological comments. Ann Chir Gynaecol 45 (Suppl) 1-107, 1956

28. Wyngaarden JB, Holmes EW: Clinical gout and the pathogenesis of hyperuricemia in McCarty DJ (ed): Arthritis and Allied Conditions, 9th Ed, Philadelphia, Lea & Febiger 1979, pp 1193-1209

Hugh Smythe

20

"Fibrositis" and Soft-tissue Pain Syndromes: The Clinical Significance of Tender Points

Many of 17 percent of adults who complain of musculoskeletal pain have none of the well-defined syndromes of degenerative or inflammatory joint disease. The pain is distressing, but examination reveals no swollen joints, no injured or damaged tissues. In the study of such patients, localized points of acute tenderness may be found, and these are both the mystery and the solution. There is a large class of pain syndromes characterized by the presence of these tender sites. The two most common members of this class are the referred pain syndromes, and the so-called "fibrositis" syndrome.

In the referred pain syndromes, pain arising from a deep central source is felt in another, more peripheral site. Pain originating deep within the neck is commonly referred to the shoulders and arms, and pain from the low back may be felt in the buttocks and legs. Diagnosis of such syndromes may be difficult, and regional clusters of tender points can be valuable markers. A special kind of enhanced pain sensitivity has developed in the involved segments as part of the neurological response to chronic regional pain, and the tenderness must not be misunderstood to imply inflammation. Under the microscope the tissues are perfectly normal, and the tenderness is due to an alteration of pain message transmission, not to local disease.

The enhancement of pain transmission may be central rather than segmental, with effects that are general rather than regional. When there is a wide distribution of tender points, with diffuse aching, stiffness, and exhaustion, the clinical descriptive term, "fibro-sitis syndrome," is used. The tender points are markers of the presence of a pain amplifica-tion syndrome (Table 20-1).

PAIN AMPLIFICATION SYNDROMES

The term "amplification" implies that the increase in pain or tenderness has resulted from altered neurophysiological mechanisms, independent of psychological influences. The effect is selective, not diffuse. Certain sites become tender but background pain

PRINCIPLES OF PHYSICAL MEDICINE AND REHABILITATION
IN THE MUSCULOSKELETAL DISEASES

Table 20-1

Pain Amplification Syndromes

Group 1: Tenderness at fibrositic sites.
 Referred pain syndromes
 Fibrositis syndrome
 Experimental sleep deprivation
 Narcotic withdrawal
 Others
Group 2: Tenderness of different distribution
 Reflex dystrophies
 Tender shins of steroid therapy

threshold is unaltered.[17] The tenderness is quite pronounced; typically 50 percent greater than the tenderness of an inflamed rheumatoid joint, best demonstrated when both conditions coexist in the same patient. It still remains difficult for patients and their physicians to accept that there is not a local inflammatory lesion, particularly in the absence of full definition of the pain mechanism. It is frustrating also that technology in the form of biochemistry, histology, and radiology has so far been of so little help. The best evidence comes from a careful examination of the clinical findings.

The Point Count

The clinician must have a systemic and effective approach to the examination of the peripheral joints, of the spine, and of the nonarticular regions. There must be a practiced familiarity with the sites in which tenderness is likely to occur, and a technique that measures the quantity of tenderness, allowing for differences among individuals in general responses to pain stimulus. One approach is to do a "point count," analogous to the joint count used in assessing changes in the severity of peripheral joint inflammation. The basic idea is simple enough, and to the novice examiner there are only two methodological problems: where to press, and how hard to press.

A list of 14 sites at which tenderness may be found has been published,[1] and is reviewed in Table 20-2 and Figure 20-1. This list is not all inclusive and certainly not immutable. The firmness of pressure is determined by using as reference sites clinically "silent" areas—the lower ribs, the forearm or thigh muscles, the fat pad lateral to the knee. For humanity as well as precision, one works at the threshold of tenderness, reducing the stimulus for generally tender individuals. Pressure over the target site should be

Table 20-2

The Point Count: 14 Tender Sites

Low cervical: anterior aspects of intertransverse spaces C5-7
Trapezius: midpoint of upper fold
Costochondral: just lateral to 2nd junction, on upper surface
Supraspinatus: above scapular spine, near medial border
Lateral Elbow: "tennis elbow" site, 4 cm distal to epicondyle, in lateral intermuscular septum, moves with radius, deep to extensor to long finger
Low lumbar: interspinous ligaments L4-S1
Gluteus medius: deep in upper outer buttocks
Medial fat pad: over ligament, proximal to joint line

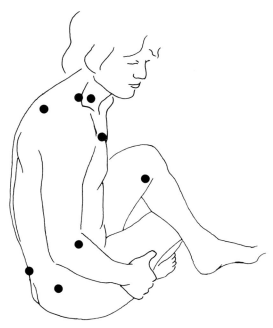

Fig. 20-1. Fourteen Tender Points. The tenderness can be quite localized. Skill and care in this assessment is rewarded. (Text, Table 20–1.)

somewhat less firm, about 80 percent of the pressure over adjacent nontender areas, and the site scored positive only if very distant tenderness is reported. This comparison of two sites, target and reference, may have to be done with some care, as the patient often assumes that the exquisite tenderness is due to deliberate roughness, and must be assured that the pressure on the target site is in fact less than on the reference area.

Numerical methods help. The use of a simple dolorimeter to record the pressure used, is of value clinically as well as in investigation. The quantity of tenderness may also be scored in terms of the number of tender points, and the distribution of these points examined for clues as the underlying mechanisms. A small number of points, clustered in a single region, unassociated with diffuse aching stiffness and fatigue, suggests a referred pain syndrome. A large number of tender sites, spread widely and symmetrically, with systemic symptoms, suggests the fibrositis syndrome. The absence, presence, number and distribution of these points is of such help in clarifying otherwise ill-defined pain syndromes that it is urged that some variation of this count be taught and used as part of the standard routine clinical examination (Fig. 20-2).

Referred Pain and Associated Phenomena

When a finger is injured, the patient can accurately localize the site of the pain and identify the nature of the stimulus. He can summon up an image of the finger, and draw a picture of the part and the site of injury. This kind of detailed knowledge of the position and environment of the hand is essential to function, and a large area of cerebral cortex is assigned to this task.

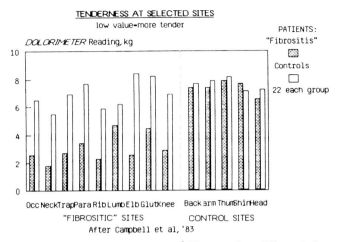

TENDERNESS AT SELECTED SITES
low value=more tender

DOLORIMETER Reading, kg

PATIENTS:
"Fibrositis"

Controls

22 each group

"FIBROSITIC" SITES   CONTROL SITES

After Campbell et al,'83

Fig. 20-2. Dolorimeter readings.[2] There is clear differentiation between normal and fibrositic subjects in the readings at fibrositic sites, and clear separation between fibrositic and control sites, But no excess tenderness of fibrositic subjects at control sites.

However, we have no comparable need for information about deeply lying structures, and no similar cortical mechanism exists. We have no body image of these deeply lying structures, and pain arising in them cannot therefore be accurately located. The pain must be referred; misinterpreted as arising in other structures, usually muscular areas and bony prominences sharing the same nerve supply and familiar enough to be included in the body image. This misinterpretation is very persistent; the brain continues to insist that the problem is in the leg even after the intellect has understood that the real trouble is in the low back. The spread of pain is not dependent on nerve root compression, and the electric numbness in the fourth and fifth fingers produced by trauma to the ulnar nerve is not a good general illustration of the nature of referred pain. The areas to which pain is referred often develop secondary reflex changes, misguided but protective in intent. These include deep tenderness and hyperesthesia, circulatory changes, and muscular splinting with inhibition of voluntary movement. These changes are enhanced by chilling, sleep deprivation, tension, and fatigue.

Quality of Referred Pain

The quality of referred pain is determined more by the site to which it is referred than by the nature of the original pain stimulus. Anginal pain is not localized to the myocardium, as we have no body image of the heart muscle. It may be felt in the precordial region, where it is appreciated as a heaviness or a crushing pressure. It may be referred to the shoulder region, where it is felt as a deep ache, perhaps exacerbated by a draft. It may be referred to the forearm or hand, which may be described as dead, numb, woody, or swollen. The same pain, arising in the same area of heart muscle, and traveling by the same pathways to association areas in the cerebral cortex, may simultaneously give three very different kinds of sensory impression to the patient struggling to find words to accurately describe the nature of the distress.

Pain Equivalents

The qualities of deadness, numbness, or swelling associated with distal referral should be particularly noted, as they are common to many pains referred distally in the limbs, and commonly are misinterpreted as evidence of neural involvement. Similarly, the patient may be absolutely convinced that the part is swollen, pointing to a perfectly normal fatty fullness, so that it is mistakenly accepted that an inflammatory process has been present.

Clustered Distribution of Referred Tenderness

Tenderness (hyperalgesia) in areas to which pain is referred is part of all the classic descriptions of referred pain.[8-11] These accounts placed emphasis on the development of skin tenderness, cutaneous hyperalgesia. Deep referred tenderness is much more common than skin tenderness. The sites that become tender are the sites described above, i.e., exactly the same sites that become tender in the fibrositis syndrome. The distribution is asymmetric, and clustered in the often broad region of reference of the deep primary site. Pathology in any deep structure, visceral or musculoskeletal, can give rise to referred pain, but the neck and low back are the origin in the great majority of cases.

The Cervical Syndrome as a Source of Referred Pain

The neck is vulnerable for a variety of reasons, of which the most important are compressive and shearing stresses arising in the unsupported arch of the cervical spine during sleep. Its importance as a source of referred pain and reflex dystrophic disorders has been much underestimated, because few observers know where to find the tenderness, including this one until a few years ago. The interspinous ligaments, posterior joints, and muscles are relatively nontender, and indeed massage of these structures often feels good to the patient with a stiff neck. The real tenderness is in the front of the lower neck, quite precisely located in the anterior aspects of the interspinous ligaments between C5 and C7. The dolorimeter can sample this by pressing through the lower sternomastoid muscle, but the tip of the examiner's thumb is more subtle, as it can be insinuated behind the muscle, well centrally to accurately localize the sites of maximum tenderness. The patient is usually unaware of this tenderness, and has to be convinced that the examiner is not deliberately trying to hurt. The dolorimeter can help convince the patient and third parties that the tenderness is very real, and greater than at any other site tested.

Neck pain, referred pain or pain equivalents, neck tenderness, and referred tenderness at characteristic sites make up the cervical syndrome; loss of range of movement occurs only in late, severe cases. But sometimes the patient minimizes or even denies neck pain, and presents with headache, or pain about the shoulder region, lateral elbow, anterior chest, or interscapular region. They may complain of pain and numbness of the hands, especially at night. The strong temptation is to make a local diagnosis, such as tennis elbow, or costochondritis. Systematic point counts reveal the multiple, clustered distribution of tender points, (Fig. 20-3), with unsuspected but marked asymmetrical tenderness deep in the neck, indicating the presence of a silent cervical syndrome. Microtrauma may have produced an undocumented inflammatory process at the tennis elbow site but once marked tenderness has also been shown in the lower neck, and in the midtrapezius and costochondral junctions, and the lateral elbow tenderness is found to be maximum at precisely the site affected in referred pain syndromes, then why add an additional diagnosis? At least concede that measures to help the neck are appropriate if

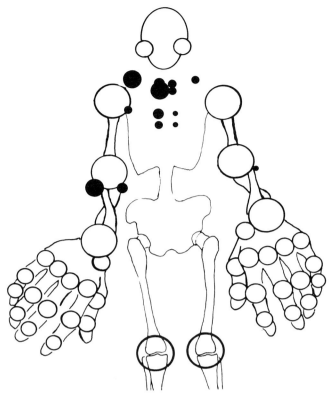

Fig. 20-3. A clustered distribution of tender points in a patient with a cervical strain syndrome; assymetrical and concentrated in one region.

local measures fail. Knowledge of additional sites is helpful in the analysis of these cases. Two common ones are the tip of the coracoid, (giving rise to frequently erroneous diagnoses of bicipital tendinitis), and the medial elbow.

The Low Back Syndrome

The low back syndrome may be similarly defined, consisting of low back pain, referred pain or pain equivalents, low back tenderness, and referred tenderness. Again, this diagnosis is easy when back pain is prominent, or when there is a band of referred pain extending continuously from buttock to posterolateral thigh, calf, and foot. Referred symptoms may differ so markedly in quality from the back pain, or be separated from it in time or distribution that the diagnosis is not obvious, again a silent low back syndrome. Furthermore, in the low back there is no access to the deep spinal structures, and there is no lumbar equivalent to the low anterior neck tenderness. We must make do with the interspinous ligament tenderness, and with the characteristic pattern of multiple, asymmetric distant referred tenderness. Gluteus medius tenderness is nearly always present, and often more marked than the interspinous tenderness. The medial fat pad tenderness is even better, because it is not central to an area of pain, and is totally unsuspected by the patient. Tenderness here does not result from knee joint pathology, and it may be important to demonstrate to the patient the absence of stress pain or tenderness in the knee, in contrast to the asymmetrical and marked tenderness of the fat pad. The patient often has a conviction that there is arthritis in the knee, reaffirmed by the brain's stubborn refusal to relate the knee region pain to the back, so that the evidence and its interpretation must be demonstrated with care to the patient. Again, knowledge of additional characteristic sites may be very helpful in establishing the multiplicity and asymmetry of unsuspected points. The insertion of soleus into Achille's tendon, and in the medial instep the origin of the short flexor muscle to the great toe are two additional sites commonly affected.

The "Fibrositis Syndrome"

When multiple regions are chronically involved, with diffuse aching and stiffness, and a wide distribution of tender points, the clinical descriptive term, "fibrositis syndrome" is used (Table 20-3).

The Rheumatic Pain Syndrome

The pain or aching in the rheumatic pain syndrome is widespread, poorly circumscribed, and deep, referred to muscles or bony prominences. When central, it has an aching character; when peripheral, pain may be replaced by pain equivalents, with swelling, stiffness, or numbness. The stiffness is an increase of a sense of tissue tension or of muscular effort required toward the extremes of range. These symptoms are concentrated in the broad areas of reference of the cervical and lumbar segments and tend to shift with time, so that the patients recurrently present with "new" sites of complaints. The stiffness is worse in the morning, and is increased by weather changes, cold, tension, fatigue, or excess use. Simple analgesics are disappointing, but heat, massage, or a holiday may give relief.

The Wide Distribution of Tender Points

The individual tender points are precisely the same in fibrositis as in referred pain syndromes, and the difference lies in the number of points, the widespread distribution, and the association with other general manifestations. Many of the points are unknown to the patient, and are situated in areas with little cortical representation or emotional significance. The pattern is impossible to fabricate. Dolorimetry can be helpful; in psychogenic pain syndromes the tenderness is diffuse or variable, while in fibrositis it is predictable, focal, and constant. Old[17,18] and new[7] studies may describe subtle pathologies, but

Table 20-3
Cardinal Features of Fibrositis

A rheumatic pain syndrome
A wide distribution of tender points
The sleep disturbance
The irritable everything syndrome
The personality

they have failed to show any local inflammation. The tenderness should be appreciated as an alteration in neurological function, not the result of immunological or other damage.

The Sleep Disturbance

The exhaustion may be most disabling, and not clearly related to lack of rest. It is often marked in the morning, and paralyzes as well as punishes initiative. The patients emphasize their exhaustion, but may minimize their sleep disturbance. They may have been light sleepers for years, and relate their frequent and prolonged wakefulness to pain. Virtually all arise feeling unrefreshed (this is the key question to ask), more exhausted than at bedtime the night before. After stress, they may spend whole nights without sleep (Table 20-4).

Key studies have provided evidence of a specific disturbance in sleep physiology. In the first,[13] 10 fibrositic subjects showed a decrease in stages 3 and 4 slow wave sleep, with intrusion of a rapid alpha rhythm, as determined by computer analysis of the energy-frequency spectra (Fig. 20-3), and all showed an overnight increase in tenderness measured by dolorimeter. These observations have since been confirmed and extended in a large number of other patients. High energy bursts of alpha intruding into slow-wave sleep was described by Hauri as alpha-delta sleep,[5] and its association with aching, fatigue, and stiffness described.[4] This more florid pattern can be read by eye, and was recognized in 8 of 26 chronic pain patients.[21]

In another study, experimental reproduction of aspects of the fibrositis syndrome were achieved in healthy university students.[14] After control nights, for three nights they were deprived either of rapid eye movement (REM), or stage 4 non-REM sleep by a buzzer, supplemented when necessary by hand arousal. The buzzer caused a rapid alpha rhythm to appear in the electroencephalogram (EEG) superimposed on the slow wave pattern, mimicking the pattern seen in the fibrositis patients (Fig. 20-4). No increase in tenderness was associated with REM deprivation, but disturbance of slow wave non-REM sleep was associated with a marked overnight increase in tenderness scores and symptoms of anorexia, overwhelming physical tiredness, and heaviness.

The Irritable Everything Syndrome

Fibrositis patients do not simply report pain, they express it in urgent verbal and body language. Pressure on a tender point may result in a dramatic twisting total body response, the leap sign. The perception of sensations other than pain is also much

Table 20-4
Symptoms of Sleep Disturbance*

Symptom	Fibrositis group (n = 22)	Control group (n = 22)
Waking with aching, stiffness	100%	23%
Tired during the day	100	41
Waking tired	95	32
Waking frequently	68	59
Difficulty falling asleep	36	23
Waking early	36	36

*(From Campbell SM, Clark S, Tindall EA, et al: Clinical characteristics of fibrositis. Arth Rheum 26:817–824, 1983, with permission.)

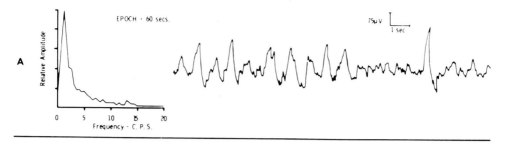

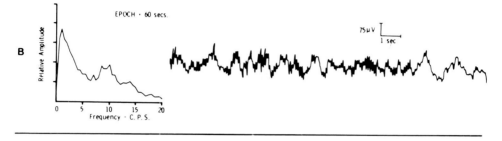

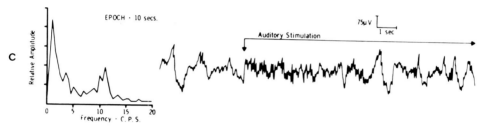

Fig. 20-4. EEGs with computer analysis of frequency spectra during deep non-REM sleep in (A) a normal subject, (B) a fibrositic subject, (C) a normal subject disturbed by a buzzer. Note the alpha intrusion in (B) and (C), indicated by energy at about 10 cycles per second.[13]

enhanced in "fibrositis" patients. They may be hypersensitive to cold, noise, and environmental irritants of all kinds, and to internal stimuli such as drug effects, cough, bladder fullness. The irritable bowel syndrome may be the gastrointestinal (GI) manifestation of fibrositis.[23] They have often had inappropriate investigation and therapy because of headaches, chest pain, urinary frequency. As with the tenderness, the hypersensitivity is widespread but not general. Patients with rheumatoid arthritis and fibrositis have much more tenderness at their points than their joints.

THE FIBROSITIS PERSONALITY

These patients set high standards, as demanding of themselves as of others. They are caring, honest, tidy, committed, moral, industrious. Their vices are their virtues carried to excess. They hate to complain, they respectfully doubt, they forgivably fail to comply, they loyally reject. Their perfectionism can be trying, but they are often very effective in their chosen field of activity and have unusual loyalty from employers and family. Queen

Victoria's husband, Prince Albert was classic; "excessively conscientious on quite minor matters."[6] "Fibrositics" are not abnormal, just characteristic. They deeply resent any suggestion that they are using their illness as a crutch, as they drive themselves harder than most, and dislike other crutches, such as alcohol and prescribed medication. They are not depressed,[1,20] and the concept of "masked depression" may have arisen because of the response of "fibrositic" symptoms to tricyclic medication.

THE ASSOCIATION OF FIBROSITIS AND OTHER DISEASES

Therapy is often determined by the urgency of the patient's complaints, and not by the severity of the underlying disease. Patients with rheumatoid arthritis, cervical or lumbar disk disease, or a whole host of other conditions may have amplification of their symptoms by fibrositic mechanisms. The point count allows rapid recognition of this complication and avoidance of the excess of therapy that might otherwise follow. Moldofsky and Chester identified a subgroup of paradoxical responders among hospitalized rheumatoid patients, identified by worsening mood with improving disease.[12] When first admitted, these patients seemed cheerful and cooperative, but they became depressed, complaining and agitated as treatment progressed. They were more likely to receive prolonged hospitalization, extensive investigation, and hazardous medical and surgical therapies, with increased morbidity and even mortality. Almost half the hospitalized rheumatoid patients showed "the squeaky wheel gets the grease" pattern, and on examination the fibrositic sites were characteristically more tender than their swollen joints.

Prevalence, Classification, and Nomenclature

The number of tender points recorded in an unselected group of rheumatic disease patients is shown in Figure 20-5. Clearly the prevalence of fibrositis will be dependent on the point count criterion chosen. In published studies, the criteria have varied from 4 of 53 points[23] to 12 of 14.[13] The 20 percent with four or more points will include a majority with simple referred pain syndromes, without the exhaustion, stiffness, and personality associated with large numbers of points, and it seems inappropriate to apply the same name, be it "fibromyalgia" or "fibrositis" to these very different groups. These archaic names are probably beyond rehabilitation, and Moldofsky has suggested the Rheumatic Pain Modulation Syndrome[15] for the generalized syndrome associated with nonrestorative sleep. The referred pain syndromes associated with tender points can simply be named according to the source pathology. "Localized fibrositis" disappears into "tender point."

One may wish to reserve judgment, but there seems to be little need for the concept of secondary fibrositis. The data collected by Wolfe[15] and Moldofsky[16] suggest that the fibrositic symptoms seen in patients with rheumatoid or osteoarthritis are identical in pathogenesis and manifestation to "primary fibrositis," and rarely a polymyalgic extension of the underlying disease.

Treatment

In fibrositis, multiple factors combine to produce the symptom complex, and explanations may involve: referred pain and reflex responses, mechanical stresses in neck and low back, the sleep disturbance, the irritable everything syndrome, and attitudes and expecta-

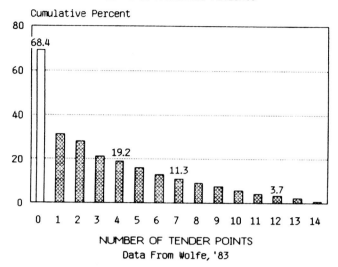

Fig. 20-5. Number of tender points found in unselected rheumatic disease patients.[22] The estimated prevalence of fibrositis or fibromyalgia is very sensitive this criterion. In general, patients with fatigue and stiffness will tend to have more, diffusely distributed points; and those with referred pain will have fewer, clustered points.

tions. The pain is neurological but not neurotic in origin. The distress arises from an interaction between segmental and central factors, with referred pain and reflex tenderness, aggravated and prolonged by tension and sleep deprivation.

Recommendations

Simple analgesic methods can do much to break the vicious cycles described above. These may include enteric-coated aspirin, 600 to 900 mg four times daily for continuous, background pain relief, with added propoxyphene, 65 mg, or codeine, 15 mg, sparingly as needed for peaks. Since no inflammation is involved, anti-inflammatory drugs are not indicated. Prednisone has been found to be ineffective in the fibrositis syndrome.[3] Heat, liniments, massage, or other counter-irritant therapy give real if short-lived relief.

MECHANICAL STRESSES IN NECK AND LOW BACK

The vast majority of mechanical problems affecting the spine arises in the lower neck, or two lower lumbar levels. The key to success in treating the neck is support for the arch of the cervical spine during sleep. A pair of cervical ruffs, made by enclosing 8 × 24-inch gauze pads within tubes of 3-inch stockinette, tied loosely in front, is quite effective for acute therapy. However, many patients stop wearing their ruffs when they begin to feel better, and so fail to prevent the next attack. Neck support pillows are cooler and more comfortable for prolonged use.

The low back is at the extreme range of hyperextension in the standing position in virtually all patients with low back problems, and many have such weak abdominal muscles that they can neither improve their posture nor use a positive intra-abdominal pressure to spare their back. Weak abdominal muscles should be recognized and corrected by specific progressive sit-up exercises, with hips and knees bent to eliminate the lumbar lordosis, and feet held. Avoid straight leg raising or push-ups, which strongly compress the hyperextended lower spine. The safe posture for the low back is that of an athlete with knees bent and back flat, not the erect ideal of parents or teachers.

The Sleep Disturbance

Oxazepam, 15 mg, or flurazepam, 15–30 mg, may be used as night sedatives, but do not restore the normal sleep pattern. Tricyclic agents such as imipramine or amitryptiline, 10 to 75 mg early in the evening, are more effective, at the cost of more side-effects. All the tricyclics currently available are too longlasting, with 30-hour half-lives. "Fibrositic" patients tend to be very sensitive to the hangover somnolence associated with these drugs, and they are best reserved for crises.

Attitudes and Expectations

These patients are often perfectionistic, with high standards of performance for themselves, their families, and their therapist. They are particularly resentful of any suggestion that they are quitters or fakers. They have often been unusually effective, but at too high a cost.

Tension normally and necessarily accompanies major effort. Consider an athlete preparing for a 4-minute mile, or an actress for a first night, or a student facing a final examination. The mother who must guide three explosive children while protecting a civilized moment for herself and her husband, and the loyal but unappreciated office worker, have less dramatic but more chronic and equally demanding roles. The defect in patients with fibrositis is not the build-up of tension, but the failure to "get out from under."

Tension and aching are built-in reaction patterns for such patients; and complete long-term freedom from symptoms is unlikely. The anatomical prognosis is excellent, and the prospect of partial relief is also good. The patients should continue to be involved; they are not helped by restricting activities, and it is extremely important that work patterns not be interrupted. We set realistic goals, and keep investigation and treatment patterns simple. Do not interrupt employment for medical care. Advise tension-dissipating routines, such as exercise, saunas, massage, cocktails, or a holiday. The activities should be social, and pleasure rather than duty. A night out, a weekend away, or other part-time escape from four walls or imprisoning interpersonal situations may often have to be specifically prescribed.

Fitness

There is accumulating evidence that a most effective way of controlling the pain is to achieve a high degree of general fitness, especially cardiopulmonary fitness. With other joint diseases, joint protection must be stressed, and caution used in exercise. With fibrositis, exercise is strongly urged, even at the cost of early increase in pain.

Responsibility

Despite (or because) of their perfectionism, fibrositic patients often comply poorly. They don't use their neck supports, don't do their situps, don't take their prescribed medications (all for the best of reasons), don't get involved in fitness activities, don't adjust their schedules and attitudes, and return for the second appointment feeling no better. This makes it easy for the doctor. All that need be done is to go over the ground again, assure them that they will not improve until they follow the appropriate program, and assure them also that the responsibility for improvement is theirs. This is not the time to prescribe tricyclic drugs, a strategy which makes the doctor primarily responsible for all outcomes, good and bad. The therapist points the way, and is a forgiving friend and counselor, wary of the temptation to become healer, accepting the crucial transfer of responsibility. It is the patient's job to improve.

REFERENCES

1. Clark F, Campbell FM, Forehand ME, et al: Clinical characteristics of fibrositis II: a blinded controlled study using standard psychological tests. Arthritis Rheum 28:132–137, 1985
2. Campbell SM, Clark S, Tindall EA, et al: Clinical characteristics of fibrositis. Arth Rheum 26:817–824, 1983
3. Clark S, Tindall E, Bennett RB: A double blind crossover study of prednisone in the treatment of fibrositis. (Abstract). Arth Rheum 27 (Suppl):S76, 1984(Abstr)
4. Hauri P: The sleep disorders. The Upjohn Co., Kalamazoo, 1977, p. 51
5. Hauri P, Hawkins DR: Alpha-delta sleep. Electroencephalogr Clin Neurophysiol 34:233, 1973
6. James, RR: Prince Albert. Knopf, New York, 1984
7. Kalyan-Raman UP, Kalyan-Raman K, Yunus MB, Masi AT: Muscle pathology in primary fibromyalgia syndrome: a light microscopic, histochemical and ultrastructural study. J Rheumatol 11:808–813, 1984
8. Kellgren JH: Observations on referred pain arising from muscle. Clin Sci 3:174–190, 1938
9. Kellgren JH: On distribution of pain arising from deep somatic structures with charts of segmental pain areas. Clin Sci 4:35–46, 1939
10. Kellgren JH: Deep pain sensibility. Lancet 1:943–949, 1949
11. Lewis T, Kellgren JH: Observations relating to referred pain, visceromotor reflexes and other associated phenomena. Clin Sci 4:47–71, 1939
12. Moldofsky H, Chester WJ: Pain and mood patterns in patients with rheumatoid arthritis. Psychosomat Med 32:309–318, 1970
13. Moldofsky H, Scarisbrick P, England R, et al: Musculoskeletal symptoms and non-REM sleep disturbance in patients with "fibrositis syndrome" and healthy subjects. Psychosomat Med 37:341–351, 1975
14. Moldofsky H, Scarisbrick P: Induction of neurasthenic musculoskeletal pain syndrome by selective sleep stage deprivation. Psychosomat Med 38:35–44, 1976
15. Moldofsky H: Rheumatic pain modulation syndrome: The interrelationships between sleep, central nervous system serotonin, and pain. Adv Neurol 33:51–57, 1982
16. Moldofsky H, Lue F, Smythe H: Alpha EEG sleep and morning symptoms in rheumatoid arthritis. J Rheum 10:373–379, 1983
17. Simons DG: Muscle pain syndromes—Part 1. Am J Phys Med 54:289–311, 1975
18. Simons DG: Muscle pain syndromes—Part 2. Am J Phys Med 55:15–42, 1976
19. Smythe HA, Moldofsky H: Two contributions to understanding of the "fibrositis" syndrome. Bull Rheum Dis 28:928–931, 1977
20. Smythe HA: Problems with the MMPI. J Rheumatol 11:417–418, 1984
21. Wittig RM, Zorick FJ, Blumer D, et al: Disturbed sleep in patients complaining of chronic pain. J Nerv Ment Dis 170:429, 1982
22. Wolfe F, Cathey MA: Prevalence of primary and secondary fibrositis. J Rheumatol 10:965–968, 1983
23. Yunus M, Masi AT, Calabro JJ, et al: Primary fibromyalgia (fibrositis): Clinical study of 50 patients with matched normal controls. Semin Arth Rheum 11:151–171, 1981

Index